# Vaccine Protocols

# METHODS IN MOLECULAR MEDICINE™

## John M. Walker, SERIES EDITOR

96. **Hepatitis B and D Protocols:** *Volume 2, Immunology, Model Systems, and Clinical Studies*, edited by *Robert K. Hamatake and Johnson Y. N. Lau, 2004*

95. **Hepatitis B and D Protocols:** *Volume 1, Detection, Genotypes, and Characterization*, edited by *Robert K. Hamatake and Johnson Y. N. Lau, 2004*

94. **Molecular Diagnosis of Infectious Diseases,** *Second Edition*, edited by *Jochen Decker and Udo Reischl, 2004*

93. **Anticoagulants, Antiplatelets, and Thrombolytics,** edited by *Shaker A. Mousa, 2004*

92. **Molecular Diagnosis of Genetic Diseases,** *Second Edition*, edited by *Rob Elles and Roger Mountford, 2003*

91. **Pediatric Hematology:** *Methods and Protocols*, edited by *Nicholas J. Goulden and Colin G. Steward, 2003*

90. **Suicide Gene Therapy:** *Methods and Reviews*, edited by *Caroline J. Springer, 2003*

89. **The Blood–Brain Barrier:** *Biology and Research Protocols*, edited by *Sukriti Nag, 2003*

88. **Cancer Cell Culture:** *Methods and Protocols*, edited by *Simon P. Langdon, 2003*

87. **Vaccine Protocols,** *Second Edition*, edited by *Andrew Robinson, Michael J. Hudson, and Martin P. Cranage, 2003*

86. **Renal Disease:** *Techniques and Protocols*, edited by *Michael S. Goligorsky, 2003*

85. **Novel Anticancer Drug Protocols,** edited by *John K. Buolamwini and Alex A. Adjei, 2003*

84. **Opioid Research:** *Methods and Protocols*, edited by *Zhizhong Z. Pan, 2003*

83. **Diabetes Mellitus:** *Methods and Protocols*, edited by *Sabire Özcan, 2003*

82. **Hemoglobin Disorders:** *Molecular Methods and Protocols*, edited by *Ronald L. Nagel, 2003*

81. **Prostate Cancer Methods and Protocols,** edited by *Pamela J. Russell, Paul Jackson, and Elizabeth A. Kingsley, 2003*

80. **Bone Research Protocols,** edited by *Miep H. Helfrich and Stuart H. Ralston, 2003*

79. **Drugs of Abuse:** *Neurological Reviews and Protocols*, edited by *John Q. Wang, 2003*

78. **Wound Healing:** *Methods and Protocols*, edited by *Luisa A. DiPietro and Aime L. Burns, 2003*

77. **Psychiatric Genetics:** *Methods and Reviews*, edited by *Marion Leboyer and Frank Bellivier, 2003*

76. **Viral Vectors for Gene Therapy:** *Methods and Protocols*, edited by *Curtis A. Machida, 2003*

75. **Lung Cancer:** *Volume 2, Diagnostic and Therapeutic Methods and Reviews*, edited by *Barbara Driscoll, 2003*

74. **Lung Cancer:** *Volume 1, Molecular Pathology Methods and Reviews*, edited by *Barbara Driscoll, 2003*

73. **E. coli:** *Shiga Toxin Methods and Protocols*, edited by *Dana Philpott and Frank Ebel, 2003*

72. **Malaria Methods and Protocols,** edited by *Denise L. Doolan, 2002*

71. **Haemophilus influenzae Protocols,** edited by *Mark A. Herbert, Derek Hood, and E. Richard Moxon, 2002*

70. **Cystic Fibrosis Methods and Protocols,** edited by *William R. Skach, 2002*

69. **Gene Therapy Protocols,** *Second Edition*, edited by *Jeffrey R. Morgan, 2002*

68. **Molecular Analysis of Cancer,** edited by *Jacqueline Boultwood and Carrie Fidler, 2002*

67. **Meningococcal Disease:** *Methods and Protocols*, edited by *Andrew J. Pollard and Martin C. J. Maiden, 2001*

66. **Meningococcal Vaccines:** *Methods and Protocols*, edited by *Andrew J. Pollard and Martin C. J. Maiden, 2001*

METHODS IN MOLECULAR MEDICINE™

# Vaccine Protocols

## Second Edition

Edited by

## Andrew Robinson
## Michael J. Hudson

*Health Protection Agency,*
*Centre for Applied Microbiology and Research,*
*Porton Down, Salisbury, Wiltshire, UK*

and

## Martin P. Cranage

*Department of Cellular and Molecular Medicine,*
*St. George's Hospital Medical School, London, UK*

**Humana Press** ✳ Totowa, New Jersey

© 2003 Humana Press Inc.
999 Riverview Drive, Suite 208
Totowa, New Jersey 07512

**www.humanapress.com**

This publication is printed on acid-free paper. ∞
ANSI Z39.48-1984 (American Standards Institute) Permanence of Paper for Printed Library Materials.

Production Editor: Kim Hoather-Potter.
Cover design by Patricia F. Cleary.

Cover illustration: From Figs. 1 and 4 in Chapter 20 "Severe Combined Immunodeficient (SCID) Mice in Vaccine Assessment," by Michael J. Dennis.

For additional copies, pricing for bulk purchases, and/or information about other Humana titles, contact Humana at the above address or any of the following numbers: Tel.: 973-256-1699; Fax: 973-256-8341; E-mail: humana@humanapr.com; or visit our Website at www.humanapress.com

Printed in the United States of America. 10 9 8 7 6 5 4 3 2 1

E-ISBN 1-59259-399-2

Library of Congress Cataloging in Publication Data

Vaccine protocols/edited by Andrew Robinson, Michael J. Hudson, and Martin P. Cranage.--2nd ed.
      p.;cm.--(Methods in molecular medicine; 87)
  Includes bibliographical references and index.
  ISBN 1-58829-140-5 (alk. paper)
  ISSN: 1543-1894
    1. Vaccines--Laboratory manuals. I. Robinson, Andrew. II. Hudson, Michael J. III. Cranage, Martin P. IV. Series.
    [DNLM: 1. Vaccines. 2. Drug Design. 3. Genetic Techniques. 4. Research Design. QW 525 V116 2003]
  QR189.V2513 2003
  615'.372--dc21

2003044968

# Preface

Vaccine research and development is advancing at an unprecedented pace, with an increasing emphasis on rational design based upon a fundamental understanding of the underlying molecular mechanisms. The aim of this volume is to provide a selection of contemporary protocols that will be useful to both novice and advanced practitioner alike. The variety of procedures required to design, develop, produce, and assess a vaccine is immense and covers aspects of chemistry, biochemistry, molecular biology, cell biology, and immunology. No single volume can hope to cover these topics exclusively. Rather, here we attempt to provide a methods sourcebook focusing on hands-on practical advice. Complementary and background information may be found in other volumes in the *Methods in Molecular Medicine* series. Of particular interest are volumes on *Dendritic Cell Protocols, Interleukin Protocols, Vaccine Adjuvants,* and *DNA Vaccines.*

Since the publication of the first edition of *Vaccine Protocols* there have been major advances, particularly in the areas of bacterial genomics, antigen-specific T-cell quantification, genetic manipulation of vaccine vectors, the harnessing of natural molecules concerned with the regulation of immune responses, and the burgeoning field of DNA vaccinology. Hence, the extensive revision of this edition with new chapters on live viral vaccine vectors, attenuated bacterial vectors, immunomodulators, MHC-peptide tetrameric complexes, and the identification of vaccine candidates by genomic analysis. Additionally, chapters from the first edition have been updated to accommodate state-of-the-art methods in vaccinology. We have maintained the overall structure of the book to comprise essentially three basic chapter types. First, those describing in detail the development and production of vaccines using specific techniques, including genetic manipulation of viruses or bacteria to produce live attenuated vaccines, vaccine vectors, or inactivated toxins and the production of synthetic peptides and conjugate vaccines. Second, chapters describing more general techniques for vaccine formulation and delivery and assessment of immune responses. Finally, a few chapters review the critical areas of scale-up to manufacture, vaccine quality assurance, and clinical trials in order to prime the reader with the relevant background information. Together with a general overview of vaccines, the present volume on *Vaccine Protocols* should provide valuable and relevant practical information to all those seeking to produce improved or novel vaccines.

*Andrew Robinson*
*Michael J. Hudson*
*Martin P. Cranage*

# Contents

Preface ............................................................................................................................ v

Contributors ................................................................................................................... ix

1  Overview of Vaccines
   **Gordon Ada** .......................................................................................................... *1*

2  Temperature-Sensitive Mutant Vaccines
   **Craig R. Pringle** .............................................................................................. *19*

3  Live Viral Vectors: *Construction of a Replication-Deficient
   Recombinant Adenovirus*
   **Anthony R. Fooks** ........................................................................................... *37*

4  Live Viral Vectors: *Vaccinia Virus*
   **Caroline Staib and Gerd Sutter** ............................................................... *51*

5  Live Viral Vectors: *Semliki Forest Virus*
   **Gunilla B. Karlsson and Peter J. Liljeström** ........................................ *69*

6  Development of Attenuated *Salmonella* Strains That Express
   Heterologous Antigens
   **Frances Bowe, Derek J. Pickard, Richard J. Anderson,
   Patricia Londoño-Arcila, and Gordon Dougan** ..................................... *83*

7  Expression and Delivery of Heterologous Antigens
   Using Lactic Acid Bacteria
   **Mark A. Reuter, Sean Hanniffy, and Jerry M. Wells** ...................... *101*

8  Synthetic Peptides
   **Michael J. Francis** ....................................................................................... *115*

9  Genetic Detoxification of Bacterial Toxins
   **Mariagrazia Pizza, Maria Rita Fontana, Vincenzo Scarlato,
   and Rino Rappuoli** ........................................................................................ *133*

10 Preparation of Polysaccharide-Conjugate Vaccines
   **Carla C. A. M. Peeters, Patrick R. Lagerman, Odo de Weers,
   Lukas A. Oomen, Peter Hoogerhout, Michel Beurret,
   Karen M. Reddin, and Jan T. Poolman** ................................................. *153*

11 Adjuvant Formulations for Experimental Vaccines
   **Duncan E. S. Stewart-Tull** ...................................................................... *175*

12 Incorporation of Immunomodulators into Plasmid DNA Vaccines
   **Linda S. Klavinskis, Philip Hobson, and Andrew Woods** ............ *195*

13  Microencapsulation of Vaccine Antigens
    **David H. Jones** ................................................................ 211

14  Lyophilization of Vaccines: *Current Trends*
    **Gerald D. J. Adams** .......................................................... 223

15  Stimulation of Mucosal Immunity
    **David J. M. Lewis and Christopher M. M. Hayward** ...................... 245

16  Induction and Detection of T-Cell Responses
    **Kingston H. G. Mills** ......................................................... 255

17  Construction of MHC Class I-Peptide Tetrameric Complexes
    for Analysis of T-Cell-Mediated Immune Responses
    **Rachel V. Samuel and Tomáš Hanke** ................................. 279

18  Assessment of Functional Antibody Responses
    **Ray Borrow and Paul Balmer** ............................................. 289

19  The Use of Complete Genome Sequences in Vaccine Design
    **Nigel J. Saunders and Sarah Butcher** ............................... 301

20  Severe Combined Immunodeficient (SCID) Mice
    in Vaccine Assessment
    **Michael J. Dennis** .......................................................... 313

21  Clinical Trials
    **Paddy Farrington and Elizabeth Miller** ........................... 335

22  Assuring the Quality and Safety of Vaccines:
    *Regulatory Expectations for Licensing and Batch Release*
    **Elwyn Griffiths and Ivana Knezevic** ............................... 353

23  DNA Vaccination: *An Update*
    **Douglas B. Lowrie** ......................................................... 377

24  From Vaccine Research to Manufacture:
    *A Guide for the Researcher*
    **Nigel Allison and Howard S. Tranter** .............................. 391

Index ........................................................................................ 409

# Contributors

GORDON ADA • *Division of Cell Biology, John Curtin School of Medical Research, Australian National University, Canberra, Australia*

GERALD D. J. ADAMS • *Gerald Adams Consultancy, Salisbury, United Kingdom*

NIGEL ALLISON • *Health Protection Agency, Centre for Applied Microbiology and Research, Porton Down, Salisbury, Wiltshire, United Kingdom*

RICHARD J. ANDERSON • *Centre for Molecular Microbiology and Immunology, Department of Biological Sciences, Imperial College, London, United Kingdom*

PAUL BALMER • *Vaccine Evaluation Department, Manchester Medical Microbiology Partnership, Manchester Royal Infirmary, Manchester, United Kingdom*

MICHAEL BEURRET • *Laboratory for Vaccine Development and Immune Mechanisms, National Institute of Public Health and Environmental Protection, Bilthoven, The Netherlands*

RAY BORROW • *Vaccine Evaluation Department, Manchester Medical Microbiology Partnership, Clinical Sciences Building, Manchester Royal Infirmary, Manchester, United Kingdom*

FRANCES BOWE • *Centre for Molecular Microbiology and Immunology, Department of Biological Sciences, Imperial College, London, United Kingdom*

SARAH BUTCHER • *The University of Oxford Bioinformatics Centre, The Sir William Dunn School of Pathology, University of Oxford, Oxford, United Kingdom*

MICHAEL J. DENNIS • *Health Protection Agency, Centre for Applied Microbiology and Research, Porton Down, Salisbury, Wiltshire, United Kingdom*

GORDON DOUGAN • *Centre for Molecular Microbiology and Immunology, Department of Biological Sciences, Imperial College, London, United Kingdom*

PADDY FARRINGTON • *Department of Statistics, Open University, Walton Hall, Milton Keynes, United Kingdom*

MARIA RITA FONTANA • *IRIS, Chiron Srl, Via Fiorentina 1, Siena, Italy*

ANTHONY R. FOOKS • *Veterinary Laboratories Agency, New Haw, Addlestone, Surrey, United Kingdom*

MICHAEL J. FRANCIS • *Schering Plough Animal Health, Harefield, Uxbridge, United Kingdom*

ELWYN GRIFFITHS • *World Health Organization, Geneva, Switzerland*

TOMÁŠ HANKE • *MRC Human Immunology Unit, Weatherall Institute of Molecular Medicine, The John Radcliffe, Oxford, United Kingdom*

SEAN HANNIFFY • *Institute of Food Research, Norwich Research Park, Colney, Norwich, United Kingdom*

CHRISTOPHER M. M. HAYWARD • *Department of Cellular and Molecular Medicine, St. George's Hospital Medical School, London, United Kingdom*

PHILIP HOBSON • *Department of Immunobiology, Guy's, King's, and St. Thomas' School of Medicine, London, United Kingdom*

PETER HOOGERHOUT • *Laboratory for Vaccine Development and Immune Mechanisms, National Institute of Public Health and Environmental Protection, Bilthoven, The Netherlands*

DAVID H. JONES • *ID Biomedical Corp of Quebec, Montreal, Quebec, Canada*

GUNILLA B. KARLSSON • *Microbiology and Tumor Biology Center, Karolinska Institutet, Stockhom, Sweden; and Department of Vaccine Research, Swedish Institute for Infectious Disease Control, Solna, Sweden*

LINDA S. KLAVINSKIS • *Department of Immunobiology, Guy's, King's, and St. Thomas' School of Medicine, London, United Kingdom*

IVANA KNEZEVIC • *World Health Organization, Geneva, Switzerland*

PATRICK R. LAGERMAN • *Laboratory for Vaccine Development and Immune Mechanisms, National Institute of Public Health and Environmental Protection, Bilthoven, The Netherlands*

DAVID J. M. LEWIS • *Department of Cellular Molecular Clinical Medicine, St. George's Hospital Medical School, London, United Kingdom*

PETER J. LILJESTRÖM • *Microbiology and Tumor Biology Center, Karolinska Institutet, Stockholm, Sweden; and Department of Vaccine Research, Swedish Institute for Infectious Disease Control, Solna, Sweden*

PATRICIA LONDOÑO-ARCILA • *Acambis plc., Peterhouse Technology Park, Cambridge, United Kingdom*

DOUGLAS B. LOWRIE • *National Institute for Medical Research, The Ridgeway, Mill Hill, London, United Kingdom*

ELIZABETH MILLER • *Immunisation Division, Health Protection Agency, Communicable Disease Surveillance Centre, London, United Kingdom*

KINGSTON H. G. MILLS • *Immune Regulation Research Group, Department of Biochemistry, Trinity College, Dublin, Ireland*

LUKAS A. OOMEN • *Laboratory for Vaccine Development and Immune Mechanisms, National Institute of Public Health and Environmental Protection, Bilthoven, The Netherlands*

CARLA C. A. M. PEETERS • *Laboratory for Vaccine Development and Immune Mechanisms, National Institute of Public Health and Environmental Protection, Bilthoven, The Netherlands*

DEREK J. PICKARD • *Centre for Molecular Microbiology and Immunology, Department of Biological Sciences, Imperial College, London, United Kingdom*

MARIAGRAZIA PIZZA • *IRIS, Chiron Srl, Via Fiorentina, Siena, Italy*

JAN T. POOLMAN • *GlaxoSmithKline Biologicals SA, Rixensart, Belgium*

CRAIG R. PRINGLE • *Biological Sciences Department, University of Warwick, Coventry, United Kingdom*

RINO RAPPUOLI • *IRIS, Chiron Srl, Via Fiorentina, Siena, Italy*

KAREN M. REDDIN • *Health Protection Agency, Centre for Applied Microbiology and Research, Porton Down, Salisbury, United Kingdom*

MARK A. REUTER • *Institute of Food Research, Norwich Research Park, Colney, Norwich, United Kingdom*

RACHEL V. SAMUEL • *MRC Human Immunology Unit, Weatherall Institute of Molecular Medicine, The John Radcliffe, Oxford, United Kingdom*

NIGEL J. SAUNDERS • *The Sir William Dunn School of Pathology, University of Oxford, Oxford, United Kingdom*

VINCENZO SCARLATO • *IRIS, Chiron Srl, Via Fiorentina, Siena, Italy*

CAROLINE STAIB • *GSF Institute of Molecular Virology and Institute of Virology, Technical University Munich, Munich, Germany*

DUNCAN E. S. STEWART-TULL • *Division of Infection and Immunity, IBLS, Joseph Black Building, University of Glasgow, Glasgow, United Kingdom*

GERD SUTTER • *GSF Institute of Molecular Virology and Institute of Virology, Technical University Munich, Munich, Germany*

HOWARD S. TRANTER • *Health Protection Agency, Centre for Applied Microbiology and Research, Porton Down, Salisbury, United Kingdom*

ODO DE WEERS • *Laboratory for Vaccine Development and Immune Mechanisms, National Institute of Public Health and Environmental Protection, Bilthoven, The Netherlands*

JERRY M. WELLS • *Institute of Food Research, Norwich Research Park, Colney, Norwich, United Kingdom*

ANDREW WOODS • *Department of Immunobiology, Guy's, King's, and St. Thomas' School of Medicine, London, United Kingdom*

# 1

## Overview of Vaccines

### Gordon Ada

## 1. Patterns of Infectious Processes

Most vaccines are designed as a prophylactic measure to stimulate a lasting immune response so that on subsequent exposure to the particular infectious agent, the extent of infection is reduced to such an extent that disease does not occur (*1*). There is also increasing interest in designing vaccines that may be effective as a therapeutic measure, immunotherapy.

There are two contrasting types of infectious processes.

### 1.1. Intracellular vs Extracellular Patterns

Some organisms, including all viruses and some bacteria, are obligate intracellular infectious agents, as they only replicate inside a susceptible cell. Some parasites, such as plasmodia, have intracellular phases as part of their life cycle. In contrast, many bacteria and parasites replicate extracellularly. The immune responses required to control the different patterns of infections may therefore differ.

### 1.2. Acute vs Persistent Infections

In the case of an acute infection, exposure of a naive individual to a sublethal dose of the infectious agent may cause disease, but the immune response generated will clear the infection within a period of days or weeks. Death occurs if the infecting dose is so high that the immune response is qualitatively or quantitatively insufficient to prevent continuing replication of the agent so that the host is overwhelmed. In contrast, many infections persist for months or years if the process of infection by the agent results in the evasion or subversion of what would normally be an effective immune control reaction(s).

Most of the vaccines registered for use in developed countries, and discussed briefly in the next section, are designed to prevent acute human infections.

From: *Methods in Molecular Medicine, Vol. 87: Vaccine Protocols, 2nd ed.*
Edited by: A. Robinson, M. J. Hudson, and M. P. Cranage © Humana Press Inc., Totowa, NJ

**Table 1**
**Currently Registered Viral and Bacterial Vaccines**

| Viral | Bacterial |
|---|---|
| **Live, attenuated** | |
| Vaccinia (smallpox) | BCG |
| Polio (OPV) | *Salmonella typhi* (Ty21a) |
| Yellow fever | |
| Measles | |
| Mumps | |
| Rubella | |
| Adeno | |
| Varicella | |
| **Inactivated, whole organism** | |
| Influenza | *Vibrio cholerae* |
| Rabies | *Bordetella pertussis* |
| Japanese encephalitis | *Yersinia pestis* |
| Hepatitis A | *Coxiella burnetii* |
| **Subunit** | |
| Influenza | *Borrelia burgdorferi* |
| Hepatitis B (Hep B) | *Salmonella typhi* VI |
| | *B. pertussis* (acellular) |
| **Carbohydrate** | *Neisseria meningiditis* (A, C, Y, W135) |
| | *Streptococcus pneumoniae* |
| **Conjugates** | *Haemophilus influenzae,* type b |
| | *Streptococcus pneumoniae* |
| | *Neisseria meningiditis* (C) |
| **Toxoids** | |
| | *Corynebacterium diphtheriae* |
| | *Clostridium tetani* |
| **Combinations** | |
| Measles, mumps, rubella (MMR) | Diphtheria, tetanus, pertussis whole organism (DTPw) |
| | Diphtheria, tetanus, pertussis acellular (DTPa) |
| | DTPa, Hib, Hep B |

## 2. Types of Vaccines

Almost all of the vaccines in use today are used against viral or bacterial infections (**Table 1**). They are mainly of three types—live attenuated agents; inactivated, whole agents; and parts of an agent—subunit, polysaccharides, carbohydrate/conjugate preparations, and toxoids.

## 2.1. Live, Attenuated Microorganisms

Some live viral vaccines are regarded by many as the most successful of all human vaccines (*see* **Subheading 4.**), with one or two administrations conferring long-lasting immunity. Four general approaches to develop such vaccines have been used.

1. One approach, pioneered by Edward Jenner, is to use a virus that is a natural pathogen in another mammalian host as a vaccine in humans. Examples of this approach are the use of cowpox and parainfluenza viruses in humans, and the turkey herpes virus in chickens. More recently, the use of avipox viruses, such as fowlpox and canarypox, which undergo an abortive infection in humans, is being used in humans as vectors of DNA coding for antigens of other infectious agents *(2)*.
2. The polio, measles, and yellow fever vaccines are typical of the second approach. The wild-type viruses are extensively passaged in tissue culture/animal hosts until an acceptable balance is reached between loss of virulence and retention of immunogenicity in humans.
3. Type 2 polio virus is a naturally occurring attenuated strain that has been highly successful. More recently, rotavirus strains of low virulence have been recovered from children's nurseries during epidemics *(3)*.
4. A fourth approach has been to select mutants that will grow at low temperatures but very poorly above 37°C (*see* Chapter 2). The cold-adapted strains of influenza virus grow at 25°C and have mutations in four of the internal viral genes *(4)*. Such strains were first described in the late 1960s, and have since been used successfully in Russia and have undergone extensive clinical trials in the United States.

In contrast to the these successes, bacillus Calmette-Guérin (BCG) for the control of tuberculosis was for many years the only example of a live attenuated bacterial vaccine. Although still widely used in the WHO Expanded Programme of Immunization (EPI) for infants, it has yielded highly variable results in adult human trials. In general, it has proven more difficult to make highly effective attenuated bacterial vaccines, but with increasing examples of antibiotic resistance occurring, there is now a greater effort. A general approach is to selectively delete or inactivate part or groups of genes (*see* **ref. 5**; Chapter 9). Salmonella strain Ty21a has a faulty galactose metabolism, and strains with other deletions are being made. The latest approach is to sequence the bacterial genome, and this has now been done for many different bacteria (*see* Chapter 19).

Genetic modifications also show promise for complex viruses. Thus, 18 open reading frames have been selectively deleted from the Copenhagen strain of vaccinia virus, including six genes involved in nucleotide metabolism, to form a preparation of very low virulence, yet one that retains immunogenicity *(6)*. This approach has also been tried with simian immunodeficiency virus (SIV), first with deletion of the *nef* gene *(7)* and more recently with portions (the V2 and V3 loops) of the *env* gene *(8)*.

Live attenuated vaccines have the potential to stimulate a wide range of immune responses that may be effective in preventing or clearing a later infection in most recipients.

## 2.2. Inactivated Whole Microorganisms

Viruses and bacteria can be treated to destroy their infectivity (inactivation) and the product used with varying efficacy as a vaccine (**Table 1**). Compared to attenuated preparations, inactivated preparations must be given in larger doses and administered more frequently. The viral vaccines are generally effective in preventing disease, and the relatively low efficacy of the influenza viral vaccine is partly the result of the continuing antigenic drift to which this virus is subject *(9)*. In contrast, the only bacterial vaccine of this nature still in wide use is the whole-cell pertussis vaccine that is reasonably effective, but has been replaced in many developed countries by the subunit (acellular) vaccine in order to avoid the adverse effects attributed to the whole-cell vaccine *(10)*.

Inactivated whole vaccines generally induce many of the desirable immune responses, particularly the infectivity-neutralizing antibody. Generally, they do not induce a class I MHC-restricted cytotoxic T-cell response, which has been shown to be the major response required to clear intracellular infections caused by many viruses and some bacteria and parasites.

## 2.3. Subunit Vaccines

The generation of antibody that prevents infection by both intra- and extracellular microorganisms has been regarded as the prime requirement of a vaccine. The epitopes recognized by such antibodies are usually restricted to one or a few proteins or carbohydrate moieties that are present at the external surface of the microorganism. Isolation (or synthesis) of such components formed the basis of the first viral and bacterial subunit vaccines. Viral vaccines were composed of the influenza surface antigens, the hemagglutinin and neuraminidase, and the hepatitis B-surface antigen (HBsAg). Bacterial vaccines contain the different oligosaccharide-based preparations from encapsulated bacteria (*see* Chapter 10). In the latter case, immunogenicity was greatly increased, especially for the children under 2 yr of age, by coupling the haptenic moiety (the carbohydrate) to a protein carrier, thereby ensuring the involvement of T-helper (Th) cells in the production of different classes of immunoglobulin (Ig), particularly IgG. This approach has become increasingly more popular in recent years *(11,12)*. The two bacterial toxoids, tetanus, and diphtheria, represent a special situation in which the primary requirement was neutralization of the toxin secreted by the invading bacteria. Whereas this has traditionally been done by treatment with chemicals, it is now being achieved by genetic manipulation (*see* Chapter 9).

HBsAg exists as such in the blood of hepatitis B virus (HBV)-infected people, and infected blood was the source of antigen for the first vaccines. Production of the antigen in yeast cells transfected with DNA coding for this antigen initiated the era of genetically engineered vaccines *(13)*. Up to 17% of adults receiving this vaccine are poor or nonresponders, and this is a result of their genetic make-up and/or their advanced age *(14)*. A second genetically engineered subunit preparation from *B. burgdorferi* to control lyme disease is now available *(15)*.

## 3. Vaccine Safety

All available data concerning the efficacy and safety of candidate vaccines are reviewed by regulatory authorities before registration (*see* Chapter 22). At that stage, potential safety hazards which occur at a frequency greater than about 1/5,000 doses should have been detected (*see* Chapter 21). Some undesirable side effects occur at much lower frequencies, which are seen only during immunosurveillance following registration. The Guillain-Barré syndrome occurs after administration of the influenza vaccine at a frequency of about 1 case per million doses; but following the mass vaccination of people in the United States with the swine influenza vaccine in 1976–1877, the incidence was about 1 case/60,000 doses *(16)*. The incidence of encephalopathy after measles infection is about 1 case per 1000 doses, but only 1 case per million doses of measles vaccine *(17)*. In the United States, the use of OPV resulted in about one case of paralysis per million doses of the vaccine, because of reversion to virulence of the type 3 virus strain. The Centers for Disease and Control (CDC) Advisory Committee on Immunization Practices and the American Academy of Pediatrics (AAP) recommended that only the IPV be used in the United States after January 1, 2000 *(18)*.

Following successful vaccination campaigns that greatly reduced disease outbreaks, the low levels of undesirable side-effects following vaccination gain notoriety. The evidence bearing on causality and specific adverse health outcomes following vaccination against some childhood viral and bacterial diseases, mainly in the United States, has been evaluated by an expert committee of the Institute of Medicine (IOM) *(19)*. The possibility of adverse neurological effects was of particular concern, and evidence for these as well as several immunological reactions, such as anaphylaxis and delayed-type hypersensitivity, was examined in detail. In the great majority of cases, there was insufficient evidence to support a causal relationship, and where the data were more persuasive, the risk was considered to be extraordinarily low.

Measles has provided an interesting example of vaccine safety. The experience of the WHO EPI shows that the vaccine is very safe *(20)*. Although natural measles infection induces a state of immunosuppression, even immunocompromised children rarely show this effect after vaccination *(19)*. In developing countries, the EPI schedule is to give the vaccine at 9 mo of age. This delay is meant to allow a sufficient drop in the level of maternally derived antibody so that the vaccine can take. In some infants, this decay occurs by 6 mo, resulting in many deaths from measles infection in the ensuing 2–3 mo. "High-titer" vaccines were therefore developed, which could be given at 6 mo of age. Trials in several countries showed the apparent safety and efficacy of the new vaccine, but after WHO authorized its wider usage, some young girls in disadvantaged countries died, leading to the withdrawal of the vaccine *(21)*. One possibility is that the high-titer vaccine caused a degree of immunosuppression sufficient to allow infections by other infectious agents.

Even after using great care in developing a vaccine, unexpected effects can occur after the vaccine has been registered for use. A rotavirus vaccine, registered for use in the United States in 1998, was withdrawn in 1999 after administration to 1.5 million

**Table 2**
**Efficacy in the USA of Some Childhood Vaccines**[a]

| Disease agent | Before vaccination | | After vaccination | |
|---|---|---|---|---|
| | Number of cases (yr) | Vaccine (yr)* | Number of cases (1997) | Decrease in disease incidence (%) |
| Diphtheria | 206,919 (1921) | 1942 | 5 | 99.99 |
| Measles | 894,134 (1941) | 1963 | 135# | 99.98 |
| Mumps | 152,209 (1971) | 1971 | 612 | 99.6 |
| Rubella | 57,686 (1969) | 1971 | 161 | 97.9 |
| Pertussis | 265,269 (1952) | 1952 | 5519 | 97.9 |
| Poliomyelitis | | | | |
| (paralytic) | 21,269 (1952) | 1952** | 0 | 100 |
| (total) | 57,879 | | | |
| *H. influenzae* | 20,000 | (1984) | 165 | 99.2 |
| (Hib) | | 1984 | | |

[a]As measured by the decrease in incidence of disease some time after the vaccine was introduced compared to the incidence during an epidemic prior to vaccine availability.

*Year of introduction of the vaccine.

** IPV, Salk vaccine in 1952; OPV, Sabin vaccine in 1963.

# A two-dose schedule for measles vaccination was introduced after an epidemic in 1989–1991. The 135 cases in 1997 were all introduced by visitors to the United States.

Data kindly provided by the Centers for Disease Control and Prevention, Atlanta, and Summary of notifiable diseases, United States. 1998; MMWR. 47; no. 53.

children, because of an unacceptable level—about one case per 10,000 recipients in some areas—of the condition intussusception *(22)*.

It is particularly difficult to attribute causality to the onset of diseases that may occur many months after vaccination. When such claims are made, national authorities or WHO establish expert committees to review the evidence. There have been claims—sometimes in the medical literature but often from anti-vaccination groups—that a vaccine can cause sudden infant death syndrome (SIDS), multiple sclerosis, autism, asthma, or a specific allergy. There is no sound medical, scientific or epidemiological evidence to support these claims. For example, at least eleven different investigations have found no evidence that inflammatory bowel disease and autism occur as a result of measles, mumps, rubella (MMR) vaccination *(23,24)*.

## 4. Efficacy

Many countries keep yearly records of disease incidence and the Centers for Disease Control and Prevention (CDC) in Atlanta have kept records from as early as 1912. The incidence of cases of some common childhood infectious diseases during a major epidemic is compared in **Table 2** with the incidence in 1997, some years after the introduction of the vaccine. Although derived in relatively ideal conditions, as all

**Table 3**
**Necessary and Desirable Factors for an Infectious Disease**
**to be Eradicated by Vaccination**

| Factor | Disease | | |
|---|---|---|---|
| | Smallpox | Poliomyelitis | Measles |
| 1. Infection is limited to humans. | Yes | Yes | Yes |
| 2. Only one or a few strains (low antigenic drift). | Yes | Yes | Yes |
| 3. Absence of subclinical/carrier cases. | Yes | Yes | Yes |
| 4. A safe, effective vaccine is available. | Yes* | Yes* | Yes |
| 5. Vaccine is heat-stable. | Yes | No | No |
| 6. Virus is only moderately infectious.** | Yes | High | Very high |
| 7. There is a simple marker of successful vaccination. | Yes | No | No |

*The levels of side effects after vaccination were/are acceptable at the time.

**The level of vaccine coverage to achieve herd immunity and prevent transmission varied from (usually) 80% for smallpox and is about 95% for measles.

the infections are acute and each agent shows little (if any) antigenic drift, the data show that vaccines can be extraordinarily effective *(20)*. Equally impressive is the reduced incidence of one infectious disease in the United Kingdom—a 92–95% reduction in toddlers and teenagers respectively, within 12 mo of the introduction in 1999 of a new *N. meningiditis* C vaccine (*see* **ref. 11**; Chapter 21).

One of the greatest public health achievements in the twentieth century was the global eradication of smallpox. Announced to the World Health Assembly (WHA) in 1980, 3 yr after the last case of indigenous smallpox in the world was treated, the goal took 10 yr to achieve after formation of the Special Programme for Smallpox Eradication by WHO *(25)*. Following the successful elimination of indigenous poliomyelitis in the Americas in 1991, the WHA announced the goal of global eradication by the year 2000. The elimination of indigenous poliomyelitis has now also been achieved in the European and Western Pacific regions, and global eradication is now planned by 2005 *(26)*.

Prevention of transmission of measles infection has been achieved in several smaller countries, including Finland, as well as in the United States and Canada, following the introduction of a two-dose vaccination schedule.

**Table 3** lists necessary and desirable properties for an infectious disease to be eradicated by vaccination. Although the first four factors are critical, the other three factors contribute to the ease or difficulty of the task. If the Smallpox Eradication Programme had failed, it is unlikely that the other eradication programs would have been initiated.

## 5. Opportunities for Improved and New Vaccines

There are over 70 infectious agents—viruses, bacteria, parasites, and fungi—that cause serious disease in humans *(27)*. There are registered vaccines against 25 infectious agents (nearly 40 different vaccines) and approx 14 other candidate vaccines have entered or passed phase II clinical trials. Vaccine development is at an earlier

**Table 4**
**Some Opportunities for Improved and New Vaccines**

| Improved | New |
|---|---|
| **Viral** | |
| Japanese encephalitis | Corona |
| Polio | Cytomegalo |
| Rabies | Dengue |
| Measles | Epstein-Barr |
| Influenza | Hantan |
| | Hepatitis C |
| | Herpes |
| | HIV-1, 2 |
| | HTLV |
| | Papilloma |
| | Parainfluenza |
| | Respiratory syncytial |
| | Rota |
| **Bacterial** | |
| Cholera | Chlamydia |
| *M. tuberculosis* | *E. coli* |
| | *H. ducreyi* |
| | *M. leprae* |
| | *N. gonorrhoeae* |
| | Shigella |
| **Others** | |
| | Malaria |
| | Filariasis |
| | Giardia |
| | Schistosomiasis |
| | Treponema |

stage with most of the other viruses and bacteria *(28)*. **Table 4** lists some examples of when improved vaccines are required, and other examples of vaccine development at an advanced stage.

## 6. New Approaches to Vaccine Development

### 6.1. Anti-Idiotypes

The advantages of this approach include the fact that the anti-idiotype should mimic both carbohydrate and peptide-based epitope; and the conformation of the epitope in question. The potential advantages of the former point have disappeared following the recent successes of carbohydrate/protein conjugate vaccines *(11,12)*. The use of this technology may be largely restricted to very special situations, such as identifying the nature of the epitope recognized by very rare antibodies that neutralize a wide spectrum of human immunodeficiency virus (HIV)-1 primary isolates *(29)*.

### 6.2. Oligo/Polypeptides (see also *Chapter 8*)

The sequences may contain either B-cell epitopes or T-cell determinants, or both. Sequences containing B-cell epitopes may either be conjugated to carrier proteins, which act as a source of T-helper cell determinants, or assembled in different ways to achieve particular tertiary configurations. Some of the obvious advantages of this approach are that the final product contains the critical components of the antigen and avoids other sequences that may mimic host sequences, and thus potentially induce an autoimmune response. Multiple Antigenic Peptide Systems (MAPS) are more immunogenic than individual sequences *(30)*, and the immunogenicity of important "cryptic" sequences may sometimes be enhanced by the deletion of other segments *(31)*. New methods of synthesis offer the possibility of more closely mimicking the conformational patterns in the original protein.

This approach is likely to be applicable, especially for some bacterial and parasitic vaccines. However, the first peptide-based candidate vaccine that underwent efficacy trials in malaria endemic regions yielded disappointing results *(32)*. A preparation composed of polymers of linked peptides from group A streptococcus, which was effective in a mouse model *(33)*, is currently undergoing clinical trials.

### 6.3. Transfection of Cells with DNA/cDNA Coding for Foreign Antigens

This is now a well-established procedure. Three cell types have been used: prokaryotes; lower eukaryotes, mainly yeast; and mammalian cells—either primary cells (e.g., monkey kidney), cell strains (with a finite replicating ability), or cell lines (immortalized cells such as Chinese Hamster Ovary cells [CHO]). Each has its own advantages. As a general rule, other bacterial proteins should preferably be made in transfected bacterial cells, and human viral antigens, especially glycoproteins, in mammalian cells, because of the substantial differences in properties, such as post-translational modifications in different cell types.

### 6.4. Live Viral and Bacterial Vectors

**Table 5** lists the viruses and bacteria mostly used for this purpose. Of the viruses, the greatest experience has been with vaccinia and its derivatives such as the highly attenuated modified vaccinia virus Ankara (*see* Chapter 4). These have a wide host range, possess many different promoters, and can accommodate DNA coding for up to 10 average-sized proteins. The avipox viruses, canary and fowlpox, undergo abortive replication in mammals, making them very safe to use as vectors. Adeno (*see* Chapter 3) and polio viruses, and Salmonella (*see* Chapter 6) are mainly used for delivery via a mucosal route, although vaccinia and BCG have been administered both orally and intranasally.

Making such chimeric vectors has also been an effective way to evaluate the potential role of different cytokines in immune processes (*see* Chapter 12). Inserting DNA coding for a particular cytokine as well as that for the foreign antigen(s) results in the synthesis and secretion of the cytokine at the site of infection so its maximum effect should be displayed. Thus, IL-4 and IL-12 have been shown to have dominant effects

**Table 5**
**Some Viruses and Bacteria Currently Used Experimentally as Vectors
of RNA/DNA Coding for Antigens from Other Infectious agents**

| Infectious agents for humans | |
|---|---|
| Viruses (RNA genome) | Influenza, picorna viruses (polio, mengoviruses) |
| | Rhino, Semliki Forest, Venezuelan equine encephalitis |
| (DNA genome) | Poxviruses* (vaccinia, Ankara, NYVAC), adeno,* herpes simplex, Vesicula stomatitis |
| Bacteria BCG* | *Brucella abortis, Lactococcus lacti, Listeria monocytogenes, Salmonella typhi** |
| Avian infections[#] | Fowlpox,* canarypox* |
| Insect | Baculovirus* |

*Vectors most widely studied.
[#]Avian viruses undergo an abortive infection in humans.

in inducing a humoral or cell-mediated immune response, respectively. Incorporating DNA coding for IL-4 into the genome of ectromelia virus greatly increased the virulence of this virus for otherwise resistant mice, and even if the latter had been immunized before challenge *(34)*.

### 6.5. "Naked" DNA

The most fascinating and exciting of the recent approaches to vaccine development has been the injection of plasmids containing the DNA coding for antigen(s) of interest, either directly into muscle cells or as DNA-coated tiny gold beads into the skin, using a "gene gun" *(35; see* Chapter 23). In the latter case, some beads are taken up by Langerhan's (dendritic) cells, and during passage to the draining lymph nodes, the expressed foreign protein(s) is processed, appropriate peptide sequences attach to MHC molecules and the complex is expressed at the cell surface. These complexes are recognized by naïve, immunocompetent T-cells in the node, and activation of these cells occurs. A basically similar process occurs following muscle injection. In subhuman primates, this procedure primarily induces a "type 1" T-cell response resulting in both an antibody and cell-mediated response, with both CD4+ and CD8+ effector T-cells, rather similar in many respects to the response following an acute infection. One advantage is that the response occurs in the presence of specific antibody to the encoded antigen.

## 7. Properties and Functions of Different Components of the Immune System

### 7.1. Classes of Lymphocytes

Our knowledge of the properties of lymphocytes—the cell type of major importance in vaccine development—has increased enormously in recent years *(36)*. The

**Table 6**
**Properties and Functions of Different Components of the Immune System**

| | | | Stages of infectious process | | | |
|---|---|---|---|---|---|---|
| Type of response | Cytokine profile | Type of infection | Prevent | Limit | Reduce | Clear |
| **Innate** | | I | – | ++ | + | – |
| | | E | – | ? | ? | – |
| **Adaptive** | | I | +++ | ++ | ++ | +/– |
| **Antibody** | | E | +++ | +++ | +++ | +++ |
| CD4+TH2 | IL-3,4,5,6,10,13 | I | | | | |
| | | E | | | | |
| CD4+Th1 | IL-2, IFNγ, TNFα | I | – | ++ | ++ | +? |
| | | E | – | ++ | ++ | ++ |
| CD8+CTLs | IFNγ, TNFβ, TNFα | I | – | +++ | +++ | +++ |
| | | E | – | – | – | – |

I, intracellular infection; E, extracellular infection; IL, interleukin; IFN, interferon; TNF, tumor necrosis factor.

major role of B-lymphocytes is the production of antibodies of different isotypes and, of course, specificity. The other class of lymphocytes, the T-cells (so called because they mature in the thymus), consist of two main types. One, with the cell-surface marker CD4, exist in two subclasses, the Th-1 and Th-2 cells (h = helper activity). The major role of Th-2 cells is to help B-cells differentiate, replicate, in the form of plasma cells, secrete antibodies of a defined specificity, and of different subclasses: IgG, IgE, and IgA. This is facilitated by the secretion of different cytokines (interleukins, or ILs) which are listed in **Table 6**. Th-1 cells also have a small but important role in helping B-cells produce antibody of various IgG subtypes, but the overall pattern of cytokine secretion is markedly different. Factors such as IFN-γ, TNF-α, and TNF-β have several functions, such as anti-viral activity and upregulation of components (e.g., MHC antigens) on other cells, including macrophages that can lead to their "activation" and, if infected, greater susceptibility to recognition by T-cells. Th-1 cells also mediate (via cytokine secretion) delayed-type hypersensitivity (DTH) responses that may have a protective role in some infections.

The other type of T-cell has the cell-surface marker CD8, and its pattern of cytokine secretion is similar to that of CD4+Th-1 cells, although they generally mediate DTH responses rather poorly. As primary effector cells in vivo, CD8+ T-cells recognize and lyse cells infected either by a virus or by some bacteria and parasites—hence the name cytotoxic T-lymphocytes (CTLs). An important aspect of this arm of the immune response is that susceptibility of the infected cell to lysis occurs shortly after infection and many hours before infectious progeny is produced, thus giving a "window of time" for the effector cell to find and destroy the infected cell *(37)*.

## 7.2. Recognition Patterns

Both CD4 and CD8 T-cells recognize a complex between the MHC molecule and a peptide from a foreign protein. In the former case, the peptide, which is derived from antigen being degraded in the lysosomes, complexes with a class II MHC antigen. In the second case, the peptide is derived from newly synthesized antigen in the cytoplasm, and binds to class I MHC antigen. These complexes are expressed at the cell surface and are recognized by the T-cell receptor. Since nearly all cell types in the body express class I MHC molecules, the role of CD8+ CTLs has been described as performing a continuous molecular audit of the body *(38)*.

## 7.3. Roles of Different Immune Responses

**Table 6** ascribes particular roles to specific antibody and to the T-cell subsets. Some general conclusions regarding adaptive immune responses are:

1. Specific antibody is the major mechanism for preventing or greatly limiting an infection.
2. CTLs are the major mechanism for controlling and finally clearing most (acute) intracellular infections *(39)*. Generally, they would not be formed during an extracellular infection. There are only a few, rather special examples of antibody clearing an intracellular infection *(40,41)*.
3. Antibody should clear an extracellular infection with the aid of activated cells expressing Fc or complement receptors such as macrophages, which can engulf and often destroy antibody-coated particles. Th-1 cells are important for the activation of such cells.
4. Th-1 cells may contribute to the control and clearance of some intracellular infections. For example, IFNγ has been shown to clear a vaccinia virus (a poorly virulent pathogen for mice) infection in nude mice *(42)*.

## 7.4. The Selective Induction of Different Immune Responses

During an acute model infection such as murine influenza, the sequence of appearance in the infected lung of adaptive responses is: first, CD4+ Th-cells, then CD8+ CTLs, and finally antibody-secreting cells (ASCs). The CTLs are largely responsible for virus clearance, and it is believed that the subsequent decline in CTL activity, which occurs shortly after infectious virus can no longer be recovered *(43)*, is a result of the short half-life of these cells. However, it has now been found that if IL-4 formation is "artificially" induced very early after infection, CTL formation is substantially suppressed *(44)*. Thus, the early decline in CTL activity, which occurs as IgG-antibody-secreting cells are increasing in number, may be the result, at least in part, of the production of IL-4 which favors a Th-2 response. The important point is that a large pool of memory CTLs has already been formed by the time CTL-effector activity disappears. These memory cells persist, and are rapidly activated if the host is exposed to the same or closely related infectious agent at a later time. In contrast, in other systems, IL-12 has been found to favor a Th-1 type response *(45)*.

It is now recognized that, as well as affecting the magnitude and persistence of immune responses to non-infectious preparations, adjuvants can also greatly influence the type of immune response (*see* Chapter 11). Some adjuvants, such as alum and cholera toxin and its B subunit, favor CD4+ Th-2 responses. Water-in-oil emulsions, such as Freund's complete and incomplete adjuvant and lipopolysaccharide (LPS), favor a Th-1 response. A variety of delivery systems is available for the induction of CTL responses *(46)*.

## 8. Some Factors That Affect the Ease of Development of Vaccines

Although the new technologies are making it more likely that attempts to develop vaccines to an increasing number of infectious agents will be successful, many other factors may influence the final outcome. Some of these factors are:

1. The simpler the agent, the greater the chance that important protective antigens will be identified.
2. The occurrence of great antigenic diversity in the pathogen can be a major hurdle, especially in the case of RNA viruses, because escape mutants (antigenic drift) may readily occur.
3. Integration of DNA/c.DNA into the host-cell genome is likely to lead to lifelong infection, which it is difficult for a vaccine to prevent/overcome.
4. If a sublethal natural infection does not lead to protection from a second infection, an understanding of the pathogenesis of the infection and how the normal protective responses (antibody, cell-mediated) are subverted or evaded is important.
5. The ready availability of an inexpensive animal model that mimics the natural human disease can be very helpful.

## 9. Promising Developments

Despite these constraints, there are also some promising recent developments.

### 9.1. Combination Vaccines

Vaccine delivery is a major cost component in vaccination programs. Combining vaccines so that three or more can be administered simultaneously results in considerable savings, so there are determined efforts to add further vaccines to DPaT and MMR, such as DPaT-hepatitis B-*H. influenzae* type b. There must be compatibility and no interference by one component on another. There is the risk of antigenic competition that occurs at the T-cell level, and the likelihood of such interference is difficult to predict. However, in the case of mixtures of carbohydrate/protein conjugates, using the same carrier protein should remove this risk. Individual components in mixtures of live viral vaccines, such as MMR, should not interfere with the take of other components. The use of the same vector—e.g., the same poxvirus, in mixtures of chimeric constructs—should also minimize this difficulty. Again, vaccination with DNA also offers the prospect of great advantages. Other than the possibility of antigenic competition, it is expected that combination of different DNA vaccines should not be subject to these other constraints.

Two other recent developments should facilitate vaccine availability and uptake. One is the application of the vaccine directly to prewashed skin using a powerful adjuvant such as cholera toxin, a technique known as transcutaneous immunization *(47)*. The second is the ability to produce some antigens (and also antibodies) in plants so that simply eating say the fruit of the plant containing the antigen would result in vaccination *(48)*.

## 9.2. Mixed Vaccine Formulations: The Prime/Boost Approach

Immunization of vaccinia-naïve volunteers with an HIV gp160/vaccinia virus construct followed by boosting with a recombinant gp 160 preparation gave higher anti-gp160 antibody titers compared to using either preparation for both priming and boosting *(49)*. Mice that were immunized with a chimeric DNA preparation and later boosted with chimeric fowlpox both expressing influenza hemagglutinin (HA), gave anti-HA titers up to 50-fold higher than those found after two injections of the same preparation *(50)*. This approach is now being vigorously pursued to induce very high and persistent specific CTL responses to HIV-1, SIV, Ebola virus, *M. tuberculosis*, and plasmodia antigens, with very encouraging results in mice and/or monkeys *(51)*. Clinical trials are now underway to determine whether humans respond as well as lower primates to this approach.

## 9.3. The Genomic Analysis of Complex Infectious Agents

Whole-genome sequencing of complex microbes such as bacteria and parasites is poised to revolutionize the way vaccines are developed (*see* Chapter 19). This enables the characterization of potential candidate proteins that might be recognized by infectivity-neutralizing antibodies, and which ones may provide important T-cell determinants. In one recent example, mice immunized with six of 108 proteins from *S. pneumoniae*, which had been identified from the DNA sequence as having appropriate structural characteristics, were protected from disease when later challenged with this organism *(52)*.

## References

1. Plotkin, S. A. and Orenstein, W. A., eds. (1998) Vaccines, 3rd ed., W. B. Saunders Co., Philadelphia, PA, pp. 1–1230.
2. Cadoz, M., Strady, A., Meigner, B., et al. (1992) Immunization with canarypox virus expressing rabies glycoprotein. *Lancet* **339,** 1429–1432.
3. Clark, H. F., Glass, R. I., and Offit, P. A. (1998) Rotavirus vaccines, in *Vaccines*, 3rd ed., (Plotkin, S. A. and Orenstein, W. A., eds.) W. B. Saunders Co., Philadelphia, PA, pp. 987–1005.
4. Maassab, H. F., Herlocher, M. L., and Bryant, M. L. (1998) Live influenza virus vaccine, in *Vaccines*, 3rd ed., (Plotkin, S.A. and Orenstein, W.A., eds.) W. B. Saunders Co., Philadelphia, PA, pp. 909–927.
5. Levine, M. M. (1998). Typhoid fever vaccines, in *Vaccines*, 3rd ed., (Plotkin, S. A. and Orenstein, W. A., eds.) W. B. Saunders Co., Philadelphia, PA, pp. 781–814.
6. Tartaglia, J., Perkus, M. E., and Taylor, J. (1992) NYVAC: a highly attenuated strain of vaccinia virus. *Virology*, **188,** 217–232.
7. Daniel, M. D., Kirchhoff, F., Czajak, S., et al. (1992) Protective effects of a live attenuated SIV vaccine with a deletion in the nef gene. *Science* **258,** 1938–1940.
8. Cohen, J. (2001) AIDS vaccines show promise after years of frustration. *Science* **291,** 1686–1688.

9. Daly, J. M., Wood, J. M., and Robertson, J. S. (1998) Cocirculation and divergence of human influenza viruses, In: *Textbook of Influenza* (Nicholson, K. G., Webster, R. G., and Hay, A. J.).Blackwell Science Ltd., Oxford. UK, pp. 168–180.

10. Edwards, K. M., Decker, M. D., and Mortimer, E. A. (1998) Pertussis vaccine, in *Vaccines* 3rd ed., (Plotkin, S. A. and Orenstein, W. A., eds.) W. B. Saunders Co., Philadelphia, PA, pp 293–344.

11. Ramsay, M. E., Andrews, N., Keezmarsk, E. B., and Miller, E. (2001) Efficacy of meningococcal serogroup C conjugate vaccine in teenagers and toddlers in England. *Lancet* **357,** 195–196.

12. Lin, F. Y. C., Ho, V. A., Khiem, H. B., et al. (2001) The efficacy of a Salmonella Vi conjugate vaccine in two-to-five-year-old children. *N. Engl. J. Med.* **344,** 1263–1269.

13. Hilleman, M. R. (1992) Vaccine perspectives from the vantage of hepatitis B. *Vaccine Res.* **1,** 1–15.

14. Egea, E., Iglesias, A., Salazar, et al. (1991) The cellular basis for the lack of antibody response to hepatitis B vaccine in humans. *J. Exp. Med.*, **173,** 531–542.

15. Keller, D., Koster, F. T., Marks, D. H., et al. (1994) Safety and immunogenicity of a recombinant outer surface protein A Lyme vaccine. *J. Am. Med. Assoc.* **271,** 1764–1768.

16. Langmuir, I. D., Bregman, D. J., Kurland, L.D., et al. (1984) An epidemiological and clinical evaluation of Guillain-Barre syndrome reported in association with the administration of swine influenza vaccine. *J. Epidemiol.* **119,** 841–879.

17. Weibel, R. E., Casuta, V., Bessor, D. E., et al. (1998) Acute encephalopathy followed by permanent brain injury or death associated with further attenuated measles vaccines. *Pediatrics* **101,** 383–387.

18. Levin, A. (2000) Vaccines today. *Ann. Intern. Med.* **133,** 661–664.

19. Stratton, K. R., Howe, C. J., and Johnston, R. B. (1994). Adverse events associated with childhood vaccines. Evidence bearing on causality. Institute of Medicine, National Academy Press, Washington D.C., pp. 1–464.

20. Galaska, A. M., Lauer, B. A., Henderson, R. H., and Keja, J. (1984) Indications and contraindications for vaccines used in the expanded programme of immunization. *Bull. WHO* **62,** 357–366.

21. Halsey, N. A. (1993) Increased mortality following high titer measles vaccines: too much of a good thing. *Pediatr. Infect. Dis.*, **12,** 462–465.

22. Murphy, T.V., Gargiullo, P. M., Nassoudi, M. S., et al. (2001) Intussusception among infants given an oral rotavirus vaccine. *N. Engl. J. Med.*, **344,** 564–572.

23. Amin, J. and Wong, M. (1999) Measles, mumps, rubella immunization, autism and inflammatory bowel diseases: update. *Communicable Disease Intelligence* **23,** 222.

24. Elliman, D., and Bedford, H. (2001) MMR vaccine: the continuing saga. *Br. Med. J.* **322,** 183–184.

25. Fenner, F., Henderson, D. A., Arita, I., Jesek, Z., and Ladnyi, I. D. (1988) Smallpox and its eradication. World Health Organization, Geneva, 1–1460.

26. Department of Vaccines and Biologicals. World Health Organization. (2000) Key elements for improving supplementary immunization activities for polio eradication. Geneva, 1–30.

27. Ada, G. and Ramsay, A. (1997) *Vaccines, Vaccination and The Immune Response.* Lippincott-Raven, Philadelphia, PA, pp. 1–247.

28. Division of Microbiology and Infectious Diseases, National Institutes of Health. (2000) The Jordan Report. Accelerated Development of Vaccines, pp. 1–173.

29. Saphire, E. O., Parren, P. W. H. I., Pantophlet, R., et al. (2001) Crystal structure of a neutralizing human IgG against HIV-1: a template for vaccine design. *Science* **293,** 1155–1159.

30. Tam, J. P. (1988) Synthetic peptide vaccine design: synthesis and properties of a high density multiple antigenic peptide system. *Proc. Natl. Acad. Sci. USA* **85,** 5409–5413.

31. D'Alessandro, U., Leach, A., Diakeley, C. J., et al. (1995) Efficacy trial of a malaria vaccine SPf66 in Gambian infants. *Lancet* **346,** 462–467.

32. Pruksakorn, S., Currie, B., Brandt, E., et al. (1994) Towards a vaccine for rheumatic fever: identification of a conserved target epitope on M protein of group A streptococci. *Lancet* **344,** 639–642.

33. Brandt, E. R., Sriprakash, K. S., Hobb, R. I., et al. (2000) New multi-determinant strategy for a group A streptococcal vaccine designed for the Australian aboriginal population. *Nat. Med.* **6,** 455–459.

34. Jackson, R. J., Ramsay, A. J., Christensen, C. D., et al. (2001) Expression of mouse interleukin-4 by a recombinant ectromelia virus suppresses cytolytic lymphocyte responses and overcomes genetic resistance to mousepox. *J. Virol.* **75,** 1205–1210.

35. McDonnell, W. M. and Askari, F. K. Molecular medicine; DNA vaccines. (1995) *N. Engl. J. Med.* **324,** 42–45.

36. Delves, P. J. and Roitt, I. M. (2000) The immune system. *N. Engl. J. Med.* **343,** Part 1, 37–49. Part 2, 108–117.

37. Jackson, D. C., Ada, G. L., and Tha Lha, R. (1976) Cytotoxic T cells recognize very early, minor changes in ectromelia virus-infected target cells. *Aust J. Exp. Biol. Med. Sci.* **54,** 349–363.

38. Geisow, M. J. (1991) Unravelling the mysteries of molecular audit: MHC class I restriction. *Tibtech* **9,** 403–404.

39. Ada, G. (1994) Twenty years into the saga of MHC-restriction. *Immunol. Cell Biol.* **72,** 447–454.

40. Taylor, G. (1994) The role of antibody in controlling and/or clearing virus infections, in *Strategies in Vaccine Design.* (Ada, GL. ed.), Landes, Austin, TX, pp. 17–34.

41. Griffin, D. E., Levine, B., Tyor, W. B., and Irani, D. N. (1992) The immune response in viral encephalitis. *Semin. Immunol.* **4,** 111–1191.

42. Ramshaw, I. R., Ruby, J., Ramsay, A., et al. (1992) Expression of cytokines by recombinant vaccinia viruses: a model for studying cytokines in virus infections in vivo. *Immunol. Rev.* **127,** 157–182.

43. Ada, G. L. (1990) The immune response to antigens: the immunological principles of vaccination. *Lancet* **335,** 523–526.

44. Sharma, D. P., Ramsay, A. J., and Maguire, D. J., et al. (1996) Interleukin 4 mediates down regulation of antiviral cytokine expression and cytotoxic T lymphocyte responses and exacerbates vaccinia virus infection in vivo. *J. Virol.* **70,** 7103–7107.

45. Afonso, L. C. C., Scharton, T. M., Vieira, L. Q., et al. (1994) The adjuvant effect of interleukin-12 in a vaccine against Leishmaniasis major. *Science* **263,** 235–237.

46. Allsopp, C. E. M., Plebanski, M., Gilbert, S., et al. (1996) Comparison of numerous delivery systems for the induction of cytotoxic T lymphocytes by immunization. *Eur. J. Immunol.* **26,** 1951–1959.

47. Glenn, G. M., Taylor, D. N., Li, X., et al. (2000) Transcutaneous immunization: a human vaccine delivery strategy using a patch. *Nat. Med.* **6,** 1403–1406.

48. Hammond, J., McGarvey, P., Yusibov, B. eds. (1999) Plant biotechnology. New procedures and applications. *Cont. Top. Microbiol. Immunol.* **240,** 1–196.

49. Graham, B. S., Matthews, T. J., Belshe, R. B., et al. (1993) Augmentation of human immunodeficiency virus type-1 neutralizing antibody by priming with gp160 recombinant vaccinia and boosting with rgp160 in vaccinia naïve adults. *J. Infect. Dis.* **167,** 533–537.

50. Leong, K. H., Ramsay, A. J., Morin, M. J., et al. (1995) Generation of enhanced immune responses by consecutive immunization with DNA and recombinant fowlpox virus, in *Vaccines '95.* (Brown, F., Chanock, R., Ginsberg, H., and Norrby, E., eds.), Cold Spring Harbor Laboratory Press, pp. 327–331.

51. Ada, G. (2001). Vaccines and vaccination. *N. Engl. J. Med.* 355.

52. Wizemann, T. M., Heinrichs, J. H., Adamou, J., et al. (2001) Use of a whole genome approach to identify vaccine molecules affording protection against *Streptococcus pneumoniae* infection. *Infect. Immun.* **69,** 1593–1598.

# 2

# Temperature-Sensitive Mutant Vaccines

## Craig R. Pringle

## 1. Introduction

Many live virus vaccines derived by empirical routes exhibit temperature-sensitive (ts) phenotypes. The live virus vaccines that have been outstandingly successful in controlling poliomyelitis are the prime example of this phenomenon. The three live attenuated strains developed by Albert Sabin were derived from wild-type isolates by rapid sequential passage at high multiplicity of infection (MOI) in monkey tissue in vitro and in vivo, a regimen that yielded variants of reduced neurovirulence. Concomitantly, the three vaccine strains developed ts characteristics, a phenotype that correlated well with loss of neurovirulence. The reproductive capacity at supraoptimal (40°C) temperature, the *rct* phenotype, proved to be a useful property for monitoring the genetic stability of the attenuated virus during propagation, vaccine production, and replication in vaccinees. Nucleotide sequencing of the genome of the poliovirus type 3 attenuated virus and its neurovirulent wild-type progenitor (the Leon strain), revealed that only ten nucleotide changes, producing three amino acid substitutions, differentiated the attenuated derivative from its virulent parent despite its lengthy propagation in cultured cells. One of the three coding changes, a serine-to-phenylalanine substitution at position 2034 in the region encoding VP3, conferred the ts phenotype. A combination of nucleotide sequencing of virus recovered from a vaccine-associated case of paralysis and assay in primates of the neurovirulence of recombinant viruses prepared from infectious cDNA established that two of the ten mutations in the type three vaccine strain were associated with the loss of neurovirulence. The mutation conferring temperature-sensitivity was one of these mutations *(1)*.

Since all three independently modified poliovirus vaccines exhibit temperature-sensitivity, it is likely that ts mutations in general may be attenuating by diminishing reproductive potential without appreciable loss of immunogenicity. However, it is not clear why temperature-sensitivity *per se* should adversely affect replication of poliovirus in the central nervous system (CNS), while allowing replication to proceed nor-

From: *Methods in Molecular Medicine, Vol. 87: Vaccine Protocols, 2nd ed.*
Edited by: A. Robinson, M. J. Hudson, and M. P. Cranage © Humana Press Inc., Totowa, NJ

mally in the gut. Since the restrictive temperature in the case of the poliovirus vaccines is above normal in vivo temperature, it is possible that a mild febrile response following initial infection is sufficient to limit the amount of virus leaving the gut epithelium and to reduce the likelihood of access of the virus to the CNS.

The potential of ts mutants as live virus vaccines is more obvious in the case of infections by the respiratory route, since the mean temperature of the nares and the upper respiratory tract is likely to be significantly lower than that of the lower respiratory tract. Thus, virus replication can proceed unrestricted in the nasopharyngeal epithelium, inducing both local and systemic immune responses, and causing minimal discomfort to the host. Temperature-sensitive mutants employed in this way must have sufficient genetic stability to ensure that the host organism can mount an effective immune response before virus penetrates into the lower respiratory tract. Experimental ts mutant vaccines have been developed for a number of human respiratory viruses, and these have shown promise in experimental animals and in volunteer trials *(2)*. None has been approved for clinical use because of uncertainties regarding their genetic stability and concern about their semi-empirical mode of development. However, ts mutant vaccines for respiratory diseases are gaining favor again as a result of the increasing ease with which the genomes of viruses can be manipulated in a controlled manner by recombinant DNA technology. The over-riding advantage of live virus vaccines is their inherent property of auto-amplification and their ability to induce a balanced immune response *(2)*.

Although the genomes of single-stranded and double-stranded DNA viruses and those of positive-stranded RNA viruses are amenable to manipulation by standard recombinant DNA methodology, until recently the introduction of specific mutations by reverse genetics was not possible in the case of negative-stranded RNA viruses. However, appropriate methodology has been developed now for genetic engineering of the genomes of both segmented genome negative-stranded RNA viruses *(3)* and non-segmented negative-stranded RNA viruses *(4)*. The existence of an infectious DNA copy of the wild-type viral genome is a prerequisite for implementation of reverse genetics. The current strategy requires also the prior existence of an empirically derived attenuated (usually ts) vaccine virus, which can be utilized as a model for the identification of the genetic determinants of virulence. Recently, the first successful incorporation of a foreign gene into the genome of the double-stranded RNA virus, reovirus type 3, has been reported *(5)*. It remains to be seen whether this approach can be generalized into a method of reverse genetics applicable to other mammalian double-stranded RNA viruses.

The first part of this chapter describes three approaches that have been used successfully to produce experimental ts attenuated viruses, and the second part provides an example of a reverse genetics approach for insertion of attenuating mutations into a viral genome, which can serve as a model.

## 1.1. Classical Empirical Approach

Three approaches have been used successfully to produce experimental ts attenuated viruses. The first approach involves continuous passage of a virulent virus at gradually reduced temperatures to produce a strain that is no longer able to replicate efficiently at supraoptimal or physiological temperatures. Cold-adapted (ca) viruses with potential as vaccines have been derived for influenza virus and several paramyxoviruses. The rationale behind this approach is that spontaneous ts mutants will accumulate and gradually diminish the pathogenic potential of the virus. The advantage of this procedure is that the process is progressive. It can be monitored continuously and terminated when the appropriate degree of attenuation has been obtained. The accumulation of spontaneous mutations is likely to achieve better genetic stability because the final phenotype is the product of many small incremental changes rather than a few major changes, which may be subject to reversion at high frequency. Such a ca virus may exhibit a reduced capacity to multiply at normal body temperature in addition to its extended low-temperature range. However, this is not always observed, and virus may become attenuated without becoming temperature-adapted. Such attenuated viruses are described as cold-passaged (cp) virus, or (cp/ts), where they exhibit a ts phenotype *(6–8)*.

The second approach is sequential passage of virus in the presence of a mutagen in order to accelerate the accumulation of mutants. This method could be combined with passage at low temperature to enhance the selection of ts mutants, but it has been used mainly at normal incubation temperatures to optimize virus replication (important in the case of base analog mutagens) and to maximize the yield of mutants. A Rift Valley fever virus vaccine has been derived in this manner using 5-fluorouracil (5-FU) as the mutagen *(9)*.

The third approach is direct isolation of single spontaneous or induced ts mutations. Individually, such mutants are generally too unstable genetically to be suitable as vaccines. Greater stability can be achieved by isolating several ts mutants. The isolation of multiple ts mutants is achieved by isolation of single ts mutants sequentially at progressively reduced restrictive temperatures, as described below.

The protocols outlined in the following sections have been used in the generation of an experimental human respiratory syncytial virus vaccine *(10,11)*, but they are generally applicable with minor modification. Human respiratory syncytial virus (order *Mononegavirales*, family *Paramyxoviridae*, subfamily *Paramyxovirinae*, genus *Pneumovirus*) has a narrow host range, grows to low titer, and is intolerant of extremes of heat and pH. Thus, modification of the protocols listed here for use with other viruses usually entail no more than a relaxation of some of the specific restrictions and a change of cell substrate.

## 2. Materials

### 2.1. General Virology and Mutagenesis

1. A class II laminar flow safety cabinet, located in a dedicated laboratory with restricted access.
2. Disposable gloves, gowns, and face masks.
3. A minimum of two $CO_2$-gassed incubators.
4. A circulating water bath able to maintain temperature within +/– 0.2°C.
5. A refrigerated bench centrifuge.

6. A UV-microscope.
7. A liquid nitrogen storage cylinder.
8. Tissue-culture-grade sterile disposable plastic ware: 150 cm$^2$, 75 cm$^2$ and 25 cm$^2$ flasks with vented caps; 50-mm Petri dishes; 6-well cluster plates, 96-well flat-bottomed plates; 1-mL, 5-mL, and 10-mL disposable pipets; plugged narrow-bore Pasteur pipets; screw-capped freezer vials.
9. Glasgow Minimum Essential Eagle's Medium (GMEM) or equivalent, supplemented with 200 m$M$ glutamine, antibiotics (100 ug/mL streptomycin and 100 U/mL penicillin). Used with 10% mycoplasma-free fetal calf serum (FCS) for cell propagation, with 1% FCS for maintenance of infected cell cultures and as a diluent.
10. Cell freezing medium; GMEM 70%, glycerol 10%, FCS 20%.
11. Versene (EDTA) and versene/trypsin solutions for cell transfer; used at a concentration of 0.5 g porcine trypsin plus 0.2 g EDTA per L.
12. Neutral red stain.
13. Agar or agarose.
14. DAPI stain (*see* **Note 5**).
15. MRC-5 human diploid embryonic lung cells (ATCC No. CCL 171).

## 2.2. Reverse Genetics

1. An infectious full-length cDNA clone of the wild-type viral genome.
2. A vaccinia virus recombinant expressing the T7 RNA polymerase, or, when available, susceptible mammalian cells stably expressing the T7 RNA polymerase.
3. Support plasmids expressing the essential proteins for replication and encapsidation of the viral genome.
4. Susceptible cells able to support virus replication and encapsidation, and expression of the vaccinia virus T7 RNA polymerase recombinant and the support plasmids.
5. Standard reagents and equipment for recombinant DNA manipulation.
6. Specific primers for polymerase chain reaction (PCR) synthesis.
7. Thermal cycler for PCR synthesis (*see* **Note 6**).

## 3. Methods
## 3.1. General Methodology

All experimental operations should be conducted according to appropriate safety regulations/guidelines in a class III facility in which all equipment and reagents are dedicated solely to vaccine development. There should be no exchange of materials or reagents with other laboratories during the course of the project. The virus isolates, media, and cell cultures should be stored in dedicated refrigerators, preferably housed within the containment area. Gowns, gloves, and perhaps special footwear should be worn at all times. Staff used on the project should not be assigned during the same working day to other tasks that could bring them into contact with other viruses and cells. Visitors should be kept from the working area.

### 3.1.1. The Cell Substrate

Use a cell substrate approved for vaccine development and production from the outset. A diploid cell line is mandatory in the case of vaccines destined for ultimate use in humans. The MRC-5 cell line is appropriate for most purposes. MRC-5 cells grow slowly and achieve confluence at low density; their useful life may extend up to about 40 passages. Beyond this time, there is a progressive retardation of growth rate.

1. Establish an adequate cell bank at the outset from a low-passage seed to ensure an adequate supply of cells for the entire enterprise. MRC-5 cells can be propagated in growth medium consisting of Eagle's medium with non-essential amino acids (Glasgow formulation), supplemented with antibiotics (100 U/mL penicillin and 100 μg/mL streptomycin) and FCS. The concentration of foetal calf serum is the critical factor (*see* **Note 1**). FCS is preferred because of its content of growth factors and the absence of inhibitory substances and antibodies present in adult animal sera (*see* **Note 2**). Newborn or other animal sera may be suitable for some purposes (*see* **Note 3**). Heat-treat sera for cell culture (30 min at 56°C) before use to destroy complement and other nonspecific inhibitory substances.

2. Propagate MRC-5 cells as monolayer cultures by seeding $1 \times 10^6$ cells into a large (150 cm$^2$) tissue culture-grade plastic flask with vented lid. Incubate in a 5% $CO_2$-gassed incubator at 35–37°C. Confluence should be achieved within 4–5 d, providing a yield of 5–10 $\times 10^6$ cells.

3. Harvest cells by removing the incubation medium and washing the monolayer with 20 mL 0.2% (v/v) versene solution. Incubate in the presence of 20 mL versene without calcium and magnesium for 5–10 min at room temperature, then wash with 20 mL trypsin/versene solution followed by incubation in the presence of 2.5 mL trypsin/versene at 37°C until the cells detach. If the cells do not detach within 5 min, decant and add fresh trypsin/versene.

4. For continued propagation of cells, seed large (150 cm$^2$) flasks at a density of $2.5 \times 10^6$/mL. Use small (25 cm$^2$) flasks for virus production and 50-mm-diameter plastic Petri dishes for virus infectivity assay, both seeded at $1 \times 10^6$ per mL. Seed multi-well plates with $2.5 \times 10^6$ cells distributed proportionally.

5. Establish a cell bank. To do this amplify low-passage MRC-5 cells by 1:1 splits, prepare a cell suspension containing $2.0 \times 10^6$ cell per mL in a storage medium consisting of Eagle's growth medium containing 10% glycerol and 20% FCS (*see* **Note 4**). Distribute aliquots of 1.5 mL into 1.8-mL screw-capped freezer vials and freeze the vials slowly (at approx 1°C per min) from room temperature to –70°C. Transfer the vials to the vapor phase of a liquid nitrogen storage cylinder.

6. Screen cell cultures for the presence of extraneous agents. Check visually and by subculture for the presence of fungi and yeasts. Inoculate samples of fluids into broth culture for the detection of bacteria. Use DAPI-staining of cells for detection of mycoplasma (*see* **Note 5**). More detailed treatments of this topic can be found in reviews by Knight *(12)* and Gwaltney et al. *(13)*.

### 3.1.2. Temperature Control

The accurate control of temperature of incubation is essential. The greatest control can be achieved by total immersion of cultures in a circulating water bath maintaining temperature with an accuracy of at least ± 0.2°C. Screw-capped glass medicinal flat bottles are generally superior to plastic flasks for this purpose. Petri dishes can be placed in plastic containers, which are gassed and sealed before submergence.

However, it is possible to obtain satisfactory temperature control using many commercial cell culture fan-assisted incubators, provided there is adequate attention to humidification, preheating of reagents and containers, and control on access.

### 3.1.3. Virus Source

It is important to initiate vaccine development with a recent virus isolate that has relevance to current epidemiological circumstances. The virus should originate from material isolated from a patient or a diseased animal, and be inoculated directly into the vaccine-approved cell substrate (*see* **Note 7**). It is preferable to inoculate the clinical specimen into cell culture, or into antibiotic-containing transport medium with subsequent inoculation into cell culture in the laboratory. After inoculation, the transport medium should be held at low temperature, unfrozen. Delay between sampling and isolation into cell culture should be kept to a minimum.

1. Establish a genetically homogeneous stock by propagation from single plaques. To do this, isolate virus from individual plaques appearing on cell monolayers infected at limiting dilution. The time of incubation and the temperature will depend on the particular virus. For respiratory syncytial virus, incubate at 37°C under a 0.9% (v/v) agar (or agarose, because the growth of some viruses is inhibited by impurities in commercial agar) overlay for 5–7 d. Visualize the plaques by addition of a 0.05% (v/v) neutral red-containing agar overlay at d 4 or 5 (*see* **Note 8**). Pick plaques into 1 mL growth medium from monolayers with single plaques whenever possible, by inserting a sterile Pasteur pipet through the agar overlay and removing an agar plug and attached cells. Resuspend the sample and after dilution plate immediately onto fresh monolayers, without intervening freeze-thawing. Many viruses are sensitive to freeze-thawing, and in the case of respiratory syncytial virus, a preferential loss of ts virus was observed *(14)*.
2. Repeat the cycle of infection and plaque picking at least three times; exceptionally, in the case of an avian pneumovirus (*Turkey rhinotracheitis virus*), it was necessary to carry out ten sequential re-isolations before homogeneous stocks of two distinct plaque morphology mutants were obtained from a mixed parental stock *(15)*.
3. Amplify the final plaque isolate by sequential passage in small (25 cm²), medium (75 cm²), and large (150 cm²) flask cultures to achieve the final volume of virus-containing supernatant required. Pool the fluids from the final passage in large flask cultures and clarify by low-speed centrifugation in a refrigerated bench centrifuge. Distribute into freezer vials as 1-mL aliquots and store frozen in the vapor phase of a liquid nitrogen storage cylinder.
4. Test several randomly selected aliquots of this stock virus for the presence of fungal, mycoplasmal, and bacterial contaminants by inoculation into appropriate detection media. Freedom from adventitious cytopathic viral agents can be verified by prolonged incubation of MRC-5 cells inoculated with the triple-cloned stock virus rendered non-infectious by exposure to specific neutralizing antiserum. The absence of known viral pathogens can be ensured by inoculation of appropriate susceptible cells and screening by immunofluorescence using specific monoclonal antibodies (MAbs). An updated consideration of likely pathogens is given by Gwalteny et al. *(13)*.

### 3.1.4. Mutagenization

Decide whether to attempt isolation of spontaneously occurring mutants or to employ mutagens to induce mutations and thus enhance the frequency of recovery of mutants *(16)*. RNA viruses have high mutation rates because viral RNA-dependent RNA polymerases lack proofreading capability. As a consequence, ts mutants can be isolated without mutagen treatment in the case of viruses that achieve moderate to high progeny virus titers during growth in cultured cells. In the case of viruses that do not grow to high titer, such as respiratory syncytial virus, it may be essential to use mutagens. Even in the case of a virus such as Rift Valley fever virus, which does grow to moderate titers, it may be expedient to use mutagens to accelerate modification of the virus during propagation in vitro (*see* **Subheading 3.5.**). Mutagenization is obligatory in the case of DNA-containing viruses.

1. Choose an appropriate mutagen. Chemical mutagens are more controllable than ionizing or non-ionizing radiation, and are preferred. In the case of easily purified viruses that grow to high titer, it is feasible to carry out the mutagen treatment in vitro by exposing purified virus or nucleic acid to the mutagenic agent for varying periods of time. The mutagen is usually added to virus-infected cells to induce mutations, predominantly by causing mis-incorporation of nucleotides during replication. 5-bromodeoxyuridine (BUDR) and 5-fluorouracil (5-FU) are the first choice for DNA-containing viruses and for RNA-containing viruses, respectively (*see* **Note 9**).

2. Determine the concentration of mutagen required to enhance the yield of mutants. To do this, inoculate replicate susceptible cell monolayers with the plaque-purified virus at a ratio of 1 pfu per cell. After adsorption, remove the virus inoculum by three changes of medium, and then add a range of concentrations of a base analog mutagen (e.g., 5-FU or 5-BUDR) made up in normal incubation medium. In the case of the mutagenization of RNA-containing viruses with 5-FU, final concentrations in the range of 10–500 µg per mL are appropriate. At these concentrations, the viability of MRC-5 cells is not seriously affected for several days.

3. Then incubate the mutagen-exposed infected cell cultures at a suboptimal temperature (30–33°C) until cytopathic effect is maximal in cultures containing no mutagen (*see* **Note 10**). Harvest the supernatant fluids and clarify by low-speed centrifugation.

4. Remove the mutagen by dialysis for 18–24 h against changes of normal incubation medium (with antibiotics, but without serum).

5. Determine the reduction in virus yield by assay of residual infectivity at both *permissive* and *restrictive* temperatures (*see* **Subheading 3.2.**). Identify the minimum mutagen concentration at which there is a measurable increase in the difference between the infectivity titers at permissive and restrictive temperatures of incubation (*see* **Subheading 3.2.**). Use this mutagen concentration as the initial treatment, and subsequently adjust in response to the yields of mutants obtained. The protocol described is designed to limit the frequency of isolation of multiple mutations so that the majority of the ts mutants isolated are the consequence of single base changes (*see* **Note 11**).

## 3.2. Isolation of TS Mutants Following Mutagen Treatment

To avoid the re-isolation of mutant virus originating from the same mutational event, several mutagenic treatments of wild-type virus should be carried out independently with only one ts mutant isolated from each treatment. The isolation of ts mutants of respiratory syncytial virus by three methods is described here as examples. As a preliminary step to all three methods, first establish appropriate permissive and restrictive temperatures as follows. Assay the wild-type unmutagenized virus for plaque-forming ability on monolayers of susceptible cells incubated at a range of temperatures between 30°C and 42°C. The *permissive temperature* should be the lowest temperature of incubation at which the virus yield does not depart significantly from the mean, and the *restrictive temperature* should be the highest incubation temperature at which the titer does not differ by more than 1 $\log_{10}$ unit from the mean.

### 3.2.1 Screening After Pre-Amplification

1. Plate out the mutagen-treated virus at limiting dilution on MRC-5 monolayers in 50-mm plastic Petri dishes, or six-well cluster plates. Aspirate off the inoculum and add an agar-containing overlay. Incubate the infected monolayers at the predetermined permissive temperature until macroscopic plaques are clearly visible. Add a second agar overlay containing neutral red stain, but no serum, and allow it to solidify. Incubate at the permissive temperature for an additional 24–48 h, avoiding exposure to light.

2. Choose monolayers with single or a few well-dispersed plaques for plaque picking (*see* **Note 12**). Plaque picking is accomplished by inserting a narrow bore (~1-mm diameter) sterile cotton wool-plugged Pasteur pipet into the agar above the plaque. Withdraw an agar plug and expel it directly onto a fresh cell monolayer or into a storage vial containing a small volume of growth medium. It is not necessary to scrape the monolayer; sufficient infectivity will be present in cells attached either to the base of the agar plug, or as virus that has diffused into the agar.

3. The screening of the plaque-picked isolates for temperature-sensitivity can be carried out either after preliminary amplification to provide a reference stock, or directly by inoculation onto replicate monolayers that are then incubated at the permissive and restrictive temperatures. The pre-amplification of plaque-picked virus is generally a more efficient and reliable procedure, although time-consuming and expensive in terms of consumables. Inoculate each plaque isolate directly onto a monolayer of susceptible cells in a small (25 cm$^2$) screw-capped flask. Adsorb for 1 h at permissive temperature; then add 3 mL of maintenance medium without removal of the inoculum. Incubate at the permissive temperature until the cytopathic effect is extensive. The advantage of this procedure is that screening and the isolation of clones can be carried out at different times.

4. To screen the amplified isolates for temperature-sensitivity, inoculate two sets of monolayers of susceptible cells in 96-well flat-bottomed cluster plates and adsorb at room temperature for 30 min. Then add maintenance medium and incubate one set of plates at permissive temperature and one set at restrictive temperature until the cytopathic effect is extensive in control wells simultaneously infected with wild-type virus (*see* **Note 13**). Those isolates that fail to produce cytopathic effect on monolayers incubated at restrictive temperature are putative ts mutants.

5. To ensure the absence of any carry-over of wild-type virus, initiate second and third cycles of cloning of these putative ts mutants by plating out and re-isolation of single plaques.

6. Verify and quantify temperature-sensitivity by determining plaque counts for the triple-cloned virus at restrictive and permissive temperatures. Those mutants that differ by less than three $\log_{10}$ units are unlikely to be useful, and should be discarded unless none better can be isolated.

### 3.2.2. Screening Without Amplification

An alternative procedure, which is more economical in time and consumables, is screening without pre-amplification. This follows the procedure outlined in the previous section, with the difference that fluid from the storage vial containing the agar plug is inoculated directly onto duplicate assay plates for incubation at the two temperatures. This procedure is the preferred one, in which the yield of infectious virus from a single plaque is appreciable (>1000 pfu). In the case of viruses for which the yield may be low (<100 pfu), this procedure is prone to error and the number of false-positives can be high. Putative ts mutants, however, must undergo the same triple cloning and verification procedure to provide a substrate for the next round of mutagenesis.

### 3.2.3. Screening by Replica Plating

An accelerated version of the preceding method is to bypass the isolation step by inoculating the agar plug in equal proportions directly into two corresponding wells in duplicate 96-well blocks. One block is then incubated at permissive temperature, and the other block at restrictive temperature. Since no virus has been stored, the block incubated at permissive temperature serves as the repository of the isolates as well as the assay control block. When a potential mutant is identified, virus is recovered from the corresponding well of the block incubated at permissive temperature, and subjected to triple cloning as previously described. This method is fast and economical, but vulnerable to losses by fortuitous contamination, since a single contaminated well entails loss of the remaining 92 isolates.

Sectored plates can substitute for multi-well plates. These are prepared as follows.

1. Allow 2.5 mL of agar overlay to solidify in 50-mm Petri dishes containing confluent monolayers of MRC-5 cells. Mark the plates into sectors on the underside with indelible ink.
2. Inoculate picked plaques onto duplicate sectored plates. Insert the Pasteur pipet through the agar overlay and expel half of the plug onto one plate. Inoculate the other half of the plug similarly onto the corresponding sector of a duplicate plate.
3. After a period of 30 min at permissive temperature in a humidified incubator for adsorption, add a second agar-containing overlay of 2.5 mL to seal the plates. Incubate one of each pair of plates at permissive temperature, and the other at restrictive temperature.
4. Absence of cytopathic effect at the restrictive temperature indicates a putative ts mutant. Produce an amplified stock by propagation of virus from the control plate incubated at permissive temperature.

This procedure is rapid and less vulnerable to losses by contamination than the multi-well plate method. It has the advantage that plaque morphology differences can be screened simultaneously with temperature-sensitivity.

### 3.3. Establishment of Mutant Stocks and Determination of Mutant Phenotype

The protocols outlined in the following sections include verification of the temperature-sensitivity of putative mutants and the growth of triple-cloned stocks.

It is also necessary to undertake some preliminary characterization of the phenotype of the first harvest of mutants in order to select a suitable mutant to form the parental virus for the next round of mutagenesis. Properties of relevance are a matter for intuitive decision for each particular infectious agent, and no general guidance can be given here; detailing of methodology is inappropriate (*see* **ref. 17** for methods of phenotyping for a respiratory syncytial virus).

In the case of respiratory syncytial virus, it was found that the mutants that showed most promise in trials in adult volunteers were those with an RNA-positive phenotype and thus able to support viral protein (antigen) synthesis at the restrictive temperature.

In general, mutants with RNA-negative phenotypes, although showing dramatic reduction in pathogenicity, did not induce good immune responses in adult volunteers *(10,11)*.

### 3.4. Vaccine Development by Sequential Selection of Multiple TS Mutants

The following protocol is generalized, with specific details for respiratory syncytial virus inserted for illustration *(10,11)*.

### 3.4.1. Isolation of the Primary Series of (Putative Single) TS Mutants

1. Establish permissive and restrictive temperatures and prepare a triple-plaque purified stock of the parental virulent virus as described in **Subheadings 3.1.3.** and **3.1.4.**, respectively. In the case of respiratory syncytial virus, the initial restrictive temperature was 39°C, and a permissive temperature of 31°C was used throughout.
2. Carry out mutagen treatment as described in **Subheading 3.1.4.** Respiratory syncytial virus was mutagenized by infection of MRC-5 cells at a multiplicity of approx 1, followed by incubation in maintenance medium (Eagle's medium plus glutamine, antibiotics, and 1% (v/v) FCS) supplemented with 100 µg/mL 5-FU (*see* **Note 14**).
3. Plate out at limiting dilution samples of the supernatant fluids of several independently mutagenized cultures.
4. Carry out plaque picking and screening for temperature-sensitivity as described in **Subheading 3.2.** It was observed in the case of respiratory syncytial virus that yields of ts mutants were improved by avoiding freeze-thawing.
5. Determine the phenotypes of at least five mutants originating from independently mutagenized cultures as described in **Subheading 3.3.** In the case of respiratory syncytial virus, the single mutant with the greatest temperature restriction at 39°C (e.g., the ratio of plaques at 39°C/plaques at 31°C), in conjunction with an RNA-positive phenotype, was identified as the most suitable parental virus for the next round of mutagenesis. A stock of this mutant, designated *ts1A*, was prepared by triple-cloning and amplification as described in **Subheading 3.1.3.**

### 3.4.2. Isolation of a Secondary Series of (Putative Double) TS Mutants

1. Mutagenize the primary series ts mutants, *ts1A* in the case of respiratory syncytial virus, as outlined in **Subheading 3.1.4.** For the second round of mutagenesis, choose a mutagen with a different chemical specificity from that used in the first round of mutagenesis. The mutagen used in isolation of the candidate respiratory syncytial virus vaccine double-mutant *tsIB* was an acridine derivative, known as ICR 340 *(10)*.
2. Incorporate the mutagen into standard maintenance medium at an appropriate concentration (10 µg/mL ICR 340 for respiratory syncytial virus) and incubate the mutant-infected cells in its presence until cytopathic effect (CPE) is far advanced in control unmutagenized cultures. Again avoid freeze-thawing (*see* **Note 15**).
3. Plate out the mutagenized virus at limiting dilution and pick plaques from plates incubated at permissive temperature as before (*see* **Subheading 3.3.**). In the case of viruses of moderate to good stability, growing to reasonable titer, the mutagen should be removed by dialysis against maintenance medium before inoculation and plaque picking.
4. Pick isolated plaques, or preferably plaques from single-plaque plates, and screen for temperature-sensitivity. In the case of respiratory syncytial virus, screening for temperature-sensitivity was carried out at a restrictive temperature arbitrarily chosen as one degree below that used for selection of the first mutant, in this case, 38°C.

5. Determine the phenotypes of at least five mutants from independently mutagenised cultures as described before in **Subheading 3.3.** In the case of respiratory syncytial virus, the single mutant with the greatest temperature restriction at 38°C, in conjunction with an RNA-positive phenotype at that restrictive temperature, was identified as the most suitable parental virus for the next round of mutagenesis. A stock of this mutant, designated *ts1B*, was prepared by triple-plaque purification and amplification as described in **Subheading 3.1.3.**

### 3.4.3. Isolation of a Tertiary Series of (Putative Triple) TS Mutants

1. Mutagenize the secondary ts mutant, designated mutant *ts1B* in the case of respiratory syncytial virus, as outlined in **Subheading 3.1.3.** Choose a mutagen of a different specificity from that used in the preceding mutagenesis. However, in the case of the respiratory syncytial virus project, 5-FU was used again because experience has shown that this mutagen is the most reliable and consistent for RNA viruses *(16)*.
2. Plate out independently mutagenized lots of the second series mutant (mutant *ts1B*) at limiting dilution and incubate the plates at permissive temperature.
3. Pick well-dispersed plaques, preferable plaques from single-plaque plates, and screen for temperature-sensitivity at a third restrictive temperature. In the case of respiratory syncytial virus, this was arbitrarily chosen as 1°C below (37°C) that used for selection of the second series mutant. The single mutant with the greatest temperature restriction at 37°C, in conjunction with an RNA-positive phenotype at that restrictive temperature, was selected as the third series (putative triple) mutant, which represented the endpoint of the project.
4. Produce a stock of this mutant, designated *ts1C* in the case of respiratory syncytial virus, by three sequential re-isolations from single plaques and amplification (*see* **Subheading 3.1.3.**) for subsequent evaluation as a candidate vaccine *(10,11,18)*.

### 3.5. Modification of Virus by Continuous Mutagenization

A successful protocol for continuous mutagenization has been described for Rift Valley fever virus (Family *Bunyaviridae*, Genus *Bunyavirus*) by Caplen et al. *(9)*. The following is a brief outline of their method, modified to permit accumulation of ts mutations.

1. Infect monolayers of MRC-5 cells at a multiplicity of 0.1 pfu/cell. Remove unadsorbed virus by several washes with growth medium and finally replace with growth medium containing 10% (v/v) FCS and 200 µg/mL 5-FU (*see* **Note 16**). Incubate the infected cultures for 3–4 h at 33°C in a 5% $CO_2$-gassed incubator. Remove unadsorbed or desorbed virus by discarding the culture fluid and replacing it with fresh medium containing the same concentration of 5-FU.
2. Harvest the culture supernatants after a further 48–72 h incubation at 33°C.
3. Titrate the yield of infectious virus on MRC-5 cell monolayers by incubation for 4 d at 33°C under a 0.5% agarose overlay containing a reduced concentration (4%) of FCS before application of a second 0.5% agarose overlay containing 0.01% neutral red stain.
4. After incubation for a further 18–24 h, pick two large well-separated plaques and inoculate onto fresh MRC-5 cell monolayers in screw-capped flasks.
5. Harvest the fluid from these infected cultures after 48–72 h incubation at 33°C, and clarify by low-speed centrifugation. Store the clarified supernatant at –70°C.
6. Assay these yields for plaque formation at a predetermined restrictive (38–40°C) and permissive (31–33°C) temperature.

7. Initiate the next round of infection and mutagenesis using the virus that exhibits the greatest differential between the assays at the permissive and restrictive temperatures.
8. Continue this procedure as long as there is evidence of an increase in temperature-sensitivity without decline in yield at the permissive temperature (*see* **Note 17**).

A control series of plaque isolations, propagated under identical conditions but in the absence of mutagen, is required to properly evaluate the progress of mutagenization and the accumulation of ts virus.

### 3.6. Modification by Passage at Low Temperature

There are many routes to achieving modification of virus by passage at low temperature. Since these are determined to a large extent by the host range and biological properties of specific viruses, it is not appropriate to present a protocol here.

The reader is referred to the literature on the derivation of ca experimental influenza A virus (Family *Orthomyxoviridae*) vaccines. Here, there is the added dimension of utilization of subunit reassortment. A ca virus has been used successfully as a donor of attenuating genes for the construction of other attenuated influenza A viruses *(19)*.

### 3.7. Evaluation of Vaccine Potential of Modified Virus

The evaluation of the vaccine potential of any virus modified by the procedures described here, or by any other methodology, is a problem of great complexity, and is beyond the scope of this chapter. Each virus poses a different set of challenges, and specific solutions must be sought without regard to precedent.

The normal path to authenticating the merits of a candidate human vaccine is through evaluation in whatever animal models are available, through volunteer trials in sero-positive individuals, ultimately to trials in sero-negative individuals *(2,6,20,21)*.

### 3.8. Reverse Genetic Approaches

#### 3.8.1. Overall Strategy

The ability to produce infectious virus from cDNA provides an alternate route for production of precisely characterized attenuated viruses. The evaluation of empirically derived candidate vaccines identifies the sites of attenuating mutations, and such mutations can be introduced by reverse genetics into other related viruses that may possess more appropriate antigenic characteristics, or to enhance the genetic stability of existing candidate vaccine strains *(22,23)*.

Paradoxically, the technique of reverse genetics has been exploited to greatest extent in the case of the negative-strand RNA viruses, long the most inaccessible to controlled genetic modification by site-specific mutagenesis. In the case of negative-strand RNA viruses, the genomic and the anti-genomic RNA are not infectious, and the minimal replicative unit is the nucleocapsid, which contains the nucleocapsid (N) protein tightly bound to the RNA, together with the phosphoprotein (P) and the polymerase (L) protein, which are less tightly bound. The basic strategy, developed first for rabies virus *(4)*, involves providing genes encoding the essential nucleocapsid components, N, P, and L, in cells together with a cDNA producing the anti-genome.

This strategy depends on intracellular synthesis of T7 RNA polymerase, which is most conveniently supplied by a vaccinia virus recombinant, to direct the synthesis of mRNAs encoding the components of the viral nucleocapsid complex and a copy of the cloned genome (usually as the +ve sense anti-genome) terminated with a ribozyme sequence to achieve precise termination of the transcript. The intracellularly synthesized nucleocapsid proteins (N, P, and L, supplied by support plasmids) mediate the replication of both the +ve sense antigenomic RNA and transcribe –ve sense genomic RNA, which also results in the production of the remaining virus structural proteins and packaging of functional nucleocapsids. The infectious progeny virus is separated from the vaccinia-T7 recombinant and propagated for analysis of phenotype. This general procedure is applicable to all negative-strand RNA viruses, varied only by the inclusion of any additional essential nucleocapsid components when applicable *(25)*.

Since all of these operations involve nucleotide sequence-specific components and primers and standard recombinant DNA methodology, a generalized protocol is inappropriate. Instead, two protocols for critical stages common to all strategies are presented in detail.

### 3.8.2. Site-Directed Mutagenesis

Site-directed mutagenesis is performed using standard recombinant DNA technology involving oligonucleotide-directed mutagenesis of an infectious cDNA clone of the virus genome. This is achieved by a polymerase chain reaction (PCR), in which one of the primers encodes the desired mutation as a mismatch to the wild-type sequence. If the mutation is close to a naturally occurring restriction enzyme cleavage site, the replacement of the wild-type sequence with the mutation is straightforward. If there is no appropriate cleavage site, then the PCR fragment containing the mutation can be joined to other PCR fragments that extend the sequence to a usable cleavage site, either by overlapping PCR or by direct ligation (*see* **Note 16**). Overlapping PCR utilizes two sets of primers, in which one of each set includes complementary sequences at their 5'-termini, and two separate PCR reactions are performed, followed by ligation of the products (**refs.** *22,23*, and *24* provide examples of how these protocols are integrated into the complete procedure, including the substitution of commercial kits in place of the following protocols).

#### 3.8.2.1. SITE-SPECIFIC MUTAGENESIS BY OVERLAPPING PCR

1. Overlapping PCR utilizes two sets of primers in which one of each set includes complementary sequences at their 5'-termini.
2. Two separate PCR reactions are performed using cDNA as the template. The following is a reliable procedure, which uses Gibco Taq polymerase and the buffers supplied by the manufacturer.
3. PCR reaction mix (on ice):
    a. 10 µL 10X buffer.
    b. 3 µL $MgCl_2$.
    c. 2 µL detergent (1% w-1) (optional).
    d. 2 µL 10 m*M* dNTP mix (*see* **Note 18**).
    e. 1 µL primers (~0.4 µg).

   f.  4 µL cDNA.

   g.  79 µL sterile distilled water.

   h.  0.4 µL Taq polymerase.

4. The amounts of primer or cDNA employed may be different, in which case the amount of sterile distilled water should be adjusted so that the final volume remains 100 µL. The 10X buffer, MgCl$_2$, and detergent are supplied ready-made with the Taq enzyme (*see* **Note 19**).

5. Use the appropriate program on the PCR thermal cycler. Use 1-min extension times for each kilobase to be amplified.

6. To check if your PCR has worked, run a sample on an agarose gel with an appropriate ladder for calibration. Different concentrations of agarose are required to resolve different size fragments: 2% gel for fragments <500 bp; 1% gel for fragments 500 bp-3K; 0.7% gel for fragments >3K.

7. The products can be purified by agarose gel electrophoresis to remove unincorporated primers. Alternatively, cut out the PCR product from the agarose gel using a clean scalpel blade.

8. Use a Qiagen gel extraction kit to purify the PCR product.

9. PCR is performed a second time using only the outside set of primers. PCR reactions should be carried out using thin-walled tubes.

10. The product of this reaction is then inserted into the plasmid carrying the cDNA copy of the viral genome using appropriate restriction enzyme sites.

### 3.8.2.2. PCR LIGATION

1. Two PCR reactions are performed using cDNA as the template.

2. Purify the PCR products by agarose gel electrophoresis.

3. Add 1 m*M* ATP reaction buffer (*see* **Subheading 3.8.2.1.**) to each PCR product. Raise the temperature to 70°C and then add 50 U of T4 polynucleotide kinase. Incubate at 37°C in a 50 µL vol for 30 min.

4. Mix 5 µL of each phosphorylated primer (adjusted to approx equimolar proportions) with 400 U of T4 DNA ligase, and leave for 15 min at room temperature.

5. Use 1 µL of this ligation reaction as the template for a PCR with appropriate external primers and insert the product into a plasmid carrying the virus genome copy using convenient restriction sites.

### 3.8.3. Transfection

The second critical stage is the recovery of the mutagenized virus from the infectious cDNA clone. A reliable method using Lipofectace (Gibco-BRL) is described here.

1. In a 12-well tissue-culture-plate seed cells (in this example, Hep-2 cells) per well in GMEM supplemented with fetal bovine serum (FBS) at a final concentration of 10%. Incubate at 37°C for 18–24 h (*see* **Note 20**). The goal is to obtain 50–75% confluent monolayers. (NB: Since transfection efficiency is sensitive to culture confluence, it is important to maintain a standard seeding protocol from experiment to experiment *see* **Note 21**).

2. Prepare the following solutions in separate polypropylene tubes: Solution A: For each transfection, dilute 1 µg plasmid DNA in 50 µL serum-free Optimem (Gibco-BRL). Solution B: For each transfection, dilute 4 µL Lipofectace (Gibco-BRL) reagent in 50 µL serum-free Optimem (Gibco-BRL).

3. Combine the two solutions, mix gently by pipetting up and down and incubate at room temperature for 15 min. The solution may appear cloudy; however, this will not affect the transfection.
4. Aspirate medium from the cells.
5. For each transfection, add 400 µL serum-free Optimem (Gibco-BRL) to each tube containing the lipid-DNA complexes. Mix gently and overlay the diluted complex onto the cells.
6. Incubate the cells for 5 h at 37°C.
7. Add 500 µL GMEM (10% FBS) without removing the transfection mixture. If toxicity is a problem, remove the transfection mixture and replace with normal medium. Replace medium with fresh medium at 18–24 h following the start of transfection.
8. Assay cell extracts for virus activity 48–72 h after the start of transfection.

## 4. Notes

1. Normally a concentration of 10% (v/v) is adequate, but sera of different origin may vary in suitability, and each batch should be tested before use. For most viruses optimal yields are obtained with optimally growing cells. Assay of virus concentration by plaque formation is best achieved at concentrations of FCS, which maintain viability but restrict growth (0.5–1%).
2. FCS originating from the United Kingdom and other European countries should not be used for vaccine development and production because of the risk of contamination by the bovine spongiform encephalopathy (BSE) prion.
3. For example, adult sheep serum has good growth-stimulating properties and is a good substitute if the presence of antibody is not a concern. However, the serum must originate from scrapie-free animals.
4. Care should be taken to remove any residual trypsin by sedimentation of the cells from the transfer medium prior to resuspension in storage medium.
5. Seed sterile degreased cover slips in 30-mm sterile Petri dishes with approx $10^5$ cells per dish. Grow to subconfluence and fix in methanol. Treat with a solution of 1 µg/mL DAPI (4,6 diamidino-2-phenylindole) for 15 min at 37°C. Remove stain and wash in methanol. Examine by fluorescence microscopy. Uncontaminated cells have brightly fluorescing nuclei but unstained cytoplasm, whereas mycoplasmal-contaminated cells show cytoplasmic and surface fluorescence.
6. In all cases of PCR-mediated mutagenesis, the reaction should be performed with proofreading polymerases and a low cycle number (<25) to limit misincorporation. (If PCR machine is not of the heated lid variety, put a drop of mineral oil on top of the mix to prevent evaporation during the PCR.)
7. It is important before initiating the process of vaccine development to verify by whatever means available that the isolate retains the characteristic pathogenic properties of the wild-type virus.
8. Neutral red has a photodynamic inactivating effect on virus. Consequently, the overlaid monolayers and any solutions containing neutral red should not be exposed to light more than is necessary.
9. 5-fluorouridine or 5-azacytidine can be used as alternative mutagens for RNA viruses, and nitrous acid, hydroxylamine, ethyl methane sulphonate, ethyl ethane sulphonate, N-methyl-N-nitro-N-nitrosoguanidine, and proflavine and other acridines are alternative mutagens for DNA and RNA viruses *(16)*.

10. In the case of respiratory syncytial virus, it was observed that a concentration of 50 μg per mL 5-FU or above inhibited cytopathic effect and reduced virus yield.

11. A concentration of mutagen which reduced the yield of progeny virus from respiratory syncytial virus-infected MRC-5 cells at permissive temperature to approx 1% of normal was found to give yields of ts mutants at frequencies in the range 1–5%.

12. Plaque picking is intended to recover progeny virus originating from a single infectious particle. In practice, this cannot be achieved reliably when there is more than one plaque on the monolayer, because there is always a fluid layer between the cell monolayer and the overlying agar allowing lateral diffusion of released virus. Nonetheless, this is not a serious concern with highly cell-associated viruses and plaques can be picked from plates with several plaques. It should be remembered, however, that virus-infected cells can extend beyond the boundary of the visible lytic plaque.

13. Each cluster plate should contain two uninoculated cell control wells and two wild-type virus infected wells. Thus, 92 isolates can be screened on each pair of multi-well plates.

14. 5-FU (Sigma, London) can be made up as a stock solution of 1 mg/mL in sterile distilled water, filtered through a 0.22-mu filter, and stored frozen as aliquots at –20°C.

15. If an interruption is unavoidable, even thermosensitive viruses such as respiratory syncytial virus can be stored at an accurately maintained +4°C for a few days without serious loss of infectivity.

16. The concentration of 5-FU used by Caplen et al. *(9)* was that required to reduce the virus yield $10^2–10^3$-fold.

17. Modification of the pathogenetic properties of Rift Valley fever virus required 16–18 cycles of mutagenesis.

18. 10 m*M* dNTP mix is prepared as follows: 5 μL 100 m*M* dATP; 5 μL 100 m*M* dTTP; 5 μL 100 m*M* dGTP; 5 μL 100 m*M* dCTP; 30 μL $H_2O$. Make sure to use dNTPs and not ddNTPs. Label the dNTP stock and store it at –20°C.

19. When setting up PCR reactions, use the PCR-grade Gilson micropipets and barrier filter tips to avoid contamination. Aways include a negative control.

20. For 6-well plates or 35-mm dishes, the amount of DNA and lipofectace should be multiplied by 2.5.

21. For transfection of other cell lines using Lipofectace or Lipofectamine, the amount of DNA and lipid used for transfection should be determined separately. By keeping the amount of DNA constant (2 μg is a good starting point), different amounts of Lipofectace or Lipfectamine should be used (e.g., 1, 2, 4, 6, 8, and 10 μL of each in the first instance).

## References

1. Almond, J. W. (1987) The attenuation of poliovirus neurovirulence. *Annu. Rev. Microbiol.* **41,** 153–180.

2. Murphy, B. R., Hall, S. L., Kulkarni, A. B., Crowe, Jr. J. E., Collins, P. L., Connors, M., et al. (1994) An update on approaches to the development of respiratory syncytial virus (RSV) and parainfluenza virus type 3 (PIV3) vaccines. *Virus Res.* **32,** 13–36.

3. Garcia-Sastre, A. and Palese, P. (1993) Genetic manipulation of negative-strand RNA virus genomes. *Annu. Rev. Microbiol.* **47,** 765–790.

4. Schnell, M. J., Mebatsoin T., and Conzelmann, K-K. (1994) Infectious rabies viruses from cloned cDNA. *EMBO J.* **13,** 4195–4203.

5. Roner, M. R. and Joklik, W. K. (2001) Reovirus reverse genetics: Incorporation of the CAT gene into the reovirus genome. *Proc. Natl. Acad. Sci. USA* **98**, 8036–8041.

6. Crowe, Jr., J. E. (1995) Current approaches to the development of vaccines against disease caused by respiratory syncytial virus (RSV) and parainfluenza virus (PIV). A meeting report of the WHO Programme for Vaccine Development. *Vaccine* **13**, 415–421.

7. Juhasz, K., Whitehead S. S., Bui, P. T,, Biggs, J. M., Boulanger, C. A., Collins, P. L., et al. (1997) The temperature-sensitive (ts) phenotype of a cold-passaged (cp) live attenuated respiratory syncytial virus vaccine candidate, designated cpts530, results from a single amino acid substitution in the L protein. *J. Virol.* **71**, 5814–5819.

8. Crowe, J. E., Bui, P. T., Silber, G. R., Elkins, W. R., Chanock, R. M., and Murphy, B. R. (1995) Cold-passaged, temperature-sensitive mutants of human respiratory syncytial virus (RSV) are highly attenuated, immunogenic, and protective in seronegative chimpanzees, even where RSV antibodies are infused shortly before immunization. *Vaccine* **13**, 847–855.

9. Caplen, H., Peter, C. J., and Bishop, D. H. L. (1985) Mutagen-directed attenuation of Rift valley fever virus as a method for vaccine development. *J. Gen. Virol.* **66**, 2271–2277.

10. McKay, E., Higgins, P., Tyrrell, D., and Pringle, C. R. (1988) Immunogenicity and pathogenicity of temperature-sensitive modified respiratory syncytial virus in adult volunteers. *J. Med. Virol.* **25**, 411–421.

11. Pringle, C. R., Filipiuk, A. H., Robinson, B. S., Watt, P. J., Higgins, P., and Tyrrell, D. A. J. (1993) Immunogenicity and pathogenicity of a triple temperature-sensitive modified respiratory syncytial virus in adult volunteers. *Vaccine* **11**, 473–478.

12. Knight, V. (l964) The use of volunteers in medical virology. *Prog. Med. Virol.* **6**, 1–26.

13. Gwaltney, Jr., J. M., Hendley, O., Hayden, F. G., McIntosh, K., Hollinger, F. B, Melnick, J. L., et al. (1994) Updated recommendations for safety-testing of viral inocula used in volunteer experiments on rhinovirus colds. *Prog. Med. Virol.* **39**, 256–263.

14. Gimenez, H. B. and Pringle, C. R. (1978) Seven complementation groups of respiratory syncytial virus temperature-sensitive mutants. *J. Virol.* **27**, 459–464.

15. Ling, R. and Pringle, C. R. (1988) Turkey rhinotracheitis virus: in vivo and in vitro polypeptide synthesis. *J. Gen. Virol.* **69**, 917–923.

16. Leppard, K. N. and Pringle, C. R. (1996) Virus Mutants, in *Virology Methods Manual* (Kangro, H. and Mahy, B. W. J., eds.), **11**, 231–248, Academic Press Ltd., London.

17. Pringle, C. R. (1985) Pneumoviruses, in *Virology; A Practical Approach* (Mahy, B. W. J., ed.), pp. 95–118, IRL Press, Oxford, and Washington, D.C.

18. Tolley, K. P., Marriott, A. C., Simpson, A., Plows, D. J., Matthews, D. A., Longhurst, S. J., et al. (1996) Identification of mutations contributing to the reduced virulence of a modified strain of respiratory syncytial virus. *Vaccine* **14**, 1637–1646.

19. Pringle, C. R. (1990) The Genetics of Viruses, in *Topley and Wilson's Principles of Bacteriology, Virology and Immunity*, 7th ed., Vol. 4 (Collier, L. H. and Timbury, M. C., eds.), Edward Arnold, London, Melbourne, and Auckland, pp. 69–104.

20. Watt, P. J., Robinson, B. S., Pringle, C. R., and Tyrrell, D. A. J. (1990) Determinants of susceptibility to challenge and the antibody response of adult volunteers given experimental respiratory syncytial virus vaccines. *Vaccine* **8**, 231–236.

21. Murphy, B. R. (1993) Use of lived attenuated cold-adapted influenza A reassortant virus vaccines in infants, children, young adults and elderly adults. *Infect. Dis. Clin. Pract.* **2,** 176–181.

22. Partin, N. T., Chiu, P., and Coelingh, K. (1997) Genetically engineered live attenuated Influenza A vaccine candidates. *J. Virol.* **71,** 2772–2778.

23. Whitehead, S. S., Firestone, C-Y., Karron, R. A., Crowe, J. E., Elkins, W. R., Collins, P. L., et al. (1999). Addition of a missense mutation present in the L gene of respiratory syncytial virus (RSV) *cpts*530/1030 to RSV vaccine candidate *cpts*248/404 increases its attenuation and temperature sensitivity. *J. Virol.* **73,** 871–877.

24. Bin, R. B., Ma, C-H., Kristoff, T., Cheng, X., and Jin, H. (2002) Identification of temperature sensitive mutations in the phosphoprotein of respiratory syncytial virus that are likely involved in its interaction with the nucleoprotein. *J. Virol.* **76,** 2871–2880.

25. Marriott, A. C. and Easton, A. J. (1999) Reverse genetics of the *Paramyxoviridae. Adv. Virus Res.* **53,** 321–340.

# 3

## Live Viral Vectors

*Construction of a Replication-Deficient Recombinant Adenovirus*

### Anthony R. Fooks

## 1. Introduction

Throughout the last century, conventional vaccination strategies have advanced significantly, and vaccine application has resulted in the reduction of the disease burden on a global scale. Despite these obvious successes, many human and veterinary diseases remain intractable with the use of conventional technologies. Novel approaches to vaccine design are now needed to tackle those pathogens for which conventional technologies have failed to generate efficacious vaccines.

Since genetic engineering techniques have become widespread, it has become possible to create new vaccine candidates by design. The development of one such group of candidate vaccine "carriers" includes the use of genetically modified live viral vectors *(1,2)*. The basis for using genetically modified recombinant viruses as potential vaccine vectors involves the incorporation of specific genes from a pathogenic organism into the modified genome of a proven, safe nonpathogenic or attenuated virus *(3)*.

Recombinant adenoviruses that are being considered as vaccine vectors can either be replication-competent or replication-deficient (*see* **ref. *4*; Table 1**). These viruses have a wide host range, and attenuated adenoviruses have already been used as vaccines with few side effects. A live, replication-competent adenovirus vaccine based on serotypes 4 and 7 was licensed for human use in 1980. The virus is capable of replication in the intestines of the recipients, but does not cause clinical disease. The vaccine is safe, non-reactogenic, and efficacious, and confers protection against acute respiratory disease. The vaccine is administered in enteric-coated capsules as a niche vaccine to US military recruits and their family members *(5,6)*.

From: *Methods in Molecular Medicine, Vol. 87: Vaccine Protocols, 2nd ed.*
Edited by: A. Robinson, M. J. Hudson, and M. P. Cranage © Humana Press Inc., Totowa, NJ

Table 1
**Relative Properties of Replication-Competent and Replication-Deficient Adenoviruses as Live Viral Vectors**

| | Adenoviral vectors | |
|---|---|---|
| | Replication-competent adenoviruses | Replication-deficient adenoviruses |
| High-level expression | Yes[a] | Yes[a] |
| Expression of authentic recombinant proteins | Yes | Yes |
| Expression of host viral proteins | Yes | No[b] |
| Oncogenic potential | Yes[c] | No[c] |
| Long-term protein expression in vitro | No (lytic) | Yes |
| Ease of scale-up | Yes | Yes |
| Gene-therapy use in animal models | Yes (50) | Yes (51) |
| Vaccination use in animal models | Yes (52) | Yes (53) |

[a]High-level expression is dependent on the promoter.

[b]Breakthrough of host viral proteins may occur at very high multiplicities of infection (in vitro).

[c]Certain adenovirus genotypes can exhibit transforming properties. However, adenovirus type 5 serotype is a non-transforming adenovirus (54).

## 1.1. First-Generation (E1⁻) Adenovirus Vectors

The development of adenovirus vectors as vehicles for vaccine research has been widely studied, and various methods for the production of adenovirus vectors have been proposed (7–25). Researchers are also promoting the usefulness of adenovirus vectors in gene-delivery protocols for therapeutic purposes.

Successful results have been obtained in rodents using replication-deficient recombinant adenoviruses as immunizing agents for tick-borne encephalitis virus NS1 protein (26), measles virus nucleoprotein (27,28), hemagglutinin (HA), and fusion proteins (29,30). It has also been shown that immune responses and protection were elicited in different animal models after the oral administration of adenovirus vectors expressing heterologous proteins. These include the measles virus nucleoprotein, HA, and fusion proteins (30,31); hepatitis B virus surface antigen (HBVsAg) in chimpanzees (32) and humans (33); vesicular stomatatis virus glycoprotein (8); PRV gp50 protein (34); the rabies virus glycoprotein in mice, dogs (35), and foxes (36,37); the respiratory syncytial virus fusion glycoprotein and attachment glycoprotein in dogs (38); and the Simian immunodeficiency virus (SIV) Gag-protein (39). Other immunogenicity studies using adenovirus vectors have included their use in stimulating the production of inflammatory cytokines *(40)* and in the induction of T-cell responses for hepatitis C virus *(41)* and human immunodeficiency virus (HIV), respectively *(42,43)*.

The main advantages of adenovirus vectors as gene delivery vehicles include:

1. Capable of infecting a wide range of cell types in vivo *(44)* and eliciting an immune response against the desired protein;
2. Ability to infect and achieve gene expression by infecting a single cell regardless of cellular replication;
3. Administration of the constructs by injection, oral, or aerosol vaccination with efficient gene delivery into human cells;
4. Induction of strong systemic and local mucosal immune responses *(45,46)*;
5. Genetically stable to ensure that reversion to a virulent phenotype is precluded;
6. Mutated genome to confer a deficiency in virus replication, especially in target cells *(47)*, since non-expression of the viral genome prevents immune clearance of infected cells;
7. Removal of deleterious regions of the virus genome;
8. Ability to carry large gene inserts;
9. High-level expression of the desired immunogen under the control of a strong, well-characterized promoter;
10. Relative ease of construction *(48)*;
11. Can be propagated to high-titer virus stocks (>$10^{10}$ pfu/mL) *(49)*.

## 1.2. Inflammatory Response Directed at the Adenovirus Vector

The major disadvantages in the use of adenoviral vectors for vaccine delivery remains the inflammatory immune responses elicited against the vector backbone, although in some circumstances, the inflammatory response may be partially directed toward the transgene *(55)*. Following such an inflammatory response, rapid clearance of the adenovirus vector occurs, thereby reducing its therapeutic potential. In addition, re-administration of the adenovirus vector as a delivery tool is not feasible. The requirement to eliminate this response has in part promoted the move toward vectors with more of the adenoviral genes removed ("*gutless adenovirus vectors*"). Refinements of the vector by removing more of the viral genome to eliminate immune responses to the vector backbone may be critical in overcoming the safety and toxicity issues for clinical use. Second-generation vectors with deletions in the E1, E2B, and E4 regions exhibit decreased immunogenicity when compared with the first-generation E1a/E1b-deleted vectors *(56)*. Such deletions require the provision *in trans* of the viral genes using a helper-cell line. Further deletions of viral genes have been achieved using the *Cre-Lox* system to remove approx 25 Kb of the viral genome *(57,58)*. These vectors require the use of an E1⁻ deleted helper virus to propagate virus particles in a permissive cell line, although a potential drawback is the contamination with helper virus at a level of up to 1% *(59)*.

Further research is still required to reveal optimal strategies for repeated adenovirus delivery and maximize long-term gene expression in the presence of immunological memory responses to the vector. It is also important to specifically address safety issues before these approaches are successfully used in the clinic; these include the prevention of pro-inflammatory responses to the vector and evaluations of the optimal route of virus inoculation. The continued use of adenovirus vectors as a vaccine-delivery vehicle for therapeutic genes underscores the need for continued fundamental research into virus interactions with the human immune system.

## 2. Materials

1. For research purposes only: Plasmid pMVI00 (transient expression vector; *see* **Note 1**) and pMV100 containing the β-galactosidase (β-gal) reporter gene (pMV35) can be obtained from The Centre for Applied Microbiology and Research (CAMR, Porton Down, UK).
2. Plasmid pMV60 (adenovirus transfer vector; *see* **Note 2**) is identical to pXCX2, except that a linker containing *Hin*dIII and *Xho*I cloning sites has been inserted at its unique *Xba*I cloning site.
3. Plasmid pJM17 (defective adenovirus vector; *60*) can be obtained from Microbix Biosystems, Inc. (Toronto, Ontario, Canada) (*see* **Note 3**).
4. All restriction and modifying enzymes were purchased from Promega (Chilworth Research Centre, Southampton, UK).
5. In many laboratories, plasmids are purified using Qiagen columns, according to the manufacturer's instructions (Qiagen, Chatsworth, CA).
6. 293 cells (human embryonic kidney cells) *(47)* and MRC5 cells (primary human fibroblasts) can be obtained from the European Culture Collection of Animal Cells (ECACC, Porton Down, UK) or from Microbix Biosystems.
7. Cells were cultured in complete Glasgow Minimal Essential Medium (GMEM) (Imperial Laboratories, Andover, UK) supplemented with 10% (v/v) fetal calf serum (FCS), (PAA, Linz, Austria), 100 mg/mL kanamycin, 0.03% (w/v) glutamine (Sigma, Poole, UK).
8. TE buffer: 0.5 m$M$ ethylenediaminetetraacetic acid (EDTA), 1 m$M$ Tris-HC1, pH 7.5: Autoclave and store at room temperature.
9. 2 $M$ Calcium chloride: Autoclave and store at room temperature.
10. 2X HBS: 280 m$M$ NaCl, 50 m$M$ HEPES, 1.5 m$M$ Na$_2$HPO$_4$, pH 7.1: The pH is very critical. Autoclave the solution, and store at –20°C for up to 6 mo.
11. TBS buffer: 137 m$M$ NaCl, 5 m$M$ KCl, 0.7 m$M$ CaCl$_2$, 0.6 m$M$ Na$_2$HPO$_4$, 25 m$M$ Tris-HCl, pH 7.4: Autoclave and store at room temperature.
12. Phosphate-buffered saline (PBS): Autoclave and store at room temperature.
13. Glutaraldehyde 0.5% (v/v) in PBS. Store at room temperature.
14. Staining solution: 3 m$M$ potassium ferrocyanide, 3 m$M$ ferricyanide, 1.3 m$M$ magnesium chloride—made up in 1X PBS. Immediately prior to use, add 100 μL of prewarmed 2% (w/v) 5-bromo-4-chloro-3-indoyl-β-D-galactopyranoside ("X-gal"; dissolved in dimethyl formamide [DMFA]). Store potassium ferrocyanide and potassium ferricyanide as 300 m$M$ stock solutions in PBS. **Note**: DMFA degrades polystyrene, and therefore should be stored in glass containers.
15. Arklone P: A site license is required from ICI Pharmaceuticals (UK) to use Arklone P for research purposes. The Arklone P phase (lower layer) must be discarded according to local health and safety regulations.

All chemicals should be evaluated and handled according to local health and safety regulations.

## 3. Methods

This chapter specifically describes the development of a recombinant adenovirus. It was assumed that readers are familiar with established molecular biological techniques *(61)*.

### 3.1. Construction of a Recombinant Vector for Expression Under the Control of the HCMV IE Promoter

As part of the cloning strategy to develop recombinant adenoviruses, the first stage requires cloning the transgene under the control of the strong HCMV IE promoter (*see* **Fig. 1**).

1. Ligate the gene of interest into the transient expression vector (pMV100) at either of the unique cloning sites (*Bam*HI or *Xba*I).
2. Transform the resulting recombinant plasmid into *E. coli* JM109.
3. Grow the bacteria on nutrient agar plates (Difco Ltd., Surrey, UK) supplemented with 50 µg/mL ampicillin at 37°C for 16 h.
4. Select single colonies and grow in 10 mL L-broth (Difco Ltd.), supplemented with 50 µg/ mL ampicillin, at 37°C in a shaking incubator at 200 rpm for 16 h.
5. Isolate the plasmid DNA from single colonies of the organism using conventional techniques.
6. Establish the presence of the transgene by restriction analysis using the unique restriction site *Hin*dIII.
7. Orient the transgene within pMV100 using the unique restriction sites *Sph*I and *Cla*I to ensure that the gene is in frame with the promoter.

### 3.2. Construction of a Recombinant Adenovirus Transfer Vector

The expression cassette containing the transgene, HCMV promoter, and terminator from pMV100 is now cloned into the adenovirus, transfer vector (pMV60) at the unique *Hin*dIII restriction site. This surrounds the cassette with adenovirus flanking regions, which are required for recombination into the replication-deficient adenovirus. If a *Hin*dIII site is present in the transgene, a partial digest can be used to clone the cassette.

1. Ligate the cassette containing the transgene (from **Subheading 3.1.**) into the transfer vector (pMV60) at the unique *Hin*dIII cloning site.
2. Transform the resulting plasmid into *E. coli* JM109.
3. Isolate the plasmid DNA from single colonies of the host organism (*see* **Subheading 3.1.**).
4. Establish the presence of the cassette by restriction analysis using the unique *Hin*dIII restriction site.
5. Orient the transgene within pMV60 using the restriction site *Sph*I.
6. Purify the plasmid DNA using either commercially available methods (*see* **Subheading 2.**, **item 5**—e.g., Qiagen columns) or CsCl purification protocols. It is important to ensure that the purified plasmid DNA is of a high quality for the subsequent transfection procedures.

### 3.3. Cotransfection of 293 Cells to Produce Recombinant Adenovirus

To produce the recombinant adenovirus, 293 cells are cotransfected with both the transfer vector containing the transgene and the replication-deficient adenovirus genome, which is present on the plasmid pJM17. Homologous recombination results in the insertion of the CMV IE promoter expression cassette into the adenovirus vector (which requires a high transfection frequency). The recombination event reduces the

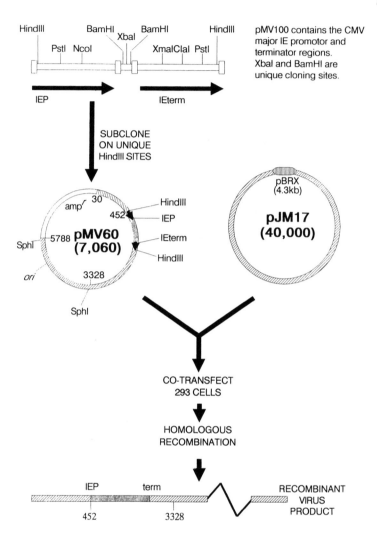

Fig. 1. Diagram of the adenovirus construction, which involves placing the gene (shaded areas) under the control of the HCMV IE promoter (IEP) and terminator (IE term) by cloning into the vector pMV100. The CMV cassette containing the transgene is then cloned into the plasmid pMV60 at a unique *Hind*III site to surround the gene/cassette with adenovirus-flanking regions (hatched areas). The resultant plasmid is then cotransfected with pJM17 in 293 cells. On homologous recombination, the prokaryotic vector (pBRX) in pJM17 is replaced with the gene/cassette, reducing the overall size of the adenovirus genome in pJM17 and producing a recombinant virus.

overall size of the vector by deleting the "stuffer" region pBRX and the adenovirus E1 region, permitting packaging of the adenovirus genome (*see* **Fig. 1**). This can be achieved using commercially available methods (e.g., transfection, DOTAP, and lipofectin), and details of these are readily available from the manufacturers. Here we describe the calcium phosphate precipitation method *(62)*, which is currently used with consistent success in many laboratories.

1. Grow 293 cells as monolayers in growth media (*see* **Subheading 2.**, **item 7**). Gas cells with 5% $CO_2$/95% air (BOC) and incubate at 37°C. Change media when acid pH becomes evident by color changes (red-yellow) within the medium.
2. Seed 293 cells produced in **step 1** into 25-$cm^2$ flasks ($2 \times 10^6$/mL) or 18-$cm^2$ Petri dishes ($1.5 \times 10^6$/mL) 24 h before transfection to produce monolayers that are 80% confluent. It is recommended that the cotransfection procedure be performed in duplicate, using appropriate controls. One particularly important control is pMV35 expressing β-gal (*see* **Subheading 2.**, **item 1**), to evaluate the transfection frequency (*see* **Note 4**).
3. Dissolve plasmid DNA (20 µg; with a molar ratio 5:1 with pJM17) in 420 µL of TE buffer in a 10-mL polypropylene centrifuge tube.
4. Gently vortex the DNA solution while adding dropwise 60 µL of 2 *M* $CaCl_2$ (*see* **Note 5**).
5. Add 480 µL of 2X HBS to a separate polypropylene centrifuge tube.
6. Gently vortex the 2X HBS while adding dropwise the DNA/calcium chloride solution.
7. Allow the precipitate to form for 15–30 min at room temperature.
8. Visualize the precipitate formation using a light microscope (×40).
9. Without removing the cell medium, add the solution containing the precipitate dropwise to the cell monolayer produced in **step 2**.
10. Re-examine the appearance of the precipitate on the cell monolayer using a light microscope. If the precipitate flocculates on the cells, wash the monolayer with prewarmed media to remove excess precipitate before incubation.
11. Gas (5% $CO_2$/95% air) the treated 293 cells and incubate for 16 h at 37°C.
12. Discard the spent medium and wash the monolayers once with 3 mL Tris-buffered saline (TBS) buffer and once with 3 mL complete medium, and replace with fresh media.
13. Gas the cells with a mixture of 5% $CO_2$/95% air and incubate at 37°C until plaques can be visualized (usually 6–10 d). Cells transfected with pMV100 with the β-gal gene (*see* **step 2**) are removed after 24 h of incubation and treated as described in **Subheading 3.4.**, to determine the transformation frequency.
14. If no plaques are visualized, change media when pH falls.
15. Harvest the medium after the formation of plaques and store at –80°C. The next stage for this procedure is to separate the recombinant virus by amplification and plaque assay (*see* **Note 6**).

### 3.4. Estimation of Transfection Efficiency

1. Wash the β-galactosidase-transfected cell monolayer (*see* **Subheading 3.3.**) once with PBS.
2. Fix the cells with 3 mL 0.5% (v/v) glutaraldehyde in PBS for 15 min at room temperature.
3. Wash the cells with IX PBS.
4. Add 3 mL of freshly prepared staining solution to the cell monolayer.
5. Incubate at 37°C for 16 h.
6. Examine using light microscope (×40) to estimate the number of blue-stained cells.

### 3.5. Virus Purification and Plaque Assay of Recombinant Adenovirus

It is essential to purify the recombinant adenovirus to homogeneity by isolating a single replication-deficient adenovirus containing the transgene. This also removes

any parental defective adenoviruses that may have been present in the initial culture. The same method is used to titrate the purified recombinant adenovirus *(49)*.

1. Seed 293 cells in 24-well trays to produce monolayers that are 80% confluent.
2. Make 10-fold dilutions of the harvested medium produced from the transfected cells in
   **Subheading 3.3.** in prewarmed fresh growth media.
3. Remove the media from the 24-well trays and discard.
4. Add 1 mL of the diluted virus solution to each well.
5. Incubate the cells for 6 d in a 5% $CO_2$/95% air atmosphere at 37°C.
6. Examine the cell monolayers for cytopathic effect (CPE; cell rounding or lysis) using a
   light microscope. Plaques or CPE should appear after 7–10 d; however, it may be necessary to incubate for longer periods, which will require feeding the cells with fresh media.
7. Determine the end point dilution where the virus has caused CPE.
8. Harvest the end point wells containing the virus.
9. Clarify the supernatant by centrifugation ($1000g$ for 10 min at 4°C), and store at –80°C.
10. Repeat this procedure twice to ensure purification of the recombinant virus.
11. Calculate the virus titers by the Spearman-Karber end point determination *(63)*.

### 3.6. Propagation of Recombinant Adenovirus Stocks

Adenovirus recombinants are propagated in 293 cells to provide a large source of
viral material. The resultant virus can be titrated using the method described in **Subheading 3.5.**

1. Seed 293 cells in a 175-$cm^2$ flask to produce cells that are 80% confluent as described in
   **Subheading 3.3.**
2. Dilute 5 mL of the recombinant virus in 15 mL of media and inoculate into a flask from
   **step 1**. Allow the virus to adsorb onto the cell monolayer for 2 h at 37°C after gassing
   with 5% $CO_2$/95% air.
3. Wash the cell monolayer 1X with prewarmed PBS.
4. Add prewarmed growth media, gas with 5% $CO_2$/95% air, and incubate at 37°C until CPE
   is evident in 100% of the monolayer.
5. Remove the cells by gentle agitation into the media.
6. Pellet the cells by centrifugation at $2000g$ at 4°C for 10 min.
7. Discard the supernatant and gently wash the pellet in 2 mL cold PBS.
8. Pellet the cells by centrifugation at $2000g$ at 4°C for 10 min.
9. Discard the supernatant and gently wash the pellet in 2 mL cold PBS.
10. Extract the virus by mixing the cells vigorously with an equal volume of Arklone P.
11. Centrifuge at $2000g$ at 4°C for 10 min.
12. Remove the aqueous phase (upper layer), which contains the virus, repeat from **step 10**,
    combine the prepared virus, and store in 1-mL aliquots at –80°C. Note that adenoviruses
    may loose titer by exposure to $CO_2$, and thus appropriate precautions should be used for
    their transportation *(64)*.

Alternatively, recombinant adenovirus vectors may be grown on 911 cells derived
from human embryonic retinoblasts, transformed with a defined region of E1 from the
adenovirus serotype 5 genome *(65)*. These cells produce up to three times more adenovirus vector compared to the quantity produced in 293 cells.

The reader may also consider further purification of the recombinant adenovirus stock
using standard methods of isopycnic gradient centrifugation with caesium chloride.

## 4. Notes

1. Plasmid pMV100 (a transient expression vector) contains the HCMV IE promoter and terminator with two unique cloning sites (*Xba*I or *Bam*HI) on the CMV cassette (**Fig. 1**). PMV100 has the polylinker of pUC 19 replaced by a fragment containing the CMV IE promoter (−299 to +69) and its associated polyadenylation signal (+2757 to +3053). Nucleotide-sequence numbering of the HCMV IE promoter has been previously described (*66,67*). For a gene to be inserted into the vector, either of the two restriction sites must be present in its flanking regions. If these sites are not available, the chosen restriction sites must be inserted by a subcloning strategy, which could include blunt-end ligation, site-directed mutagenesis, or PCR cloning (*61*).

2. Plasmid pMV60 (adenovirus transfer vector) was derived from pXCX2 (*68*), and contains the unique cloning *Hind*III site (*69*), which is used to construct the adenovirus recombinants (*see* **Fig. 1**). The *Hind*III linker in pMV60 is located between regions, with homology from either side of the genome. The nucleotide regions of the areas of homology of the human adenovirus type 5 genome are at nucleotides 30 and 420, and between 3328 and 5788. Regions of the adenovirus genome that share homology with the replication-deficient adenovirus surround the unique cloning sites.

3. Plasmid pJMl7 (defective adenovirus vector) contains the genome of adenovirus type 5 dl309, with the prokaryotic vector pBRX (size 4.3 kb) inserted into the Ela gene, resulting in the deletion of the E1 gene. The Ela gene between bp 402 and 3328 shares regions of homology with the adenovirus transfer vector (pMV60) between bp 30–452 and 3328–5788, to allow recombination to occur on co-transfection (*60*).

4. Using 293 cells at an early stage of growth after subculture (2 h) before cell clumping is evident may enhance transfection efficiency.

5. The success of the calcium phosphate transfection method depends on obtaining a correctly sized precipitate. If the precipitate is too small or too large, the cells will not accept the DNA. The correct precipitate forms at an optimum pH value, which is critical for the process. It is therefore important to vortex the DNA solution gently when adding the $CaCl_2$ solution in a dropwise manner.

6. **Caution**: An important safety consideration is that adenovirus vectors containing transgenes are potentially infectious in humans or other permissive cell lines. The use of recombinant virus vectors is normally carried out in accordance with local health and safety regulations, and will require the use of a class II safety cabinet. Recombinant adenoviruses containing transgenes should be individually constructed to prevent cross-contamination.

## References

1. Mackett, M., Smith, G. L., and Moss, B. (1982) Vaccinia virus: a selectable eukaryotic cloning and expression vector. *Proc. Natl. Acad. Sci. USA* **79**, 7415–7419.
2. Robinson, A. J., Nicholson, B. H., and Lyttle, D. J. (1994) Engineered viruses and vaccines, in *Synthetic Vaccines* (Nicholson, B., ed.), pp. 331–375.
3. Stephenson, J. R. (2001) Genetically modified viruses: vaccines by design. *Current Pharmaceutical Biotechnology* **2**, 47–76.
4. Graham, F. L. and Prevec, L. (1992) Adenovirus-based expression vectors and recombinant vaccines. *Biotechnology* **20**, 363–390.
5. Top, F. H., Grossman, R.A., Bartellomi, P.J., Segal, H.E., Dudding, B.A., Russell, P.K., and Buescher, E.L. (1971) Immunization with live types 7 and 4 adenovirus vaccines. I. Safety, infectivity, antigenicity, and potency of adenovirus type 7 vaccine in humans. *J. Infect. Dis.* **124**, 148–154.

6. Top, F. H., Buescher, E. L., Bancroft, W. H., and Russell, P. K. (1971) Immunization with live types 7 and 4 adenovirus vaccines. II. Antibody response and protective effect against acute respiratory disease due to adenovirus type 7. *J. Infect. Dis.* **124,** 155–160.

7. Berkner, K. L. (1988) Development of adenovirus vectors for the expression of heterologous genes. *BioTechniques* **6,** 616–629.

8. Prevec, L., Schneider, M., Rosenthal, K. L., Belbeck, I. W., Derbyshire, J. B., and Graham, F. L. (1989) Use of human adenovirus-based vectors for antigen expression in animals. *J. Gen. Virol.* **70,** 429–434.

9. Grunhaus, A. and Horwitz, M. (1992) Adenoviruses as cloning vectors. *Semin. Virol.* **3,** 237–252.

10. Imler, J. L., Chartier, C., Dieterle, A., Dreyer, D., Mehtali, M., and Pavirani, A. (1995) An efficient procedure to select and recover recombinant adenovirus vectors. *Gene Ther.* **2,** 263–268.

11. Imler, J. L. (1995). Adenovirus vectors as recombinant viral vaccines. *Vaccine* **13,** 1142–1151.

12. Rabdrianarison-Jewtoukoff, V. and Perricaudet, M. (1995) Recombinant adenoviruses as vaccines. *Biologicals* **23,** 145–157.

13. Chartier, C., Degryse, E., Gantzer, M., Dieterle, A., Pavirani, A., and Mehtali, M. (1996) Efficient generation of recombinant adenovirus vectors by homologous recombinantion in *Escherichia coli. J. Virol.* **70,** 4805–4810.

14. Fu, S. and Deisseroth, A.B. (1997) Use of the cosmid adenoviral vector cloning system for the in vitro construction of recombinant adenoviral vectors. *Human Gene Therapy* **8,** 1321–1330.

15. He, T-C., Zhou, S., da Costa, L.T., Yu, J., Kinzler, K.W., and Vogelstein, B. (1998) A simplified system for generating recombinant adenoviruses. *Proc. Natl. Acad. Sci. USA* **95,** 2509–2514.

16. Souza, D.W. and Armentano, D. (1999) Novel cloning method for recombinant adenovirus construction in *Escherichia coli. BioTechniques* **26,** 502–508.

17. Danthinne, X. and Werth, E. (2000) New tools for the generation of E1- and/or E3-substituted adenoviral vectors. *Gene Ther.* **7,** 80–87.

18. Richards, C., Brown, C. E., Cogswell, J. P., and M. P. Weiner. (2000) The admid system: generation of recombinant adenoviruses by Tn7-mediated transposition in *E. coli. BioTechniques* **29,** 146–154.

19. Oualikene, W., Lamoureux, L., Weber, J. M., and Massie, B. (2000) Protease-deleted adenovirus vectors and complementing cell lines: potential applications of single-round replication mutants for vaccination and gene therapy. *Human Gene Therapy* **11,** 1341–1353.

20. Ng, P., Parks, R. J., Cummings, D. T., Evelegh, C. M., and Graham, F. L. (2000) An enhanced system for construction of adenoviral vectors by the two-plasmid rescue method. *Human Gene Therapy* **11,** 693–699.

21. Danthinne, X. and Imperiale, M. J. (2000) Production of first generation adenovirus vectors: a review. *Gene Ther.* **7,** 1707–1714.

22. Anderson, R. D., Haskell, R. E., Xia, H., Roessler, B. J., and Davidson, B. L. (2000) A simple method for the rapid generation of recombinant adenovirus vectors. *Gene Ther.* **7,** 1034–1038.

23. Davis, A. R., Wivel, N. A., Palladino, J. L., Tao, L., and Wilson, J. M. (2001) Construction of adenoviral vectors. *Mol. Biotechnol.* **18,** 63–70.

24. Danthinne, X. (2001) Simultaneous insertion of two expression cassettes into adenovirus vectors. *BioTechniques* **30,** 612–619.

25. Mizuguchi, H., Kay, M. A., and Hayakawa, T. (2001) Approaches for generating recombinant adenovirus vectors. *Adv. Drug Deliv. Rev.* **52,** 165–176.

26. Jacobs, S. C., Stephenson, J. R., and Wilkinson, G. W. G. (1992) High level expression of the tick-borne encephalitis virus NS1 protein by using an adenovirus-based vector: protection elicited in a murine model. *J. Virol.* **66,** 2086–2095.

27. Fooks, A. R., Schadeck, E., Liebert, U. G., Dowsett, B. A., Rima, B. K., Steward, M., et al. (1995) High-level expression of the measles virus nucleocapsid protein by using a replication-deficient adenovirus vector: induction of an MHC-1-restricted CTL response and protection in a murine model. *Virology* **210,** 456–465.

28. Schadeck, E. B., Partidos, C. D., Fooks, A. R., Obeid, O. E., Wilkinson, G. W. G., Stephenson, J. R., et al. (1999) CTL epitopes identified with a defective recombinant adenovirus expressing measles virus nucleoprotein and evaluation of their protective capacity in mice. *Virus Res.* **65,** 75–86.

29. Niewiesk, S., Eisenhuth, I., Fooks, A. R., Clegg, J. C. S., Schnorr, J-J., Schneider-Schaulies, S., et al. (1997) Measles Virus induced immune suppression in the cotton rat (Sigmodon hispidus) model depends on viral glycoproteins. *J. Virol.* **71,** 7214 – 7219.

30. Fooks, A. R., Jeevarajah, D., Lee, J., Warnes, A., Niewiesk, S., ter Meulen, V., et al. (1998) Oral or parenteral administration of replication-deficient adenoviruses expressing the measles virus haemmagglutinin and fusion proteins: protective immune responses in rodents. *J. Gen. Virol.* **79,** 1027–1031.

31. Sharpe, S., Fooks, A. R., Lee, J., Hayes, K., Clegg, J. C. S., and Cranage, M. (2002) Single oral dose of replication-deficient recombinant adenovirus expressing measles virus N-protein elicits long-lived cellular and humoral immune responses in mice. *Virology* **292,** 210–216 .

32. Lubeck, M. D., Davis, A. R., Chengalvala, M., Natuk, R. J., March, J. E., Molnar-Kimber, K., et al. (1989) Immunogenicity and efficacy testing in chimpanzees of an oral hepatitis B vaccine based on live recombinant adenovirus. *Proc. Natl. Acad. Sci. USA* **86,** 6763–6767.

33. Tacket, C. O., Losonsky, G., Lubeck, M. D., Davis, A. R., Mizutani, S., Horwith, G., et al. (1992) Initial safety and immunogenicity studies of an oral recombinant adenohepatitis B vaccine. *Vaccine* **10,** 673–676.

34. Eloit, M., Gilardi-Hebenstreit, P., Tome, B., and Perricaudet, M. (1990) Construction of a defective adenovirus vector expressing the pseudorabies virus glycoprotein gp50 and its use as a live vaccine. *J. Gen. Virol.* **71,** 2425–2431.

35. Prevec, L., Campbell, J.B., Christie, B.S., Belbeck, L., and Graham, F.L. (1990) A recombinant human adenovirus vaccine against rabies. *J. Infect. Dis.* **161,** 27–30.

36. Charlton, K. M., Artois, M., Prevec, L., Campbell, J. B., Casey, G. A., Wandeler, A. I., et al. (1992) Oral rabies vaccination of skunks and foxes with a recombinant human adenovirus vaccine. *Arch. Virol.* **123,** 169–179.

37. Vos, A., Neubert, A., Pommerening, E., Muller, T., Dohner, L., Neubert, L., et al. (2001) Immunogenecity of an E1-deleted recombinant human adenovirus against rabies by different routes of administration. *J. Gen. Virol.* **82,** 2191–2197.

38. Hsu, K-H. L., Lubeck, M. D., Davis, A. R., Bhat, R. A., Selling, B. H., Bhat, B. M., et al. (1992) Immunogenicity of recombinant adenovirus-respiratory syncytial virus vaccines with adenovirus types 4, 5, and 7 vectors in dogs and a chimpanzee. *J. Infect. Dis.* **166,** 769–775.

39. Flanagan, B., Pringle, C. R., and Leppard, K. N. (1997) A recombinant human adenovirus expressing the simian immunodeficiency virus Gag antigen can induce long-lived immune responses in mice. *J. Gen. Virol.* **78,** 991–997.

40. Timofeev, A. V., Ozherelkov, S. V., Pronin, A. V., Deeva, A. V., Karhanova, G. G., Elbert, L. B., et al. (1998) Immunological basis for protection in a murine model of tick-borne encephalitis by a recombinant adenovirus carrying the gene encoding the NS1 non-structural protein. *J. Gen. Virol.* **79**, 689–695.
41. Bruna-Romero, O., Lasartte, J. J., Wilkinson, G., Grace, K., Clarke, B., Borras-Cuesta, F., et al. (1997) Induction of cytotoxic T-cell response against hepatitis C virus structural antigens using a defective recombinant adenovirus. *Hepatology* **25**, 470–477.
42. Bruce, C. B., Akrigg, A., Sharpe, S. A., Hanke, T., Wilkinson, G. W., and Cranage, M. P. (1999) Replication-deficient recombinant adenoviruses expressing the human immunodeficiency Env antigen can induce both humoral and CTL immune responses in mice. *J. Gen. Virol.* **80**, 2621–2628.
43. Yoshida, T., Okuda, K., Xin, K. Q., Tadokoro, K., Fukushima, J., Toda, S., et al. (2001) Activation of HIV-1 specific immune responses to an HIV-1 vaccine constructed from a replication-defective adenovirus vector using various combinations of immunization protocols. *Clin. Exp. Immunol.* **124**, 445–452.
44. Harrison, T., Graham, F., and Williams, J. (1977) Host-range mutants of adenovirus type 5 defective for growth in HeLa cells. *Virology* **77**, 319–329.
45. Gallichan, W. S., Johnson, D. C., Graham, F. L., and Rosenthal, K. L. (1993) Mucosal immunity and protection after intranasal immunization with recombinant adenoviruses expressing herpes simplex virus glycoprotein B. *J. Infect. Dis.* **168**, 622–629.
46. Natuk, R. J., Lubeck, M. D., Davis, A. R., Chengalvala, M., Chandra, P. R., Mizutani, S., et al. (1992) Adenoviruses as a system for induction of secretory immunity. *Vaccine Res.* **1**, 275–280.
47. Graham, F. L., Smiley, J., Russell, W. C., and Nairn, R. (1977) Characteristics of a human cell line transformed by DNA from human adenovirus type 5. *J. Gen. Virol.* **36**, 59–72.
48. Ghosh-Choudhury, G., Haj-Ahmad, Y., Brinkley, P., Rudy, I., and Graham, F. L. (1986) Human adenovirus cloning vectors based on infectious bacterial plasmids. *Gene* **50**, 161–171.
49. Graham, F. L. and Prevec, L. (1991) Manipulation of adenovirus vectors, in *Methods in Molecular Biology, vol. 7: Gene Transfer and Expression Protocols* (Murray, E. J., ed.), Humana Press, Totowa, NJ.
50. Grubb, B. R., Pickles, R. J., Ye, H., Yankaskas, J. R., Vick, R. N., Engelhardt, J. F., et al. (1994) Inefficient gene transfer by adenovirus vector to cystic fibrosis airway epithelia of mice and humans. *Nature* **371**, 802–806.
51. Rosenfeld, M. A., Chu, C. S., Seth, P., Danel, C., Banks, T., Yoneyama, K., et al. (1994) Gene transfer to freshly isolated human respiratory epithelial cells in vitro using a replication-deficient adenovirus containing the human cystic fibrosis transmembrane conductance regulator cDNA. *Hum. Gene Ther.* **5**, 331–342.
52. Hsu, K. H., Lubeck, M. D., Bhat, B. M., Bhat, R. A., Kostek, B., Selling, B. H., et al. (1994) Efficacy of adenovirus-vectored respiratory syncytial virus vaccines in a new ferret model. *Vaccine* **12**, 607–612.
53. Ganne, V., Eloit, M., Laval, A., Adama, M., and Trouve, G. (1994) Enhancement of the efficacy of a replication-defective adenovirus vectored vaccine by the addition of oil adjuvants. *Vaccine* **12**, 1190–1196.
54. Wilkinson, G. W. and Borysiewicz, L. K. (1995) Gene therapy and viral vaccination: the interface. *Br. Med. Bull.* **51**, 205–216.
55. Zheng, C., Goldsmith, C. M., O'Connell, B. C., and Baum, B. J. (2000) Adenoviral vector cytoxicity depends in part on the transgene encoded. *Biochem. Biophys. Res. Commun.* **274**, 767–771.

56. Amalfitano, A. (1999) Next-generation adenoviral vectors: new and improved. *Gene Ther.* **6**, 1643–1645.

57. Hardy, S., Kitamura, M., Harris-Stansil, T., Dai, Y., and Phipps, M. L. (1997) Construction of adenovirus vectors through Cre-*lox* recombination. *J. Virol.* **71**, 1842–1849.

58. Morsy, M. A. and Caskey, C. T. (1999) Expanded-capacity adenoviral vectors—the helper-dependent vectors. *Mol. Med. Today* **5**, 18–24.

59. Kochanek, S., Clemens, P. R., Mitani, K., Chen, H. H., Chan, S., and Caskey, C.T. (1996) A new adenoviral vector: Replacement of all viral coding sequences with 28kb of DNA independently expressing both full-length dystrophin and β-galactosidase. *Proc. Natl. Acad. Sci. USA* **93**, 5731–5736.

60. McGrory, W. J., Bautista, D. S., and Graham, F. L. (1988) A simple technique for the rescue of early region 1 mutants into infectious adenovirus type 5. *Virology* **163**, 614–617.

61. Sambrook, J., Fritsch, E. F., and Maniatis, T. (1989) *Molecular Cloning: A Laboratory Manual.* Cold Spring Harbor Laboratory, Cold Spring Harbor, NY.

62. Graham, F. L. and Van der Eb, A. J. (1973) A new technique for the assay of infectivity of human adenovirus 5 DNA. *Virology* **52**, 456–467.

63. Finney, D. J. (1971) *Statistical Methods in Biological Assay*, 2nd ed., Griffin, London.

64. Nyberg-Hoffman, C. and Anguilar-Cordova, E. (1999) Instability of adenoviral vectors during transport and its implication for clinical studies. *Nat. Med.* **5**, 955–957.

65. Fallaux, F. J., Kronenburg, O., Cramer, S. J., Houwelting, A., van Ormondi, J., Hoeben, R. C., et al. (1996) Characterisation of 911: a new helper cell line for the titration and propagation of early-region-I-deleted adenoviral viral vectors. *Human Gene Therapy* **7**, 215–222.

66. Akrigg, A., Wilkinson, G. W. G., and Oram, J. D. (1985) The structure of the major immediately early gene of human cytomegalovirus. *Virus Res.* **2**, 107–121.

67. Wilkinson, G. W. G. and Akrigg, A. (1991) The cytomegalovirus virus major immediate early promoter and its use in eukaryotic expression systems. *Adv. Gene Technic.* **2**, 287–310.

68. Spessot, R., Inchley, K., Hupel, T. M., and Bacchetti, S. (1989) Cloning of herpes simplex virus ICP4 gene in an adenovirus vector. *Virology* **168**, 378–387.

69. Wilkinson, G. W. G. and Akrigg, A. (1992) Constitutive and enhanced expression from the CMV major IE promoter in a defective adenovirus vector. *Nucleic Acids Res.* **20**, 2233–2239.

# 4

## Live Viral Vectors
### Vaccinia Virus

### Caroline Staib and Gerd Sutter

### 1. Introduction

Poxviruses are among prime candidates for generation of recombinant virus vaccines against infectious diseases and cancer. Poxvirus-based experimental vaccines have already proven to be efficient with regard to antigen delivery and the induction of antigen-specific immune responses in several animal models and first clinical trials *(1–7)*. Live vector vaccines are designed to mimic microbial infections allowing for *de novo* synthesis of vaccine antigens that appear particularly suitable for presentation via MHC-I molecules. Vaccination with these live vaccines may elicit appropriate "danger" signals to the immune system, resulting in preferential recognition and presentation of recombinant (vaccine) antigens. Additional features of poxvirus vectors include the ability to accommodate large amounts of foreign DNA, high stability, and reasonable cost of manufacturing. However, vaccinia virus—the prototype live viral vaccine—can replicate in humans, and its imperfect safety record as a smallpox vaccine was a concern for its use as a vector in clinical applications. Therefore, most of the currently evaluated recombinant vaccines are based on vectors derived from highly attenuated vaccinia viruses such as modified vaccinia virus Ankara (MVA) *(8)*, NYVAC *(9)* or avipoxviruses *(10,11)*. These viruses all share the property of replication deficiency in mammalian cells that may have contributed to the already established clinical safety of these vectors *(12–14)*. Importantly, even high dose inoculation of MVA was shown to be safe in immune-suppressed macaques, suggesting the safety of recombinant MVA vaccines in potentially immunocompromised individuals *(15)*. Moreover, MVA vector vaccines induced significant levels of humoral and cellular immune responses to vaccine antigens, and were found to be less affected by preexisting vaccinia virus-specific immunity when compared to replication-competent vaccinia virus vectors *(16)*.

Here, we describe an up-to-date methodology for the generation and characterization of recombinant MVA. The protocol includes different selection techniques for

From: *Methods in Molecular Medicine, Vol. 87: Vaccine Protocols, 2nd ed.*
Edited by: A. Robinson, M. J. Hudson, and M. P. Cranage © Humana Press Inc., Totowa, NJ

isolation of cloned viruses and optimized procedures for cell culture, virus amplification, and titration, as well as preparation of vaccine stocks.

## 2. Materials

### 2.1. Virus Strain

1. Vaccinia virus strain MVA (cloned isolate F6), 582nd CEF passage.

### 2.2. Cell Culture

1. Rabbit kidney (RK-13) cells (ATCC CCL-37).
2. Baby hamster kidney (BHK-21) cells (ATCC CCL-10).
3. Primary chicken embryo fibroblasts (CEF), freshly prepared.
4. RPMI-1640 medium (Seromed, Biochrome KG, Berlin, Germany).
5. Heat-inactivated fetal calf serum (FCS) (Seromed, Biochrome KG).
6. Antibiotics, antimycotics as streptomycin, penicillin, and amphothericin B (AB/AM) (Gibco-BRL, Grand Island, NY).
7. 6-well tissue-culture plates, T85, and T185 tissue-culture flasks (Costar, Corning, NY, USA).

### 2.3. Preparation of Primary Chicken Embryo Fibroblasts

1. Ten 11-d-old eggs.
2. RPMI-1640 supplemented with 10% FCS and 1% AB/AM.
3. Trypsin $T_D$-ethylenediaminetetraacetic acid (EDTA) (Seromed, Biochrom KG).
4. Absolute ethanol (EtOH abs) (Merck KGaA, Darmstadt, Germany, laboratory use-grade).
5. 50-mL Falcon tubes.
6. Sterile Petri dishes, 10-cm diameter (Costar).
7. T185 tissue-culture flasks.
8. Sterile instruments for dissection—e.g., scissors, forceps.
9. 10-mL syringes.
10. One sterile Erlenmeyer flask, two sterile beakers covered with two layers of gauze (wrapped in autoclave tape).

### 2.4. Virus Growth

#### 2.4.1. Amplification of MVA

1. Confluent monolayers of CEF or BHK-21 cells grown on 60 cm$^2$ dishes, T85, and T185 tissue-culture flasks (for growth conditions, *see* **Subheading 3.1.**).
2. Cell scraper.
3. 10 m$M$ Tris-HCl, pH 9.0, autoclaved (store at 4°C).

#### 2.4.2. Purification of MVA

1. Cell scraper.
2. Cup sonicator and/or sonification needle (Sonopuls HD 200, Bandelin, Germany).
3. Dounce homogenizer, glass, tight-fitting, autoclaved.
4. 10 m$M$ Tris-HCl, pH 9.0, autoclaved (store at 4°C).

5. 1 m$M$ Tris-HCl, pH 9.0, autoclaved (store at 4°C).
6. 36% sucrose in 10 m$M$ Tris-HCl, pH 9.0, sterile-filtered (store at 4°C).

### 2.4.3. Titration of MVA Determining Amount of Infectious Units per mL (IU/mL)

1. Subconfluent monolayers of CEF or BHK-21 cells grown on 6-well tissue-culture plates (for growth conditions, *see* **Subheading 3.1.**).
2. Fixing solution: 1:1 mixture of acetone:methanol (Merck KGaA), (laboratory use-grade) (store at at 4°C).
3. Phosphate-buffered saline (PBS), pH 7.5.
4. Blocking buffer: PBS pH 7.5/2% bovine serum albumin (BSA).
5. Primary antibody (1st Ab): Polyclonal rabbit anti-vaccinia antibody (IgG fraction, Biogenesis Ltd, Poole, England, Cat. No. 9503-2057) diluted 1:500–1:1000 in blocking buffer.
6. Secondary antibody (2nd Ab): horseradish peroxidase-conjugated polyclonal goat anti-rabbit antibody (IgG (H+L)) (Dianova, Hamburg, Germany, Cat. No. 111-035-114) diluted 1:1000 in blocking buffer.
7. o-dianisidine (Sigma, Deisenhofen, Germany), **Caution**: very toxic!
8. Absolute ethanol (EtOH abs) (Merck KGaA).
9. Hydrogen peroxide >30% ($H_2O_2$ >30%) (Sigma).

### 2.4.4. Titration of MVA Determining the Tissue-Culture Infectious Dose 50 (TCID$_{50}$)

1. Sub-confluent monolayers of CEF or BHK-21 cells grown on 96-well tissue culture plates (for growth conditions, *see* **Subheading 3.1.**).
2. For all additional materials, *see* **Subheading 2.4.3.**

## 2.5. Generation of Recombinant MVA

### 2.5.1. Molecular Cloning of Recombinant Gene Sequences

1. MVA-targeting vector plasmids.
2. Restriction endonucleases.
3. DNA-modifying enzymes, e.g., Klenow DNA polymerase, T4 DNA ligase.

### 2.5.2. Transfection of MVA-Infected Cells with Vector Plasmids

1. Sub-confluent monolayers CEF or BHK-21 on 6-well plates.
2. Recombinant MVA transfer vector plasmid, e.g., pIII dHR P7.5-target gene.
3. Serum-free RPMI-1640 supplemented with 1% AB/AM (store at 4°C).
4. FUGENE™ (Roche, Mannheim, Germany) (store at –20°C).

## 2.6. Isolation of Recombinant MVA (for all procedures)

1. Cup sonicator (Sonopuls HD 200).
2. RPMI-1640 medium supplemented with 5% FCS and 1% AB/AM (store at 4°C).
3. Sub-confluent monolayers of RK-13 cells, primary CEF or BHK-21 grown on 6-well plates in RPMI-1640 medium.
4. 1.5-mL Eppendorf vials.

### 2.6.1. Isolation of rMVA Screening for Transient β-Galactosidase Expression

1. X-gal solution: X-gal (5-bromo-4-chloro-3-indolyl β-D-galactoside, Roche), 4% in dimethyl formamide (DMFA, Sigma) (store at –20°C, light-sensitive, toxic).
2. 2xRPMI-1640 supplemented with 4% FCS, 2% AB/AM (store at 4°C).
3. LMP-agarose: 2% low-melting-point agarose (LMP-agarose) (Life Technologies, Karisruhe, Germany) in distilled water (store at room temperature).

### 2.6.2. Isolation of rMVA by Live Immune Detection of the Target Antigen

2.6.2.1. CONCANAVALIN-A COATED PLATES FOR LIVE IMMUNOSTAINING

1. Concanavalin-A (Con-A) (Sigma, Deisenhofen, Germany, #C-2010).
2. 10% Con-A in PBS (Con-A/PBS).

2.6.2.2. IMMUNOSTAINING

*See* **Subheading 2.4.3.** with following variations:

1. Confluent monolayers of CEF or BHK-21 cells on 6-well tissue-culture plates (for growth conditions, *see* **Subheading 3.1.**).
2. Primary antibody (1st Ab): directed against target protein and diluted in blocking buffer as appropriate.
3. Secondary antibody (2nd Ab): horseradish peroxidase-conjugated antibody binding to 1st Ab and diluted in blocking buffer.

## 2.7. Characterization of Recombinant MVA Genomes by PCR

1. Confluent RK-13, BHK-21, or CEF cells grown on 6- or 12-well culture plates.
2. 10X TEN buffer pH 7.4: 100 m$M$ Tris-HCl, 10 m$M$ EDTA, 1 $M$ NaCl.
3. DNA-grade proteinase K prepared as 1 mg/mL stock solution in 1 m$M$ CaCl$_2$ (prot K), (AGS GmbH, Heidelberg, Germany) (store at –20°C).
4. 20% sodium dodecyl sulfate in distilled water (sodium dodecyl sulfate [SDS] 20%) (DNase-free; sterile-filtered).
5. Phenol-chloroform 1:1 mixture (Applied Biosystems, Foster City, CA) (store at 4°C).
6. 3 $M$ sodium acetate in distilled water (3 $M$ NaAc) (Merck KGaA).
7. Absolute ethanol (EtOH abs) (Merck KGaA).
8. 70% ETOH in distilled water.
9. Primer 1 (MVA-III-5′) and primer 2 (MVA-III-3′) dissolved in sterile distilled water to a final concentration of 5 pmol/µL (store at –20°C): MVA-III-5′ (Primer 1): 5′-GAATGCACATACATAAGTACCGGCATCTCTAGCAGT-3′, MVA-III-3′ (Primer 2): 5′-CACCAGCGTCTACATGACGAGCTTCCGAGTTCC-3′.
10. Template DNA:
    a. Viral genomic DNA prepared as described in **Subheading 3.6.**
    b. Plasmid DNA diluted to a final concentration of 100 ng/µL.
11. PCR master kit (Roche, Mannheim, Germany) (store at –20°C).

## 2.8. From a Single Plaque Pick to a Virus Stock

1. Confluent CEF or BHK-21 cells grown on 35-mm and 60-mm Petri dishes, or in 75 cm$^2$ and 175 cm$^2$ tissue-culture flasks.
2. Cell scraper.

### 2.9. Preparation of Vaccines for Mice

1. Vaccine buffer: 120 m*M* NaCl, 10 m*M* Tris-HCl, pH 7.4, autoclaved.

## 3. Methods
### 3.1. Cell Culture

RK-13, BHK-21, and CEF cells are grown on 6-well plates, T85, or T185 flasks in RPMI-1640 medium supplemented with 2–10% heat-inactivated fetal calf serum (FCS), 100 µg/mL streptomycin, 100 IU/mL penicillin, and 25 µg/mL amphotericin B (1% AB/AM) at 37°C and 5% $CO_2$.

### 3.2. Preparation of CEF (see Notes 1 and 2)

1. Prewarm 200 mL of trypsin in a 37°C water bath.
2. Place eggs with blunt ends facing up, in order to position the air space upwards.
3. Wipe eggs with ethanol, crack eggshell with scissors, and cut it off, taking care not to damage the membrane.
4. Remove membrane and pick up embryo on legs with forceps. Transfer into a Petri dish containing 10 mL serum-free RPMI using a second pair of forceps to support embryo.
5. Remove head, wings, legs, and internal organs (scrape forceps over stomach).
6. Transfer to a second Petri dish containing 10 mL serum-free RPMI.
7. Homogenize by pressing five embryos at a time through a 10-mL syringe into an Erlenmeyer flask.
8. Add 100 mL 37°C trypsin and trypsinize by stirring for 10 min at room temperature using a magnetic stirrer.
9. Fill cell suspension through gauze into beaker. Take care not to transfer remaining embryo clumps.
10. Fill up Erlenmeyer flask with remaining clumps to 100 mL with 37°C trypsin. Stir for 10 min at room temperature.
11. Pass whole content through gauze of a second beaker and pool filtrates in 250-mL centrifuge bottle.
12. Spin for 10 min at 1800*g* and 4°C.
13. Remove supernatant, resuspend by pipetting vigorously (10–15 times) in 10 mL of supplemented RPMI, then add 90 mL RPMI to wash cells.
14. Centrifuge 10 min at 1800*g*.
15. Prepare 20 T185 culture flasks, fill with 40 mL of RPMI.
16. Resuspend cell pellet in 5 mL RPMI (pipetting 10–15 times), then transfer to 50-mL Falcon tube and fill up to a final volume of 20 mL.
17. Add 1 mL of cell suspension to each T175 flask.
18. Incubate for 3–4 d at 37°C until monolayers are confluent.
19. Split at ratio of 1:4 for 6-well plates (2 mL/plate), 12-well plates (1 mL/plate) or T175 flasks.

### 3.3. Virus Growth (see also Note 3)
#### 3.3.1. Amplification of MVA (see Notes 4–9)

This protocol can be used to amplify parental MVA or to grow stocks of recombinant MVA (rMVA). If titered MVA starting material is available for amplification, use a multiplicity of infection (MOI) of 0.01 to 0.1 IU/cell for all infections. Either

CEF or BHK-21 cells can be used for virus amplification, although growth in chicken cells yields a higher virus output. Remove growth medium from cells before adding virus material to allow for efficient infection of cell monolayers (*see also* **Note 4**).

1. Infect cell monolayers of 10–40 175-cm$^2$ tissue-culture flasks by inoculating each flask with 5-mL virus suspension (0.01–0.1 IU/cell).
2. Allow virus adsorption for 1 h at 37°C.
3. Gently rock flasks in 20-min intervals.
4. Add 30 mL RPMI/2% FCS /1% AB/AM per flask.
5. Incubate at 37°C for 2 d or until cytopathic effect (CPE) is obvious.
6. Remove approx 25 mL medium from each flask.
7. Scrape cells in leftover medium, and transfer to 50-mL centrifuge tubes.
8. Centrifuge 10 min at 1800*g* and 4°C.
9. Discard medium, resuspend, and combine cell pellets in 10 m*M* Tris-HCl, pH 9.0. Use approx 1 mL per T175 culture flask.
10. Freeze-thaw virus material 3×—(i.e., on dry ice and in a 37°C water bath). Vortex in between.
11. Homogenize the material using a cup sonicator (*see* **Notes 5–7**). Fill cup of sonicator with ice-water (50% ice), place tube containing virus material in ice-water, and sonicate at maximal power for 1 min. Repeat 3×, take care to avoid heating of the sample by replenishing ice in cup. Store virus material at –80°C as crude material or until further purification (*see* **Subheading 3.3.2.**).

### 3.3.2. Purification of MVA

Crude stock preparations of MVA can be semi-purified from cell debris and recombinant proteins by ultra centrifugation through a sucrose cushion (*see* **Note 10**).

1. Transfer virus material to a dounce homogenizer and dounce 5 × 5 times on ice. Allow suspension to cool between sets of strokes.
2. Transfer virus suspension to 50-mL Falcon tube and centrifuge 5 min at 1800*g* and 4°C.
3. Collect supernatant in 50-mL Falcon tube, resuspend pellet in 10 mL of 10 m*M* Tris-HCl, pH 9.0 and repeat **steps 1–3**. Pool supernatants.
4. Prepare 36% sucrose cushions by filling half volume of an ultracentrifuge tube—e.g., SW 28 with sucrose. Overlay with equal volumes of virus suspension.
5. Spin 60 min at 30,000*g* and 4°C.
6. Discard supernatant (cell debris and sucrose) and resuspend pelleted virus material in 1 m*M* Tris-HCl, pH 9.0. Use about 1 mL per ten cell-culture flasks.
7. Store at –80°C.

### 3.3.3. Titration of MVA Determining Amount of Infectious Units per mL (IU/mL)

To titrate the infectivity of MVA stock preparations, foci of MVA infected cells are visualized by specific immunoperoxidase-staining of cells containing vaccinia viral antigens (*see* also **Notes 11–13**).

1. Thaw virus material and homogenize in cup sonicator as described in **Subheading 3.3.1.**, **step 11**.
2. Make 10-fold serial dilutions (ranging from $10^{-1}$ to $10^{-9}$) of virus material in 3 mL RPMI/ 2% FCS /1% AB/AM.

3. Plate on CEF or BHK-21, 6 wells, 1 mL of virus suspension per well in duplicates. Use $10^{-4}$ to $10^{-9}$ dilutions.
4. Incubate for 48 h at 37°C.
5. Remove medium from infected tissue-culture plates. Fix and permeabilize cells with 1 mL fixing solution per well for 2 min at room temperature.
6. Remove fixing solution and air-dry fixed monolayers.

The following incubations are carried out at room temperature on a rocking device:

7. Add 1 mL first antibody solution (1st Ab) per well and incubate for 1 h.
8. Remove first Ab and wash 3× with 1 mL PBS per well for 5 min each.
9. Add 1 mL second antibody solution (2nd Ab) per well and incubate for 45–60 min.
10. Remove second Ab and wash 3× with 1 mL PBS per well for 5 min each.
11. Prepare substrate solution in two steps as follows:
    Make saturated dianisidine solution in 500 µL EtOH abs. (transfer flock of dianisidine to tube), mix by vortexing for 2 min. Centrifuge for 30 s at top speed at room temperature. Use supernatant only. Prepare final substrate solution for peroxidase-staining by adding 240 µL saturated dianisidine solution to 12 mL PBS in a 15-mL conical centrifuge tube. Mix by vortexing, add 12 µL $H_2O_2$ >30%, gently mix again, and use immediately.
12. Add 1 mL of substrate solution per well and leave 15–30 min to clearly visualize stained viral foci.
13. To determine the titer count viral foci in a suitable dilution. Count in both wells of the dilution and calculate the mean. To express titer as IU/mL, multiply the counted number of foci by the dilution. Wells with 20–100 viral foci generate the most accurate results.

### 3.3.4. Titration of MVA Determining the Tissue-Culture Infectious Dose 50 (TCID$_{50}$)

To titrate the infectivity of MVA stock preparations, foci of MVA infected cells are visualized by specific immunoperoxidase-staining of cells containing vaccinia viral antigen (*see* **Note 14**).

1. After thawing, homogenize MVA stock virus preparation by sonication as described in **Subheading 3.3.1., step 11**.
2. Make 10-fold serial dilutions (ranging from $10^{-1}$ to $10^{-9}$) of virus material in RPMI/2% FCS /1% AB/AM.
3. Add 100 µL of each dilution in replicates of eight to sub-confluent cell monolayers grown in 96-well plates using a multipipet and incubate at 37°C for 48 h.
4. Remove medium from infected tissue-culture plates. Fix and permeabilize cells with 200 µL fixing solution per well for 2 min at room temperature.
   The following incubations are carried out at room temperature on a rocking device:
5. Add 100 µL first antibody solution (1st Ab) per well and incubate for 1 h.
6. Remove first Ab and wash 3× with 200 µL PBS per well. For each washing step, allow to incubate with PBS for 10 min. Add 100 µL second antibody solution (2nd Ab) per well and incubate for 45–60 min.
7. Remove second Ab and wash 3× with 200 µL PBS per well.
8. Prepare substrate solution as described in **Subheading 3.3.3., step 11**.
9. Add 100 µL of substrate solution per well and leave for 15–30 min to clearly visualize stained viral foci.
10. Observe 96-well plate under microscope and count all wells positive in which viral foci can be detected. Calculate titer according to the method of Kaerber (*17*) (*see* **Note 14** for

**Table 1**
**MVA Transfer Vectors**

| Vector | Insertion site | Screening/selection | Reference |
|---|---|---|---|
| PIIIdHR-P7.5, pIIIdHR-sP | Del III | Transient K1L | *(18)* |
| PIIIdHR-PH5 | Del III | Transient K1L | *(23)* |
| PVIdHR-PH5 | Del VI | Transient K1L | *(23)* |
| PIILZ-P7.5 | Del II | Stable β-galactosidase | *(19)* |
| PIILZdel-P7.5 | Del II | Transient β-galactosidase | *(20)* |
| PLW7 (sP), pLW9 (PH5) | Del III | Immunostaining | *(21)* |
| PMC03 (sP) | Del III | β-glucuronidase | *(22)* |
| PIIIgptex-dsP | Del III | Immunostaining | *(4)* |
| PIIIgpt-dsP | Del III | Stable gpt | *(4)* |

calculation example). First, determine the endpoint dilution that will infect 50% of the wells that were inoculated by calculating in the following way:

$$\log_{10} \text{ 50\% endpoint dilution} = x - d/2 + (d \text{ S } r/n)$$

$x$ = highest dilution in which all 8 wells (8/8) are counted positive.
$d$ = the $\log_{10}$ of the dilution factor ($d = 1$ when serial 10-fold dilutions are used).
$r$ = number of positive wells per dilution.
$n$ = total number of wells per dilution ($n = 8$ when dilutions are plated out in replicates of eight).

## 3.4. Generation of Recombinant MVA

### 3.4.1. Molecular Cloning of Recombinant Gene Sequences

Recombinant genes that should be transferred into the MVA genome are sub cloned into MVA plasmid vectors such as listed in **Table 1**.

DNA-fragments containing the coding sequence of the gene of interest, including authentic start (ATG) and stop (TAA/TAG/TGA) codons, are cloned into the multiple cloning site of the respective vector to generate the MVA transfer vector plasmid. The correct orientation of the recombinant gene is determined by the direction of promoter-specific transcription. Prepare stocks of transfer plasmid DNA (*see* **Note 15**) for generation of recombinant MVA (*see* **Subheading 3.4.2.**).

### 3.4.2. Transfection of MVA-Infected Cells with Vector Plasmids

Recombinant plasmids are transfected into MVA infected cells and homologous recombination between MVA and plasmid DNA generates a recombinant virus.

1. Grow CEF or BHK-21 cell monolayers to 80% confluence in 6-well tissue-culture plates. Use one well per transfection.
2. Discard medium and overlay cells with RPMI/2% FCS/1% AB/AM containing MVA at a MOI of 0.01 (e.g., an inoculum of $1 \times 10^4$ IU MVA in 1-mL medium for one well with $1 \times 10^6$ cells). Incubate for 90 min at 37°C.

3. 15–30 min post-infection, start preparing FUGENE/plasmid DNA-mix as described by the manufacturer in serum-free medium (Roche Diagnostics) using 1.5 µg plasmid DNA.
4. Add FUGENE/plasmid DNA-mix directly into the medium. Incubate for 48 h at 37°C.
5. Harvest cell monolayer with a cell scraper and transfer cells and medium into 1.5-mL microcentrifuge tubes. Store transfection harvest at –20 to –80°C.

## 3.5. Isolation of Recombinant MVA (rMVA) (see also Note 16)

### 3.5.1. Transient Host Range Selection

This technique relies on stringent growth selection of MVA on rabbit kidney RK-13 cells (**Fig. 1**). Vector plasmids contain the vaccinia virus K1L gene flanked by segments of MVA-DNA that direct integration into the viral genome precisely at the site of a naturally disrupted MVA gene sequence (e.g., deletion III, *18*). rMVA expressing the recombinant antigen and transiently co-expressing K1L coding sequences are cloned by consecutive rounds of plaque purification in RK-13 cell monolayers selecting for K1L-specific cell aggregates. The K1L expression cassette is designed to contain repetitive DNA sequences that allow for deletion of the marker gene from the recombinant MVA genome under nonselective growth conditions, e.g., by additional rounds of plaque purification on CEF or BHK-21 cells.

1. Freeze-thaw transfection harvest three times (3×) and homogenize in a cup sonicator. For use refer to **Subheading 3.3.1.**, **step 11**.
2. Make four 10-fold serial dilutions ($10^{-1}$ to $10^{-4}$) of the virus suspension in RPMI/2% FCS /1% AB/AM medium.
3. Remove growth medium from sub-confluent RK-13 cell monolayers grown in 6-well plates and infect with 1 mL diluted virus suspension per well. Incubate at 37°C for 48–72 h (*see* **Note 17**).
4. Select typical cell aggregates of MVA/K1L infected RK-13 cells under a microscope. Mark foci with a permanent marker on the bottom of the culture well.
5. Add 0.5 mL RPMI/2% FCS /1% AB/AM medium to sterile microcentrifuge tubes.
6. Pick marked foci in a 20-µL volume by aspiration with an air-displacement pipet. Scrape and aspirate cells together with medium and transfer material to the tube containing 0.5 mL medium. Pick 5–15 foci, each time using new tips and placing in a separate tube.
7. Freeze-thaw, sonicate, and replate virus material obtained from plaque picks as described in **steps 1–3** or store at –80°C. Proceed as in **steps 4–7**.
8. Repeat as described in **steps 1–7** until clonally pure rMVA/K1L is obtained (usually requires 2 to 4 rounds of plaque purification). Use PCR analysis of viral DNA to monitor for absence of wild-type MVA (*see* **Subheading 3.6.**).
9. Continue plaque purification on CEF or BHK-21 cell monolayers, selecting for MVA specific foci. Repeat steps as described in **steps 1–7**. Use PCR analysis of viral DNA to monitor for absence of K1L selection cassette (*see* **Subheading 3.6.** and **Note 30**; usually requires 3 to 5 rounds of plaque purification).
10. Amplify (*see* **Subheading 3.7.**) and analyze (*see* **Subheading 3.6.**) the cloned rMVA.

### 3.5.2. Isolation of rMVA Screening for Transient β-Galactosidase Expression

rMVA expressing the recombinant antigen and transiently co-expressing β-galactosidase coding sequences (rMVA/LZ) are cloned by consecutive rounds of plaque

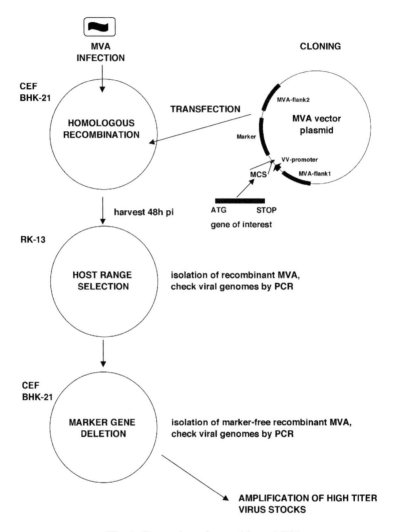

Fig. 1. Generation of recombinant MVA.

purification in CEF/BHK-21 cell monolayers stained with X-gal, selecting blue foci
*(19)*. To remove the reporter gene from rMVA an additional round of plaque purification is carried out, screening for nonstained viral foci in the presence of X-gal.

1. Freeze-thaw transfection harvest 3× and homogenize in cup sonicator. For use, refer to
   **Subheading 3.3.1., step 11**.
2. Make four 10-fold serial dilutions ($10^{-1}$ to $10^{-4}$) of the virus suspension in RPMI/ 2%
   FCS /1% AB/AM medium.
3. Remove growth medium from confluent-cell monolayers grown in 6-well plates and infect
   with 1 mL diluted virus suspension per well. Incubate at 37°C for 2 h.

4. Melt 2% LMP-agarose, and keep at 37°C until needed. Prewarm 2× RPMI /4% FCS/2% AB/AM medium; maintain at 37°C until needed.
5. 2 h after infection of cell monolayers mix equal amounts of 2% LMP-agarose and 2× RPMI.
6. Remove inoculum from cells and overlay cell monolayers with 1 mL of RPMI/LMP-agarose mixture. Allow agar to solidify at room temperature, and incubate for 48 h at 37°C.
7. Prepare second agarose overlay containing X-gal as described in **steps 4** and **5** by mixing equal amounts of 2% LMP-agarose and 2× RPMI medium supplemented with 1/100 vol of X-gal solution. Add to each well 1 mL of the RPMI/LMP-agarose/X-gal mixture, allow to solidify at room temperature, and incubate for 4–12 h at 37°C.
8. Add 0.5 mL RPMI/2% FCS /1% AB/AM medium to sterile microcentrifuge tubes.
9. Pick blue foci of cells infected with recombinant MVA by inserting the tip of a sterile cotton-plugged Pasteur pipet through agarose onto stained viral foci. Scrape and aspirate cells together with agarose plug by squeezing a rubber bulb on Pasteur pipet, and transfer to the tube containing 0.5 mL medium. Pick 5–15 foci, using separate pipets, and placing in separate tubes.
10. Freeze-thaw, sonicate, and replate virus material obtained from plaque picks as described in **steps 1–6** or store at –80°C. Proceed as in **steps 7–9**.
11. Repeat as described in **steps 1–9** until clonally pure rMVA/LZ is obtained (usually requires 5 to 10 rounds of plaque purification). Use PCR analysis of viral DNA to monitor for absence of wild-type MVA (*see* **Subheading 3.6.**, **Note 18**).
12. Continue plaque purification in the presence of X-gal, now selecting *nonstaining* viral foci. Repeat steps as described in **steps 1–9** until all viral isolates fail to produce any blue foci in the presence of X-gal.
13. Amplify (*see* **Subheading 3.7.**) and analyze (*see* **Subheading 3.6.**) the cloned rMVA.

### 3.5.3. Isolation of rMVA by Live Immune Detection of the Target Antigen

This is an alternate protocol that allows selection of recombinant MVA if an antibody that works in immunostaining specific for the recombinant gene product is available. The live immunostaining will enable the specific detection of cells that are infected with rMVA and produce the antigen of interest. In this approach no selective pressure is used and it works best for surface proteins. CEF or BHK-21 cells should be plated on culture wells that have been pretreated with Concanavalin-A, which allows for tighter attachment of the monolayer to the plates during staining procedure (*see* **Note 19**).

#### 3.5.3.1. Concanavalin-A Coated Plates for Live Immunostaining

1. Add 1 mL of Con-A/PBS solution to each well of a 6-well plate. Leave for 1 h at room temperature.
2. Rinse each well with 1 mL PBS and let plates dry in hood (sterile!).
3. Store in plastic bag at room temperature—it will be stable for months.
4. When needed, plate cells in the usual manner.

#### 3.5.3.2. Immunostaining

1. Freeze-thaw transfection harvest 3× and homogenize in a cup sonicator. For use, *see* **Subheading 3.3.1.**, **step 11**.
2. Make four 10-fold serial dilutions ($10^{-1}$ to $10^{-4}$) of the virus suspension in RPMI/2% FCS /1% AB/AM medium.

3. Remove growth medium from sub-confluent CEF or BHK-21 cell monolayers grown in 6-well plates pretreated with Con-A, and infect with 1 mL diluted virus suspension per well. Incubate at 37°C for 48–72 h. Use one cell monolayer as mock-infected control.

4. Dilute antibody in PBS/3% FCS. Optimum dilution must be determined. Usually start with 1:500. Add 1 mL diluted antibody (first Ab) per well and incubate for 1 h at room temperature, rocking gently.

5. Remove first Ab and wash 2× with 2 mL PBS per well.

6. Dilute appropriate anti-species antibody conjugated to peroxidase (second Ab) 1:1000 in PBS/3% FCS.

7. Add 1 mL second antibody dilution (second Ab) per well and incubate for 30–45 min at room temperature, rocking gently.

8. Remove second Ab and wash 2× with 2 mL PBS per well.

9. Prepare substrate solution as described in **Subheading 3.3.3., step 11**.

10. Add 1 mL of substrate solution per well. Incubate for up to 30 min at room temperature until foci of stained cell can be detected. Continue to monitor staining under microscope.

11. Add 0.5 mL RPMI/2% FCS /1% AB/AM medium to sterile microcentrifuge tubes.

12. Pick stained foci in a 20 µL vol by aspiration with an air-displacement pipet. Scrape and aspirate cells together with supernatant and transfer material to the tube containing 0.5 mL medium. Pick 5–15 foci, each time using new tips and placing in separate tube.

13. Freeze-thaw, sonicate, and replate virus material obtained from plaque picks as described in **steps 1–3** or store at –80°C. Proceed as in **steps 4–13**.

14. Repeat as described in **steps 1–13** until clonally pure rMVA is obtained. Use PCR analysis of viral DNA to monitor for absence of wild-type MVA (*see* **Subheading 3.6.**).

15. Amplify (*see* **Subheading 3.7.**) and analyze (*see* **Subheading 3.6.**) the cloned rMVA.

## 3.6. Characterization of Recombinant MVA Genomes by PCR (see also Notes 20–30)

MVA-DNA is analyzed by PCR using oligonucleotide primers, which are designed to amplify DNA fragments at the specific insertion site used within the MVA genome. Thus, genomes of rMVA and wild-type MVA can be easily identified and distinguished in DNA preparations from infected cell cultures. Elimination of wild-type MVA during plaque purification of rMVA can be monitored, and correct insertion of foreign DNA within the MVA genome can be determined. An example of a PCR analysis follows for using deletion III of MVA as insertion site and transient K1L selection to generate recombinant viruses. Primers MVA-III-5′ and MVA-III-3' anneal to template MVA-DNA sequences adjacent to insertion site III and PCR will produce DNA fragments that are specific for wild-type MVA, rMVA/K1L co-expressing the *K1L* marker gene, or for the final rMVA. Expected fragments will be:

Wild-type MVA: 0.7 kb corresponding to empty deletion III
rMVA/K1L : 2.2 kb (Del III+K1L) + x kb (recombinant gene sequence)
rMVA: 0.95 kb (rMVA/K1L -K1L) + x kb (recombinant gene sequence)

The amplification product for wild-type MVA has a defined size of 0.7 kb, indicating that no foreign DNA is inserted into insertion site III. The expected mol wt of the PCR product for rMVA/K1L can be calculated by adding the size of the recombinant insert to 2.2 kb (empty MVA and K1L marker cassette). DNA extracted from cells infected with wild-type MVA and plasmid DNA from pIII dHR P7.5-recombinant gene are used as control templates. The size of the PCR fragment that is specific for the final recombinant virus rMVA results from the mol wt of rMVA/K1L being reduced by 1.35 kb DNA, corresponding to the desired loss of K1L reporter gene sequences.

1. Infect cell monolayer of one well in 6-well/12-well plate with 1 mL of $10^{-1}$ dilution of the virus suspension obtained from the last round of plaque purification, and incubate for 3 d at 37°C.
2. Discard medium, harvest cell monolayer in 400 μL distilled water, and transfer into 1.5 mL microcentrifuge tube.
3. Add 50 μL 10X TEN pH 7.4, and freeze-thaw 3×.
4. Mix by vortexing, microcentrifuge at 1800$g$ for 5 min at room temperature to remove cellular debris.
5. Transfer supernatant into fresh 1.5 mL microcentrifuge tube. Add 50 μL prot K and 23 μL SDS 20%.
6. Vortex and incubate for 2 h at 56°C.
7. Extract suspension twice with phenol-chloroform: add equal volume of phenol-chloroform 1:1, mix and microcentrifuge at top speed for 5 min at room temperature, and pipet supernatant into new 1.5-mL microcentrifuge tube.
8. Add 1/10 vol 3 $M$ NaAc and 2 vol of EtOH abs, mix gently, and cool for 15 min at –80°C. Centrifuge at top speed for 15 min at 4°C.
9. Aspirate supernatant, wash DNA pellet with EtOH 70%, air-dry for 10 min, and resuspend in 50 μL distilled water.
10. Prepare PCR reaction mix on ice by adding 39 μL double-distilled water, 5 μL primer 1, 5 μL primer 2, 1 μL template DNA, and 50 μL PCR master mix to obtain total volume of 100 μL.
11. Perform PCR as follows:
    Step 1: Denaturation at 94°C for 2 min.
    Step 2: Cycle 1–30: Denaturation at 94°C for 30 s.
            Annealing at 55°C for 40 s.
            Elongation at 72°C for 3 min.
    Step 3: Final elongation at 72°C for 7 min.
    Storage at 4°C.
12. Use 20-μL aliquot of each PCR reaction to perform agarose gel electrophoresis, visualize amplified DNA fragments, and determine mol wts in comparison to double-stranded DNA standards (e.g., 1-kb DNA Ladder, Gibco-BRL).

### 3.7. From a Single Plaque Pick to a Virus Stock

1. Infect confluent CEF- or BHK-21 cell monolayer grown in a 35-mm-diameter tissue-culture dish, adding to the medium 250 μL virus suspension of isolated rMVA obtained from the last passage of plaque purification, and incubate at 37°C for 2 d or until cytopathic effect (CPE) is obvious.
2. Discard medium, harvest cell monolayer in 1 mL RPMI/ 2% FCS /1% AB/AM, transfer into 1.5-mL microcentrifuge tube, freeze-thaw, and sonicate as described in **Subheading 3.3.1.**, **step 11**, and proceed to **step 3** below or store at –20 to –80°C as first passage of rMVA.
3. Infect cell monolayer grown in a 60-mm-diameter tissue-culture dish, by adding to 1 mL medium 0.5-mL virus suspension obtained from first passage of rMVA. Allow virus to adsorb for 1 h at 37°C, add 2 mL RPMI/2% FCS /1% AB/AM and incubate at 37°C for 2 d or until CPE is obvious.

4. Scrape cells, transfer to 15-mL conical centrifuge tube, centrifuge 5 min at 1800$g$, discard medium and resuspend cells in 2 mL RPMI/2% FCS/1% AB/AM, freeze-thaw and sonicate as described in **step 2**, and proceed to **step 5** or store at –20 to –80°C as second passage of rMVA.

5. Infect cell monolayer in 75-cm$^2$ tissue-culture flask by adding 0.5 mL of virus material from second passage of rMVA and 1.5 mL RPMI/2% FCS/1% AB/AM. Allow virus adsorption for 1 h at 37°C, rocking flask at 20-min intervals. Overlay with 10 mL RPMI/2% FCS/1% AB/AM, and incubate at 37°C for 2 d or until CPE is obvious.

6. Scrape cells, transfer to 15-mL conical centrifuge tube, centrifuge 5 min at 1800$g$, discard medium, and resuspend cells in 5 mL RPMI/2% FCS/1% AB/AM, freeze-thaw and sonicate as described in **step 2**, and proceed to **step 7** or store at –20 to –80°C as third passage of rMVA.

7. Infect cell monolayer in 175-cm$^2$ tissue-culture flask with 2 mL of virus material from the third passage of rMVA. Allow virus adsorption for 1 h at 37°C, rocking flask at 20-min intervals, add 30 mL RPMI/2% FCS/1% AB/AM, and incubate at 37°C for 2 d or until CPE is obvious.

8. Scrape cells in medium, transfer to 50-mL conical centrifuge tube, centrifuge 5 min at 1800$g$, discard medium, and resuspend cells in 15 mL RPMI/2% FCS/1% AB/AM, freeze-thaw and sonicate as described in **step 2**, and store at –20 to –80°C as fourth passage of rMVA.

In order to amplify high-titer vaccine preparations follow **Subheading 3.3.1.**

### 3.8. Preparation of Vaccines for Mice

For immunization experiments with new MVA vectors, we suggest to evaluate $10^6$ to $10^8$ IU of vaccine as single dose per mouse. Vaccine volumes will differ depending on the route of immunization:

- intranasal (in): 30 μL
- intramuscular (im): 100 μL (50 μL into each *M. tibialis cran.*)
- subcutaneous (sc): 100μL
- intraperitoneal (ip): 500 μL
- intravenous (iv): 250 μL

1. Dilute the amount of MVA needed in vaccine buffer either freshly before use, or store in aliquots at –80°C until needed.

2. Prepare extra volumes. There is some loss of vaccine material in the needle and syringe.

3. Always transport virus material on ice, vortex, and prewarm before inoculation—e.g., using water bath or hands.

## 4. Notes
### 4.1. Preparation of CEF

1. Use 11-d-old embryonated eggs, 10-d-old eggs are still small, 12-d-old embryos may have already developed feathers.

2. When the shell membrane is opened, check for viability of the embryo by monitoring the blood vessels on the chorioallantoic membrane.

### 4.2. Virus Growth

3. For all steps, when using virus, always sonicate for 30 s in cup sonicator after thawing.

### *4.3. Amplification of MVA*

4. When infecting cell monolayers grown in larger tissue-culture flasks (e.g., 185-cm$^2$ flasks), avoid drying of the cell monolayer by rocking flask by hand at 20-min intervals.
5. In order to homogenize virus material most efficiently after amplification, we recommend use of a sonication needle instead of the cup sonicator.
6. For use, place tube containing virus material in small beaker with ice water and plunge needle into virus suspension.
7. Sonicate 4× for 15 s at maximal power. Take care to avoid heating of the sample.
8. Having obtained a rMVA stock virus, the following procedures are recommended:

   a. Titer the virus stock on CEF or BHK-21 cell monolayers (*see* **Subheadings 3.3.3. or 3.3.4.**).
   b. Analyze clonal purity and genomic stability of rMVA by PCR (*see* **Subheading 3.6.**) or Southern blot analysis of viral DNA.
   c. Characterize synthesis of recombinant antigen by specific immunostaining of cell foci infected with virus expressing recombinant gene(s) (*see* **Subheading 3.3.3.**, but substitute first Ab with antigen-specific Ab), by immunoblot analysis of lysates from rMVA-infected cells, or by immunoprecipitation of the target antigen made during rMVA infection following labeling with radioactive amino acids.

9. It is recommended to prepare a first virus stock as *primary* stock, which is used to amplify *working* stocks of rMVA.

### *4.4. Purification of MVA*

10. If after amplification virus material has been homogenized using a sonification needle, there is no need for douncing. Proceed as follows:

    a. Transfer virus suspension to 50-mL Falcon tube and centrifuge 5 min at 1800 $g$ and 4°C.
    b. Discard pellet and continue purification with supernatant as described in **Subheading 3.3.2., step 4.**
    c. In order to obtain highly purified viruses, material obtained from **Subheading 3.3.2., step 6** can be centrifuged through a 25%–40% sucrose gradient for 50 min at 28000$g$ and 4°C. Harvest virus band. To discard sucrose, fill with >3 vol 1 m$M$ Tris-HCl, pH 9.0, and pellet virus material at 38000$g$ for 1 h at 4°C. Resuspend in 1 m$M$ Tris-HCl, pH 9.0, and store at –80°C.

### *4.5. Titration of MVA*

11. Before titration, virus material *must* be homogenized by sonication. Sonicate aliquots of maximal 1.5-mL virus suspension as described in **Subheading 3.3.1., step 11.**
12. Alternatively, after fixing of cell monolayers, incubation with blocking buffer can be done overnight at 4°C.
13. To remove small clumps of o-dianisidine, filter the PBS/dianisidine mix through a 0.2-μm filter into a new tube before adding the $H_2O_2$ >30%.
14. Determining Tissue-Culture Infectious Dose 50—Example for calculating TCID$_{50}$: Given that all 8 wells are counted positive in dilution $10^{-7}$, $x$ is 7. Additionally, 5 infected wells are found in dilution $10^{-8}$, and the number of infected wells in dilution $10^{-9}$ (the highest dilution in which positive wells can be found) is 2. Then, the log 50% endpoint dilution would be: $7 - 1/2 + (8/8 + 5/8 + 2/8) = 7 - 0.5 + (1.875) = 7 + 1.375 = 8.375$. As the endpoint dilution that will infect 50% of the wells inoculated is $10^{-8.375}$ the recip-

rocal of this number yields the titer in terms of infectious dose per unit volume. As the inoculum added to an individual well was 0.1 mL, the titer of the virus suspension would therefore be: $10^{8.375}$ TCID$_{50}$/0.1 mL = $10^{9.375}$ TCID$_{50}$/mL.

## 4.6. Molecular Cloning of Recombinant Gene Sequences

15. For best transfection efficiencies prepare clean, supercoiled DNA either by centrifugation through cesium chloride gradients or by using plasmid purification kits (Qiagen GmbH, Hilden, Germany).

## 4.7. Isolation of Recombinant MVA

16. For either selection technique, keep the following in mind:
    a. Because of its highly host-restricted nature, MVA does not produce the rapid CPE accompanied by destruction of the cell monolayer seen with standard strains of vaccinia (e.g., Western Reserve, Copenhagen) in mammalian cells. Plaque formation is only observed in CEF or BHK-21 cells, or when providing K1L expression in RK-13 cells.
    b. When picking rMVA plaques, it is preferable to choose well-separated viral foci from wells infected with highest dilutions. This will drastically reduce the number of plaque passages needed to isolate clonally pure rMVA.

17. Transient host range selection:
    a. In order to distinguish rMVA-specific RK-13 aggregates, it may be helpful to use mock and wild-type MVA-infected control wells for comparison.
    b. To allow for most efficient plaque cloning, it may be helpful to perform plaque passages under agar (for overlay, follow **Subheading 3.5.2., steps 4–6**).

18. Transient β-galactosidase screening: As the expression cassette of the *lacZ* marker gene is designed to be efficiently deleted from the rMVA genome, non-staining MVA foci may be observed during plaque purification even after all wild-type MVA has been successfully eliminated. To avoid unnecessary plaque passages, it is important to confirm the absence of parental MVA by PCR analysis.

19. Screening by Live Immunodetection:
    a. The staining results will only be as good as the antibody. When weakly staining antibodies are used, this procedure can be difficult. The first round of picking for the recombinant is the most difficult, as recombinant foci may be small (1–4 cells) because of the large amount of wild-type MVA present. In subsequent passages, foci will be larger and easier to pick.
    b. For detection of intracellular target antigens, it may be helpful to freeze-thaw culture plates before staining (incubate at –80°C without medium for 1–2 h).

## 4.8. Characterization of Recombinant MVA DNA by PCR

20. Virus material harvested from cell monolayers grown in 6-well/12-well plates and infected for 24 h with an MOI of 10 IU per cell will yield a good amount of viral DNA for PCR.
21. To monitor the presence of wild-type MVA during plaque purification, viral DNA sufficient for PCR analysis is isolated from cell monolayers infected with the $10^{-1}$-dilution of virus suspensions plated out for plaque passage.
22. If infectivity is to low, a second round of amplification may be necessary. Harvest amplification, freeze-thaw, sonicate, and re-plate on cell monolayers.
23. Avoid sonication of infected tissue-culture material to be used for DNA extraction because unpackaged viral DNA will be destroyed and lost for analysis.

24. DNA precipitation may be done on dry ice for 15 min or at −20°C for 30 min.
25. Carefully air-dry the pelleted DNA material to remove all ethanol.
26. Always use DNA of wild-type MVA and respective plasmid as control templates for PCR analysis.
27. As DNA preparations might contain variable quantities of viral DNA, the amount of template DNA used for PCR may be optimized.
28. PCR conditions (temperatures and number of cycles) may be optimized according to the size of the expected fragment to be amplified. Conditions as stated in the protocol have been used for amplification of up to 4 kb DNA inserted into the MVA genome.
29. If template DNA is derived from mixed virus populations on RK-13 cells containing both, rMVA/K1L as well as wild-type MVA, PCR may preferentially amplify the fragment for wild-type MVA because of its smaller size, and rMVA/K1L may not be detectable. A signal for rMVA may also be detected, as the K1L marker cassette is designed to be efficiently deleted from recombinant genomes, and this process already occurs in RK-13 cells.
30. Check for efficient deletion of the K1L marker cassette from virus genomes by K1L-specific PCR using the following primers and 55°C annealing temperature: K1L-int-1: 5'-TGA TGA CAA GGG AAA CAC CGC-3', K1L-int-2: 5'-GTC GAC GTC AAT TAG TCG AGC-3'.

## Acknowledgments

This work was supported by the European Community Grants BIO4-CT98-0456, QLK2-CT-2002-01867 and by the Deutsche Forschungsgemeinschaft.

## References

1. Zavala, F., Rodrigues, M., Rodriguez, D., Rodriquez J. R., Nussenzweig, R. S., and Esteban, M. (2001) A striking property of recombinant poxviruses: efficient inducers of in vivo expansion of primed CD8(+) T cells. *Virology* **280**, 155–159.
2. Moss, B. (1996) Genetically engineered poxviruses for recombinant gene expression, vaccination and safety. *Proc. Natl. Acad. Sci. USA* **93**, 11,341–11,348.
3. Rosenberg, S. A. (1997) Cancer vaccines based on the identification of the genes encoding cancer regression antigens. *Immunol. Today* **18**, 175–182.
4. Sutter, G., Wyatt, L. S., Foley, P. L., Bennink, J. R., and Moss, B. (1994) A recombinant vector derived from the host range-restricted and highly attenuated MVA strain of vaccinia virus stimulates protective immunity in mice to influenza virus. *Vaccine* **12**, 1032–1040.
5. Hirsch, V. M., Fuerst, T. R., Sutter, G., Carroll, M. W., Yang, L. C., Goldstein, S., et al. (1996) Patterns of viral replication correlate with outcome in simian immunodeficiency virus (SIV)-infected macaques: effect of prior immunization with a trivalent SIV vaccine in modified vaccinia virus Ankara. *J. Virol.* **70**, 3741–3752.
6. Schneider, J., Gilbert, S. C., Blanchard, T. J., Hanke, T., Robson, K. J., Hannan, C. M., et al. (1998) Enhanced immunogenicity for CD8+ T cell induction and complete protective efficacy of malaria DNA vaccination by boosting with modified vaccinia virus Ankara. *Nat. Med.* **4**, 397–402.
7. Amara, R. R., Villinger, F., Altman, J. D., Lydy, O'Neil, S. P., Staprans, S. I., Montefiori, D. C., Xu, Y., et al. (2001) Control of a mucosal challenge and prevention of AIDS by a multiprotein DNA/MVA vaccine. *Science* **292**, 69–74.

8. Sutter, G. and Moss, B. (1992) Nonreplicating vaccinia vector efficiently expresses recombinant genes. *Proc. Natl. Acad. Sci. USA* **89,** 10,847–10,851.

9. Tartaglia, J., Perkus, M. E., Taylor, J., Norton, E. K., Audonnet, J-C., Cox, W. I., et al. (1992) NYVAC: a highly attenuated strain of vaccinia virus. *Virology* **188,** 217–232.

10. Taylor, J., Weinberg, R., Languet, B., et al. (1988) Recombinant fowlpox virus inducing protective immunity in non-avian species. *Vaccine* **6,** 497–503.

11. Taylor, J., Trimarchi, C., Weinberg, R., Languet, B., Guillemin, F., Desmettre, P., et al. (1991) Efficacy studies on a canarypox-rabies recombinant virus. *Vaccine* **9,** 190–193.

12. Meyer, H., Sutter, G., and Mayr, A. (1991) Mapping of deletions in the genome of the highly attenuated vaccinia virus MVA and their influence on virulence. *J. Gen. Virol.* **72,** 1031–1038.

13. Drexler, I., Heller, K., Wahren, B., Erfle, V., and Sutter, G. (1998) Highly attenuated modified vaccinia virus Ankara replicates in baby hamster kidney cells, a potential host for virus propagation, but not in various human transformed and primary cells. *J. Gen. Virol.* **79,** 347–352.

14. Carroll, M. W. and Moss, B. (1997) Host range and cytopathogenicity of the highly attenuated MVA strain of vaccinia virus: propagation and generation of recombinant viruses in a nonhuman mammalian cell line. *Virology* **238,** 198–211.

15. Stittelaar, K. J., Kuiken, T., de Swart, R. L., van Amerongen, G., Vos, H. W., Niesters, H. G. M., et al. (2001) Safety of modified vaccinia virus Ankara (MVA) in immune-suppressed macaques. *Vaccine* **19,** 3700–3709.

16. Ramirez, J. C., Gherardi, M. M., Rodriguez, D., and Esteban, M. (2000) Attenuated modified vaccinia virus Ankara can be used as an immunizing agent under conditions of preexisting immunity to the vector. *J. Virol.* **74,** 7651–7655.

17. Kaerber, G. (1931) Beitrag zur kollektiven Behandlung pharmakologischer Reihenversuche. *Arch. Exp. Pathol. Pharmakol.* **162,** 480.

18. Staib, C., Drexler, I., Ohlmann, M., Wintersperger, S., Erfle, V., and Sutter, G. (2000) Transient host range selection for genetic engineering of modified vaccinia virus Ankara. *BioTechniques* **6,** 1137–1142, 1144–1146, 1148.

19. Sutter, G., Ohlmann, M., and Erfle, V. (1995). Non-replicating vaccinia vector efficiently expresses bacteriophage T7 RNA polymerase. *FEBS Lett.* **371,** 9–12.

20. Drexler, I., Antunes, E., Schmitz, M., Wolfel, T., Huber, C., Erfle, V., et al. (1999) Modified vaccinia virus Ankara for delivery of human tyrosinase as melanoma-associated antigen: induction of tyrosinase- and melanoma-specific human leukocyte antigen A*0201-restricted cytotoxic T cells in vitro and in vivo. *Cancer Res.* **59,** 4955–4963.

21. Wyatt, L. S., Shors, S. T., Murphy, B. R., and Moss, B. (1996) Development of a replication-deficient recombinant vaccinia virus vaccine effective against parainfluenza virus 3 infection in an animal model. *Vaccine* **14,** 1451–1458.

22. Carroll, M. and Moss, B. (1995) *E. coli* beta-glucuronidase (GUS) as a marker for recombinant vaccinia viruses. *BioTechniques* **19,** 352–355.

23. Staib, C., Löwell, M., Erfle, V., and Sutter, G. (2003) Improved host range selection for recombinant modified vaccinia virus Ankara. *BioTechniques* **34,** (in press).

# 5

## Live Viral Vectors
### *Semliki Forest Virus*

## Gunilla B. Karlsson and Peter Liljeström

## 1. Introduction

A continuously expanding body of data supports the use of recombinant viral vectors as vehicles in vaccination. Studies have shown that when antigen-expressing viral vectors are used alone or in boosting following a naked DNA prime, the T- and B-cell responses elicited are both broader and of a higher order of magnitude than following immunization with DNA alone *(1–6)*. The mechanisms underlying the efficiency of live viral vectors probably lie in their replicative nature. Although in most cases the vectors are attenuated or "suicidal," resulting in nonproductive infections (e.g., no spread of progeny virus in the vaccinee), the vectors replicate inside the target cell, mimicking an authentic virus infection and resulting in the activation of innate anti-viral responses in the antigen-expressing cell. Live viral vectors thus come with built-in immuno-stimulatory properties much like a live attenuated virus vaccine, giving these platforms an advantage over strategies using conventional plasmid DNA to express antigen. Another characteristic of many viral vaccine vectors is that they induce apoptosis in the target cell. This may contribute to the generation of a specific immune response caused by uptake of antigen-loaded apoptotic bodies by dendritic cells and consequent activation of a specific response through cross-presentation. Further studies are required to formally demonstrate to what extent such mechanisms contribute to the activity of live viral vectors. It will be important to learn more about how the different viral vectors work in relation to each other and what other mechanisms are involved.

The two viral vectors systems that have been studied the most extensively are poxvirus vectors and adenovirus vectors *(1–6)*. Next in line are vector systems built on alphaviruses *(7–9)*. Although not yet tested in humans, data from preclinical models are rapidly accumulating and human trials are likely to be initiated in the near future. Alphaviruses for which vector systems have been developed include Semliki Forest

From: *Methods in Molecular Medicine, Vol. 87: Vaccine Protocols, 2nd ed.*
Edited by: A. Robinson, M. J. Hudson, and M. P. Cranage © Humana Press Inc., Totowa, NJ

virus (SFV; *10–19*), Sindbis virus *(20–24)* and Venezuelan equine encephalitis virus (VEE; *25–27*). Significant human disease has only been associated with VEE *(28)*. This chapter focuses on the use of SFV vectors as a vaccine platform.

## 1.1. Alphavirus Biology

Alphaviruses, which are members of the *Togaviridae* family, have small single-stranded RNA genomes of positive polarity, and the packaged genome is both capped and poly-adenylated. The genomic RNA serves as an mRNA immediately upon release in the infected cell, and allows the synthesis of a polyprotein encoding the viral replicase (the viral non-structural proteins nsp 1–4). The replicase complex produces a negative-strand RNA that acts as a template for the production of new genomic RNAs for packaging. In addition, a subgenomic promoter is exposed on the negative-strand RNA, driving the production of a subgenomic RNA species corresponding to the 3' one-third of the viral genome. This transcript encodes the structural proteins of the virus, which are synthesized as a polyprotein precursor ($NH_2$-C-p62-6K-E1-COOH). In SFV, a sequence at the 5' end of the capsid gene functions as a translational enhancer, providing high-level production of the structural proteins *(29)*. When the enhancer element is fused to an antigen of interest in the vector, antigen expression is increased by about 10-fold.

## 1.2. The SFV Vector System

In the SFV vectors, the replicase gene and the 5' and 3' sequences needed for replication are intact, and the structural genes are replaced by the foreign antigen of interest. The risk of generating anti-vector immunity is low, since no structural genes are encoded by the vector. Pre-existing immunity to SFV has only been reported in limited geographic locations in man, and is expected to be rare globally *(30)*.

For SFV, three vaccination strategies have been developed. One method relies on the packaging of recombinant vectors into viral particles using a helper system followed by infection of target cells, and the other two methods are based on direct transfection of target cells, either by using naked DNA encoding the SFV replicon placed downstream of an RNA polymerase II-dependent promoter (layered DNA), or by using in vitro transcribed RNA encoding the SFV replicon. All three approaches result in the delivery of a self-replicating SFV vector into target cells, with expression of foreign genes being driven from the highly efficient viral sub-genomic promoter (**Fig. 1**). A common feature of these three strategies is that genetic manipulations (insertion of antigens or other desired elements) are performed on a plasmid backbone containing a cDNA copy of the SFV replicon. Methods for the production of recombinant SFV RNA and particles and protocols for in vitro infection and analysis of recombinant gene expression, as well as the design of the SFV-layered DNA vectors, are described in greater detail in the following section.

The SFV system is suicidal; thus, transmission of infectious particles from cells targeted by the vector cannot occur. Suicidal vaccine strategies have the benefit that concerns sometimes associated with genetic vaccinations, such as the potential integration of the transgene into the chromosome, or induction of tolerance resulting from prolonged expression of the antigen, are circumvented *(31)*.

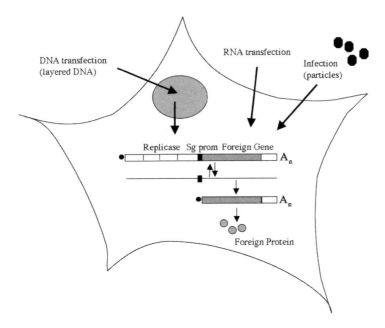

Fig. 1. Methods to deliver self-replicating SFV vectors into mammalian cells. The three methods; DNA transfection using the layered DNA constructs, RNA transfection with in vitro transcribed vector RNA, and infection with recombinant particles, all result in the delivery of the self-replicating antigen-expressing vector into the cell. Only the layered DNA transfections are dependent on RNA polymerase II driven transcription in the cell nucleus. Sg prom, the 26S subgenomic promoter; $A_n$, polyadenylation sequence.

## 2. Materials

### 2.1. Plasmids

The plasmids required for the methods described in this chapter have recently been reviewed *(16)*. Briefly, the pSFV1 and pSFV10 vectors, as well as the Helper-C (S219A) and Helper-S2 split helper constructs used for packaging SFV particles, are pGEM-based and confer ampicillin resistance. They contain a SP6 promoter to drive synthesis of RNA in vitro, and unique restriction endonuclease sites that allow linearization of the plasmids are present immediately downstream of the poly A sequence in the viral 3' end (*Spe* I for pSFV1 and the two helper constructs, *Nru* I for pSFV10) (**Fig. 2**).

1. pSFV1: pSFV1 encodes a functional replicase gene, including an intact packaging signal. The structural genes encoded by the subgenomic RNA in the wild-type SFV genome have been removed in the vector constructs to allow expression of foreign proteins or antigens in this position (*see* **Note 1**). The subgenomic transcript starts 31 nucleotides upstream of the Bam HI restriction endonuclease site (**Fig. 2A**).
2. pSFV10: In the pSFV10 vector, several silent point mutations in the replicase gene have been introduced to remove recognition sites for useful cloning enzymes such as *Rsr* I, *Xho* I, and *Not* I. A versatile poly-linker, that contains these enzyme sites and others, has

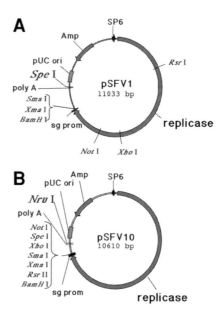

Fig. 2. Molecular constructs. (**A**) pSFV1. (**B**) pSFV10. Sg prom, the 26S subgenomic promoter; poly A, SFV polyadenylation sequence; Amp, ampicillin resistance gene; SP6, the SP6 prokaryotic promoter; CMV prom, CMV promoter.

been introduced, allowing insertion of foreign genes in this position. The 3' SFV sequence between the polylinker and the poly A sequence has been trimmed from 888 nucleotides (in pSFV1) to 459 (in pSFV10) (**Fig. 2B**).

The development of the SFV split-helper system has been described in detail *(32)*. Briefly, Helper-C (S219A) and Helper-S2 were constructed by deleting 6091 bases of the replicase gene (*Acc* I [308] to *Acc* I [6399]). The resulting RNA molecules cannot be packaged into particles, as a region at the end of nsP1 required for this function is removed by the deletion. Both Helper-C (S219A) and Helper-S2 retain the 5' and 3' sequences needed for RNA replication.

3. Helper-C (S219A): An artificial stop codon was introduced immediately downstream of the natural cleavage site between capsid and spike, after the ultimate 3' residue of the capsid protein (a tryptophan residue). The capsid gene was further modified to abolish its natural protease activity by mutating serine 219 to alanine (agt [S] to gcc [A]) at the core of the enzyme active site (**Fig. 3A**).

4. Helper-S2: The translational enhancer region corresponding to the first 34 amino acids of the capsid gene was included in the Helper-S2 construct to obtain similar levels of protein from spike Helper construct as the capsid Helper construct. A short sequence encoding autoprotease 2A of the foot-and-mouth-disease virus (FMDV) was inserted in frame between the enhancer sequence and the spike protein *(32)*. This allows cleavage of the spike proteins from the short coding capsid sequence and generates a p62 protein, which starts from the second amino acid (Ala) of the natural sequence (**Fig. 3B**).

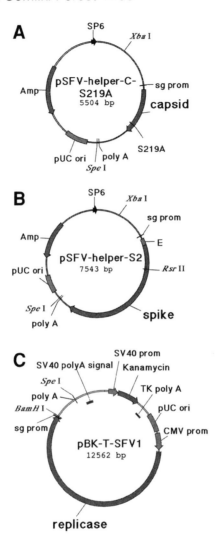

Fig. 3. Molecular constructs. (**A**) pSFV-helper-C-S219A, (**B**) pSFV-helper-S2, and (**C**) pBK-T-SFV1. Sg prom, the 26S subgenomic promoter; poly A, SFV polyadenylation sequence; Amp, ampicillin resistance gene; SP6, the SP6 prokaryotic promoter; CMV prom, CMV promoter; E, capsid enhancer linked to the 2A autoprotease.

5. pBK-T-SFV1: The SFV sequence was placed downstream of the immediate early cytomegalovirus (CMV) promoter in pBK-CMV (Stratagene). The CMV promoter drives the expression of the SFV replicon, allowing replication of the vector and expression of foreign genes from the viral subgenomic promoter once the RNA polymerase II-generated mRNA has been transported into the cytoplasm and the nsp1-4 genes have been expressed (**Fig. 3C**).

## 2.2. Apparatus and Reagents

1. Electroporator and electroporation cuvets (0.2 or 0.4 cm) are available from BioRad (Hercules, CA).
2. SP6 RNA polymerase, $^{35}$S-methionine, m7 (5′) ppp (5′) G, and rNTP mix are available from Amersham BioSciences (Uppsala, Sweden).
3. RNasin (an RNase inhibitor) can be obtained from Promega (Madison, WI).
4. BHK-21 cells are available from American Type Culture Collection (ATCC, Manassas, VA).

## 2.3. Solutions and Cell Culture Medium

1. TBE gel buffer (1X) for agarose gels: 50 m$M$ Tris base, 50 m$M$ $H_3BO_3$, 2.5 m$M$ ethylenediaminetetraacetic acid (EDTA). pH will be 8.3; do not adjust.
2. 5X TD solution: 20% Ficoll 400, 25 m$M$ EDTA, pH 8.0, 0.05% bromophenol blue, 0.03% xylene cyanol.
3. 10X SP6 buffer: 400 m$M$ HEPES-KOH, pH 7.4, 60 m$M$ MgAc, 20 m$M$ spermidine-HCl.
4. TNE buffer: 50 m$M$ Tris-HCl, pH 7.4, 100 m$M$ NaCl, 0.5 m$M$ EDTA.
5. Phosphate buffered saline (PBS) without $Mg^{2+}$ and $Ca^{2+}$, G-MEM, Trypsin-EDTA and Eagle's Minimum Essential Medium (E-MEM) can be obtained from Invitrogen (Paisley, UK).
6. BHK-21 medium: G-MEM containing 5% fetal calf serum (FCS), 10% tryptose phosphate broth, 10 m$M$ HEPES, 2 m$M$ L-glutamine, 0.1 U/mL penicillin (optional), 0.1 μg/mL streptomycin (optional).
7. Starvation medium: methionine and cysteine-free MEM is available from Sigma (St. Louis, MO). Add 2 m$M$ L-glutamine, 10 m$M$ HEPES.
8. Chase medium: E-MEM containing 2 m$M$ L-glutamine, 10 m$M$ HEPES, 150 μg/mL unlabeled methionine and cysteine.
9. 1X lysis buffer: 1% NP-40 (use 10% stock), 50 m$M$ Tris-HCl, pH 7.6, 150 m$M$ NaCl, 2 m$M$ EDTA.
10. Mowiol mounting medium: mix 6 g glycerol and 2.4 g Mowiol (Calbiochem, San Diego, CA) in 6 mL $H_2O$ thoroughly. Incubate at room temperature for 2 h. Add 12 mL 0.2 $M$ Tris pH 8.5. Incubate at 50°C to dissolve the Mowiol. Clarify by centrifugation at 5000$g$ for 15 min. Aliquot and store at –20°C.

## 3. Methods

## 3.1. Preparation of RNA In Vitro for Production of Recombinant SFV Particles

For technical tips related to the preparation of RNA *see* **Note 2** and **Fig. 4**.

1. Linearize 5 μg of the vector plasmid (based on pSFV1 or pSFV10) and 5 μg each of the two split-helper plasmids, by digesting with the appropriate restriction enzymes (*Spe* I for pSFV1 and the split-helper constructs, *Nru* I for the pSFV10 vector). Phenol-extract and ethanol-precipitate the DNA. Resuspend the DNA in $H_2O$ to obtain a final concentration of 1.5 μg/5 μL.
2. Set up in vitro transcription reactions for each plasmid: 5 μL DNA (1.5 μg), 5 μL 10X SP6 buffer, 5 μL 50 m$M$ dithiothreitol (DTT), 5 μL 10 m$M$ m$^7$G(5')ppp(5')G, 5 μL rNTP mix, 23 μL $H_2O$, 1.5 μL RNasin (50 U), 0.5 μL (30 U) SP6 RNA polymerase.
3. Incubate at 37°C for 60–90 min, then take a 1-μL aliquot into 10 μL of $H_2O$, add 3 μL of DNA gel-loading solution (5XTD) and run sample on a 0.5% agarose gel to check the RNA. The quality of the RNA should be as shown in **Fig. 4**. Use lambda DNA (e.g.,

A     B     C

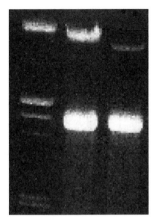

DNA template

RNA transcript

Fig. 4. A typical agarose gel analysis of SFV transcripts, in which 1 μL of a standard in vitro transcription mixture was analyzed on a 0.8% agarose gel (commonly used for DNA restriction-fragment analysis). A. Lambda DNA (*Hin*d III + *Eco*R I) restriction fragments were used as markers (although not as true mol wt indicators). Lanes B and C show transcripts of the same linearized DNA template; where in lane B the amount of template per transcription mixture is significantly greater than in the sample in lane C. This shows that if the correct protocol is used, the amount of template per defined amount of units SP6 is saturated; i.e., both transcription reactions yield the same amount of RNA.

*Eco*RI + *Hin*dIII) cut) as marker. This protocol yields approx 50 μg RNA per construct, which is the amount used for one electroporation.

4. Freeze the remainder in aliquots at –80°C.

## 3.2. Transfection of BHK-21 Cells by Electroporation

The transfection efficiency is critical for obtaining high-titer viral stocks (*see* **Note 3**).

1. Grow BHK-21 cells to late log phase in complete BHK medium.
2. Wash cells once with PBS (without $Mg^{2+}$ and $Ca^{2+}$).
3. For a 75 cm$^2$ bottle, add 2 mL of trypsin and incubate at 37°C until the cells detach (about 1 min), then briefly pipet cell solution back and forth to ensure that a single-cell suspension is obtained (monitor by microscope). Stop trypsinization by adding 10 mL of BHK-21 medium.
4. Harvest cells by centrifugation for 5 min at 400*g*, and resuspend cells in 10–20 mL PBS (without $MgCl_2$ and $CaCl_2$).
5. Harvest cells as in 4, and resuspend in phosphate-buffered saline (PBS) (without $MgCl_2$ and $CaCl_2$) to get $10^7$ cells/mL.
6. Transfer 0.8 mL of cell suspension to an Eppendorf tube containing the RNAs to be transfected. For virus packaging use 50 μL of RNA from each of the three plasmids (vector and the two split helpers). Mix thoroughly by pipetting, and transfer the mixture to a 0.4-cm electroporation cuvet.

7. Pulse twice at 850 V/25 μF at room temperature. The time constant after the pulse should be 0.4.
8. Dilute transfected cells 10–20-fold in complete BHK-21 medium and rinse the cuvet with the same medium to collect all cells. Seed cells from one electroporation into one 75-cm² flask or cells from three electroporations into one 225-cm² flask. It takes about 1 h for the cells to reattach to the dish.
9. Incubate the transfected BHK-21 cells in a 5% $CO_2$ incubator for 24 h at 33°C to allow the cells to assemble and release virus particles (*see* **Note 4**).
10. Collect and clarify the medium containing the recombinant SFV particles by centrifuging at 40,000$g$ for 30 min at +4°C to remove remaining cells and cell debris. Aliquot and freeze the supernatant quickly on dry ice or in liquid nitrogen. Store at –80°C.

### 3.3. Purification and Concentration of SFV Particles

To concentrate and purify recombinant virus from the medium of transfected BHK-21 cells, the particles are sedimented by ultracentrifugation through a sucrose cushion (*see* **Note 5** for safety considerations).

1. Transfer the viral supernatant to ultracentrifuge tubes (two 35-mL Beckman 25 × 89 mm tubes are suitable for a viral supernatant resulting from three electroporations). Add 5 mL 20% sucrose with a pipet through the supernatant down into the bottom of the tube. Fill the tube to the top with viral supernatant or medium. Balance the tubes carefully and spin at 140,000$g$ for 90 min at 4°C.
2. Tilt the tube and aspirate the entire medium and sucrose fraction, without touching the bottom of the tube. Add 250–500 μL TNE buffer per tube, and resuspend the virus pellet from the bottom of the tube.
3. Filter the concentrated virus stock through a 0.22-μm filter, using a small syringe.
4. Aliquot and freeze the purified virus stock quickly, and store at –80°C.

### 3.4. Infection of Target Cells

To obtain full infection of most cell types, such as BHK-21 cells, a multiplicity of infection (MOI) of approx 10–20 is required. For example, from a virus stock of $10^9$ infectious particles per mL, use 10 μL of virus stock diluted in a total volume of 500 μL to infect $0.5 \times 10^6$ cells in a 35-mm well (a 1:50 dilution of the virus). In general, the virus must be diluted 25–100×, depending on the titer of the stock and infectability of the target cells, to achieve full infection. The following is a standard protocol for in vitro infection of target cells.

1. Wash 80–100% confluent cells thoroughly with PBS.
2. Thaw recombinant virus preparation quickly (room temperature), then dilute as needed in E-MEM containing 0.2% bovine serum albumin (BSA), 2 m$M$ L-glutamine and 20 m$M$ HEPES.
3. For a 35-mm plate, apply 500 μL of virus solution (diluted as required from the frozen stock) on the cells and incubate at 37°C for 45 min–1 h.
4. Remove the virus solution, add 3 mL complete BHK-21 medium (or other suitable medium required for the experiment), and continue incubation as required.

### 3.5. Titer Determination of Recombinant Virus Particles

Use different dilutions of the virus stock to infect cells. Detect protein expression by immunofluorescence, using a primary antibody with specificity for the heterologous protein expressed by the vector.

1. Grow cells on glass cover slips to approx 70% confluency.
2. Infect the cells with different dilutions of the recombinant virus stock diluted in E-MEM containing 0.2% BSA, 2 m*M* glutamine, and 20 m*M* HEPES. Allow 10–16 h for expression of the protein of interest.
3. Rinse cover slips twice with PBS, then fix cells in –20°C methanol for 5 min.
4. Remove methanol and wash cover slips 3× with PBS.
5. Block nonspecific binding by incubating with PBS containing 0.5% gelatin and 0.2% BSA (30 min at room temperature).
6. Replace blocking buffer with same buffer containing primary antibody. Incubate at room temperature for 30 min.
7. Wash 3× with PBS, then bind secondary antibody as in **step 5**.
8. Wash 3× with PBS and 1× with water, drain and let cover slip air-dry.
9. Mount on glass slide using 10–20 µL Mowiol 4–88 containing 2.5% DABCO (1,4-diazobicyclo-[2.2.2]-octane). (The DABCO will reduce fading of fluorescein isothiocyanate [FITC])
10. Count twenty fields of a dilution for which individual positive cells can be clearly identified (usually the 1:10,000 or the 1:100,000 dilution) to obtain a reliable average value per field. Virus titer is determined based on the dilution factor and a microscope-specific constant (depending on size of eye field, lens used, and area of the dish), according to the following formula: (average value counted cells) × (constant) × (dilution factor) = infectious U/mL.

### 3.6. Analyses of Protein Expression by Metabolic Labeling of Cells

The following protocol is given for 35-mm tissue-culture plates (80–100% confluent). *See* **Note 6** for technical comments.

1. Aspirate growth medium and wash cells twice with 3 mL PBS prewarmed to 37°C, then overlay cells with 2 mL starvation medium and incubate plates at 37°C (5% $CO_2$) for 30–45 min.
2. Aspirate medium and replace with 500 µL of the same containing 50–100 µCi/mL of $^{35}$S-methionine, incubate for appropriate pulse time at 37°C.
3. Remove pulse medium and wash cells once with 2 mL of chase medium, then overlay cells with 2 mL of chase medium and incubate for required chase time.
4. Remove medium and wash cells with 3 mL ice-cold PBS, add 300 µL of lysis buffer and incubate on ice for 10 min.
5. Resuspend cells and transfer solution into an Eppendorf tube, spin at max speed in an Eppendorf centrifuge for 5 min to pellet unbroken cells, nuclei, and cellular debris. Transfer supernatant to a fresh tube and store at –80°C.
6. Assay for protein expression by sodium dodecyl sulfate polyacrylamide gel electrophoresis (SDS-PAGE) and autoradiography.

### 3.7. Immunizations Using SFV Particles

Recombinant SFV particles have been used to immunize a variety of model animals including mice *(11)*, rabbits *(18)*, chickens *(31)*, sheep *(19)*, and nonhuman primates *(12)*. Comprehensive dose-titration experiments have not been performed for all these animal species, but doses ranging from $10^6$ particles (mice), $10^7$ (chicken and rabbits), $10^8$ particles (monkeys), or $10^9$ particles (sheep) are sufficient to elicit strong immune responses. A good boost effect is usually observed (up to three boosts have been tested), suggesting that generation of neutralizing activity against the particles is not a major concern.

Several immunization routes may be used for SFV particle-based vaccines, including intraperitoneal (ip), intranasal (in), subcutanous (sc), intravenous, (iv), and intradermal (id). Intramuscular (im) immunization is not commonly used, as it has been shown to work less effectively *(14)*. The authors use sc or ip as the primary route for most vaccination studies.

The SFV split-helper system used for particle production was developed for maximal safety. *See* **Note 7** for more details related to this.

### 3.8. Immunizations Using SFV RNA

To prepare recombinant vector RNA for immunization, follow the protocols in **Subheading 3.1.** and **3.2.**, omitting the split-helper plasmids. The SFV-vector RNA is relatively stable, and thus it is not necessary to be overprotective when handling this RNA.

### 3.9. Immunizations Using SFV-Layered DNA

Immunization with SFV-layered DNA is performed according to standard plasmid DNA vaccination protocols, and the preferred routes of administration are id and im. Several studies have reported that 10–1000-fold less layered DNA plasmid is required to obtain strong immune responses against a given antigen, as compared to when the same antigen is expressed from a conventional DNA vaccination vector *(13,21,23)*, making this system particularly interesting in studies in which large numbers of subjects are vaccinated.

## 4. Notes

1. A variety of foreign genes have been expressed using the pSFV1 and pSFV10 vectors. Larger genes, such as Lac Z, are readily expressed without affecting the viral titers. Vectors containing double sub-genomic promoters, expressing two foreign genes from the same vector, have also been constructed successfully. The efficiency of packaging may become compromised as the total length of the inserted cDNA increases, ultimately resulting in decreased viral titers.
2. Spermidine is present in the SP6 buffer, so the reaction mixture should be set up at room temperature to avoid precipitation of the DNA. For one in vitro transcription reaction using 30 U of SP6 RNA polymerase, a total of 1.5 µg of linear DNA is required. Under the conditions decribed, the transcription mixture is saturated for DNA and yields approx 50 µg of RNA. Although the gel is non-denaturing and thus does not reflect the mol wt of the RNA produced, it is nevertheless useful for checking the quality and quantity of the RNA. The RNA band should be defined (no smearing) and relatively thick in comparison

to the DNA bands (*see* **Fig. 4**). If necessary, RNA samples of known concentration can be run for comparison.

3. Using this protocol, a transfection efficiency near 100% can be obtained in BHK-21 cells. The optimal electroporation parameters must be determined on a case-by-case basis if other cell types are used, as they are likely to vary greatly between different cell types. To optimize the electroporation protocol on a new cell type, it is necessary to compare differences in voltage, capacitance, time constant of electrical pulse, and the number of pulses given to identify the optimal conditions. If other cell types are to be used, it is important to check their ability to support virus-particle formation. This can be achieved by performing an infection with wild-type SFV.

4. Incubation of the BHK-21 cells at 37°C gives, on average, a 10-fold lower titer than incubation at 33°C, probably because the onset of apoptosis is delayed when the cells are cultured at the lower temperature. A second harvest can be performed at 48 h after transfection if fresh media is placed on the cells after the 24-h harvest time point. The second harvest can yield as high titers as the first one, doubling the total amount of virus that can be obtained from each transfection. The anticipated titre from $10^7$ BHK-21 cells is $10^9$–$10^{10}$ infectious recombinant particles.

5. As with all recombinant viral systems, caution should be used when handling viral supernatants, especially when concentrating virus using high-speed ultracentrifugation because of the risks of aerosol formation. The SFV split-helper system has been designed to minimize the risk of recombination (*32*), and thus far the appearance of replication-proficient viruses (RPVs) has not been reported. Nevertheless, all work using these systems should be carried out in biosafety level 2 laminal flowhoods according to standard biosafety level 2 practices.

6. Metabolic labeling experiments of cells expressing foreign proteins from the SFV vectors are easy to analyze, as the vector RNA replication results in a general shut-off of host protein synthesis, dramatically reducing the background of labeled host proteins. The labeling can be done already at 4–6 h after RNA transfection or infection. However, in order to achieve maximum labeling of vector-expressed proteins and to ensure minimum labeling of host proteins, it is recommended that 8–9 h should elapse before adding the radioactivity. If the cells have been infected with a high MOI, achieving full infection of the cell population, it is possible to visualize the vector-expressed protein as the major species on an SDS gel. When the antigen is introduced into cells by transfection of DNA encoding the SFV replicon (layered DNA), the radioactivity can be added around a similar time point. However, since in most cases it is not possible to achieve 100% transfection of the cell population using methods such as Lipofectamine, immunoprecipitation prior to analysis by SDS gel may help the analysis.

7. Two issues related to the safety of genetic or recombinant viral vaccines are: persistence of the nucleic acid in the tissue following immunization and the risk of generating infectious recombinant virus when high-titer virus supernatants are used. These issues are discussed briefly here. The persistence in the tissue of SFV particles as well as layered DNA has been investigated following vaccination of mice and chickens (*31*). These studies show that the recombinant constructs do not cross the placental barrier, and they do not persist in the tissue long-term. In particular, the recombinant SFV particles were cleared rapidly from the site of injection while still inducing potent immune responses, suggesting that this approach holds significant promise to be developed as a safe vaccine platform. The split-helper approach used here has been developed to minimize the risk of generating replication proficient virus. The theoretical frequency of restoring infectious

virus has been estimated to be less than 1 in $10^{-17}$, a number that is too small to test experimentally *(31)*. However, thus far, disease caused by replicating virus has not been detected in any vaccinated animals despite extensive use of these vectors in several independent laboratories.

## References

1. Moss, B. (1996) Genetically engineered poxviruses for recombinant gene expression, vaccination and safety. *Proc. Natl. Acad. Sci. USA* **15**, 11,341–11,348.
2. Schneider, J., Gilbert, S. C., Blanchard, T.J., Hanke, T., Robson, K. J., Hannan, C. M., et al. (1998) Enhanced immunogenicity for CD8+ T cell induction and complete protective efficacy of malaria DNA vaccination by boosting with modified vaccinia virus Ankara. *Nat. Med.* **4**, 397–402.
3. Amara, R. R., Villinger, F., Altman, J. D., Lydy, S. L., O'Neil, S. P., Staprans, S. I., et al. (2001) Control of a mucosal challenge and prevention of AIDS by a multiprotein DNA/ MVA vaccine. *Science* **292**, 69–74
4. Hel, Z., Tsai, W. P., Thornton, A., Nacsa, J., Giuliani, L., Tryniszewska E., et al. (2001) Potentiation of simian immunodeficiency virus (SIV)-specific CD4(+) and CD8(+) T cell responses by a DNA-SIV and NYVAC-SIV prime/boost regimen. *J. Immunol.* **167**, 7180–7191
5. Shiver, J. W., Fu, T-M., Chen, L., Casimiro, D. R., Davies M-E., Evans, R. K., et al. (2002) Replication-incompetent adenoviral vaccine vector elicits effective anti-immunodeficiency-virus immunity. *Nature* **415**, 331–334
6. Gilbert, S. C., Schneider, J., Hannan, C. M., Hu, J. T., Plebanski, M., Sinden, R., et al. (2002) Enhanced CD8 T cell immunogenicity and protective efficiency in a mouse malaria model using recombinant adenoviral vaccine in heterologous prime-boost immunisation regimes. *Vaccine* **20**, 1039–1045
7. Strauss, J. H. and Strauss, E. G. (1994) The alphaviruses: gene expression, replication, and evolution. *Microbiol. Rev.* **58**, 491–562.
8. Frolov I., Hoffman T.A., Prágai B. M., Dryga S. A., Huang H. V., Schlesinger S., et al. (1996) Alphavirus-based expression vectors: strategies and applications. *Proc. Natl. Acad. Sci. USA* **93**, 11,371–11,377.
9. Schlesinger, S. (2001) Alphavirus vectors: development and potential therapeutic applications. *Expert Opin. Biol. Ther.* **1**, 177–91.
10. Liljeström, P. and Garoff, H. (1991) A new generation of animal cell expression vectors based on the Semliki Forest virus replicon. *Biotechnology* **9**, 1356–1361.
11. Zhou, X., Berglund, P., Rhodes, G., Parker, S. E., Jondal, M., and Liljeström, P. (1994) Self-replicating Semliki Forest virus RNA as recombinant vaccine. *Vaccine* **12**, 1510–1514.
12. Mossman, S. P., Bex., F., Berglund, P., Arthos, J., O'Neil, S. P., Riley, D., et al. (1996) Protection against lethal simian immunodeficiency virus SIVsmmPBj14 disease by a recombinant Semliki Forest virus gp160 vaccine and by a gp120 subunit vaccine. *J. Virol.* **70**, 1953–1960.
13. Berglund, P., Smerdou, C., Fleeton, M. N., Tubulekas, I., and Liljeström, P. (1998) Enhancing immune responses using suicidal DNA vaccines. *Nat. Biotechnol.* **16**, 562–565.
14. Berglund, P., Fleeton, M. N., Smerdou, C., and Liljeström, P. (1999) Immunization with recombinant Semliki Forest virus induces protection against influenza challenge in mice. *Vaccine* **17**, 497–507
15. Atkins, G. J., Sheahan, B. J., Liljestrom, P. (1999) The molecular pathogenesis of Semliki Forest virus: a model virus made useful? *J. Gen. Virol.* **80**, 2287–2297.

16. Smerdou, C. and Liljeström, P. (2000) Alphavirus vectors: from protein production to gene therapy. *Gene Ther. Reg.* **1,** 33–63.
17. Fleeton, M. N., Chen, M., Berglund, P., Rhodes, G., Parker, S. E., Murphy, M., et al. (2001) Self-replicative RNA vaccines elicit protection against influenza A virus, respiratory syncytial virus, and a tickborne encephalitis virus. *J. Infect. Dis.* **183,** 1395–1398.
18. Lemiale, F., Brand, D., Lebigot, S., Verrier, B., Buzelay, L., Brunet, S., et al. (2001) Immunogenicity of recombinant envelope glycoproteins derived from T-cell line-adapted isolates or primary HIV isolates. *J. AIDS* **26,** 413–422.
19. Morris-Downes, M. M., Sheahan, B. J., Fleeton, M. N., Liljeström, P., Reid, H. W., and Atkins, G. J. (2001) A recombinant Semliki Forest virus particle vaccine encoding the prME and NS1 proteins of louping ill virus is effective in a sheep challenge model. *Vaccine* **19,** 3877–3884.
20. Xiong, C., Levis, R., Shen, P., Schlesinger, S., Rice, C. M., and Huang, H. V. (1989) Sindbis virus: an efficient, broad host range vector for gene expression in animal cells. *Science* **243,** 1188–1191.
21. Hariharan, M. J., Driver, D.. A., Townsend, K., Brumm, D., Polo, J. M., Belli, B. A., et al. (1998) DNA immunization against Herpes Simplex Virus: enhanced efficacy using a Sindbis virus-based vector. *J. Virol.* **72,** 950–958.
22. Ying, H., Zaks, T. Z., Wang, R. F., Irvine, K. R., Kammula, U. S., Marincola, F. M., et al. (1999) Cancer therapy using a self-replicating RNA vaccine. *Nat. Med.* **5,** 823–827.
23. Leitner, W. W., Ying, H., Driver, D. A., Dubensky, T. W., and Restifo, N. P. (2000) Enhancement of tumor-specific immune response with plasmid DNA replicon vectors. *Cancer Res.* **60,** 51–55.
24. Vajdy, M., Gardner, J., Neidleman, J., Cuadra, L., Greer, C., Perri, S., et al. (2001) Human immunodeficiency virus type 1 Gag-specific vaginal immunity and protection after local immunizations with sindbis virus-based replicon particles. *J. Infect. Dis.* **15,** 1613–1616.
25. Pushko, P., Parker, M., Ludwig, G. V., Davis, N. L., Johnston, R. E., and Smith, J. F. (1997) Replicon-helper systems from attenuated Venezuelan equine encephalitis virus - Expression of heterologous genes in vitro and immunization against heterologous pathogens *in vivo. Virology* **239,** 389–401.
26. Caley, I. J., Betts, M. R., Davis, N. L., Swanstrom, R., Frelinger, J. A., and Johnston, R. E. (1999) Venezuelan equine encephalitis virus vectors expressing HIV-1 proteins: vector design strategies for improved vaccine efficacy. *Vaccine* **17,** 3124–3135.
27. Harrington, P. R., Yount, B., Johnston, R. E., Davis, N., Moe, C., and Baric, R. S. (2002) Systemic, mucosal, and heterotypic immune induction in mice inoculated with Venezuelan equine encephalitis replicons expressing Norwalk virus-like particles. *J. Virol.* **76,** 730–742.
28. Rosenbloom, M., Leikin, J. B., Vogel, S. N., and Chaudry, Z. A. (2002) Biological and chemical agents: a brief synopsis. *Am. J. Ther.* **9,** 5–14.
29. Sjöberg, E. M., Suomalainen, M., and Garoff, H. (1994) A significantly improved Semliki Forest virus expression system based on translation enhancer segments from the viral capsid gene. *Bio/Technology* **12,** 1127–1131.
30. Mathiot, C. C., Grimaud, G., Garry, P., Bouquety, J. C., Mada, A., Daguisy, A. M., et al. (1990) An outbreak of human Semliki Forest virus infections in Central African Republic. *Am. J. Trop. Hyg.* **42,** 386–393.
31. Morris-Downes, M. M., Phenix, K. V., Smyth, J., Sheahan, B. J., Lileqvist, S., Mooney, D. A., et al. (2001) Semliki Forest virus-based vaccines: persistence, distribution and pathological analysis in two animal systems. *Vaccine* **19,** 1978–1988.
32. Smerdou, C. and Liljeström, P. (1999) Two-helper RNA system for production of recombinant Semliki forest virus particles. *J. Virol.* **73,** 1092–1098.

# 6

## Development of Attenuated *Salmonella* Strains That Express Heterologous Antigens

**Frances Bowe, Derek J. Pickard, Richard J. Anderson, Patricia Londoño-Arcila, and Gordon Dougan**

## 1. Introduction

The ability of attenuated strains of *Salmonella* to express foreign antigens—which then induce humoral, secretory, and cellular immune responses following oral ingestion—has made them attractive as a system for delivering heterologous antigens to the mammalian immune system. More recently, *Salmonella* has also been successfully used as a means of delivering DNA vaccines to intracellular sites *(1)*. A number of attenuated *Salmonella* hosts are available, and these have been fully characterized. In using *Salmonella* as a delivery system, some consideration must be given to the desired final outcome, as this can be influenced by the host strain chosen. The balance of humoral vs cell-mediated immunity stimulated, for example, can depend on the nature of the attenuating lesion. It has been observed that some mutants stimulate antibody preferentially, and others generate strong humoral and cell-mediated immunity *(2)*. Once an appropriate host has been selected, DNA capable of driving the expression of heterologous antigens can be introduced into *Salmonella* vaccine strains using a variety of approaches. In general, there are two common methods of expressing a foreign antigen in salmonellae: from plasmid vectors or from the bacterial chromosome. Since there are many similarities in the cellular and molecular biology of *Escherichia coli* and *Salmonella*, most of the genetic manipulations required to construct expression cassettes can be carried out in *E. coli*. The resulting constructs can then be introduced into the vaccine strains using simple transformation or other similar techniques. However, the laboratory manipulation of *Salmonella* strains should be undertaken using techniques that do not lead to the accumulation of undefined genetic lesions, which may compromise the growth and immunogenicity of *Salmonella* in vivo. With this in mind, we will describe appropriate techniques for manipulating *Salmonella* with the goal of constructing effective oral vaccines.

From: *Methods in Molecular Medicine, Vol. 87: Vaccine Protocols, 2nd ed.*
Edited by: A. Robinson, M. J. Hudson, and M. P. Cranage © Humana Press Inc., Totowa, NJ

## 1.1. Plasmid Vectors

In general, bacterial plasmids used for expression in *Salmonella* contain replication origins that are functional in *E. coli*. Derivatives of well-known plasmids, many of which are commercially available, can be used for construction of expression vectors, but only modifications that do not favor the accumulation of plasmid-free bacteria in vivo can ultimately be introduced into *Salmonella*. Overexpression of many foreign proteins in *Salmonella* can be toxic for the bacteria and lead to the accumulation of more vigorous, plasmid-free bacteria in the population. This toxicity is believed to be caused by a vastly increased metabolic burden on the cell, and can be exacerbated by use of plasmids that are large or have high copy numbers. Thus, the level of the immune response induced against the heterologous antigen depends both on the persistence of the carrier *Salmonella* strain and the stable expression of the antigen in vivo.

A number of approaches have addressed the problem of potential plasmid instability. Many groups have taken advantage of a system developed by Nakayama et al. *(3,4)*, which utilizes a plasmid expression vector harboring the gene encoding aspartate β-semialdehyde dehydrogenase, an enzyme that is essential for the viability of bacteria. This vector can then be introduced into *Salmonella* vaccine strains harboring lesions in the host *asd* gene encoding the enzyme; thus, loss of the plasmid results in cell death.

Galen et al. have developed a noncatalytic plasmid maintenance system to stabilize plasmids in *Salmonella typhi (5)*. It is based on a postsegregational killing strategy involving the *hok-sok* plasmid addiction system from pR1. Hok is a pore-forming protein whose expression is lethal. Its synthesis is prevented by the hybridization of *sok* anti-sense mRNA to *hok* mRNA. The key to the system is that *sok* mRNA is more susceptible to degradation by nucleases than *hok* mRNA, and therefore its concentration is dependent on constitutive transcription by the expression plasmid. Loss of the plasmid leads to a drop in *sok* mRNA levels, which in turn allows translation and synthesis of Hok. To further enhance stability, plasmid partition functions have also been incorporated into the plasmid.

Tijhaar and colleagues have developed another approach in which the expression plasmid carries an invertible $\gamma P_L$ promoter, which can only drive expression in one orientation. Since the promoter is inverted at random, there is always a subpopulation of bacteria harboring the plasmid, but not expressing the antigen. This population can disseminate in the host and continually segregate antigen-producing bacteria *(6)*.

Galen et al. have speculated that, in the future, toxicity of foreign antigens may also be avoided by expanding a number of approaches that have recently yielded very promising results—e.g., designing stabilized expression vectors that allow secretion or surface display of the expressed antigen. Such plasmids would utilize export systems that are endogenous to the host strain, such as the type III secretion system of *S. typhimurium (7)*. It may also be desirable to co-express immune modulators, an approach that has already been applied successfully *(8)*.

Plasmid stability is highly dependent on the level of expression of the foreign antigen, which in turn is influenced by the promoter used to drive its expression. Our group has been investigating the use of inducible promoters that can be switched on by specific environments that the *Salmonella* encounter within the host. Using these promoters, the deleterious effects associated with constitutive expression of foreign proteins can be avoided. Furthermore, promoters can be chosen which influence the nature of the immune response *(9)*. We have investigated several regulated promoters, including *spv*, *dps*, and the *nirB* promoter. The *nirB* promoter was initially identified in *E. coli*, and is naturally used to express NADH-dependent nitrite reductase. In *E. coli*, *nirB* is induced by nitrites in the environment or by anaerobic conditions *(10)*. A modified version of the *nirB* promoter, which can be induced by anaerobiosis but not nitrites *(11)*, was used to express the tetanus toxin fragment C (tetC) in *S. typhimurium (12)*. Analysis of the in vivo stability of *S. typhimurium* strains expressing the tetC gene using either *tac* or *nirB* promoters from homologous plasmids showed that the latter was much more stable. Both strains induced protection against a tetanus challenge after oral inoculation. However, two doses of the vaccine strain using the *tac* promoter were required to ensure complete protection, as opposed to only one with the strain expressing the antigen from *nirB (12)*.

spv and *dps* are promoters induced in the stationary phase. *dps* is derived from the DNA protective system, and is induced in response to oxidative stress. *SpvA* drives expression of the *spv* genes on the virulence plasmid of *S. typhimurium*. The *spv* operon is essential for systemic spread of infection in mice. We have compared the ability of these promoters to control expression of *tetC* in an attenuated *S. typhimurium* strain (*aroA*) during growth in vitro *(13)*. We found that the spv promoter was more strongly induced in culture and following uptake by macrophages in vitro. We also compared antibody responses generated to *tetC* following immunization of mice. Both dps and spv induced anti-tetC-specific antibodies in mice following one oral immunization. However, the level of antibody detected was higher among mice immunized with the dps construct, which may reflect the fact that, unlike the spv construct, it is stably maintained in vivo. Thus, the expression level a of foreign antigen taken alone is not the best predictor of immunogenicity in vivo.

## 1.2. Expression of Heterologous Antigens From the Chromosome (a)

An alternative strategy to achieve the stable expression of heterologous antigens in vaccine strains of *Salmonella* is inserting the foreign gene sequence directly into the bacterial chromosome. This eliminates the problem of plasmid segregation and the need for suitable selectable markers *(14,15)*. We describe two methods for doing this. The first is the classic technique, which has been used for a number of years. It involves cloning the gene of interest into an appropriate suicide vector containing flanking regions of homology to a host gene and recombining it into the chromosome using homologous recombination. The host gene of choice for the integration site can vary. One approach is to integrate the foreign gene within an open reading frame for a host gene required for growth in vivo. Using this approach, a new attenuating mutation can be introduced into the vaccine strain, which may increase the safety of the strain by decreasing the possibility of reversion to the wild-type phenotype. The target gene should be chosen carefully to avoid impairment of the ability of the strain to survive in host tissues above the level for which adequate immunity can be induced using a single oral immunization. Two different *Salmonella* genes that have been used as a target for foreign gene insertion are *his (15)* and *aroC (14)*. Once the host gene to be used to drive chromosomal insertion has been identified, it is necessary to clone the gene sequence into a suitable vector. A detailed restriction map of the target gene is also required to determine the cloning strategy for inserting the gene encoding the heterologous antigen. The foreign gene should be inserted into the target gene downstream of a suitable promoter; constitutive promoters have most frequently been used for this purpose. The DNA cassette containing the interrupted target gene, promoter, and the foreign gene should then be cloned into a suicide vector, such as pGP704, which is shown in **Fig. 1** *(16)*. This vector has a mobilization origin from R6K, an antibiotic-resistance gene, and a deletion in the *pir* gene, which is required for plasmid replication. As a result, the plasmid can only be maintained in specially constructed bacterial strains in which the *pir* gene has been incorporated into the chromosome, such as *E. coli* SY327 or SM10. If the *pir* gene is not present on the chromosome, as is the case for all wild-type *Salmonella*, the plasmid cannot be replicated.

The *Salmonella* strain is transformed with the suicide vector pGP704 carrying the foreign DNA cassette. The suicide vector should integrate into the bacterial chromosome by homologous recombination. The resulting single crossover events can be recovered because these bacteria will be resistant to the antibiotic. A further recombination event, thus a double crossover, should result in the loss of antibiotic resistance and either the foreign gene or the wild-type target gene.

## 1.3. Expression of Antigens From the Chromosome (b)

A more recent system of creating deletions in specific genes of enteric organisms was developed by Datsenko et al. *(17)* and is a one-step inactivation procedure based on polymerase chain reaction (PCR). This system has the advantage over other gene disruption techniques in that it can be used with not only a PCR product derived from cloned genes and containing an antibiotic marker, but also with PCR products resulting from the use of hybrid PCR oligo primers generated from a novel antibiotic cassette and the gene to be disrupted. The oligonucleotides required to generate these particular PCR products are composed of two components: 50 bases of DNA homologous to each end of the gene to be disrupted (to facilitate homologous recombination), along with 20 bases derived from a novel specialised antibiotic cassette that can be removed using the directly repeated FLP recognition targets (FRT) that flank this cassette on either side. This is achieved using a vector (pCP20) that encodes a recombinase enzyme that recognizes the FRT sites and consequently removes the DNA region internal to these sites. The deletion is left intact while removing the antibiotic marker, which may be detrimental if left in the genome for some procedures (e.g., construction of live vaccines for use in humans).

The technique requires the introduction of a specialized plasmid, pKD46, into the host bacterium. This plasmid contains an ampicillin-resistance gene along with an arabinose inducible promoter that drives a RED recombination fragment consisting of lambda phage genes Gam, Bet and Exo. Gam inhibits RecBCD exonuclease V activity such that Bet and Exo can promote homologous recombination between DNA ends.

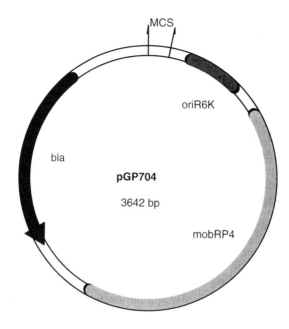

Fig. 1. Suicide Vector pGP704.

After introduction of this plasmid into the host strain, the PCR fragment or cloned gene (plus antibiotic marker) can be introduced by electroporation. Further steps allow for recovery of the host strain containing the disrupted gene, the loss of the RED plasmid by temperature shift and the optional loss of the antibiotic resistance cassette if it is flanked by directly repeated FRT (FLP recognition target) sites. These vectors are described in **Table 1**.

### 1.4. Introduction of Plasmid DNA into Salmonella

Vectors should be introduced into *Salmonella* vaccine strains using methodologies that reduce the frequency of selection for transformants with modified cell surfaces, particularly rough mutants, that grow poorly in vivo. Direct transformation of smooth *Salmonella*, using techniques such as electroporation, enriches for transformants with altered lipopolysaccharide (LPS) side chains. Thus, for the procedures described in **Subheadings 1.2.** and **1.3.**, vectors are normally introduced initially into an intermediate laboratory *Salmonella* that is restriction-negative, modification-competent, and *galE*. (This is not necessary for the inactivation system based on PCR described in **Subheading 1.3.**). A suitable strain for this purpose is LB50I0 *(18)*. The presence of the *galE* mutation renders the bacteria semi-rough and more readily transformable. However, LB*50I0* can still be infected by P22 bacteriophage. The transformed strain of LB50I0 can then be used as a host to create a P22 lysate that is used to introduce the plasmid or integrated mutation and foreign gene into the *Salmonella* vaccine strain by transduction. P22 utilizes the side chain of LPS as a receptor, and thus P22 transductants are

**Table 1**
**Vectors Used for One-Step PCR Inactivation of Chromosomal Genes**

| Plasmid name | Vector details |
|---|---|
| pKD46 | Ampicillin-resistant. Carries the RED recombinase system. |
| pKD3 | Chloramphenical-resistant. Replicates in pir+ve strains only such as *E. coli* SY327.Contains an rbs-start site to allow gene expression downstream of the mutation. Also has stop codons in all six reading frames. |
| pKD4 | Kanamycin-resistant, otherwise details as for pKD3. |
| pKD13 | Kanamycin-resistant. Replicates in pir+ve strains. Has no rbs site, but has stop codons in 4/6 reading frames. |
| pCP20 | Ampicillin-resistant. Carries the FRT recombinase enzyme. |

usually fully smooth. **Figure 2** shows a schematic representation of the development of *Salmonella* vaccine strains that express foreign antigens.

## 2. Materials

### 2.1. Transformation of Salmonella by Electroporation

1. Special equipment: Gene pulser; electroporation cuvets.
2. L-broth/agar: for 1 L of medium, add 10 g bacto-tryptone, 5 g bacto-yeast extract, and 10 g NaC1 to 950 mL of deionized water. Adjust pH to 7.0 and sterilize by autoclaving. For solid medium, add 15 g of bacto-agar/L of broth before sterilization.
3. Glycerol/water solution: 10% (v/v) glycerol in double-distilled water. Sterilize by autoclaving.
4. Glucose stock: Prepare a 1 *M* glucose solution in double-distilled water and sterilize by filtration through a 0.22-μm filter. Add to L-broth before use.

### 2.2. Transduction of Salmonella Using P22 Lysates

1. L-broth/agar, as in **Subheading 2.1.**
2. T2 buffer: 1.5 g/L $KH_2PO_4$; 4.0 g/L NaCl; 5.0 g/L $K_2SO_4$, 3.0 g/L $Na_2HPO_4 \cdot 2H_2O$, 0.12 g/L $MgSO_4 \cdot 7H_2O$, 0.011 g/L $CaC1_2 \cdot 6H_2O$, 0.01 g/L gelatin.
3. TGMS buffer: 10 mL 1 *M* Tris-HC1, pH 7.4, 2.47 g $MgSO_4$, 1 g gelatin, 5.844 g NaC1, make up to 1 L with distilled water.
4. Top agar: Prepare L-broth as in **Subheading 2.1.** Add 7 g of bacto-agar/L of broth before sterilization.
5. 5 m*M* EGTA: Add 95.1 g of EGTA to 200 mL distilled water and dissolve by adjusting to pH 8.0 with 2 *M* NaOH. Make up to 500 mL with sterile distilled water, and sterilize by autoclaving. Store at room temperature.
6. Chloroform.

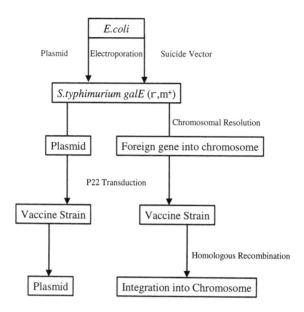

Fig. 2. Development of *Salmonella* vaccine strains expressing heterologous antigens by introduction of plasmid DNA.

## 2.3. Integration of Foreign Genes into the Bacterial Chromosome (a) Special Equipment: Spectrophotometer; Colony Transfer Pads for Replication of Plates

1. L-broth/agar: as in **Subheading 2.1.**
2. Ampicillin: Prepare a stock solution of 50–100 mg/mL in distilled water. Sterilize by filtration through a 0.22-μm filter. Store at –20°C.
3. 0.1 *M* phosphate-buffered saline (PBS): 0.2 g/L KC1, 0.2 g/L KH$_2$PO$_4$, 1.136 g/L Na$_2$HPO$_4$, and 8 g/L NaC1. Adjust pH to 7.2.

## 2.4. Integration of Foreign Genes into the Bacterial Chromosome (b)

1. *DpnI* enzyme.
2. Taq polymerase.
3. Incubating ovens for 30°C and 37°C (and possibly 43°C.)
4. Ampicillin, kanamycin, and chloramphenicol antibiotics.
5. 100 m*M* arabinose.
6. SOC recovery medium. For 100 mL of medium, add 2 g of backtotryptone, 0.5 g of yeast extract, 1 mL of 1 *M* NaC1 and 0.25 mL of 1 *M* KC1 to 97 mL of H$_2$O. Autoclave to sterilize. Add 1 mL each of 1 *M*, filter-sterilized stocks of MgCl$_2$ and MgSO$_4$. Add 1 mL of 2 *M* glucose and filter the complete medium through a 0.2 μ filter. The pH should be 7.0.

### 2.5. Screening by PCR

1. Special equipment: Thermal cycler, wooden toothpicks sterilized by autoclaving, agarose gel electrophoresis apparatus, suitable power supply, and materials for preparing and staining DNA agarose gels *(19)*.
2. Sense and anti-sense oligonucleotide primers. Prepare stock solution at 20 μ*M*, Store at −20°C.
3. 10X PCR buffer: 100 m*M* Tris-HC1, pH 8.3, 500 m*M* KC1, 15 m*M* MgC1$_2$, 0.01% (w/v) gelatin.
4. Deoxynucleotide mixture: 1.25 m*M* of each deoxynucleotide triphosphate: d-ATP, d-GTP, d-CTP, and d-TTP.
5. *Taq* DNA polymerase.

### 2.6. Detection of Expression of Heterologous Antigens Using Sodium Dodecyl Sulfate-Polyacrylamide Gel Electrophoresis (SDS-PAGE)

1. Special equipment and materials: Spectrophotometer; SDS-PAGE apparatus and reagents to make the gel according to Sambrook et al. *(19)*.
2. L-broth, as in **Subheading 2.1.**
3. SDS-PAGE loading buffer: 100 m*M* Tris-HCl, pH 6.8, 700 m*M* β-mercaptoethanol, 3% (w/v) SDS, 10% (v/v) glycerol, 1 mg/mL bromphenol blue. Store at room temperature.

### 2.7. Lipopolysaccharide Gels

1. Special equipment: SDS-PAGE apparatus and a suitable power supply.
2. SDS-PAGE reagents, as described in *Methods in Molecular Biology*, vol. 32 and **ref. *19***.
3. Proteinase K solution (1 mg/mL): freshly prepared in distilled water.
4. Gel-fixing solution: 40% (v/v) methanol, 5% (v/v) acetic acid in double-distilled water; store at room temperature.
5. Silver-staining reagents required: concentrated ammonia, 0.1 *M* NaOH, 20% (w/v) AgNO$_3$ in double-distilled water. *See* **step 4**, **Subheading 3.5.3.1.** for the preparation of this reagent.
6. Oxidizing solution: 0.7% (w/v) periodic acid, 40% (v/v) ethanol, 5% (v/v) acetic acid in double-distilled water; prepare fresh.
7. Formaldehyde developer: 50 mg citric acid, 0.5 mL of 37% (v/v) formaldehyde in 1 L of double-distilled water; prepare fresh.

## 3. Methods

### 3.1. Introduction of Foreign DNA into Salmonella

Foreign DNA can be introduced into *Salmonella* by conjugation, transformation, transduction, and electroporation. Electroporation is the preferred and most common method for introducing foreign DNA into the intermediate *Salmonella* strains. The foreign DNA should then be transduced into the vaccine strain in order to avoid selection of LPS mutants.

### 3.1.1. Transformation of Salmonella by Electroporation

During electroporation, a voltage is applied through a suspension of bacterial cells in a nonconductive solution. The applied voltage allows the DNA to cross the membranes into the cytoplasm of the salmonellae.

### 3.1.1.1. PREPARATION OF ELECTROCOMPETENT CELLS (*SEE* **NOTE 1**)

1. Grow 30 mL of culture of *S. typhimurium* LB50I0 in L-broth until midlog growth is achieved ($A_{650}$ 0.3–0.6).
2. Harvest the culture by centrifuging at 3000g in a benchtop centrifuge.
3. Wash the cells by discarding the supernatant and resuspending the pelleted cells in 10 mL of sterile ice-cold 10% (v/v) glycerol/water solution.
4. Harvest the cells as in **step 2** and resuspend the pellet in sterile ice-cold 10% (v/v) glycerol/water solution (300–400 µL) to a final concentration of approx $1 \times 10^{10}$ cells/mL. This suspension can be stored for future use by freezing 60-µL aliquots at –70°C.

### 3.1.1.2. ELECTROPORATION

1. Prior to electroporation, aliquot 1 mL of L-broth enriched with 20 m*M* glucose into a microcentrifuge tube for each electroporation.
2. Add approx 200 ng of plasmid DNA or 1 µg of suicide vector DNA contained in a maximum volume of 5 µL of sterile water to 60 µL of electrocompetent cell suspension (*see* **Note 2**).
3. Transfer the DNA/bacterial suspension to an ice-cold sterile position cuvet and electroporate using the following conditions: 1.75 kV; 25 µF; 600 Ω (*see* **Notes 3** and **4**).
4. Immediately transfer the bacterial suspension into 1 mL of the broth (prepared as in **step 1**) using a long loading tip. Incubate the broth for 1.5–2 h without shaking at 37°C.
5. After incubation, plate out 200 µL of the broth on selective agar and grow overnight at 37°C.

## 3.1.2. Transduction of Salmonella Using P22 Lysates

As mentioned previously, this is the method of choice for introducing foreign DNA into *Salmonella* vaccine strains following transformation of the intermediate strain (*see* **Note 5**).

### 3.1.2.1. P22 LYSATE PREPARATION

1. Grow the intermediate *Salmonella* strain (LB50I0), containing the gene encoding the foreign antigen inserted in either a plasmid or the chromosome, overnight in L-broth with antibiotic selection at 37°C in an orbital shaker (200 rpm).
2. Prepare serial dilutions of a standard P22 (HT int-ve) bacteriophage stock ranging from $10^{-1}$ to $10^{-6}$ in T2 or TGMS buffer.
3. Add 100 µL of the overnight culture to 10 µL of each P22 serial dilution. Allow the phage to infect the *Salmonella* by incubating the mixture for 30–45 min at 37(C (*see* **Note 6**).
4. Following the incubation, add 3 mL of melted top agar to the bacteria/phage mixture, and spread immediately onto an L-agar plate containing the appropriate antibiotic. Once the top agar has set, incubate the plates at 37°C for 4–6 h until the plaques become visible.
5. Select the plate containing the phage dilution that gives semiconfluent plaques (*see* **Note 7**). Add 3 mL of T2 or TGMS buffer to this plate, and harvest by scraping off the top agar layer into a 15-mL centrifuge tube. Then add 50 µL of chloroform. Vortex the mixture, and shake for 30 min in order to lyse the bacteria, thus releasing the phage.
6. Centrifuge at 15,000g for 15 min at 4°C until a clear supernatant is produced.
7. Remove any residual bacteria from the supernatant by filtration through a 0.22-µm cellulose acetate filter.

8. This P22 phage stock is now ready for further transductions into *Salmonella* vaccine strains. The P22 stock should be stored in a glass container at 4°C with 50 µL of chloroform as a preservative.

### 3.1.2.2. P22 Bacteriophage Transduction

1. Grow the recipient *Salmonella* vaccine strain overnight in an orbital shaker (200 rpm) at 37°C.
2. Prepare serial dilutions of P22 lysate (prepared in **Subheading 3.1.2.1.**) of $10^{-1}$–$10^{-4}$ in T2 or TGMS buffer.
3. Add 100 µL. of the overnight culture to 10 µL of neat P22 lysate and each serial dilution. Mix and incubate at 37°C for 25 min to allow the phage to infect the bacteria.
4. Add 1 mL of L-broth containing 5 m*M* EGTA, and incubate for 1 h at 37°C to allow adequate expression of any antibiotic resistance genes that have been inserted into the recipient strain.
5. Spread 100-µL aliquots of each bacteria/phage mixture onto L-agar plates containing 5 m*M* EGTA and the appropriate antibiotic. Incubate overnight at 37°C.
6. The colonies isolated after overnight growth will contain phage, as shown by their crenated appearance. Therefore, they should be packaged twice on L-agar containing 5 m*M* EGTA to ensure that the phage particles are completely eliminated. The transduced isolates are then ready for further analysis.

## 3.2. Integration of Foreign Genes into the Bacterial Chromosome (a)

1. Electroporate the suicide vector pGP704 containing the inserted foreign gene into an intermediate *Salmonella* strain following the protocol given in **Subheading 3.1.**. Include ampicillin at 30 µg/mL in the L-agar plates used in the final stage of the electroporation protocol.
2. Select one colony only and inoculate into 25 mL of L-broth without antibiotic selection. Grow at 37°C overnight in an orbital shaker.
3. Following overnight incubation, reinoculate 25 mL of fresh L-broth with 250 µL of the overnight culture. Grow this culture at 37°C in an orbital shaker.
4. After 8 h, determine the concentration of the culture by comparing the optical density (OD) at 650 nm with a calibration curve (*see* **Note 8**). Make serial dilutions of the culture in PBS to obtain a suspension that contains 1000–2000 CFU/mL. Plate out 200 µL of this dilution on 10–20 L-agar plates *without* ampicillin and grow overnight at 37°C.
5. Following overnight growth, replicate these master plates onto L-agar plates containing ampicillin at 30 µg/mL and grow overnight at 37°C (*see* **Note 9**).
6. Examine the colonies on the L-agar ampicillin plates and compare them to the master plates. Colonies that have not grown on the ampicillin plates should be restreaked from the master plate onto both L-agar plates with and without ampicillin to confirm that they are sensitive to the antibiotic.
7. The colonies that are confirmed to be ampicillin-sensitive are double crossovers (*see* **Note 10**) and the presence of the inserted gene can be determined using PCR (*see* **Subheading 3.5.1.**) and Southern blotting.
8. P22 lysates of the intermediate strain containing the foreign gene should be prepared and used to introduce the foreign gene into a suitable *Salmonella* vaccine strain (*see* **Subheading 3.1.2.**).

### 3.3. Integration of Foreign Genes into the Bacterial Chromosome (b)(i)

The following is a description of one-step inactivation of chromosomal genes in an enteric strain using a plasmid containing an antibiotic resistance gene marker (e.g., *aph-T*) inserted into the gene to be disrupted (e.g., *htrA*, *tviB*, *aroC*, or *hisG*).

1. Prepare and gel-purify the DNA to be electroporated into the *selected host strain*. The gene to be inactivated is first cloned into a suitable vector. This can be a PCR vector such as pGEM-T or a pir-negative vector (cloning into this vector has the advantage that plasmids used cannot replicate in any wild-type strains, since they lack the pir gene required for vector replication).

   The gene to be disrupted is inactivated by insertion of an antibiotic-resistance cassette such as the *aph-T* kanamycin marker. A PCR product of this gene containing the marker is prepared. The resulting PCR product should be *DpnI* treated so as to digest any of the original template DNA, leaving purified PCR product only. This product can be gel-purified after the *DpnI* digestion. Store until required.

2. Grow up the selected host strain overnight in L-broth at 37°C.

3. Electroporate with pKD46, but ensure that the incubation is done for *all* subsequent steps at 30°C only, since the plasmid is temperature-inducible and will be lost at the higher temperature.

4. Plate out onto L-agar plates containing ampicillin. Leave 14–24 h at 30°C.

5. The next day, many ampicillin-resistant colonies should be obtained. Choose one of these isolates and replate.

6. Inoculate the chosen isolate into L-broth containing ampicillin. Shake overnight at 30°C.

7. Sub-culture strain the next morning in 25-mL L-broth (1 in a 100 dilution) containing ampicillin and *1 mM arabinose in order to induce the RED genes on pKD46*. Leave at 30°C until $OD_{600}$ reaches 0.6, and then spin down and prepare electroporation-competent cells as before.

8. Electroporate with gel purified and *DpnI*-treated PCR fragment.

9. Add SOC recovery medium and grow at 37°C for 90 min. This temperature shift is important, since pKD46 is a temperature-sensitive replicon and will therefore be lost after growth at 37°C. Plate out the electroporated cells onto selective medium (either kanamycin or chloramphenical, depending on the template plasmid used), and leave overnight at 37°C.

10. Select colonies that are resistant to the chosen marker and are also ampicillin-sensitive. Confirm that the gene chosen has been disrupted using PCR or by phenotypic testing. If colonies tested are still ampicillin resistant, plate out a number of isolates at 43°C and leave overnight. Re-test to verify loss of the ampicillin resistance.

### 3.4. Integration of Foreign Genes into the Bacterial Chromosome (b)(ii)

The following is a description of one-step gene inactivation using "hybrid PCR oligos" consisting of 50 bases of flanking DNA from the gene to be disrupted and 20 bases either side from a specialized antibiotic cassette.

1. Prepare and gel-purify the PCR cassette to be electroporated into the *selected host strain*. This specialized cassette has already been briefly described. It is amplified by PCR using a "hybrid oligo" primer. This consists of 36–50 bases of DNA homologous to the gene to be disrupted at both the 5' and 3' ends, and internal to these, are sequences of 20 bases that

serve as primers to the antibiotic cassettes constructed by Datsenko et al. in plasmids pKD3 (CmR), pKD4 (KmR) or pKD13 (kmR) (*see* **Table 1. Note**: For primer designs of "hybrid oligos," *see* **ref.** *17* for full details). These plasmids serve as the template DNA. The use of these particular cassettes is an advantage if removal of the antibiotic-resistance gene is required, since all three are flanked by FRT (FLP recognition) sites, which allows removal using a FLP recombinase carried on a plasmid (*see* **Subheading 3.4.1.** for this procedure). The PCR reactions yield product sizes of 1.1-, 1.6-, or 1.4 kbp from these plasmids, respectively. The PCR products are treated with *DpnI* and gel-purified prior to use.

2. Grow up the *selected host strain* overnight and follow the procedure above (**steps 2–10** inclusive from **Subheading 3.3.**). Thus, selected colonies that are resistant to the chosen marker and also ampicillin-sensitive are recovered. Confirmation that the gene chosen has been disrupted is carried out using PCR or by phenotypic testing. If colonies tested are still ampicillin-resistant because of the presence of pKD46, a number of isolates are plated out at a higher temperature of 43°C and left overnight. The isolates are re-tested to verify their ampicillin sensitivity and thus loss of pKD46 vector.

### 3.4.1. Curing of the Strains of the Antibiotic Cassettes Using a Helper Plasmid Carrying a FLP Recombinase

1. This helper plasmid system is only able to remove the antibiotic cassettes used in method b (ii), since they are flanked by FRT (FLP recognition) sites on either side. The helper plasmid, pCP20, carries such a recombinase that specifically recognizes FRT sites. pCP20 is electroporated into isolates recovered after removal of pKD46 as described previously. After addition of SOC recovery medium, the cells are allowed to grow at 30°C for 90 min before plating out onto L-agar ampicillin plates and left overnight at 30°C.

2. Colonies isolated from the ampicillin plates are then re-grown at 43°C, and the majority lose the FRT-flanked resistance genes and the FLP helper plasmid simultaneously at this stage.

3. The resulting colonies are screened by colony PCR and for antibiotic sensitivity. The colonies can then be stored until needed.

### 3.5. Characterization of Recombinant Salmonella Strains

Recombinant strains of *Salmonella* should be characterized in vitro before they can be used as potential vaccine strains. The in vitro characterization that is required is dependent on the vaccine strain used, the type of expression system, and the nature of the heterologous antigen that is expressed. Initially, the presence of the recombinant DNA within the vaccine strain should be established. Once this has been done, the heterologous strain can be further characterized: The expression and localization of the antigen can be measured; the effect of expression of the foreign antigen on the growth and stability of the strain should be determined, and the integrity of the LPS can be determined.

### 3.5.1. Screening of Recombinant Strains by PCR

In our laboratory we use a PCR-based method to screen recombinant *E. coli* or *Salmonella* strains that have been transformed with the appropriate DNA. This method allows the screening of a large number of bacterial colonies obtained directly after transformation within 1 d of work.

This screening method requires the use of a pair of sense and anti-sense synthetic oligonucleotides to be used as primers (*see* **Note 11**). These can be derived from:

1. The inserted recombinant gene.
2. The DNA sequences flanking the 5' and 3' ends of the inserted gene.
3. The sense primer from a region flanking the inserted gene and the anti-sense primer from within the cloned gene, or vice versa (*see* **Note 12**).

1. Prepare a PCR mixture that contains all the necessary components for the reaction except for the enzyme. The components of the PCR reaction should be optimized for amplification of each specific DNA sequence. Nevertheless, the following mixture can be used initially:
    a. 63 µL double-distilled water.
    b. 10 µL 10X concentrated PCR buffer.
    c. 16 µL deoxynucleotide mixture.
    d. 5 µL of a 20 µ$M$ solution of sense primer (final concentration should be 1 µ$M$).
    e. 5 µL of a 20-µ$M$ solution of anti-sense primer (final concentration should be 1 µ$M$).

2. Use a sterile toothpick to collect a small amount of bacteria from the recombinant colony of choice and resuspend into the PCR mixture by vortexing. Repeat for a different colony, and resuspend the bacteria in the same tube. Bacteria from up to five different colonies can be pooled into the same PCR reaction. Prepare a negative control reaction using a colony from the untransformed bacterial strain and a blank reaction containing no DNA.
3. Lyse the bacteria to release the DNA by incubating the mixture at 100°C for 10 min. Let cool for a further 10 min and then spin tubes for a few seconds in a benchtop microcentrifuge.
4. Add 2.5 U of Taq polymerase contained in 1 µL of diluted PCR buffer. Spin the tubes for a few seconds in a bench microcentrifuge and add 50–100 µL of mineral oil to each tube to prevent evaporation.
5. Carry out the amplification reaction in a thermal cycler as follows: Incubate for 1 min at 94°C, and then repeat 30 cycles of 20 s at 94°C, 1 min at 55°C, and 1 min at 74°C. Finally, incubate for 6 min at 74°C (*see* **Note 13**).
6. Take 5–10 µL of each reaction and analyze by agarose gel electrophoresis. Include a DNA mol wt standard in the gel. To visualize the amplified DNA fragments, stain the gel with ethidium bromide.
7. If primer combination (1) is used, recombinant colonies carrying the gene of interest can be identified by the appearance of an amplified fragment of the expected size. With primer combination (2), the presence of the foreign gene can be determined by comparing the size of the fragments amplified from the recombinant colonies with the fragment amplified from the parental strain. Finally, if the primer combination (3) is used, the appearance of an amplified fragment of the correct size will indicate that the recombinant strain carries the foreign gene in the expected orientation.
8. Identify the pools of colonies containing recombinant plasmids and repeat the process with individual colonies.

### 3.5.2. Expression of Heterologous Proteins

As mentioned previously, foreign antigens can be expressed in *Salmonella* using constitutive promoters, such as *lac* or *tac* (which, in contrast, are inducible in *E. coli*), or promoters that are potentially inducible in vivo, such as *nirB* (**3**). If constitutive promoters are used, induction of expression is not necessary. The method of induction with inducible promoters, however, is specific for the promoter used. The *nirB* promoter, for example, can be induced by lowering the oxygen tension of the culture or by heat shock at 42°C.

### 3.5.2.1. DETECTING THE EXPRESSION OF THE HETEROLOGOUS ANTIGEN

SDS-PAGE and Western blotting provide effective methods for determining both the presence and level of expression of a foreign antigen in a recombinant *Salmonella* vaccine strain (*see* **Notes 14** and **15**).

Samples of bacterial culture can be prepared for SDS-PAGE by the following method:

1. Dilute an overnight culture of the recombinant strain 1:100 into fresh broth with appropriate antibiotic. If an inducible promoter is used, follow the appropriate protocol for induction. Otherwise, grow the culture at 37°C in an orbital shaker for 4–8 h.
2. Determine the OD of the culture at 650 nm ($A_{650}$). Freeze at least 1 mL of the culture immediately at –20°C for further analysis.
3. Thaw the frozen culture samples and pellet by centrifugation for 3 min at top speed in a microcentrifuge.
4. Based on the original $A_{650}$ reading of the culture (**step 2**), resuspend the pellet in SDS-PAGE loading buffer to an OD equivalent to 10 U ($A_{650}$).
5. Boil the samples for 5 min, and centrifuge for 10 min at top speed in a microcentrifuge tube. Load 7.5 µL of each sample onto an SDS-PAGE minigel (6 × 8 cm). Following electrophoresis, the proteins can be visualized directly within the gel using Coomassie blue stain, or, after electrophoresis transfer to nitrocellulose, by Western blotting with a suitable specific antibody.

## 3.5.3. Determining Whether the LPS is Intact

Electroporation of *Salmonella* can select for strains of bacteria that have defective LPS. Lesions in the LPS can lead to further attenuation of *Salmonella* strains in vivo. Therefore, the integrity of the LPS should be determined before these strains are used for vaccination experiments.

A quick method for determining whether the LPS of a strain is defective is agglutination of the strain using polyclonal antiserum against the O antigens and observing the general colony morphology (*see* **Note 16**). However, this method does not give a full profile of the LPS. To achieve this, it is necessary to analyze the LPS by SDS-PAGE.

### 3.5.3.1. ANALYSIS OF LPS USING SDS-PAGE

The following method for the analysis of LPS is based on the method of Tsai and Frash *(20)*.

1. Resuspend a sweep of colonies from an overnight streaked LB-agar plate in 0.25 mL of sterile distilled water contained in a 1-mL plastic vial. Add 1 mL of SDS-PAGE sample buffer, and boil the vials for 5 min before the addition of 0.1 mL of proteinase K (1 mg/ mL). Incubate the samples for 1 h at 60°C, and then load 25 µL of each sample onto a 12 × 15 cm 10% SDS-polyacrylamide gel (*see* **Note 17**).
2. The gel should be run using a cooling system or preferably in a cold room at 4°C. Initially, run the gel at 18 V until the samples reach the top of the separating gel, then increase voltage to 30 V (*see* **Note 18**). Electrophoresis is completed when the Bromphenol blue tracking dye has run off the bottom of the gel; this should occur after approx 6 h.

3. Following electrophoresis, fix the gel by soaking overnight in 200 mL of fixing solution in a clean glass dish. Once the gel is fixed, oxidize the LPS for 5 min by replacing the fixing solution with 200 mL of oxidizing solution. Perform three 15-min washes in a second dish using 500–1000 mL of distilled water for each wash.

4. Prepare the silver-staining reagent as follows: Add 2 mL of concentrated ammonia to 28 mL of 0.1 *M* NaOH, and then add 5 mL of 20% (w/v) silver nitrate solution while stirring rapidly. A transient brown precipitate will form during this process, but it should disappear within seconds. Make this solution up to a final volume of 150 mL with distilled water. **Caution**: This solution should be discarded immediately after use, since it may become explosive when dry!

5. To stain the LPS in the gel, drain the water from the gel, add 150 mL of freshly prepared silver-staining reagent, and agitate vigorously on a stirring platform (approx 70 rpm) for 10 min. Following staining, perform three 10-min washes in a second dish using 500–1000 mL of distilled water for each wash.

6. Replace the water with 200 mL of formaldehyde developer. The LPS in the gel will be stained dark brown within 2–5 min. The development of the gel should be terminated when the LPS bands have reached a desired intensity or when the clear gel background becomes discolored.

7. **Figure 3** compares the LPS profiles of a *S. typhimurium* vaccine strain with intact LPS and a *galE* mutant of *S. typhimurium*, which has defective LPS. When the LPS is intact, a ladder of LPS fragments can be observed on the gel, whereas only low mol wt fragments are observed in strains with defective LPS.

## 4. Notes

### 4.1. Introduction of Foreign DNA into Salmonella

#### 4.1.1. Transformation of Salmonella by Electroporation

1. Care should be taken to ensure that all the reagents used for electroporation and the preparation of electrocompetent cells are kept on ice at <4°C throughout this procedure.

2. Both positive and negative controls should be set up during the electroporation. The intact parental plasmid provides a suitable positive control, and should give confluent growth on selective L-agar plates after overnight growth. Parental plasmid, cut at one or two restriction endonuclease sites, can be used as a negative control.

3. The cell suspension may arc during electroporation. This occurs because either the electrocompetent cells or the DNA solution are conductive. To overcome this problem, the electrocompetent cells and DNA should be prepared to ensure that they do not contain any contaminating salts.

4. Electroporators, such as the Bio-Rad (Hercules, CA) Gene Pulser, give a time constant for each electroporation. For an effective electroporation, the time constant should fall between 10.5 and 12.5 ms. If the time constant is above this range, repeat the electroporation using a larger quantity of DNA.

#### 4.1.2 Transduction of Salmonella Using P22 Lysates

5. The bacteriophage P22 can carry up to 42 kb of contiguous DNA from the host bacterial genome, and can carry both plasmid and cosmid DNA from the host.

6. When P22 gyrates of *galE*-mutant strains of *S. typhimurium*, such as LB5010, are prepared, galactose should be added to the culture after overnight growth to a final concentration of 0.4% (w/v) to facilitate the infection of the bacteria by P22. The culture should then be incubated for a further 20–30 min before the addition of the dilutions of P22 phage.

BRD 509         LB 5010

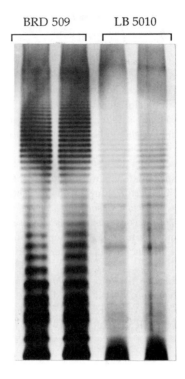

Fig. 3. LPS Profiles of BRD509, with intact LPS and LB5010, an LPS mutant.

7. Some *Salmonella* strains produce very small plaques following infection with P22. In some cases, these plaques may not be visible at all. In this case, the plate containing the lowest dilution of the P22 should be harvested.

## 4.2. Integration of Foreign Genes into the Bacterial Chromosome

8. A calibration curve of OD at 650 nm against a number of colony-forming units can be determined by making dilutions of an overnight culture in the range between $1 \times 10^7$ and $1 \times 10^9$ cells. The optical density and viable count of each dilution should be measured and compared to determine the dilution curve.
9. Replica plating is most practically carried out using replica transfer mats, which are specifically designed for this purpose.
10. The number of insertions per experiment will vary, depending on the target gene, from approx 1–50%.

## 4.3. Screening of Recombinant Strains by PCR

11. Primers should be 15–30 nucleotides long. If the primers are derived from the cloned sequences, they must be separated by approx 100 bp to facilitate the detection of the amplification products using agarose electrophoresis.
12. The primer combination 3 (*see* **Subheading 3.5.1.**) is particularly useful when the heterologous gene could have been ligated in two different orientations into the cloning site—

for example, when a single restriction site has been used for cloning. A single PCR reaction will define the orientation of the inserted DNA fragment.

13. The conditions described here can be used as a starting point for optimizing the parameters for amplification of the chosen DNA sequence. The recommended annealing temperature (55°C) can be changed according to the length and sequence of the primers used. It is important to empirically determine the optimal temperature for amplification before screening. Higher temperatures increase the specificity of the reaction, but may not allow annealing if short primers that are rich in A/T residues are used.

### 4.4. Detecting the Expression of the Heterologous Antigen

14. SDS-PAGE and Western blotting are common techniques. Therefore, the protocols for these techniques are not included in this chapter. For the relevant methods, consult a general laboratory methods manual, such as Sambrook et al. *(19)* and *Methods in Molecular Biology*, vol. 32.

15. As an empirical rule, to obtain an immune response against a heterologous antigen, the foreign antigen should be visible as a band on a Coomassie-stained gel. If a more precise measure of the level of expression is required, the Coomassie-stained gel can be scanned using a densitometer to determine the quantity of foreign antigen that is expressed as a percentage of the total bacterial-cell protein.

### 4.5. Determining Whether the LPS is Intact

16. Observing the general colony morphology of the recombinant strains gives an indication of the integrity of the LPS. Strains with intact LPS have a smooth and glossy appearance on L-agar, whereas LPS mutants have a rough appearance.

17. Since silver stain is extremely sensitive, all the apparatus used for the LPS gel should be handled with gloves and washed thoroughly with sterile distilled water followed by a rinse in methanol before use.

18. The gel should be kept as cool as possible while running. Overheating causes the LPS to degrade. If a cooling system is not available, the gel can be run at a lower voltage for a longer period of time.

## References

1. Darji, A., zur Lage, S., Garbe, A. I., Chakraborty, T., and Weiss, S. (2000) Oral delivery of DNA vaccines using attenuated *Salmonella*. *FEMS Immunol. Med. Microbiol.* **27**, 341–349.
2. Van Cott, J. L., Chatfield, S. N., Roberts, M., Hone, D. M., Hohmann, E. L., Pascual, D. W., et al. (1998) Regulation of host immune responses by modification of *Salmonella* virulence genes. *Nat. Med.* **4**, 1247–1252.
3. Nakayama, K., Kelly, S. M., and Curtiss, R. (1988) Construction of an Asd$^+$ expression-cloning vector: stable maintenance and high level expression of cloned genes in a *Salmonella* vaccine strain. *Bio/Technology* **6**, 693–697.
4. Ascon, M. A., Hone, D. M., Walters, N., and Pascual, D. W. (1998) Oral immunization with a *Salmonella typhimurium* vaccine vector expressing recombinant enterotoxigenic *Escherichia coli* K99 fimbriae elicits elevated antibody titers for protective immunity. *Infect. Immun.* **66**, 5470–5476.
5. Galen, J. E., Nair, J. Y., Wasserman, S. S., Tenner, M. K., Sztein, M. B., and Levine, M. M. (1999) Optimization of plasmid maintenance in the attenuated live vector vaccine strain *Salmonella typhi* CVD 908-htrA. *Infect. Immun.* **67**, 6424–6433.

6. Tijhaar, E. J., Zheng-Xin, Y., Karlas, J. A., Meyer, T. F., Stukart, M. J., Osterhaus, A. D. M. E., et al. (1994) Construction and evaluation of an expression vector allowing the stable expression of foreign antigens in a *Salmonella typhimurium* vaccine strain. *Vaccine* **12,** 1004–1011.

7. Galen, J. E. and Levine M. M. (2001) Can a "flawless" live vector vaccine strain be engineered? *Trends Microbiol.* **9,** 372–376.

8. al-Ramadi, B. K, Al-Dhaheri, M. H., Mustafa, N., Abouhaidar, M., Xu, D., Liew, F. Y., et al. (2001) Influence of vector-encoded cytokines on anti-*Salmonella* immunity: divergent effects of interleukin-2 and tumor necrosis factor α. *Infect. Immun.* **69,** 3980–3988.

9. Medina, E., Paglia, P., Rohde, M., Colombo, M. P., and Guzman, C. A. (2000) Modulation of host immune responses stimulated by *Salmonella* vaccine carrier strains by using different promoters to drive the expression of the recombinant antigen. *Eur. J. Immunol.* **30,** 768–777.

10. Peakman, T., Crouzet, J., Mayaux, J. F., Busby, S., Mohan, S., Harborne, N., et al. (1990) Nucleotide sequence, organisation and structural analysis of the products of genes in the *nirB-cysB* region of the *E. coli* K-12 chromosome. *Eur. J. Biochem.* **191,** 315–323.

11. Oxer, M. D., Bently, C. M., Doyle, J. G., Peakman, T. C., Charles, I. G., and Makoff, A. J. (1991) High level heterologous expression in *E. coli* using the anaerobically-activated *nirB* promoter. *Nucleic Acid Res.* **19,** 1889–1892.

12. Chatfield, S. N., Charles, I. G., Makoff, A. J., Oxer, M. D., Dougan, G., Pickard, D., et al. (1992) Use of the *nirB* promoter to direct the stable expression of heterologous antigens in *Salmonella* oral vaccine strains: development of a single-dose oral tetanus vaccine. *BioTechnology* **10,** 888–892.

13. Marshall, D. G., Haque, A., Fowler, R., Del Guidice, G., Dorman, C. J., Dougan, G., et al. (2000) Use of the stationary phase inducible promoters, spv and dps, to drive heterologous antigen expression in *Salmonella* vaccine strains. *Vaccine* **18,** 1298–1306.

14. Strugnell, R. A., Maskell, D., Fairweather, N., Pickard, D., Cockayne, A., Penn, C., et al. (1990) Stable expression of foreign antigens from the chromosome of *Salmonella typhimurium* vaccine strains. *Gene* **88,** 57–63.

15. Hone, D., Attridge, S., Van den Bosch, L., and Hackett, J. (1988) A chromosomal integration system for stabilization of heterologous genes in *Salmonella* based vaccine strains. *Pathogen. Microbiol.* **5,** 407–418.

16. Miller, V. L. and Mekalanos, J. J. (1988) A novel suicide vector and its use in construction of insertion mutations: osmoregulation of outer membrane proteins and virulence determinants in *Vibrio cholerae* requires *toxR*. *J. Bacteriol.* **170,** 2575–2583.

17. Datsenko, K. A. and Wanner, B. L. (2000) One-step inactivation of chromosomal genes in *Escherichia coli* K-12 using PCR products. *Proc. Natl. Acad. Sci. USA* **97,** 6640–6645.

18. Bullas, L. R. and Ryu, J. I. (1983) *Salmonella typhimurium* LT2 strains which are r−m+ for all three chromosomally located systems of DNA restriction and modification. *J. Bacteriol.* **156,** 471–474.

19. Sambrook, J., Fritsch, E. F., and Maniatis, T. (1989) *Molecular Cloning: A Laboratory Manual.* Cold Spring Harbor Laboratory, Cold Spring Harbor, NY., 18.49–18.54.

20. Tsai, C. M. and Frash, C. E. (1982) A sensitive silver stain for detecting lipopolysaccharides in polyacrylamide gels. *Anal. Biochem.* **119,** 115–119.

# 7

# Expression and Delivery of Heterologous Antigens Using Lactic Acid Bacteria

## Mark A. Reuter, Sean Hanniffy, and Jerry M. Wells

## 1. Introduction

There has been increasing interest in developing delivery vehicles for use as mucosally administered vaccines. *Lactobacillus lactis* is a harmless noninvasive bacterium with a history of safe use in the food industry, which makes it more acceptable than attenuated pathogens for vaccine delivery, particularly with respect to infants and partially immunocompromised individuals. A number of potential vaccine antigens has now been expressed in *L. lactis* (*1–9*), but most immunological studies have been carried out with *L. lactis*-producing tetanus toxin fragment C (TTFC) (*4,10,11*). These studies have shown that *L. lactis*-expressing TTFC can elicit antigen-specific secretory IgA and protective levels of serum antibodies—responses that were enhanced in strains that coexpress selected cytokines. Further potential exists to use lactic acid bacteria (LAB) delivery systems to prevent hypersensitivity to certain allergens or suppress atopic disease through the mucosal delivery of allergens or peptides (*12*).

For a number of reasons including those mentioned above, the expression of heterologous genes in *L. lactis* has received much attention over the last few years, and is the subject of several detailed reviews in the field (*13,14*). In this chapter, we describe the pTREX series of theta-replicating plasmid vectors derived in our laboratories using the non-self-transmissible plasmid pIL253 that carries the broad Gram-positive host replicon pAMβ1, which has been adapted for both constitutive and inducible expression of heterologous protein antigens in *L. lactis* (*15*). Although these vectors do not replicate in *Escherichia coli*, we often found them to be more structurally stable than the alternative rolling-circle replication vectors, especially when constitutive promoters or large DNA fragments were inserted into the vector.

A range of lactococcal promoters identified in our laboratory (*16*) has been incorporated into pTREX, generating a series of constitutive expression vectors containing promoters with different activities. Although constitutive expression systems generally produce less protein antigen than inducible expression systems, they have been

From: *Methods in Molecular Medicine, Vol. 87: Vaccine Protocols, 2nd ed.*
Edited by: A. Robinson, M. J. Hudson, and M. P. Cranage © Humana Press Inc., Totowa, NJ

used to construct immunogenic strains that are capable of expressing antigen in vivo. Lactococcal strains that constitutively express TTFC (pTREX1-TTFC containing the lactococcal P1 promoter) elicited high-level TTFC-specific antibody in serum that was sufficient to protect against a lethal challenge of tetanus toxin *(17)*.

In previous studies, we have developed a regulated dual-plasmid expression system in *L. lactis* based on lactose-inducible transcription of the lactose operon that utilizes the T7 bacteriophage RNA polymerase and its cognate promoter. Currently, we use the nisin-inducible expression system for high-level expression of antigen prior to immunization. Nisin is an antimicrobial peptide with a safe history of use in the food industry as a preservative. The structural gene, *nisA*, is the first gene of a cluster that encodes proteins for the modification, translocation, and immunity to nisin *(18–20)*. The gene cluster also encodes a two-component sensor and response regulator, NisK and NisR, that coregulates transcription of the nisin gene cluster. Nisin autoregulates its own expression through interaction with the membrane-bound sensor NisK, which in turn activates NisR by phosphorylation, resulting in expression from the *nisA* promoter.

Expression host strains containing the *nisK* and *nisR* genes constructed in more than one laboratory *(21,22)* have been used to induce expression of recombinant protein under the control of the *nisA* promoter by adding nisin to the growth medium. In addition to high expression levels—up to 60% of total intracellular protein *(23)*—the nisin system also offers greater flexibility because protein expression is tightly regulated and directly proportional to the addition of the inducing molecule (allowing the expression of potentially lethal genes). This system is now widely used to overexpress proteins in *L. lactis*, and has been adapted for use in other LAB, including *Leuconostoc* and *Lactobacillus* spp. *(24,25)*.

Targeting protein antigens either extracellularly or to different cellular locations in *L. lactis* may play a significant role in determining the parental immunogenicity of antigen-expressing strains when presented to the immune system. By virtue of their greater accessibility, protein antigens displayed at the bacterial surface may be more immunogenic. In terms of the dose required to elicit protection against a lethal challenge of tetanus toxin, lactococcal strains expressing cell-wall-anchored TTFC were 10–20 times more immunogenic than strains expressing alternative forms of the protein (by the subcutaneous route [sc] of administration) *(11)*. We have adapted the pTREX series further to include secretion leaders and/or cell-wall-anchoring motifs so that recombinant antigen can be targeted to different cellular locations (**Fig. 1**).

We have also investigated the potential of recombinant *L. lactis* to deliver other bioactive molecules such as cytokines to the immune system. The pTREX series was used to coexpress intracellular TTFC and fully biologically active secreted murine IL-2 or murine IL-6 in *L. lactis*. TTFC-specific immune responses were 10–15-fold higher in mice that were immunized intranasally with cytokine-expressing strains when compared to those mice immunized with strains expressing TTFC alone *(26)*. This enhanced immune response was only observed when live cells were used, indicating that lactococci were producing the cytokines in vivo.

In conclusion, we have demonstrated that mucosally administered *L. lactis* expressing a heterologous protein is capable of eliciting both local and systemic immune

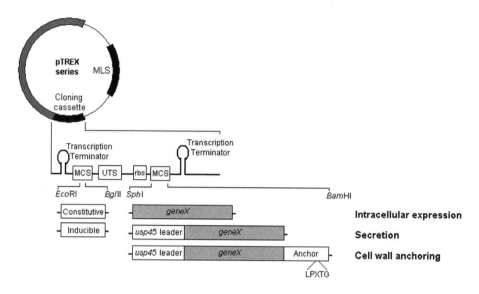

Fig. 1. Diagram showing the pTREX series of plasmids. The pTREX cloning cassette contains two multiple cloning sites (MCS). The first MCS is used to insert either constitutive or inducible promoter fragments such as the nisin-inducible *nisA* promoter. The second MCS is used to insert genes encoding the heterologous protein. Gene fusions with the leader sequence of the abundant lactococcal secreted protein Usp45 *(27)* allow secretion of the recombinant protein. The inclusion of a cell-wall-anchor sequence (such as the C-terminal-anchoring domain of *L. lactis* protease C *(11)* targets the expressed protein to the *L. lactis* cell envelope. MLS, resistance to macrolides, lincosamines and streptogramin B type antibiotics; UTS, universal translational stop sequence; rbs, ribosome binding site. All restriction enzyme sites shown are unique in pTREX.

responses. Most of this work has been performed using TTFC as a model antigen; however, the potential and applicability of *L. lactis* as a vaccine delivery system is currently being expanded to include a growing number of antigens and other therapeutic molecules. Here, we describe methods used when working with *L. lactis* with a view to using this bacterium to express and deliver heterologous proteins that can ultimately be developed to treat or prevent diseases in humans.

## 2. Materials

1. MilliQ water (sterile).
2. M17 broth and M17 broth supplemented with 2.5% glycine.
3. M17 agar (sterile 95-mL aliquots) and sterile 5-mL aliquots of 10% glucose.
4. GM17 agar supplemented with sucrose to a final concentration of 0.5 $M$ plus sterile magnesium chloride solution (1 $M$) and sterile calcium chloride solution (200 m$M$).
5. Osmotically stabilizing poration/storage (OSPS) buffer: 0.5 $M$ sucrose in 10% glycerol (*see* **Note 1**).
6. Sterile glycerol.

7. Abs ethanol and 70% ethanol.
8. TE buffer: 10 m$M$ Tris-HCl (pH 8.0), 1 m$M$ ethylenediaminetetraacetic acid (EDTA).
9. 10% (w/v) sucrose in 20 m$M$ Tris-HCl, pH 7.5.
10. Phosphate-buffered saline (PBS) buffer: 80 m$M$ Na$_2$HPO$_4$, 20 m$M$ NaH$_2$PO$_4$, 100 m$M$ NaCl, pH 7.0.
11. PBS-Tween: PBS containing 0.05% Tween 20.
12. PBS-Tween-bovine serum albumin (BSA): PBS containing 0.05% Tween 20 and 3% BSA.
13. TBS buffer: 0.15 $M$ NaCl, 0.02 $M$ Tris-HCl, pH 7.5.
14. Erythromycin (5 mg/mL stock solution).
15. Lysozyme (500 mg/mL).
16. Mutanolysin (10 U/µL).
17. Nisin (25 µg/mL solution dissolved in 0.02 $M$ HCl).
18. Trichloroacetic acid (TCA).
19. 0.01% poly-L-lysine.
20. 0.25% glutaraldehyde.
21. Nitrophenyl phosphate, 5-mg tablets.
22. Diethanolamine buffer: 48.5 mL diethanolamine, adjust pH to 9.8 using 1 $M$ HCl and add distilled water to a final volume of 500 mL.
23. Carbonate/bicarbonate buffer, pH 9.6: 0.80 g Na$_2$CO$_3$, 1.46 g NaH$_2$CO$_3$, adjust to pH 9.6 using HCl, and add distilled water to a final volume of 500 mL.
24. Cell resuspension buffer: 1.25 mL 20% casein hydrolysate, 0.5 mL 50% glucose, 10 mL $M$ sodium bicarbonate in 38.25 mL PBS.
25. Restriction endonucleases and DNA modification enzymes, such as T4 DNA ligase, or T4 DNA polymerase.
26. Taq DNA polymerase and 10X buffer.
27. dNTPs solution (dATP, dTTP, dCTP, and dGTP).
28. 106-µm glass beads (acid-washed).
29. Sodium dodecyl sulfate-polyacrylamide gel electrophoresis (SDS-PAGE) gels (pre-cast or materials necessary for their preparation).
30. SDS-PAGE loading buffer and running buffer.
31. Electro-blotting transfer buffer.
32. Commercial plasmid miniprep kit.
33. DNA electrophoresis kit, gel-loading buffer and running buffer, DNA size markers, ethidium bromide.
34. Electroporation cuvets.
35. Primers to PCR-amplify gene(s) of interest.
36. Primers that anneal either side of insert DNA for colony polymerase chain reaction (PCR) screening/sequencing.
37. Antibody that crossreacts to recombinant protein plus suitable secondary antibody (alkaline phosphatase-conjugated).

## 3. Methods

### 3.1. Construction of Expression Vector

#### 3.1.1. Purifying Plasmid DNA

Because of their thicker cell wall, Gram-positive bacteria such as *L. lactis* are generally more difficult to lyse than Gram-negative bacteria. However, plasmid DNA can be readily purified using conventional methods *(28)* or commercial kits by including an additional enzymatic lysis step. Lysozyme and mutanolysin degrade the peptidoglycan component of the lactococcal cell wall, thus facilitating cell lysis.

1. Plate a glycerol stock or agar stab of the desired strain on a GM17 agar plate supplemented with the appropriate antibiotic (*see* **Note 2**). Incubate the plates at 30°C until individual colonies have grown. This may take 2–3 d.
2. Inoculate 10 mL of GM17 broth, supplemented with the appropriate antibiotic with a single colony from the GM17 agar plate. Grow the culture overnight at 30°C without shaking.
3. The following day, harvest cells from 2 × 5 mL of culture by centrifuging at approx 15,000*g* for 2 min. Discard supernatant and resuspend the cell pellet in resuspension buffer supplemented with lysozyme and mutanolysin (to a final concentration of 5 mg/mL and 100 U/mL, respectively) (*see* **Note 3** and **Note 4**). Incubate the resuspended cells at 37°C for 15 min.
4. From this stage, follow conventional protocols or those recommended by the manufacturer if using a commercial kit.

Purified plasmid DNA can be analysed by agarose gel electrophoresis. Uncut lactococcal plasmid DNA will resolve on an agarose gel as a high mol-wt species, and must be digested with an appropriate restriction endonuclease enzyme in order to estimate its size. The method described can be scaled up when purifying large amounts of plasmid.

### 3.1.2. Molecular Biology Manipulations

Standard molecular biology techniques can be used to digest plasmid DNA with restriction endonuclease enzymes, visualize DNA on agarose gels and ligate DNA fragments *(28)*. The transformation efficiency of *L. lactis* is lower than that achieved with *E. coli* (*see* **Subheading 3.1.3.**), so it is recommended that ligated DNA be concentrated by ethanol-precipitation. The DNA pellet should be vacuum-dried and resuspended in 4 µL sterile Milli-Q water prior to transformation (*see* **Note 5**).

### 3.1.3. Preparation of Electro-Competent L. lactis

It is necessary to transform lactococcus using electroporation to achieve efficient transformation. For *L. lactis*, the transformation efficiencies are generally lower than that obtained with *E. coli*, but the following procedure should yield greater than $1 \times 10^5$ transformants per microgram of DNA, although transformation efficiencies of $5 \times 10^7$ have been reported *(29)*.

1. Plate a glycerol stock or agar stab of the desired strain on a GM17 agar plate (supplement the agar with the appropriate antibiotic if the strain contains an antibiotic-resistance marker). Incubate the plate at 30°C until individual colonies have grown. This may take 2–3 d.
2. Inoculate 10 mL of GM17 broth (supplemented with appropriate antibiotic if necessary) with a single colony from the GM17 agar plate. Grow the culture overnight at 30°C without shaking.
3. On the same day as preparation of electro-competent cells, prepare the following medium and buffer:

    a. GM17 broth supplemented with glycine to a final concentration of 2.5%.

    b. Osmotically-stabilizing poration/storage buffer (OSPS). 0.5 $M$ sucrose in 10% glycerol (*see* **Note 1**).

4. Use 1 mL of overnight culture to inoculate 50 mL of prewarmed GM17 2.5% glycine medium (again supplemented with appropriate antibiotic if necessary). Grow the culture at 30°C (without shaking) and monitor $OD_{600}$.

5. When the culture has reached an optical density (OD) of approx 0.5 (this can take up to 5 h), chill the culture on ice for 10 min.

6. Centrifuge the culture, in sterile falcon tube, at 3000$g$ for 15 min at 4°C (*see* **Note 6**). Carefully discard the supernatant and resuspend the cell pellet in 5 mL ice-cold OSPS by gentle mixing. Do not vortex the cells or resuspend using a pipet. Instead, use a sterile spreading loop or tip to loosen the cells from the tube wall. Cells should resuspend after gentle agitation.

7. Centrifuge the cells at 3000$g$ for 15 min at 4°C. Discard the supernatant and carefully resuspend the cell pellet in 5 mL ice-cold OSPS. Centrifuge again (3000$g$ for 15 min at 4°C), discard supernatant, and resuspend cells in 0.5 mL OSPS.

8. Aliquot 90 µL of cells into sterile microcentrifuge tubes and snap-freeze using either liquid nitrogen (*see* **Note 7**) or a dry ice-ethanol bath. Store cells at –70°C or use directly.

9. To transform cells, either use directly following the cell preparation or thaw the appropriate number of tubes on ice. One tube of cells is sufficient for two transformations.

### 3.1.4. Electro-Transformation of L. lactis

1. Aliquot DNA into a sterile microcentrifuge tube prechilled on ice. The volume of DNA cannot exceed 4 µL. If transforming cells with the product of a ligation reaction, include a positive control plasmid of known concentration to determine transformation efficiency. Chill the appropriate number of electroporation cuvets on ice.

2. Prepare SMG17MC outgrowth medium (GM17 broth supplemented with sucrose to a final concentration of 0.5 $M$, magnesium chloride to a final concentration of 20 m$M$, and calcium chloride to a final concentration of 2 m$M$), and chill on ice.

3. Add 40 µL of electro-competent cells to DNA. Mix briefly by tapping the tube and pipet the mixture into an electroporation cuvet. Ensure that no air bubbles remain in the electroporation chamber (these can be removed by gently tapping the cuvet). Wipe the side of the cuvet to remove any water/moisture and pulse at 2500 V (25 µFD capacitance, 200Ω resistance).

4. Place cuvette back in ice and add 960 µL ice-cold SGM17MC. Transfer resuspended cells into an ice-cold sterile microcentrifuge tube and incubate on ice for 10 min. Mix these cells with a further 9 mL of SGM17MC and incubate at 30°C for 2 h.

5. Centrifuge cells at 3000$g$ for 15 min. Remove and discard supernatant and carefully resuspend cells in 1 mL GM17 broth. If plating cells transformed with ligated DNA, plate up to $5 \times 100$ µL of cells onto GM17 agar plates supplemented with the appropriate antibiotic. If plating cells transformed with a positive control plasmid, plate a range of volumes (e.g., 10 µL, 50 µL, 100 µL, and 200 µL). To the remaining cells, add an equal volume of sterile glycerol and store cells at –20°C in case further transformants are required.

6. Incubate the agar plates at 30°C. Inspect plates the following day, although it may take 2–3 d for the colonies to become visible.

### 3.1.5. Colony PCR

Colony PCR, using primers that anneal to loci on either side of the DNA insert, can be used to screen transformants for plasmid DNA containing a DNA insert using a method adapted from that used for *E. coli (30)*. An additional 5-min incubation step at 95°C is included in the thermal cycle at the start of the program to break open the cells.

## 3.2. Assessing Expression of Cloned Genes

If using the nisin-inducible *nisA* promoter to express foreign proteins in *L. lactis*, it is necessary to transform the expression vector into a strain that contains the *nisRK* two-component regulatory genes but lacks a functional *nisA* gene; the transformation procedure is described in **Subheading 3.1.4.** Recombinant proteins expressed in *L. lactis* may be readily visible on Coomassie blue or Colloidal blue-stained SDS-PAGE gels (*see* **Fig. 2B**). However, this is dependent on the level of expression and nature of the protein being expressed, as well its cellular localization in *L. lactis*. All these factors contribute to the decision of which protein-extraction method is most suitable for analysis of recombinant protein expression. When expression of recombinant protein is not apparent using standard SDS-PAGE, it is recommended that immunoblot analysis of protein extracts, using protein-specific antibodies, be carried out.

### 3.2.1. Evaluating the Effect of Nisin on Growth

Upon induction, expression of certain heterologous proteins may have a deleterious effect on cell growth. It is therefore advisable to check that induction with nisin does not have an adverse effect on the growth characteristics of the (transformed) strain containing the expression vector. Expression from the *nisA* promoter is proportional to the amount of nisin added; therefore, the optimal nisin concentration, corresponding to optimal gene expression with minimal growth defect, can be determined.

1. From an agar plate containing the recombinant protein expression strain, pick a single colony into 10 mL GM17 supplemented with an appropriate antibiotic. Also pick a clone of the same host strain containing a plasmid without the insert (as a negative control). Grow cultures overnight at 30°C without shaking.
2. Inoculate several 10-mL aliquots of GM17 broth, supplemented with the appropriate antibiotic, with 1 mL of overnight culture (both expression strain and negative control). The number of cultures to be inoculated depends to the range of nisin concentrations to be tested. However, a control culture should always be included to which no nisin will be added.
3. Grow cultures at 30°C without shaking and monitor growth using a spectrophotometer. When cultures have reached an $OD_{600}$ of approx 0.5, induce with nisin over a range of final concentrations (for example, 0.1 ng/mL, 1 ng/mL, 10 ng/mL, and 50 ng/mL final concentration). A control culture containing no nisin should also be grown.
4. Continue to grow cultures at 30°C without shaking and monitor $OD_{600}$ for an additional 5–6 h.
5. Plot growth curves and calculate doubling times for each culture using a standard procedure. Upon the addition of nisin, growth defects in strains harboring the recombinant protein-expression vector relative to strains harboring a control plasmid, may be attributed to expression of the heterologous protein (*see* **Fig. 2A**).

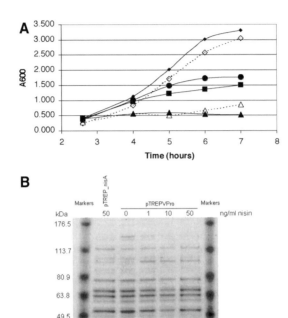

Fig. 2. Induction of a viral protease in *L. lactis* induced with nisin. (**A**) Graph showing the effect of different nisin concentrations on growth of *L. lactis* strains expressing a viral protease (◆ minus nisin, ● 1 ng/mL nisin, ■ 10 ng/mL nisin, ▲ 50 ng/mL nisin) compared to an empty vector control strain (◊ minus nisin, △ 50 ng/mL nisin). (**B**) SDS-PAGE analysis of soluble cell extracts from the final time point of the above growth experiment. Protein samples were resolved on 4–12% NuPAGE gradient gel (precast) and stained with Colloidal blue. pTREP-nisA, empty expression vector; pTREPVPro, viral protease under the control of the inducible *nisA* promoter.

## 3.2.2. Preparation of Soluble and Insoluble Protein Extracts From Whole Cells

1. Using 50-mL broths, induce cultures with a range of nisin concentrations using a scaled-up version of the experiment described in **Subheading 3.2.1.** Again, ensure that suitable controls are included. After 5–6 h growth in the presence of nisin, cells are harvested by centrifuging 10 mL of culture at 3000*g* for 15 min at 4°C. At this stage, cell pellets can be stored at –20°C and subsequently thawed on ice when extracting protein.
2. Resuspend cell pellet in 1 mL PBS and transfer suspension to a 7-mL bijoux to which 1 mL of sterile acid-washed glass beads (0.10–11 mm) have been added. Shake bijoux using a bead-beater at 1600 rpm 3 times for 1 min with 1-min intervals during which the suspension is kept on ice (*see* **Note 8**).
3. Transfer suspension samples into a 2-mL microcentrifuge tube (samples are difficult to pipet as this stage because of the glass beads). Centrifuge the tubes at <1000*g* in a microcentrifuge for 2 min to separate cellular material from glass beads and unbroken

cells. Using a pipet, carefully remove the upper layer containing cellular material (taking care to exclude any glass beads), and transfer the suspension to a fresh microcentrifuge tube. Usually, it is only possible to recover 400–500 µL of cellular suspension at this stage. This material will contain both insoluble and soluble material.

4. Centrifuge the samples at maximum speed for 5 min (the insoluble material forms a pellet). Using a pipet, carefully transfer the supernatant (soluble fraction) to a fresh microcentrifuge tube (take care not to remove insoluble material).
5. Resuspend the insoluble fraction in PBS using the same volume as that obtained for the soluble fraction. Add an equal volume of 2X SDS-PAGE sample buffer (denaturing) to both the soluble and insoluble fractions and boil for 3–5 min. Extracts can be stored at –20°C or analyzed immediately by SDS-PAGE or immunoblotting, using standard procedures *(31,32)*. To compare extracts for relative amounts of protein expression, it is recommended that approx equal amounts of protein should be loaded into each lane prior to SDS-PAGE and immnunoblot analysis. When possible, a sample containing purified recombinant protein should also be included to aid identification of the lactococcal-expressed protein.
6. To determine the level of induced protein expression over time, the experiment should be repeated using the optimal nisin concentration, taking 10-mL samples prior to and at various time points after induction with nisin. Protein extracts are prepared and analyzed by SDS-PAGE as described previously.

### 3.2.3. Preparation of Cytoplasmic (Protoplast) and Cell-Wall Protein Extracts

Depending on the expression construct used, it may be desirable to investigate the amount of recombinant protein present in the cytoplasmic, cell-wall, or culture supernatant fractions.

1. Harvest 5 mL of *L. lactis* culture (OD$_{600}$ = 1; approx $2.5 \times 10^9$ bacteria per mL) by centrifugation at 4°C for 5 min at 6000$g$ (Sigma 1K15).
2. Wash the cell pellet 3× in Tris-buffered saline (TBS).
3. Resuspend the cell pellet in 200 µL of 20 m$M$ Tris-HCl, pH 7.5, 10% w/v sucrose, and add mutanolysin (100 U/mL) and freshly prepared lysozyme (5 mg/mL) (*see* **Note 9**). Incubate the mix for 1 h at 37°C.
4. Recover cells from enzymatically released cell-wall material by gentle centrifugation (1500$g$ for 10 min).
5. Transfer supernatant containing released cell-wall extract to a new microcentrifuge tube.
6. Wash the protoplast cell pellet once in 20 m$M$ Tris-HCl, pH 7.5, 10% w/v sucrose, and resuspend in 100 µL of a 1:1 mix of 2X SDS-PAGE sample buffer and TE buffer.
7. Proteins in the supernatant containing the cell-wall fraction can be analyzed directly by SDS-PAGE by adding an equal volume of 2X SDS-PAGE sample buffer and boiling for 3–5 min. Alternatively, proteins in the supernatant can be concentrated either by phenol extraction or by trichloroacetic acid (TCA) precipitation using standard techniques *(28)*.

### 3.2.4. Preparation of a Supernatant Fraction

1. Harvest 5 mL of *L. lactis* culture (OD$_{600}$ = 1; approx $2.5 \times 10^9$ bacteria per mL) by centrifugation at 4°C for 5 min at 6000$g$ (Sigma 1K15).
2. To remove all bacteria, filter the supernatant using a sterile 0.2-µm-pore filter (low protein retention; Millisar NML Sartorius, Göttingen, Germany).

3.  Add TCA to the filtrate to a final concentration of 10–15%.
4.  Incubate on ice for 1–2 h followed by centrifugation at 10,000$g$ for 10 min.
5.  Remove supernatant and drain pellet, ensuring that no drops of TCA remain.
6.  Resuspend pellet in 50 µL of a 1:1 mix of 2X SDS-PAGE sample buffer and TE buffer, boil for 3–5 min and analyze 10–20 µL (approx the equivalent of 1 mL culture) by SDS-PAGE or immunoblotting.

### 3.2.5. Whole-Cell ELISA to Confirm Surface Expression of Heterologous Protein in L. lactis

1.  Coat the wells of a 96-well microtiter plate with 0.01% poly-L-lysine (100 µL/well) for 1 h at room temperature.
2.  Wash the plates by briefly immersing in 0.05 $M$ PBS and then shaking the contents of the plate over a collection tray.
3.  To each well, add 100 µL of freshly prepared *L. lactis* cells diluted in 0.05 $M$ PBS to an $OD_{600}$ of 0.2.
4.  For comparison, a subset of wells from the plate can be overlayed with 100 µL of the recombinant protein at different concentrations (1 mg/mL and serial dilutions thereof). Incubate the plate overnight at 4°C.
5.  Add 50 µL of 0.25% glutaraldehyde to each well and incubate at room temperature for 15 min.
6.  Wash the plates by soaking in PBS 3× briefly. Block glutaraldehyde residues by adding 100 µL of 100 m$M$ glycine buffer containing 0.1% BSA to each well and incubate at room temperature for 1 h.
7.  Wash plates 5× in PBS containing 0.05% Tween 20 and then block with 3% BSA in PBS-Tween (200 µL/well) for 2 h at 37°C
8.  Add 100 µL of protein-specific antibody (typically diluted 1/20 and 1/50) to each well and incubate at room temperature for 90 min.
9.  After washing, add 100 µL of alkaline phosphatase-conjugated goat secondary antibody) diluted 1:1000 and incubate at 37°C for 2 h.
10. Add 100 mL of alkaline phosphatase-conjugated secondary antibody, diluted 1:1000 in PBS + 0.05% Tween 20, to all wells except the secondary antibody negative control and blank wells.
11. Incubate the microtiter plate at 37°C for 2 h. Wash wells by soaking in PBS + 0.05% Tween 20 briefly 3× (followed by two 3-min soaks, and pat dry.)
12. To prepare substrate, dissolve one 5-mg tablet of nitrophenyl phosphate in 5 mL diethanolamine buffer. Add 100 µL of substrate to each well, then cover the microtiter plate with foil (the substrate is photo-sensitive) and incubate at room temperature for 30 min. Using a microtiter plate reader, measure the absorbance of each well at 405 nm.

### 3.3. Preparation of Lactococci for Immunization

1.  From an agar plate containing the recombinant protein-expression strain, pick a single colony into 10 mL GM17 supplemented with appropriate antibiotic. Also pick a strain of the identical background containing plasmid without insert (as a negative control). Grow cultures overnight at 30°C without shaking—this broth is used to inoculate overnight cultures for a series of immunizations (three consecutive oral doses or just one intra nasal dose) and a sample is taken to check for expression of the heterologous antigen.
2.  Inoculate several 10-mL aliquots of GM17 broth, supplemented with the appropriate antibiotic, with 0.2 mL of overnight culture (both expression strain and negative control). The number of cultures required depends on the number of inoculations to be carried out

(ensuring that there will be at least a twofold excess of cells). Grow cultures overnight at 30°C without shaking.

3. Dilute overnight cultures 1:5 in GM17, supplemented with appropriate antibiotics, and measure absorbance at 600 nm (ensure that the OD reading falls between 0.2 and 0.6). The volume of culture required to provide sufficient cells (usually twofold excess to allow for losses during administration to mice) is calculated based on OD $1.0 = 5 \times 10^8$ cfu/mL.

4. Centrifuge the appropriate volume of cells at $1200g$ in microfuge (or $2500g$ in Eppendorf 5810R) for 15 min and wash the cells once in sterile PBS. Centrifuge the cells again and resuspend the cell pellet in a small volume of cell resuspension buffer. The volume is measured and then extra buffer is added to make up the required total volume at $5 \times 10^{10}$ cfu/mL.

**Caution**: When working with animals all procedures should be carried out subject to the Animals (Scientific Procedures) Act, 1986 and to guidelines set out by the Home Office. Researchers should consult the relevant authorities.

### 3.3.1. Oral Inoculation of Mice with Bacteria

An inoculation regime similar to that used with microparticles has been used when orally administering the bacterium. Typically, live bacteria ($5 \times 10^9$ in 0.1-mL vol) are administered to mice intragastrically using a gavage tube without anaesthetic or adjuvant on three consecutive d (d 0, 1, and 2). This set of doses is repeated 4 wk later (d 28, 29, and 30). Five days later, a single booster dose is administered. Mice are tail bled at regular 2-wk intervals in order to monitor immune responses.

### 3.3.2. ELISA Assay for Detecting Antibodies to Lactococcal-Expressed Antigen

1. Coat the wells of a 96-well microtiter plate with 50 μL recombinant protein (1 μg/mL diluted in carbonate/bicarbonate buffer. Cover microtiter plate and leave overnight at 4°C in a plastic box containing a damp paper towel.

2. Wash plates twice by briefly immersing in a container of PBS + 0.05% Tween 20 and then shaking the contents out of the wells over paper toweling. Pat the microtiter plate dry with 2–3 taps on a paper towel.

3. To prevent nonspecific antibody binding, incubate wells with 100 μL of 3% BSA in PBS + 0.05% Tween 20 for 1 h at room temperature.

4. Wash plates 3× as described in **step 2** and pat dry.

5. Add 50 μL pre-immune serum, diluted 1:50 in PBS + 0.05% Tween 20 to wells C1, D1, E1, F1 and G1 (these enable the calculation of end point titers). Add 50 μL primary test serum to the remaining wells. Start at a dilution of 1:40 (diluted in PBS + 0.05% Tween 20) increasing in a series of double dilutions (e.g. 1:40, 1:80, 1:160 continued along a row of the microtiter plate). Do not add primary antibody to well A2, as this will serve as the primary antibody negative control. Incubate the microtiter plate at room temperature for 90 min.

6. Wash wells by briefly soaking in PBS + 0.05% Tween 20 3× followed by two 3-min soaks. Pat dry.

7. Add 50 μL of alkaline phosphatase-conjugated secondary antibody, diluted 1:3000 in PBS + 0.05% Tween 20, to all wells except A1 (secondary antibody negative control and blank). Incubate the microtiter plate at room temperature for 90 min.

8. Wash wells by soaking in PBS + 0.05% Tween 20 briefly 3× followed by two 3-min soaks and pat dry.
9. To prepare substrate, dissolve one 5-mg tablet of nitrophenyl phosphate in 5 mL diethanolamine buffer. If using all 96 wells, make up two batches of substrate. Add 100 µL of substrate to each well then cover the microtiter plate with foil (the substrate is photo-sensitive) and incubate at room temperature for 30 min. Using a microtiter plate reader, measure the absorbance of each well at 405 nm. Use well A1 as the blank.
10. Plot A405 against primary antibody dilution (log scale). End point titer is the dilution of primary antibody, giving the same absorbance as the mean of the preimmune wells.

## 4. Notes

1. Use sterile Milli-Q water to dissolve the sucrose and glycerol. Sterilize by filtration.
2. M17 broth can be purchased from Difco. Dissolve 37.25 g M17 broth (and 15 g agar for M17 agar) in 950 mL of glass-distilled water. Prepare ten 95-mL aliquots and sterilise by autoclaving. Agar can be used directly or cooled and re-melted. To use, add 5 mL 10% glucose (final glucose concentration is 0.5%) to 95 mL medium plus appropriate antibiotic. Pour plates and allow them to dry. Store unused plates at 4°C.
3. A stock solution of Lysozyme can be prepared at 500 mg/mL and stored at –20°C. A stock solution of Mutanolysin can be prepared at 10U µL and stored at –20°C.
4. When using the Qiagen plasmid miniprep kit, aliquot an appropriate amount of resuspension buffer into a bijoux and add Lysozyme and Mutanolysin. This adaptation also works for the Promega miniprep kit, and is probably adaptable to other commercial miniprep kits.
5. Typically, precipitated DNA should be resuspended in 1/10 the volume of electro-competent cells that will be used for the transformation.
6. It is important not to centrifuge the cells too hard, as this will damage them.
7. If using liquid nitrogen to snap-freeze cells, make a needle hole in the microcentrifuge lid to allow air to escape.
8. If a bead-beater is not available, samples can be vortexed using a benchtop whirlimixer.
9. Alternatively, lysostaphin, at a final concentration of 2.5 mg/mL, can be used in place of mutanolysin.

## References

1. Bermudez-Humaran, L. G., Langella, P., Miyoshi, A., Gruss, A., Guerra, R. T., Montes de Oca-Luna, R., et al. (2002) Production of human papillomavirus type 16 E7 protein in *Lactococcus lactis*. *Appl. Environ. Microbiol.* **68,** 917–922.
2. Chatel, J. M., Langella, P., Adel-Patient, K., Commissaire, J., Wal, J. M., and Corthier, G. (2001) Induction of mucosal immune response after intranasal or oral inoculation of mice with *Lactococcus lactis* producing bovine beta-lactoglobulin. *Clin. Diagn. Lab. Immunol.* **8,** 545–551.
3. Enouf, V., Langella, P., Commissaire, J., Cohen, J., and Corthier, G. (2001) Bovine rotavirus nonstructural protein 4 produced by *Lactococcus lactis* is antigenic and immunogenic. *Appl. Environ. Microbiol.* **67,** 1423–1428.
4. Wells, J. M., Wilson, P. W., Norton, P. M., Gasson, M. J., and Le Page, R.W. (1993) *Lactococcus lactis*: high-level expression of tetanus toxin fragment C and protection against lethal challenge. *Mol. Microbiol.* **8,** 1155–1162.
5. Gilbert, C., Robinson, K., Le Page, R. W., and Wells, J. M. (2000) Heterologous expression of an immunogenic pneumococcal type 3 capsular polysaccharide in *Lactococcus lactis*. *Infect. Immun.* **68,** 3251–3260.

6. Ribeiro, L. A., Azevedo, V., Le Loir, Y., Oliveira, S. C., Dieye, Y., Piard, J. C., et al. (2002) Production and targeting of the *Brucella abortus* antigen L7/L12 in *Lactococcus lactis*: a first step towards food-grade live vaccines against brucellosis. *Appl. Environ. Microbiol.* **68,** 910–916.

7. Holmes, A. R., Gilbert, C., Wells, J. M., and Jenkinson, H. F. (1998) Binding properties of *Streptococcus gordonii* SspA and SspB (antigen I/II family) polypeptides expressed on the cell surface of *Lactococcus lactis* MG1363. *Infect. Immun.* **66,** 4633–4639.

8. Iwaki, M., Okahashi, N., Takahashi, I., Kanamoto, T., Sugita-Konishi, Y., Aibara, K., et al. (1990) Oral immunization with recombinant *Streptococcus lactis* carrying the *Streptococcus mutans* surface protein antigen gene. *Infect. Immun.* **58,** 2929–2934.

9. Wells, J. M., Robinson, K., Chamberlain, L. M., Schofield, K. M., and Le Page, R. W. (1996) Lactic acid bacteria as vaccine delivery vehicles. *Antonie Van Leeuwenhoek* **70,** 317–330.

10. Robinson, K., Chamberlain, L. M., Schofield, K. M., Wells, J. M., and Le Page, R. W. (1997) Oral vaccination of mice against tetanus with recombinant *Lactococcus lactis*. *Nat. Biotechnol.* **15,** 653–657.

11. Norton, P. M., Brown, H. W., Wells, J. M., Macpherson, A. M., Wilson, P. W., and Le Page, R. W. (1996) Factors affecting the immunogenicity of tetanus toxin fragment C expressed in *Lactococcus lactis*. *FEMS Immunol. Med. Microbiol.* **14,** 167–177.

12. Kruisselbrink, A., Heijne Den Bak-Glashouwer, M. J., Havenith, C. E., Thole, J. E., and Janssen, R. (2001) Recombinant *Lactobacillus plantarum* inhibits house dust mite-specific T-cell responses. *Clin. Exp. Immunol.* **126,** 2–8.

13. Djordjevic, G. M. and Klaenhammer, T. R., (1998) Inducible gene expression systems in *Lactococcus lactis*. *Mol. Biotechnol.* **9,** 127–139.

14. Kuipers, O. P., de Ruyter, P. G., Kleerebezem, M., and de Vos, W. M. (1997) Controlled overproduction of proteins by lactic acid bacteria. *Trends Biotechnol.* **15,** 135–140.

15. Wells, J. M. and Schofield, K. M. (1996) Cloning and expression vectors for lactococci, in *Lactic acid bacteria: current advances in metabolism, genetics, and applications.* (Bozoglu, T. F. and Ray, B., eds.), NATO ASI Series. Springer-Verlag: Berlin, Germany, pp. 37–62.

16. Waterfield, N. R., Le Page, R. W., Wilson, P. W., and Wells, J. M. (1995) The isolation of lactococcal promoters and their use in investigating bacterial luciferase synthesis in *Lactococcus lactis*. *Gene* **165,** 9–15.

17. Robinson, K., Chamberlain, L. M., Schofield, K. M., Wells, J. M., and Le Page, R. W. F. (1995) Oral vaccination of mice with recombinant *Lactococcus lactis* expressing tetanus toxin fragment C elicits both secretory and protective high level systemic immune responses. *Immunology* **86: Suppl. 1,** 27.

18. van der Meer, J. R., Poolman, J., Beerthuyzen, M. M., Siezen, R. J., Kuipers, O. P., and De Vos, W. M. (1993) Characterization of the *Lactococcus lactis* nisin A operon genes *nisP*, encoding a subtilisin-like serine protease involved in precursor processing, and *nisR*, encoding a regulatory protein involved in nisin biosynthesis. *J. Bacteriol.* **175,** 2578–2588.

19. Kuipers, O. P., Beerthuyzen, M. M., Siezen, R. J., and De Vos, W. M. (1993) Characterization of the nisin gene cluster *nisABTCIPR* of *Lactococcus lactis*. Requirement of expression of the *nisA* and *nisI* genes for development of immunity. *Eur. J. Biochem.* **216,** 281–291.

20. de Vos, W. M., Kuipers, O. P., van der Meer, J. R., and Siezen, R. J. (1995) Maturation pathway of nisin and other lantibiotics: post-translationally modified antimicrobial peptides exported by gram-positive bacteria. *Mol. Microbiol.* **17,** 427–437.

21. Dodd, H. M., Horn, N., Chan, W. C., Giffard, C. J., Bycroft, B. W., Roberts, G. C., and Gasson, M. J. (1996) Molecular analysis of the regulation of nisin immunity. *Microbiology* **142,** 2385–2392.
22. de Ruyter, P. G., Kuipers, O. P., and de Vos, W. M. (1996) Controlled gene expression systems for *Lactococcus lactis* with the food-grade inducer nisin. *Appl. Environ. Microbiol.* **62,** 3662–3667.
23. de Ruyter, P. G., Kuipers, O. P., Beerthuyzen, M. M., van Alen-Boerrigter, I., and de Vos, W. M. (1996) Functional analysis of promoters in the nisin gene cluster of *Lactococcus lactis*. *J. Bacteriol.* **178,** 3434–3439.
24. Pavan, S., Hols, P., Delcour, J., Geoffroy, M. C., Grangette, C., Kleerebezem, M., and Mercenier, A. (2000) Adaptation of the nisin-controlled expression system in *Lactobacillus plantarum*: a tool to study *in vivo* biological effects. *Appl. Environ. Microbiol.* **66,** 4427–4432.
25. Kleerebezem, M., Beerthuyzen, M. M., Vaughan, E. E., de Vos, W. M., and Kuipers, O. P. (1997) Controlled gene expression systems for lactic acid bacteria: transferable nisin-inducible expression cassettes for *Lactococcus, Leuconostoc*, and *Lactobacillus spp. Appl. Environ. Microbiol.* **63,** 4581–4584.
26. Steidler, L., Robinson, K., Chamberlain, L., Schofield, K. M., Remaut, E., Le Page, R. W., and Wells, J. M. (1998) Mucosal delivery of murine interleukin-2 (IL-2) and IL-6 by recombinant strains of *Lactococcus lactis* coexpressing antigen and cytokine. *Infect. Immun.* **66,** 3183–3189.
27. van Asseldonk, M., Rutten, G., Oteman, M., Siezen, R. J., de Vos, W. M., and Simons, G. (1990) Cloning of usp45, a gene encoding a secreted protein from *Lactococcus lactis* subsp. *lactis* MG1363. *Gene* **95,** 155–160.
28. Sambrook, J., Fritsch, E. F., and Maniatis, T. (eds.) (1989) *Molecluar Cloning: A Laboratory Manual*, 2nd ed., Cold Spring Harbor Laboratory Press, Cold Spring Harbor, NY.
29. Wells, J. M., Wilson, P. W., and Le Page, R. W. (1993) Improved cloning vectors and transformation procedure for *Lactococcus lactis*. *J. Appl. Bacteriol.* **74,** 629–636.
30. Gussow, D. and Clackson, T. (1989) Direct clone characterization from plaques and colonies by the polymerase chain reaction. *Nucleic Acids Res.* **17,** 4000.
31. Laemmli, U. K. (1970) Cleavage of structural proteins during the assembly of the head of bacteriophage T4. *Nature* **227,** 680–685.
32. Towbin, H., Staehelin, T., and Gordon, J. (1979) Electrophoretic transfer of proteins from polyacrylamide gels to nitrocellulose sheets: procedure and some applications. *Proc. Natl. Acad. Sci. USA* **76,** 4350–4354.

# 8

# Synthetic Peptides

## Michael J. Francis

## 1. Introduction
### 1.1. A Brief History

Efforts to produce more stable and defined vaccines have focused on a detailed analysis of the immune response to many infectious diseases in order to identify the antigenic sites on the pathogens that are involved in stimulating protective immunity. Armed with this knowledge, it is possible to mimic such sites by producing short chains of amino acids (peptides), and to use these as the basis for novel vaccines. The earliest documented work on peptide immunization is actually for a plant virus—the tobacco mosaic virus. In 1963, Anderer (1) demonstrated that rabbit antibodies to an isolated hexapeptide fragment from the virus-coat protein coupled to bovine serum albumin (BSA) would neutralize the infectious virus in culture. Two yr later, he used a synthetically produced copy of the same peptide to confirm this observation. This was pioneering work, and it was more than 10 years before the next example of a peptide that elicited antivirus antibody appeared, following work by Sela and his colleagues (2) on a virus—MS2 bacteriophage—which infects bacteria. The emergence of more accessible techniques for sequencing proteins in 1977, coupled with the ability to readily synthesize peptides already developed in 1963, heralded a decade of intensive research into experimental peptide vaccines. The first demonstration that peptides could elicit protective immunity in vivo, in addition to neutralizing activity in vitro, was obtained using a peptide from the VP1 coat protein of foot-and-mouth-disease virus (FMDV) in 1982, with the guinea pig as a laboratory animal model (3,4). This finding was subsequently supported by the demonstration of protective immunity in cattle and pigs (5,6). Such protective immunity has also been demonstrated in dogs (7) and mink (8) following immunization with a synthetic canine parvovirus vaccine. Thus, peptides have now been used to elicit immune responses against a wide variety of pathogens, including some for which more conventional vaccine approaches have not yet proven to be successful (9).

From: *Methods in Molecular Medicine, Vol. 87: Vaccine Protocols, 2nd ed.*
Edited by: A. Robinson, M. J. Hudson, and M. P. Cranage © Humana Press Inc., Totowa, NJ

## 1.2. Advantages of Peptide Vaccines

The advantages of peptide-based vaccines are numerous. The peptides are chemically defined, can be stored as a freeze-dried powder, are stable indefinitely, and no infectious material is involved in their manufacture. Furthermore, they can be designed to stimulate an appropriate protective immune response against specific sites on an antigen and, with minor changes to the primary sequence, by using peptide mixtures or by use of conserved sequences, they can stimulate broad immunity to cover different strains or serotypes of a pathogen *(10,11)*. They also provide the opportunity to enhance the immune response by using various novel adjuvants that cannot be used with many conventional vaccines because of their labile nature *(12)*, for targeting or directing the immunogen at important sites within the body in order to elicit a predetermined immune response, and for developing delayed or triggered release systems in order to remove the requirement for booster vaccination. In addition to the more traditional routes of vaccination, synthetic peptides have been shown to be effective following intranasal (in) *(13–15)*, oral *(16)*, and transdermal delivery *(15,17)*. From the manufacturer's perspective, peptides should reduce the need for a large-scale production plant and for complex downstream processing. In essence, they offer the opportunity to move vaccines from the biological arena to the pharmaceutical arena.

A wide variety of techniques is currently available to synthesize peptides and enhance their immunogenicity for formulation as a vaccine. The choice of technique adopted will vary with—and depend on—the particular peptide being studied. It is not possible in this chapter to provide detailed protocols for all the available techniques. Thus, the methodology and techniques for peptide synthesis, choice of carrier protein and identification of Th-cell epitopes will be discussed in more general terms, identifying advantages and disadvantages of the various techniques when appropriate. The techniques for linking B-cell epitopes and Th-cell epitopes are discussed in detail (*see* **Subheading 3.4.3.**). In addition, examples of experiments to enhance the immunogenicity of an FMDV peptide by adding foreign Th-cell determinants and by forming multimeric peptides are described.

## 2. Materials

The following materials are required for the detailed protocol of methods to link B- and T-cell epitopes (*see* **Subheading 3.4.3.**).

1. Phosphate-buffered saline (PBS), pH 7.2.
2. 25% glutaraldehyde (Sigma, St. Louis, MO).
3. Distilled water.
4. m-Maleimidobenzoyl-*N*-hydroxysuccinimide ester (MBS) (Pierce Chemical Co., Rockford, IL).
5. Dimethylformamide (DMF) (Sigma).
6. 10 m*M* sodium phosphate buffer, pH 7.0.
7. 50 m*M* sodium phosphate buffer, pH 6.0.
8. Low mol wt dialysis tubing.
9. Freeze dryer.
10. Sephadex G-25 column (Pharmacia, Piscataway, NJ).
11. Bio Gel P-2 (Bio-Rad laboratories, Richmond, CA).
12. High-performance liquid chromatography (HPLC) apparatus.

## 3. Methods

### 3.1. Peptide Synthesis

Peptides required for such studies can be readily synthesized using standard solid-phase protocols involving *tert*-butoxy-carbonyl (t-Boc) *(18)* and 9-fluorenylmethoxycarbonyl (Fmoc) *(19)* chemistry. Moreover, recent developments in synthetic peptide production involving the compartmentalization of resins into small packets have greatly facilitated the production of large numbers of peptides for experimental analysis *(20)*. It is not appropriate for this chapter to discuss the methodology for such synthesis in detail, since the focus is on the application of the technology to vaccination.

### 3.2. Mimotopes

The technique commonly known as mimotope production is a novel method for producing peptides that match the binding site of an important functional antibody *(21)*. It can use either random libraries of peptides for screening *(22,23)* or the more selective process of amino acid substitution *(24)*. Such a procedure can be used to define functional discontinuous epitopes that would not normally be detected by simply referring to the linear sequence of a protein molecule. An example of this technique being successfully used to identify an 8-amino acid mimotope that will induce a protective immune response is provided by work on the parasite *Schistosoma mansoni (25)*.

### 3.3. The Use of Carrier Proteins

There is little doubt that carrier proteins still offer the most straightforward and convenient way of presenting poorly immunogenic peptides to the immune system. This may be achieved either by chemical linkage of synthetic peptides to "foreign" protein molecules or by direct linkage for expression as recombinant fusion proteins (the latter method is not discussed in this chapter). However, it should be recognized that the method used to link the peptide to the carrier could greatly influence both the quantitative and qualitative nature of the immune response observed.

The classical role of a carrier protein in immunology is to provide T-cell help for B-cell antibody production to a poor/non-immunogenic antigen or hapten. For peptide delivery, carrier proteins are also generally used to recruit T-cell help for poorly immunogenic B-cell epitopes. However, in some cases, the peptides may be immunogenic in their own right because of the presence of B- and T-cell epitopes within the same sequence, and the carrier molecule is simply acting as a polymeric delivery system. In addition, peptide carriers may act by increasing the molecular mass of the peptide, and thus improve the uptake by antigen-presenting cells (APCs). Small peptides generally have a very short half-life within the body, which may be prolonged by linkage to carrier protein.

Thus, peptide carriers may actually function in a number of different ways, but their overall role is to increase the immunogenicity of the peptide, and thus assist in producing an antibody response against the peptide in vivo.

### 3.3.1. Factors to Consider Before Coupling a Peptide to a Carrier Protein

When selecting a suitable carrier, there are a number of important points that should be considered. These are as follows:

### 3.3.1.1. Purpose of Coupling

What is the reason for coupling? Is it simply to elicit a high-titer anti-peptide antibody response or to immunize an animal against infection? Does the peptide require a carrier? This last point is well-illustrated by a study carried out with a foot-and-mouth-disease (FMD) serotype SAT2 peptide *(26)*, in which coupling of the peptide to a carrier via a carboxy-terminal cysteine residue reduced immunogenicity and abolished its ability to elicit neutralizing antibodies against the virus.

### 3.3.1.2. Nature of the Peptide

Study the primary sequence of the peptide. Is it hydrophilic or hydrophobic? Are certain residues likely to be important for its antigenicity? Will these residues be affected or masked by coupling to a carrier? Are cysteine residues that may form disulfide bridges present?

### 3.3.1.3. Choice of Carrier

It is vital to remember that an immune response will be raised against the carrier as well as the peptide. Will you use a natural or artificial carrier? Should the carrier come from the same organism as the peptide? Should it be a common protein or an unusual protein? Is there a risk of eliciting autoimmunity or hypersensitivity? Will antibodies to the carrier interfere with subsequent in vitro analysis? Is there a possibility that prepriming against the carrier has occurred?

### 3.3.1.4. Method of Conjugation

Some of the most commonly used methods of conjugation will have a significant effect on the antigenicity of many peptides (*see* **Subheading 3.3.3.**). It is therefore important to consider what effect the conjugation procedure will have and how you wish to present the peptide to the immune system. The peptide-to-carrier ratio can also be very important.

### 3.3.1.5. Method of Immunization

A number of factors can affect the qualitative and quantitative immune response following peptide-carrier immunization. These include the route of immunization, dose, choice of adjuvant, frequency, interval between primary and subsequent booster inoculations, age, and sex.

### 3.3.1.6. Species

The choice of species can have a marked effect on the nature of the anti-peptide antibodies produced. The response in laboratory animals may be very different from the response in target species for a vaccine. Differences may also be observed between different species of laboratory animal and even different strains within a species. Wherever possible, appropriate inbred strains of animals should be used.

### 3.3.2. Commonly Used Carriers

Traditional carriers include proteins, such as keyhole limpet hemocyanin (KLH) and sperm whale myoglobin (SWM). These are generally chosen because they are likely to be foreign to the species being immunized and are unlikely to elicit crossreactive or interfering antibodies. They are also well-established model immunogens and, as is the case of SWM, they have been extensively characterized. Interestingly, KLH has also been used in a number of studies in humans with no obvious side effects *(27)*. Other common carriers include albumins, such as bovine serum albumin (BSA) and ovalbumin. These appear to work well and are freely available. However, it should be noted that they are also commonly used as blocking proteins in immunoassays. Such assays would thus have to be modified for screening anti-peptide antisera generated with these carriers. Furthermore, since anti-peptide antibodies are commonly used for screening mixtures of proteins—for example, by Western blotting—the anticarrier antibodies may crossreact. This is particularly important if bovine serum is used to culture an organism and BSA is used as the carrier. Other possible carriers that have been used successfully in the past include bacterial toxoids, such as tetanus toxoid and diptheria toxoid, and other bacterial proteins used in vaccines, such as Purified Protein Derivative from BCG *(28)*. One of the reasons for this is that a preprimed human population will exist that may produce an enhanced response to the peptide or hapten linked to the same carrier *(29)*. However, other reports suggest that no prepriming occurs *(30)*, or even that active suppression may be the result *(31)*. Clearly, this must be studied on a case-by-case basis.

### 3.3.3. Coupling Methods

A wide range of methods now exist for coupling peptides to protein carriers. Perhaps the most popular method, because of its simplicity, is to use glutaraldehyde. However, this is relatively uncontrolled and may under certain circumstances involve primary reactions with α-amino groups, ε-amino groups on lysine residues, and sulfhydryl groups on cysteine residues, as well as secondary reactions with phenolic hydroxyl groups on tyrosine residues and imidazole groups on histidine residues. Therefore, if Lys, Cys, Tyr, or His residues are involved in antigenic sites on the peptide, these may be significantly altered by this coupling method. The use of heterobifunctional crosslinkers can largely overcome this problem by facilitating specific linkages. For example, the crosslinker MBS has an amino-reactive *N*-hydroxysuccinimide (NHS)-ester as one functional group and a sulfhydryl reactive group as the other. Amino groups on the carrier are acylated with the NHS-ester via the hydroxysuccinimide group, and then a peptide is introduced that possesses a free sulfhydryl group that can react with the malemide group of the coupling reagent. This may require synthesis of a specific peptide with a non-natural cysteine residue added to its carboxy- or amino-terminus, or indeed anywhere else within the sequence. By using this technique the orientation of the peptide may be altered. The effect of peptide orientation on the immune response is well-illustrated by the work of Dyrberg and Oldstone *(32)*. In this study, peptide linked via its amino-terminus elicited antibodies that would only recognize amino-linked peptide in vitro, and vice versa for the carboxy-linked peptide. A further study examined the effect of oxime, thioester, and disulfide bond formation on the biological activity of a peptide *(33)*. Thus, linkage can have a marked influence on the specificity of the antipeptide antibody response in vivo.

### 3.3.4. Guidelines for Delivery

Although it is difficult to provide any firm guidelines for peptide delivery, an attempt has been made to compare published data in order to reach a consensus *(34)*. The results of this study are as follows:

1. Peptides should be 10–15 residues long. In the experience of this author, longer peptides of 20–30 residues often make the best immunogens for vaccine purposes.
2. Peptides can be positively or negatively charged, but should be hydrophilic.
3. In this limited comparison, BSA was a better carrier than KLH, but in practice it may be worth trying a range of carriers for any given antigen, and BSA may not be the best choice (*see* **Subheading 3.3.2.**).
4. MBS is better than glutaraldehyde or carbodimide. It is also likely to be a more controlled process (*see* **Subheading 3.3.3.**).
5. Finally C- or N-terminal sequences of a protein may be the best first choice for raising antiprotein antibodies.

### 3.3.5. Potential Problems

Although chemical coupling offers a quick and convenient method for presenting peptides in a more immunogenic form, a number of potential problems should be recognized. The coupling process is often poorly defined, and the reaction is difficult to control. As a result, the reproducibility from batch to batch is likely to be poor. There is also a strong risk of actually masking important antigenic sites and of modifying the peptides during the coupling process. Problems of carrier-induced suppression and hypersensitivity to the carrier may also be encountered.

## 3.4. Methods for Adding T-Cell Epitopes to Peptides

In the past, it was generally assumed that, because of their relatively small molecular size, many synthetic peptides would behave like haptens and would require coupling to a large "foreign" protein carrier to enhance their immunogenicity. Immunization with such conjugates often resulted in the production of anti-peptide antibodies that totally failed to recognize the native protein or infectious agent because of the method of peptide-carrier linkage (*see* **Subheading 3.3.1.**).

It was the goal of many immunologists to dispense with such poorly defined carrier proteins and to produce a totally synthetic immunogen. It is now clear that synthetic peptides can be highly immunogenic in their free form, provided that they contain appropriate antibody recognition sites (B-cell epitopes) as well as sites capable of eliciting help for antibody production (Th-cell epitopes). These Th-cell epitopes must be capable of binding class II major histocompatibility complex (MHC) molecules on the surface of host antigen-presenting cells (APC) and B-cells, and of subsequently interacting with the T-cell receptor in the form of a tri-molecular complex in order to induce B-cells to differentiate and proliferate. Indeed, there are good examples—such as the

141–160 sequence from VP1 of FMDV—of peptides that contain B- and Th-cell epitopes, which undoubtedly account to a large extent for their success as immunogens *(35,36)*. However, if a free peptide is a poor immunogen or produces an immune response that is genetically restricted, appropriate Th-cell epitopes may be added.

### 3.4.1. Identification of Class II Th-Cell Epitopes

A number of Th-cell epitopes has been defined from a wide range of proteins and infectious agents. Such epitopes may be used to improve the immunogenicity of a peptide in order to raise anti-peptide antibodies for experimental purposes, despite the fact that they will come from "foreign" proteins. A good example would be the use of an H-$2^d$ restricted Th-cell epitope to facilitate the production of monoclonal antibodies (MAbs) against an important peptide sequence in Balb/c mice. Th-cell epitopes from "foreign" proteins may also be used for vaccines in situations in which protective levels of antibody must be maintained by repeated inoculation of the population at risk; for example, FMDV prophylaxis requires regular revaccination at intervals of 6–12 mo.

In situations in which memory responses are required for effective immunity, natural Th-cell epitopes from the infectious agent should be used. There are few shortcuts in identifying these sites and generally a detailed analysis of component proteins, protein fragments, and peptides, using in vitro T-cell stimulation techniques, will be required to identify appropriate sequences. However, there are now two published algorithms that appear to improve the chances of selecting appropriate peptide sequences with T-cell-stimulating activity from the primary sequence of a protein. The first, proposed by DeLisi and Berzofsky *(37)*, suggests that T-cell sites tend to be amphipathic structures—i.e., molecules that possess opposing hydrophobic and hydrophilic domains—which are frequently in the form of an α helix. The originators of this hypothesis have published a computer program to assist in the identification of amphipathic helices from the primary amino-acid sequence of a protein. The second method, proposed by Rothbard *(38)*, suggests that each T-cell epitope has within it a sequence composed of either a charged residue or glycine, followed by two hydrophobic residues, and, in many cases, the next residue is charged or polar. This algorithm has subsequently been refined to consider further residues flanking the two central hydrophobic amino acids and to suggest possible subpatterns responsible for the genetic restriction of an epitope *(39)*. Another method for identification of potential Th-cell epitopes is to study the ability of a peptide to bind to the Class II MHC antigen *(40)*. By using a variety of predictive methodologies, a broadly crossreactive Th-cell peptide has been identified from the fusion protein of measles virus *(41)* that stimulates both mouse and human lymphocytes.

### 3.4.2. Identification of Class I CTL Epitopes

Cytotoxic T-lymphocyte (CTL) epitopes are generally presented on the surface of cells in the context of Class I MHC antigen. The peptides that bind to Class I MHC antigen are typically 8–10 residues in length and representative of linear sequences on the native protein molecule. There are distinct sequence motifs that are associated with binding to Class I MHC antigen *(42)*, and these can be used to predict potential epitopes from a known protein sequence. CTL epitopes can also be identified by screening primed cell populations using sets of overlapping peptides *(43)*. Once identified, synthetic peptides representing CTL epitopes may be delivered in an appropriate manner in order to elicit an antigen-specific CTL response in vivo *(44–46)*

### 3.4.3. Methods of Linking B- and T-Cell Epitopes

Once identified, it is important that the appropriate Th-cell epitope(s) is linked to the B-cell epitope peptide to facilitate internalization by the B-cell and representation on the surface in association with class II MHC molecules. However, studies have indicated that covalent linkage of the B- and T-cell epitopes is not necessary for the generation of T-cell-dependent antibody responses to non-immunogenic B-cell epitopes, provided that they are co-immunized *(47)*. Three methods of linkage have been successfully used to date.

#### 3.4.3.1. GLUTARALDEHYDE POLYMERIZATION

The glutaraldehyde method involves copolymerization of a B-cell peptide with a T-cell peptide via their amino groups.

1. Dissolve equal weights of T-cell and B-cell peptides in phosphate-buffered saline (PBS) to produce a 2 mg/mL solution.
2. Add a stock solution of 25% glutaraldehyde (Sigma, St. Louis, MO) in water slowly with continuous stirring to yield a final concentration of 2.63 m$M$.
3. Stir the mixture overnight at room temperature in the dark.
4. Dialyze the resulting polymer extensively against distilled water, using dialysis tubing with a low-mol-wt retention capacity in order to avoid loss of the peptide.
5. The material can then be lyophilized and weighed.

The main disadvantages of this approach are the uncontrolled nature of the reaction and the risk of affecting the antigenic nature of the peptides. For example, glutaraldehyde may completely abolish the antigenicity of peptides containing key lysine residues. Nevertheless, this method has been used to link a streptococcal peptide, containing B- and T-cell epitopes, to a hepatitis B virus (HBV) peptide, which contained only a B-cell epitope, thus making the hepatitis peptide immunogenic in Balb/c mice *(48)*.

#### 3.4.3.2. CONJUGATION WITH THE HETEROBIFUNCTIONAL CROSSLINKING REAGENT MBS

The crosslinker MBS has an amino-reactive NHS-ester as one functional group and a sulfhydryl reactive group as the other. Amino groups on one peptide, A (e.g., B-cell epitope), are acylated with the NHS-ester via the hydroxysuccinimide group, and then a second peptide, B (e.g., the T-cell epitope), that possesses a free sulfhydryl group that can react with the maleimide group of the coupling reagent, is introduced. This may require the synthesis of a specific peptide with a non-natural cysteine residue added to its carboxy-terminus. Conjugation is carried out as follows.

1. Slowly add 5.7 mg of MBS (Pierce Chemical Co., Rockford, IL) in 380 µL DMF to 15 mg of peptide A in 1.5 mL of 10 m$M$ sodium phosphate buffer, pH 7.0.
2. Stir the mixture for 30 min at room temperature.

3. Separate the *m*-maleimidobenzoyl peptide (MB-peptide) from the unreacted MBS by desalting on a column of Sephadex G-25 (Pharmacia, Piscataway, NJ) in 50 m*M* sodium phosphate buffer, pH 6.0.
4. Mix the resulting MB-peptide pool with 15 mg of peptide B, possessing a carboxy-terminal cysteine, in 15 mL of PBS, pH 7.2.
5. Stir the mixture at room temperature for 3 h.
6. Desalt the final conjugate on a column of BioGel P-2 (Bio-Rad Laboratories, Richmond, CA), analyze for purity by reversed-phase HPLC, and determine its amino acid composition.

Once again, it should be noted that the presence of key lysine residues, or a natural cysteine in peptide A, or the presence of a natural cysteine within peptide B, is likely to affect the nature and final antigenicity of the conjugate produced. This method has been used to link the malaria-encoded sequence (NANP) from the circumsporozoite protein, which will elicit an antibody response in, and stimulate T-cells from, mice carrying the I-A$^b$ gene, to an amphipathic helical segment from residues 326–343 of the same protein. The resultant conjugate raised anti-(NANP) antibodies in H-2$^k$ mice that are nonresponders to the (NANP) sequence alone *(49)*.

### 3.4.3.3. COLINEAR SYNTHESIS OF B- AND TH-CELL PEPTIDES

Problems encountered with the methods covered in **Subheadings 3.4.3.1** and **3.4.3.2** . involving glutaraldehyde or MBS may be overcome by colinear synthesis of a peptide containing B- and Th-cell epitopes. This method enables a peptide to be constructed with known immunological properties. It also provides flexibility to enable the position of one epitope to be altered in relation to the other and to synthesize peptides containing a number of B- and/or T-cell epitopes. As a technique, it has been successfully used to overcome nonresponsiveness in defined strains of mice to a bovine rotavirus peptide *(50)*, a foot-and-mouth-disease virus (FMDV) peptide *(51)*, a hepatitis B virus (HBV) envelope peptide *(52)* and a measles virus peptide *(53)*. The principle of colinear synthesis combined with polymerization via disulfide bonding has been applied to what may be the first successful vaccine against malaria *(54)*.

## 3.5. An Immunization Study Using FMDV Peptides with Added Foreign Th-Cell Determinants

A good example of the colinear synthesis approach to peptide immunization is provided by work on a 20-amino acid peptide from FMDV *(51)*. This 141–160 sequence from the VP1 protein of the virus induces a protective immune response, contains B- and Th-cell epitopes, and shows an H-2$^k$-restricted response in inbred mice when inoculated with Freund's incomplete adjuvant (FIA). Therefore, it was a suitable candidate to determine whether the immune response could be broadened to other mouse strains by adding further Th-cell epitopes. From the literature, three suitable T-cell epitopes were chosen that were active in H-2$^d$ nonresponders, one from ovalbumin contained within the sequence 323–339 (OVA) and two from sperm whale myoglobin (SWM) contained within the sequences 132–148 (SWMI) and 105–121 (SWMII). Peptides were synthesized with the FMDV VP1 141–160 sequence followed at the carboxy-terminus by one of these "foreign" T-cell epitopes ending with a carboxy-terminal cysteine residue, which has been shown to enhance the immunogenicity of uncoupled FMDV peptide. As a control, a fourth peptide was synthesized with the FMDV VP1 141–160 sequence followed by a further 17 residues from VP1 and a carboxy-terminal cysteine.

Groups of eight inbred B10.BR (H-$2^k$), B10.D2 (H-$2^d$), and Balb/c (H-$2^d$) mice were inoculated intramuscularly with 0.2 mL of solutions containing 25 mmol of one of the experimental peptide preparations (FMDV 141–177 alone, FMDV 141–160 + OVA, FMDV 141–160 + SWMI, and FMDV 141–160 + SWMII) emulsified with an equal volume of FIA. Each mouse was bled before inoculation and at regular 14-d intervals for 2 mo. Reinoculation can also be carried out at this stage to study the memory response. Serum was separated from each blood sample and stored at –20°C until needed.

Anti-FMDV peptide 141–160 was determined in each sample using an indirect enzyme-linked immunosorbent assay (ELISA). The results obtained 42 d after inoculation demonstrated that all four peptides were immunogenic in the B10.BR (H-$2^k$) mice. These results were expected, because this strain had previously been shown to be a high responder to the 141–160 sequence. In contrast, the B10.D2 and Balb/c (H-$2^d$) strains failed to respond to the extended FMDV sequence alone. The addition of the further 17 natural residues from VP1 had not overcome the nonresponsiveness of these strains to the 141–160 sequence. However, each of the peptides with an added foreign T-cell epitope did induce an anti-peptide 141–160 response at 42 d in the H-$2^d$ mice Therefore, T-cell epitopes from ovalbumin and SWM were capable of overcoming genetic restriction and of helping to induce an antibody response to the FMDV peptide.

Having determined that nonresponder H-$2^d$ mice produced an anti-peptide response when inoculated with the 141–160 peptide plus a foreign T-cell epitope, it was then necessary to determine whether these antibodies had virus-neutralizing activity. Once again, the B10.BR mice responded to all the peptides, giving neutralizing antibody levels of between 1.5 and 2.3 log. However, neutralizing antibodies were only produced in the B10.D2 and Balb/c mice that had been inoculated with peptides that included OVA or SWMI T-cell epitopes. The antipeptide antibodies produced to the peptide with the SWMII T-cell epitopes did not have virus-neutralizing activity. Although these results demonstrated that virus-neutralizing antibody responses can be produced in nonresponder H-$2^d$ mice using peptides with foreign Th-cell epitopes, they also showed that the choice of epitope or its location in relation to the B-cell epitope is important. Other studies have confirmed that flanking sequences (55) and epitope polarity (56) can influence the antigenicity and immunogenicity of chimeric peptides.

### 3.6. Multimeric and Cyclic Presentation of Peptides

The FMDV peptide has also provided an excellent model for the study of peptide presentation. The peptide was known to be immunogenic in the absence of a carrier protein, provided it was polymerized either by crosslinking with glutaraldehyde or oxidized in air after addition of a cysteine residue on each terminus (57). The free peptide was also immunogenic when delivered in small unilamellar liposomes (35). A number of synthetic derivatives has since been prepared and subsequently tested for their immunogenicity. Initially, the role of a non-natural terminal cysteine residue was examined by comparing the immunogenicity in FIA of the 141–160 peptide (which contains B- and Th-cell epitopes), with that of the 141–160 peptide plus an additional C-terminal cysteine residue (141–160 Cys ), and 141–l60 Cys with an *S*-acetamido-methyl thiol-blocking group on the cysteine (141–160 Cys [Acm]) *(34)*. No primary neutralizing antibody response was seen following a 100-µg dose of the 141–160 peptide. However, the incorporation of a non-natural unblocked cysteine residue at the C-terminus resulted in a primary neutralizing antibody response. If the thiol group on the cysteine was blocked as in the 141–160 Cys (Acm) peptide, no such response was seen. Thus, the presence of a C-terminal cysteine with a free thiol group greatly enhanced the immunogenicity of free 141–160 peptide in IFA.

The presence of a free thiol cysteine residue is likely to result in the formation of peptide dimers that may have a more ordered secondary structure, cause crosslinking of B-cell receptors, and/or lead to the formation of immune complex in vivo. To test whether a fixed dimer form of the peptide was immunogenic, the monomer 141–160 Cys was crosslinked with *N*,*N*-1,-4-phenylenedimaleimide via free sulfhydryls to produce stable dimer peptides that were purified by HPLC. The immune response of guinea pigs to these crosslinked dimers was indistinguishable from that obtained with air-oxidized disulfide dimers using a 100-µg dose of each peptide in FIA. Therefore, it was concluded that the dimer form of the peptide was responsible for its increased immunogenicity and not simply the presence of a free sulfhydryl group *(58)*.

Following the observation that FMDV peptide disulfide dimers were more immunogenic than monomers, dimer peptides in the form of tandem repeats were synthesized with or without a C-terminal cysteine residue. The immunogenicity of these tandem repeats (137–162 Cys [×2] and 137–162 Gly [×2]) was compared with that of a single-copy 137–163 Cys peptide. The results of this study demonstrated that tandem repeats of the FMDV peptide were generally more immunogenic than single-copy disulfide dimers, and that the addition of a cysteine residue—which could result in the formation of disulfide tetramer structures—may also improve the response further *(58)*. The enhanced activity of similar tandem-repeat peptides from single serotypes of FMDV, as well as double serotypes (O and A), has also been reported *(26)*.

In order to exploit fully the concept of multiple-copy synthetic peptides, the Multiple Antigenic Peptide (MAP) system was studied *(59,60)*. This system provides a method for direct solid-phase synthesis of a peptide antigen onto a branching lysine backbone, and has been used to produce several polylysine octamer constructs *(61)*. Levels of neutralizing antibody responses known to protect guinea pigs against challenge infection with FMDV *(62)* were obtained following a single inoculation of 0.8–4 µg of the octameric or tetrameric form of the peptide in IFA, whereas 20 µg of the lysine dimer were required to produce a similar level of antibody *(63)*. A monomeric preparation did not evoke measurable levels of neutralizing antibody at doses up to 20 µg. On a weight-for-weight basis, octamer peptides appeared to be 25- to 50-fold more immunogenic than disulfide dimers. Another interesting feature of the MAPs was their ability to elicit significant levels of neutralizing antibodies following two inoculations with aluminum hydroxide *(63)*, the only adjuvant currently licensed for use in humans.

FMDV peptides had previously been shown to be poorly immunogenic when inoculated with this adjuvant *(36)* unless they were coupled to a protein carrier *(35)*. Therefore, in this respect, the octameric MAP was behaving like a carrier-linked peptide, possibly because of its improved adsorption to aluminum hydroxide when compared with that of the 141–160 Cys disulfide dimer. A MAP peptide has even been successfully used to immunize fish *(64)*.

In order for a peptide to be used successfully as a vaccine, it must stimulate the appropriate B-cells in order to elicit antibodies that will recognize native pathogen and neutralize its infectivity. This relies to a large extent on the peptide adopting an appropriate structure or shape that correctly mimics antigenic determinants on the pathogen. Certain linear peptides have been very successful in this respect, although the activity of these peptides can be further improved by the addition of non-natural cysteine residues to the natural sequence, the presentation of multiple copies, or the inclusion of other parts of the natural virus B-cell epitope within the same peptide. Peptides can also be fixed into a loop structure (cyclized) in order to represent more closely structured antigenic determinants on a pathogen. This has been successfully achieved for hepatitis B *(65)*, influenza *(66)*, and polio *(67)* virus peptides by placing cysteine residues at each end of the peptide and allowing the formation of a disulfide bond between them. The resultant anti-peptide antibody has an enhanced binding activity (functional affinity) for the virus. Other groups have attempted to produce more ordered structure in synthetic peptides by chemical modification of a linear sequence. Thus, by substitution of putative hydrogen bonds with covalent mimics, nucleation sites for α-helix formation or type-1 reverse turns may be created within the peptide *(68)*.

## 3.7. Conclusions

Our knowledge of peptide immunochemistry has increased greatly since the first observations in 1963 that peptides could raise neutralizing antibodies *(69)*. It is now possible to deliver structured peptides and multiple-copy peptides, to dispense with carriers by incorporating B- and Th-cell sites, and to use defined recombinant carriers that enable the immunogenicity of the peptide to approach that of the whole virus. Peptides have been produced from nearly all the major viruses *(9)* plus a number of important bacterial and parasite antigens *(70)*. In addition, synthetic peptides offer a real opportunity to develop immunotherapeutic vaccines against cancer *(71,72)* and allergy *(73)*. As our ability to screen for active peptides and to present them to the immune system in a more defined manner improves, the possibilities for their use as vaccines will further increase. When one considers their numerous potential advantages over existing products, combined with the ability to adapt a vaccine to meet specific needs, and the opportunity to move vaccines from the biological arena to the pharmaceutical arena, peptides offer significant opportunities.

It seems likely that synthetic peptide vaccines of the future will be polymeric and likely to contain defined/structured B-cell sites, Th-cell sites (class II-restricted), and possibly cytotoxic T-cell sites (class I-restricted), plus synthetic adjuvant, immunostimulants, and targeting sequences. This concept of polymeric synthetic peptide presentation has already been successfully applied in the development of a vaccine against malaria *(54)*. However, with the development of more efficient recombinant particle-based peptide systems *(74,75)*, which have not been discussed in this chapter on synthetic peptides, it seems likely that these will provide an attractive alternative route to producing defined and controlled peptide vaccines in the future.

## References

1. Anderer, F. A. (1963) Versuch zur bestimming der seralogisch terminaten gruppen des tobakmosaik virus. *Naturforsch. Tell B.* **188**, 1010–1014.
2. Langebeheim, H., Amon, R., and Sela, M. (1976) Antiviral effect of MS-2 coliphage obtained with a synthetic antigen. *Proc. Natl. Acad. Sci. USA* **73**, 4636–4640.
3. Bittle, J. L., Houghten, R. A., Alexander, H., Schinnick, T. M., Sutcliff, J. G., Lerner, R. A., et al. (1982) Protection against foot-and-mouth disease by immunization with a chemically synthesized peptide predicted from the viral nucleotide sequence. *Nature* **298**, 30–33.
4. Pfaff, E., Mussgay, M., Bohm, H. O., Schalz, G. E., and Schaller, H. (1982) Antibodies against a preselected peptide recognize and neutralize foot and mouth disease virus. *EMBO J.* **1**, 869–874.
5. DiMarchi, R., Brooke, G., Gale, C., Crocknell, V., Doel, T., and Mowat, N. (1986) Protection of cattle against foot-and-mouth disease by a synthetic peptide. *Science* **232**, 639–641.
6. Broekhuijsen, M. P., Van Rijn, J. M. M., Blom, A. J. M., Pouwels, P. H., Enger-Valk, B. E., Brown, F., et al. (1987) Fusion proteins with multiple copies of the major antigenic determinant of foot-and-mouth disease virus protect both the natural host and laboratory animals. *J. Gen. Virol.* **68**, 3137–3143.
7. Langweld, J. P. M., Casal, J. I., Osterhaus, A. D. M. E., Cotes, E., Swart, R. de., Vela, C., et al. (1994) First peptide vaccine providing protection against viral infection in the target animal: studies on canine parvovirus in dogs. *J. Virol.* **68**, 4506–4513.
8. Loangeveld, J. P. M., Kamstrup, S., Uttenthal, A., Strandbygaard, B., Vela, C., Dalsgaard, K., et al. (1995) Full protection in mink against mink enteritis virus with new generation canine poarvovirus vaccines based on synthetic peptide or recombinant protein. *Vaccine* **13**, 1033–1037.
9. Francis, M. J. (1990) Peptide vaccines for viral diseases. *Sci. Prog.* **74**, 115–130.
10. Ijaz, M. K., Attah Poku, S. K., Redmond, M. J., Parker, M. I., and Babiuk, L. A. (1991) Heterotypic passive protection induced by synthetic peptides corresponding to VP7 and VP4 of bovine rotavirus. *J. Virol.* **65**, 3106–3113.
11. Barnett, P. V., Pullen, L., Staple, R. F., Lee, L. J., Butcher, R., Parkinson, D., et al. (1996) A protective anti-peptide antibody against the immunodominant site of the A24 Cruzeiro strain of foot-and-mouth disease virus and its reacitvity with other subtype viruses containing the same minimum binding sequesce. *J. Gen. Virol.* **77**, 1011–1018.
12. Partidos, C. D., Vohra, P., Jones, D., Farrar, G., and Steward, M. W. (1997) CTL responses induced by a single immunization with peptide encapsulated in biodegradable microparticles. *J. Immunol. Methods* **206**, 143–151.
13. Delmas, A. and Partidos, C. D. (1996) The binding of chimeric peptides to GM1 gangliotides enables induction of antibody responses after intranasal immunization. *Vaccine* **14**, 1077–1082.
14. Partidos, C. D., Vohra, P., and Steward, M. W. (1996) Induction of measles virus-specific cytotoxic T-cell response after intranasal immunization with synthetic peptides. *Immunology* **87**, 179–185.

15. Partidos, C. D., Beignon, A. S., Semetey, V., Briand, J. P., and Muller, S. (2001) The bare skin and the nose as non-invasive routes for administration peptide vaccines. *Vaccine* **19**, 2708–2715.

16. Jones, D. H., Partidos, C. D., Steward, M. W., and Farrar, G. H. (1997) Oral delivery of poly (lactide-co-glycolide) encapsulated vaccines. *Behring. Inst. Mitt* **98**, 220–228.

17. Beignon, A. S., Briand, J. P., Muller, S., and Partidos, C. D. (2001) Immunization onto bare skin with heat-labile enterotoxin of *Escherichia coli* enhances immune responses to coadministered protein and peptide antigens and protects mice against lethal toxin challenge. *Immunol.* **102**, 344–351.

18. Merrifield, R. B. (1963) Solid phase peptide synthesis. 1. The synthesis of a tetrapeptide. *J. Am. Chem. Soc.* **85**, 2149–2154.

19. Chang, C. D. and Meienhofer, J. (1978) Solid-phase peptide synthesis using mild base cleavage of N-alpha-fluororenylmethyloxycarbonylamino acids, exemplified by a synthesis of dihydrosomatostatin. *Int. J. Pept. Protein Res.* **11**, 246–249.

20. Houghton, R. A. (1985) General method for the rapid solid-phase synthesis of large numbers of peptides: specificity of antigen-antibody interaction at the level of individual amino acids. *Proc. Natl. Acad. Sci. USA* **82**, 5131–5135.

21. Partidos, C. D. (2000) Peptide mimotopes as candidate vaccines. *Curr. Opin. Mol. Ther.* **2**, 74–79.

22. Devlin, J. J., Panganiban, L. C., and Devlin, P. E. (1990) Random peptide libraries: a source of specific protein binding molecules. *Science* **249**, 404–409.

23. Lam, K. S., Salmon, S. E., Hersh, E. M., Hruby, V. J., Kazmierski, W., and Knapp, R. J. (1991) A new type of synthetic peptide library for ligand-binding activity. *Nature* **354**, 82–84.

24. Geysen, H. M., Rodda, S. J., and Mason, T. J. (1986) A priori deliniation of a peptide which mimics a discontinuous antigenic determinant. *Mol. Immunol.* **23**, 709–715.

25. Arnon, R., Tarrab-Hazdai, R., and Steward, M. (2000) A mimotope peptide based vaccine against *Schistosoma mansoni*: synthesis and characterization. *Immunology* **4**, 555–562.

26. Francis, M. J., Hastings, G. Z., Clarke, B. E., Brown, A. L., Beddell, C. R., Rowlands, D. J., et al. (1990) Neutralizing antibodies to all seven serotypes of foot-and-mouth disease virus elicited by synthetic peptides. *Immunology* **69**, 171–176.

27. Dewey, M. E., Bleasdale-Barr, K. M., Bird, P., and Amlot, P. L. (1990) Antibodies of different human IgG subclasses show distinct patterns of affinity maturation after immunisation with keyhole limpet haemocyanin. *Immunology* **70**, 168–174.

28. Davies, D., Chardhri, B., Stephens, M. D., Carne, C. A., Willers, C., and Lachmann, P. J. (1990) The immunodominance of epitopes within the transmembrane protein (gp4l) of human immunodeficiency virus type 1 may be determined by the host's previous exposure to similar epitopes on unrelated antigens. *J. Gen. Virol.* **71**, 1975–1983.

29. Katz, D. H., Paul, W. E., Goidl, E. A., and Benacerraf, B. (1970) Carrier function in anti-hapten immune responses. 1. Enhancement of primary and secondary anti-hapten antibody responses by tamer pre-immunisation. *J. Exp. Med.* **132**, 261–282.

30. Gupta, S. G., Hengartner, H., and Zinkernagel, R. M. (1986) Primary antibody responses to a well-defined and unique hapten are not enhanced by pre-immunisation with carrier: analysis in a viral model. *Proc. Natl. Acad. Sci. USA* **83**, 2604–2608.

31. Herzenberg, L. A., Tokuhisa, T., and Herzenberg, L. A. (1980) Carrier-priming leads to hapten-specific suppression. *Nature* **285**, 664, 667.

32. Dyrberg, T. and Oldstone, M. B. (1986) Peptides as antigens, importance of orientation. *J. Exp. Med.* **164**, 1344–1349.

33. Zeng, W., Ghosh, S., Macris, M., Pagnon, J., and Jackson, D. C. (2000) Assembly of synthetic peptide vaccines by chemoselective ligation of epitopes: influence of different chemical linkages and epitope orientation on biological activity. *Immunology* **19**, 3843–3852.

34. Palfreyman, J. W., Aitcheson, T. C., and Taylor, P. (1984) Guidelines for the production of polypeptide specific antisera using small synthetic oligopeptides as immunogens. *J. Immunol. Methods* **75**, 383–393.

35. Francis, M. J., Fry, C. M., Rowlands, D. J., Brown, F., Bittle, J. L., Houghton, R. A., et al. (1985) Immunological priming with synthetic peptides of foot-and-mouth disease virus. *J. Gen. Virol.* **66**, 2347–2354.

36. Francis, M. J., Fry, C. M., Rowlands, D. J., Bittle, J. L., Houghton, R. A., Lerner, R. A., and Brown, F. (1987) Immune response to uncoupled peptides of foot-and-mouth disease virus. *Immunology* **61**, 1–6.

37. DeLisi, C. and Berzofsky, J. A. (1987) T-cell antigenic sites tend to be amphipathic structures. *Proc. Natl. Acad. Sci. USA* **82**, 7048–7052.

38. Rothbard, J. B. (1986) Peptides and the cellular immune response. *Ann. Inst. Pasteur* **137E**, 518–526.

39. Rothbard, J. B. and Taylor, W. R. (1988) A sequence pattern common to T cell epitopes. *EMBO J.* **7**, 93–100.

40. Berzofsky, J. A. (1993) Epitope selection and design of synthetic vaccines. Molecular approaches to enhancing immunogenicity and cross-reactivity of engineered vaccines. *Ann NY Acad. Sci.* **12**, 256–264.

41. Partidos, C. D. and Steward, M. W. (1990) Prediction and identification of a T cell determinant in the fusion protein molecule of measles virus immunodominant in mice and humans. *J. Gen. Virol.* **71**, 2099–2105.

42. Falk, K., Rotzschke, O., Stevanovic, S., Jung, G., and Rammensee, H.-G. (1991) Allele-specific motifs revealed by sequencing of self-peptides eluted form MHC molecules. *Nature* **351**, 290–296.

43. Schadeck, E. B., Partidos, C. D., Fooks, A. R., Obeid, O. E., Wilkinson, G. E., Stephenson, J. R, et al. (1999) CLT epitopes identified with a defective recombinant adenovirus expressing measles virus nucleoprotein and evaluation of their protective capacity in mice. *Virus Res.* **65**, 75–86.

44. Partidos, C. D., Delmas, A., and Steward, M. W. (1996) Structural requirements for synthetic immunogens to induce measles virus specific CLT responses. *Mol. Immunol.* **33**, 1223–1229.

45. Partidos, C. D., Vohra, P., and Steward, M. W. (1996) Priming of measles virus-specific CTL responses after immunization with a CTL epitope linked to a fusogenic peptide. *Virology* **215**, 107–110.

46. Partidos, C. D., Vohra, P., Jones, H. H., Farrar, G., and Steward, M. W. (1999) Induction of cytotoxic T-cell responses following oral immunization with synthetic peptides encapsulated in PLG microparticles. *J. Control Release* **62**, 325–332.

47. Shaw, D. M., Stanley, C. M., Partidos, C. D., and Steward, M. W. (1993) Influence of the T-helper epitope on the titre and affinity of antibodies to B-cell epitopes after co-immunization. *Mol. Immunol.* **30**, 961–968.

48. Leclerc, C., Przewlocki, G., Schutze, M., and Chedid, L. (1987) A synthetic vaccine constructed by co-polymerization of B and T cell determinants. *Eur. J. Immunol.* **17**, 269–273.

49. Good, M. F., Malay, W. F., Lunde, M. N., Margalit, H., Cornette, J. L., Smith, G. L., et al. (1987) Construction of synthetic immunogen: use of new T-helper epitope on malaria circumsporozoite protein. *Science* **235**, 1059–1062.

50. Borras-Cuesta, F., Petit-Camurdan, A., and Fedon, Y. (1987) Engineering of immuno-genic peptides by co-linear synthesis of determinants recognised by B and T cells. *Eur. J. Immunol.* **17**, 1213–1215.
51. Francis, M. J., Hastings, G. Z., Syred, A. D., McGinn, B., Brown, F., and Rowlands, D. J. (1987) Nonresponsiveness to a foot-and-mouth disease virus synthetic peptide overcome by addition of foreign helper T-cell determinants. *Nature* **330**, 168–169.
52. Milich, D. R., Hughes, J. L,, McLachlan, A., Thornton, G. B., and Moriarty, A. (1988) Hepatitis B synthetic immunogen comprised of nucleocapsid T-cell sites and an envelope B-cell epitope. *Proc. Natl. Acad. Sci. USA* **85**, 1610–1614.
53. Partidos, C. D., Stanley, C. M., and Steward, M. W. (1991) Immune response in mice following immunization with chimeric synthetic peptides representing B and T cell epitopes of measles virus protein. *J. Gen. Virol.* **72**, 1293–1299.
54. Patarroyo, M. E., Romero, P., Torres, M. L., Clavijo, P., Moreno, A., Martinez, A., et al. (1987) Induction of protective immunity against experimental infection with malaria using synthetic peptides. *Nature* **328**, 629–632.
55. Partidos, C. D., and Steward, M. W. (1992) The effects of a flanking sequence on the immune response to a B and a T cell epitope from the fusion protein of measles virus. *J. Gen. Virol.* **73**, 1987–1994.
56. Fernandez, I. M., Snijders, A., Benaissa-Trouw, B. J., Harmsen, M., Snippe, H., and Kraaijeveld, C. A. (1993) Influence of epitope polarity and adjuvants on the immunoge-nicity and efficacy os a synthetic peptide vaccine against Semliki Forest virus. *J. Virol.* **67**, 5843–5848.
57. Bittle, J. L., Worrell, P., Houghten, R. A., Lerner, R. A., Rowlands, D. J., and Brown, F. (1984) Immunization against foot-and-mouth disease with a chemically synthesized pep-tide, in *Modern Approaches to Vaccines* (Chanock, R. M. and Lerner, R. A., eds.), Cold Spring Harbor Laboratory, Cold Spring Harbor, NY, pp. 103–108.
58. Francis, M. J. (1991) Enhanced immunogenicity of recombinant and synthetic peptide vaccines, in *Vaccines: Recent Trends and Progress. NATO ASI Series: Vaccines*, vol. 215, pp. 13–23.
59. Tam, J. P. (1988) Synthetic peptide vaccine design: synthesis and properties of a high-density multiple antigenic peptide system. *Proc. Natl. Acad. Sci. USA* **85**, 5409–5413.
60. Posnett, D. N., McGrath, H., and Tam, J. P. (1988) A novel method for producing anti-peptide antibodies: production of site specific antibodies to the T cell antigen receptor β-chain. *J. Biol. Chem.* **263**, 1719–1725.
61. Tam, J. P. (1989) Multiple antigen peptide system: a novel design for peptide-based anti-body and vaccine, in *Vaccines 90: Modern Approaches to New Vaccines Including Pre-vention of AIDS* (Lerner, R. A., Ginsberg, H., Chanock, R. M., and Brown, F., eds.), Cold Spring Harbor Laboratory, Cold Spring Harbor, NY, pp. 21–25.
62. Francis, M. J., Fry, C. M., Rowlands, D. J., and Brown, F. (1988) Qualitative and quanti-tative differences in the immune response to foot-and-mouth disease virus antigens and synthetic peptide. *J. Gen. Virol.* **69**, 2483–2491.
63. Francis, M. J., Hastings, G. Z., Brown, F., McDermed, J., Lu, Y. A., and Tam, J. P. (1991) Immunological evaluation of the multiple antigen peptide (MAP) system using a major immunogenic site of foot-and-mouth disease virus. *Immunology* **73**, 249–254.
64. Riley, E. M., Young, S. C., and Secombes, C. J. (1996) Immunisation of rainbow trout Oncorhynchus mykiss with a multiple antigen peptide system (MAPS), *Vet. Immunol. Immunopathol.* **55**, 243–253.
65. Kennedy, R. C., Dressman, G. R., Sparrow, J. T., Culwell, A. R., Sanchez, Y., Ionescu-Matiu, E., et al. (1983) Inhibition of a common human anti hepatitis B surface antigen idiotype by a cyclic synthetic peptide. *J. Virol.* **46**, 653–655.

66. Schultz-Gahmen, U., Klenk, H. D., and Beyreuther, K. (1986) Immunogenicity of loop structured short synthetic peptides mimicking the antigen site A of influenza virus haemagglutinin. *Eur. J. Biochem.* **159**, 283–289.
67. Fergusen, M., Evans, D. M. A., Magrath, D. I., Minor, P. D., Almond, J. W., and Schild, G. C. (1985) Induction by synthetic peptides of broadly reactive, type specific neutralizing antibody to poliovirus type 3. *Virology* **143**, 505–515.
68. Satterthwait, A. C., Arrhenius, T., Hagopian, R. A., Zavala, F., Nussenzweig, V., and Lerner, R. A. ( 1988) Conformational restriction of peptidyl immunogens with covalent replacements for the hydrogen bond. *Vaccine* **6**, 99–103.
69. Arnon, R. and Van Regenmortal, M. H. V. (1992) Structural basis of antigenic specificity and design of new vaccines. *FASEB J.* **6**, 3265–3274.
70. Spitzer, N., Jardin, A., Lippert, D., and Olafson, R. W. (1999) Long-term protection in mice against Leishmania major with a synthetic peptide vaccine. *Vaccine* **17**, 1298–1300.
71. Minev, B. R., Chavez, F. I., and Mitchell, M. S. (1998) New trends in the development of cancer vaccines. *In Vivo* **12**, 629–638.
72. Hipp, J. D., Hipp, J. A., Lyday, B. W., and Minev, B. R. (2000) Cancer vaccines: an update. *In Vivo* **14**, 571–585.
73. Stanworth, D. R., Jones, V. M., Lewin, I. V., and Nayyar, S. (1990) Allergy treatment with a peptide vaccine. *The Lancet* **336**, 1279–1281.
74. Francis, M. J. (1991) Enhanced immunogenicity of recombinant and synthetic peptide vaccines, in *Vaccines: Recent Trends and Progress. NATO ASI Series: Vaccines*, vol. 215, pp. 13–24.
75. Francis, M. J. (1992) Use of hepatitis B core as a vehicle for presenting viral antigens. *Rev. Med. Virol.* **2**, 225–231.

# 9

## Genetic Detoxification of Bacterial Toxins

### Mariagrazia Pizza, Maria Rita Fontana, Vincenzo Scarlato, and Rino Rappuoli

## 1. Introduction

Several pathogens, such as *Corynebacterium diphtheriae*, *Clostridium tetani*, *Bordetella pertussis*, *Vibrio cholerae*, enterotoxigenic *Escherichia coli (1)*, and even some emerging pathogens, such as *Helicobacter pylori (2)*, produce potent toxins that are responsible for the pathology caused by the bacterium. In most cases the disease, and often even the infection, can be prevented by a vaccine that induces immunity against the toxin. In order to be used in vaccines, the dangerous toxins must be depleted of their toxic activity in an effective and irreversible manner. The most effective way to inactivate toxins for inclusion in vaccines was developed by Ramon in 1924 by using formaldehyde treatment at 37°C to detoxify diphtheria toxin *(3)*. This method was then used to inactivate other toxins and also viral and bacterial suspensions. Even today, widely used vaccines, such as diphtheria, tetanus, inactivated polio, and whole-cell pertussis, and even some of the newly developed acellular pertussis vaccines, are produced using formaldehyde or other chemical treatments to inactivate the toxin and/or kill the microorganisms that are present in the vaccine *(4,5)*.

Although highly effective, chemical detoxification has some drawbacks:

1. The chemical treatment modifies to a great extent the surface of the molecules so they induce immunity against structures that barely resemble the native ones.
2. The chemical reaction may be reversible and toxicity may be restored by long-term storage.
3. The production process requires handling large quantities of very dangerous material.

The era of recombinant DNA and biotechnology has provided powerful genetic tools to inactivate bacterial toxins, allowing the production of molecules that have a superior immunogenicity and none of the drawbacks of the chemically detoxified toxins. This chapter describes the construction of nontoxic derivatives of pertussis toxin (PT), cholera toxin (CT), and *E. coli* heat-labile enterotoxin (LT). The genetically detoxified PT that will be described *(6)* has been successfully evaluated in Phase II

From: *Methods in Molecular Medicine, Vol. 87: Vaccine Protocols, 2nd ed.*
Edited by: A. Robinson, M. J. Hudson, and M. P. Cranage © Humana Press Inc., Totowa, NJ

clinical trials and recently in Phase III clinical trials for use in human vaccination against pertussis *(7,8)*. The nontoxic derivatives of CT and LT are presently being tested in animal models and may be used in the future to improve vaccines against cholera and enterotoxigenic *E. coli (9,10)*. Some of these nontoxic derivatives, in addition to being good candidates for inclusion in vaccines, also have unexpected properties, since they work as mucosal adjuvants *(11)* and therefore may provide the tools to develop vaccines with innovative design that were not even considered possible up to a few years ago.

## 1.1. Pertussis, Cholera, and Heat-Labile Toxins: Structure and Strategy for their Genetic Detoxification

PT, CT, and LT belong to the adenosine diphosphate (ADP)-ribosylating bacterial toxins, a family that also includes diphtheria and *Pseudomonas* exotoxin A *(1)*. These toxins have an A-B structure, where the A subunit is an enzyme that binds NAD and transfers the ADP-ribose group on the NAD to a target guanosine triphosphate (GTP)-binding protein of eukaryotic cells, thus causing the toxic effects. The B subunit is the nontoxic portion of the toxin that serves as a carrier for the A subunit; it binds to specific receptors on the surface of eukaryotic cells and facilitates the transfer of the toxic A subunit to the cytoplasm of the target cells. In PT, CT, and LT, the A subunit is a polypeptide of 235–240 amino acids that is secreted into the bacterial periplasm by a typical signal peptide. The B moieties of LT and CT are oligomers composed of five noncovalently linked identical subunits. In the case of PT, the B oligomer is composed of the subunits S2, S3, S4, and S5 that are present in 1:1:2:1 ratio *(12)*. The B subunits are also secreted into the periplasm via signal peptide, where they assemble to form the holotoxin, containing the B oligomer and the A subunit. The three-dimensional (3D) structure of the above molecules that has been recently determined *(13,14)* shows the details and the beauty of these molecules, and makes the design of nontoxic mutants a challenging game planned at the computer and played in the laboratory.

In order to make these toxins nontoxic by genetic detoxification, it is sufficient to alter by site-directed mutagenesis the amino acids of the A subunit that are involved in enzymatic activity and replace them with other amino acids that are unable to carry out the reaction. In doing this, it is very important not to change the 3D structure of the molecule, because this is essential for the immunological properties.

Analysis of the primary structure of the A subunits of PT, CT, and LT shows that CT and LT are 80% homologous *(15)*, whereas PT shows only some stretches of amino acid homology. In the 3D structures, the A subunits of LT and CT are indistinguishable, whereas the S1 subunit of PT shows homology only in the region containing the NAD-binding and catalytic site *(16)*. Computer analysis of the structure of this region, schematically shown in **Fig. 1**, shows that it is composed of an α-helix bent over a β-strand, which creates a cavity containing the NAD-binding site. Two amino acids, a glutamic acid at the entrance of the cavity and an arginine located in the far end of the cavity, are the residues that are important in catalysis. Detoxification can be achieved either by replacing the amino acids involved in catalysis or those forming the NAD-binding cavity. Many experiments have been performed to find the optimal substitu-

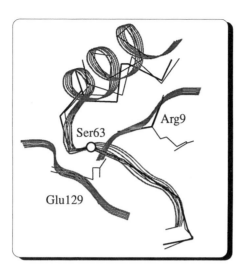

Fig 1. Schematic drawing of the structure of the active site of LT, CT, and PT. The positions of key amino acids (Arg9, Ser63, Glu129) are indicated.

tions for each of these amino acids; only some of them have been found to eliminate the toxicity without changing the immunogenicity of the molecules. This chapter describes only the following mutations: In the S1 subunit of PT, Arg9 and Glu129 will be changed to Lys and Gly, respectively *(6)*, whereas in CT and LT, Ser63 will be changed to Lys *(9)*. These mutations have been shown to produce molecules that are nontoxic but fully immunogenic.

## 1.2. Gene Structure and Mutagenesis

The genes that code for PT *(17,18)* and CT *(19)* are located on the bacterial chromosome, whereas the gene coding for LT is naturally found on a plasmid *(20)*. The three genes can now be conveniently obtained already subcloned in plasmid vectors that can be used as a starting point for mutagenesis. Alternatively, the genes can be cloned from the bacterial DNA by PCR.

Since toxins are encoded by operons that occupy very large fragments of chromosomal or plasmid DNAs, their size makes any DNA manipulation and mutagenesis difficult. To perform site-directed mutagenesis of defined amino acids, it is always convenient to identify small DNA fragments with unique restriction enzyme sites surrounding the encoded amino acids that must be mutagenized. Once a small DNA fragment has been identified, it is transferred to a plasmid to make single-stranded DNA, which is the template for site-directed mutagenesis. Techniques for mutagenesis of single-stranded DNA have been extensively described by Zoller and Smith *(21)* using defined oligonucleotides, and the resulting recombinant clones are analyzed for the presence of the mutation by hybridization with the respective primers as probes and confirmed by DNA sequencing. After mutagenesis, the mutated fragment is used to reconstitute the entire operon. Because of the complexity of the methods used, we will describe in detail only the techniques that are not in general use. DNA cloning, DNA sequencing, and mutagenesis have been fully described in detail in laboratory handbooks *(22)*.

*B. pertussis* is a bacterium that has a duplication time of 4–6 h at 35°C and requires special media to produce colonies on plates. Conversely, *V. cholerae* and *E. coli* are bacteria that grow faster and do not require special medium. Their generation times range from 20–40 min. Genetic manipulations of the toxin-encoding genes are always performed in an *E. coli* strain and then transferred to the appropriate host using conjugation between *E. coli* and *B. pertussis*, electroporation for *V. cholerae*, or transformation for *E. coli*.

## 2. Materials

### 2.1. Pertussis Toxin

#### 2.1.1. Medium and Plates

1. BG agar plates *(23)* (40 g/L Bordet-Gengou [BG] agar, 10 g/L glycerol, 30% [v/v] sterile defibrinated sheep blood) and LB agar plates *(22)* supplemented with 100 µg/mL ampicillin.
2. BG plates with 10 m$M$ MgCl$_2$.
3. BG plates containing 400 µg/mL streptomycin.
4. BG plates containing 20 µg/mL nalidixic acid, 25 µg/mL kanamycin, and 10 µg/mL gentamycin.
5. BG plates containing 20 µg/mL nalidixic acid and 10 µg/mL gentamycin.
6. Stainer and Scholte (SS) medium *(24)*.

#### 2.1.2 Plasmids and Strains

1. Plasmid pSS1129 *(25)* carrying the kanamycin cassette cloned between flanking regions of the PT gene (pSS1129/PT::Kan::PT).
2. Plasmid pSS1129 carrying the PT mutagenized encoding gene (PT-9K/129G).
3. Bluescript KS vector (Stratagene, La Jolla, CA).
4. *E. coli* SM10-competent cells *(26)*.

#### 2.1.3. Resins and Buffers

1. Hydroxylapatite (Biosepra, Villeneuve la Garenne, France).
2. Fetuin sepharose. An affinity chromatography resin obtained by coupling fetuin to CNBr-activated Sepharose 4B (Pharmacia, Uppsala, Sweden). Coupling is performed according to the manufacturer's instructions.
3. 70 m$M$ phosphate buffer, pH 6.6–7.0.
4. 250 m$M$ phosphate buffer, pH 6.6–7.0.
5. 50 m$M$ Tris-HCl, pH 7.4.
6. 50 m$M$ Tris-HCl, pH 7.4, 1 $M$NaCl.
7. 50 m$M$ Tris-HCl, pH 7.4, 0.5 $M$ NaCl.
8. Phosphate-buffered saline (PBS).

#### 2.1.4. Miscellaneous Items

1. Dialysis tubes.
2. Sterile toothpicks.
3. Dacron swab (American Scientific Products, McGraw Park, IL).

## 2.2. Heat-Labile Enterotoxin

### 2.2.1. Medium and Plates

1. Luria Bertani (LB) plates containing 100 µg/mL ampicillin *(22)*.
2. LB medium *(22)*.

### 2.2.2. Plasmids and Strains

1. Plasmid pEWD299 carrying the 2-kb *Sma*I-*Hin*dIII fragment containing the LT-encoding operon.
2. Bluescript KS (Stratagene, La Jolla, CA).
3. *E. coli* strain TG1.

### 2.2.3. Resins and Buffers

1. CPG (controlled-pore glass for chromatography, 500B, Serva, Heidelberg, Germany).
2. A5M agarose (BioRad Laboratories, Inc., Hercules, CA).
3. Sephacryl S-200 (Pharmacia).
4. 50 m$M$ Tris-HCl, pH 8.0.
5. TEAN buffer: 50 m$M$ Tris-HCl, 200 m$M$ NaCl, 1 m$M$ ethylenediaminetetraacetic acid (EDTA), 3 m$M$ NaN$_3$, pH 9.7.
6. TEAN, pH 9.7, 1 $M$ NaCl.
7. TEAN, pH 9.7, 0.2 $M$ galactose.
8. TEAN, pH 7.4.

### 2.2.4. Miscellaneous Items

1. Sonicator.
2. Amazon PMI0 ultrafilters.

## 2.3. Cholera Toxin

### 2.3.1. Plates and Medium

1. LB-plates.
2. LB-plates supplemented with 200 µg/mL ampicillin *(22)*.
3. LB-plates supplemented with 100 µg/mL ampicillin, 0.75 µg/mL polymixin, 0.75 µg/mL gentamycin.
4. LB-plates supplemented with 20% sheep blood.
5. Syncase medium (modified from **ref**. *27*): 20 g/L casamino acids, 2.5 g/L sucrose, 1.18 g/L NH$_4$Cl, 0.089 g/L Na$_2$SO$_4$; 6.27 g/L Na$_2$HPO$_4$·2H$_2$O, 6.27 g/L, K$_2$HPO$_4$·3H$_2$O, 0.042 g/L MgCl$_2$·6H$_2$O, 0.004 g/L MnCl$_2$·4H$_2$O, 0.005 g/L FeCl$_3$·6H$_2$O.
6. TYS medium: LB without NaCl supplemented with 10% sucrose.

### 2.3.2. Plasmids and Strains

1. Plasmid pJM17 carrying the 5-kb *Pst*I-*Eco*RI fragment that contains the CT-encoding operon.
2. pEMBL19.
3. pGEM3 (Promega, Madison, WI).
4. Bluescript KS (Stratagene, La Jolla, CA).
5. Plasmid p*hly*3 containing the *hly* gene (isolated from a *Vibrio* DNA library) as 3.5-Kb *Eco*RI-*Pst*I fragment cloned in Bluescript KS.

6. Plasmid pctK63 obtained by cloning in pEMBL19 vector a fragment of 1.3 kb, containing the upstream regulatory sequences and coding region of CTK63 mutant, amplified from pGEM/CTK63. The oligonucleotides used for amplification are: 5'-AACCGAA-TTCAAGGCTGTGGGTAGAAGTG-3' (forward) containing a *Eco*RI site and 5'-AAGTTAACGTCGACAAGCTTAATTTGCCATACTAATT-3' (reverse) including a *Hin*dIII restriction site.
7. CVD442, conjugative plasmid.
8. *V. cholerae* strain 0395-NT.
9. *E. coli* SM10 λpir strain.

### 2.3.3. Resins and Buffers

1. Carboxy-methyl Sepharose CL-6B (Pharmacia).
2. 2.5 g/L sodium hexametaphospate.
3. 0.1 $M$ sodium phosphate buffer, pH 8.0.
4. 10 m$M$ sodium phosphate buffer, pH 7.0.
5. 20 m$M$ sodium phosphate buffer, pH 7.5.
6. 40 m$M$ sodium phosphate buffer, pH 7.5.

### 2.3.4. Miscellaneous Items

1. Dialysis tubes.
2. Microfilters Sartocon and Sartocon minimodule (Sartorius, Goëttingen, Germany).

## 2.4. Toxicity Testing and Immunogenicity Testing

### 2.4.1. Cell Lines and Medium

1. Y1 adrenal cells *(28)*.
2. Chinese hamster ovary (CHO) cells *(29)*.
3. Y1 culture medium (nutrient mixture Ham's F-10 supplemented with 2 m$M$ glutamine, 50 mg/L gentamycin, 15% [v/v] horse serum, 2.5% [v/v] fetal bovine serum [FBS]) (Gibco-BRL, Paisley, UK).
4. Y1 assay medium: nutrient mixture Ham's F-10 supplemented with 2 m$M$ glutamine, 50 mg/L gentamycin, 1.5% (v/v) horse serum.
5. CHO culture and assay medium: Dulbecco's Modified Eagle Medium (D-MEM) (Gibco-BRL) supplemented with 2 m$M$ glutamine, 50 mg/L, gentamycin, 10% (v/v) fetal calf serum (FCS).

### 2.4.2. Buffers

1. PBS.
2. Transfer buffer: 0.025 $M$ Tris-HC1, 0.192 $M$ glycine buffer, pH 8.3, 20% (v/v) methanol.
3. Saturation buffer: phosphate buffer, pH 7.4, containing 3% (v/v) lowfat milk and 0.1% (v/v) Triton X-100 (PBMT).
4. PBS, 0.05% (v/v) Tween 20 (PBS/T).

### 2.4.3. Miscellaneous Items

1. 96-well microtiter plates.
2. Sodium dodecyl sulfate (SDS)-polyacrylamide gel.
3. Nitrocellulose filter BA-85 (Schleicher & Schuell, Damsel, Germany).

## 2.4.4. Reagents

1. Anti-mouse or anti-rabbit immunoglobulin G (IgG) conjugated to alkaline phosphatase (Sigma, St. Louis, MO).
2. Anti-mouse or anti-rabbit γ-globulins conjugated to peroxidase (Sigma).
3. Substrate for alkaline phosphatase: p-nitrophenyl phosphate (pNPP) (Sigma) at 1 mg/mL in 10% (v/v) diethanolamine buffer, pH 9.8, containing 0.5 m$M$ MgCl$_2$.
4. Substrate for peroxidase: 0.3% (w/v) 4.chloro-1-naphthol (Sigma) in methanol.

## 2.4.5. Animals

1. Mice.
2. Rabbits.

## 3. Methods

### 3.1. Pertussis Toxin

#### 3.1.1. Site-Directed Mutagenesis to Generate PT-9K/129G Mutated Operon

1. Clone the plasmid pT110 *(17)* carrying the 4690 bp *Eco*RI fragment (**Fig. 2A**) that contains the PT-encoding operon into pEMBL18 and generate two small DNA fragments, *Kpn*I-*Sal*I of 0.5 kb and *Sal*I-*Xba*I of 0.4 kb, that are suitable for mutagenesis of the S1 subunit.
2. Subclone the 0.4-kb *Sal*I-*Xba*I fragment encoding the C-terminal part of S1 into Bluescript KS vector and mutagenize using the oligonucleotide primer: 1003-(5')GCCAGATA**CCC**GCTCTGG-986, where the codon GAA of Glu129 is substituted by the codon CCC (*in bold*) of Gly.
3. Subclone the 0.5-kb *Kpn*I-*Sal*I fragment encoding for the N-terminal part of S1, including the leader peptide and the upstream region, into Bluescript KS vector (**Fig. 2A**) and mutagenize using the oligonucleotide primer: 643-(5')GAGTCATA **CTT**GTATA-626, where the codon GCG of Arg9 is changed with the codon CTT (in bold) of Lys.
4. Purify the two mutagenized fragments, *Sal*I-*Xba*I containing the 129G (Glu129 → Gly) mutation and the *Kpn*I-*Sal*I containing the 9K (Arg9 → Lys) mutation, and clone into pT110 that has been previously digested with *Kpn*I and *Xba*I to remove the wild-type S1 gene.
5. The resulting plasmid contains the mutated PT-9K/129G operon.

#### 3.1.2. Transfer of the Mutated PT Gene into the B. pertussis Chromosome

Here we describe the procedure used to manipulate a *B. pertussis* strain in order to create a mutant strain expressing the PT-9K/129G mutant. This can be achieved in two steps:

1. Replacing the chromosomal region coding for the *PT* gene by a kanamycin cassette.
2. Replacing the kanamycin cassette with the *PT* operon that has been mutagenized in *E. coli* by site-directed mutagenesis.

To transfer the genes from *E. coli* to *B. pertussis* it is necessary to use conjugative plasmids. The most commonly used are pRTP1 and pSS1129 *(25,30)*. These plasmids

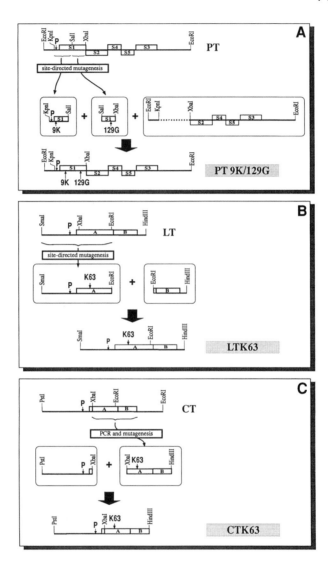

Fig 2. Schematic representation of the plasmids containing the *PT* (**A**), *LT* (**B**), and *CT* (**C**) genes and their mutations.

contain the *oriT* from the broad-host-range plasmid RK2 for conjugative transfer, a vegetative origin of replication from *ColE1*, an ampicillin-resistance gene, and the gene encoding the *E. coli* ribosomal protein S12 *(25,30)*. pSS1129 also carries a gentamycin-resistance cassette. Expression of the ribosomal protein S12 is dominant over the streptomycin resistance, and it therefore converts a streptomycin-resistant strain into a streptomycin-sensitive strain. Plasmids pRTP1 and pSS1129 are suicide plasmids that are unable to replicate in *B. pertussis*, and thus, if the recipient strain is

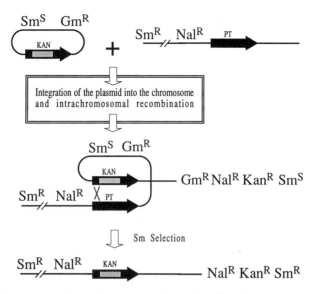

Fig. 3. Schematic representation of the events of recombination after conjugation of *B. pertussis* with *E. coli* to construct a PT-deletant strain. The black arrow indicates the wild-type *PT* gene, the gray box the kanamycin cassette. Arrow indicates the direction of transcription. Symbols: Sm, streptomycin; Nal, nalidixic acid; Gm, gentamycin; Kan, kanamycin.

subject to antibiotic selection carried by the plasmid, only the bacteria that have integrated the plasmid into the chromosome will grow. Therefore, the integration of the plasmid occurs through a single homologous recombination event, the exconjugants acquire the genetic markers of the plasmid, and a streptomycin-resistant strain becomes streptomycin-sensitive. A second event of homologous (intrachromosomal) recombination could be selected on streptomycin-containing plates. This recombination allows the selection of strains that have lost the *S12* gene and, possibly, all the genetic markers carried on the plasmid.

### 3.1.2.1. Construction of a PT-Deletion Mutant Strain (Fig. 3)

1. Digest plasmid pT110 with enzyme *Bst*EII and end-repair with Klenow enzyme. This digestion removes the entire *PT* coding region, leaving 422 bp at the 5'-end of the operon and 834 bp at the 3'-end of the operon.
2. Clone a blunt-ended kanamycin cassette between the 5'- and 3' -flanking regions of the *PT* operon.
3. Clone this new *Eco*RI recombinant DNA fragment (5'-*PT*::*Kan*::*PT*-3') into the conjugative suicide vector pSS1129 and transform into a RecA *E. coli* strain. DNA from a selected positive transformant is used to transform the conjugative strain *E. coli* SM10. (*see* **Note 1** and **Fig. 3**).
4. Spread a recipient *B. pertussis* strain on a BG plate containing 400 µg/mL streptomycin and incubate for 3 d at 35°C.
5. After 2 d, transform *E. coli* strain SM10 with the conjugative plasmid pSS1129/ *PT*::*Kan*::*PT* and incubate overnight at 37°C.
6. Collect all *B. pertussis* cells from the plate using a Dacron swab and spread uniformly on a BG plate supplemented with 10 m*M* MgCl₂. Rotate the plate by 90° and spread one colony of SM10(pSS1129/*PT*::*kan*::*PT*) freshly transformed. After 5 h of incubation at

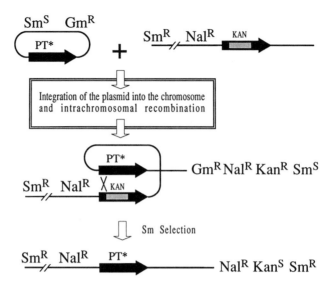

Fig. 4. Schematic representation of the events of recombination after conjugation of *B. pertussis* with *E. coli* to construct a *PT*-mutant strain. Symbols are as in **Fig. 3**.

35°C, collect all the bacteria and swab onto a BG plate supplemented with nalidixic acid to counterselect *E. coli*, and kanamycin and gentamycin to select for the integration of the plasmid into the chromosome of *B. pertussis*. Incubate the plate at 35°C for 6–7 d.

7. To select strains that have lost the plasmid and have been subjected to the second recombination event, plate the exconjugants on BG plates supplemented with streptomycin and incubate for 3 d at 35°C.

8. Analyze the bacteria grown on BG-streptomycin plates for the loss of the plasmid and the acquisition of the kanamycin resistance. To do this, streak with a toothpick each single colony on a BG plate containing kanamycin. Incubate for 3 d at 35°C. To confirm the insertion of the kanamycin cassette into the *PT* gene, perform Southern blot analyses or PCRs on chromosomal DNA extracted from kanamycin-resistant isolates. At the end, a *PT* deletion strain will be isolated.

### 3.1.2.2. INSERTION OF THE MUTATED PT OPERON INTO THE CHROMOSOME

With the same procedure described in **Subheading 3.1.2.**, the interrupted gene can be reconstituted by substituting the kanamycin cassette with a site-directed mutagenized fragment of the PT-encoding gene (**Fig. 4**).

1. Gel-purify the *Eco*RI fragment containing the PT-9K/129G produced as described in **Subheading 3.1.1., step 4** and clone into pSS1129 conjugative vector.

2. Spread *B. pertussis PT* deletion mutant strain (Km$^R$) on a BG plate containing kanamycin and incubate for 3 d at 35°C.

3. After 2 d, transform *E. coli* strain SM10 with the conjugative plasmid pSS1129 carrying the *PT* mutagenized operon (pSS 1129/PT-9K/129G) and incubate overnight at 37°C.

4. Collect all *B. pertussis* cells from the plate using a Dacron swab and spread uniformly on a BG plate supplemented with 10 m*M* MgCl$_2$. Rotate the plate by 90° and spread on top of *B. pertussis* one colony of SM10(pSS1129/PT-9K/129G), freshly transformed. After 5 h of incubation at 35°C, collect all the bacteria and swab onto a BG plate supplemented with nalidixic acid to counterselect *E. coli* and gentamycin to select for the integration of the plasmid into the chromosome of *B. pertussis*. Incubate the plate at 35°C for 6–7 d.

5. The exconjugants contain the entire plasmid integrated into the chromosome, which confers streptomycin sensitivity. In order to select for the loss of the plasmid and the second recombination event, plate the exconjugants on BG plates supplemented with streptomycin and incubate at 35°C for 3 d.

6. Analyze bacteria grown on BG-streptomycin plates for the loss of the plasmid and for the loss of the kanamycin resistance. Streak each single colony in duplicate, using a toothpick, on BG plates with and without kanamycin. Incubate for 3 d at 35°C. Colonies that have lost the kanamycin resistance should have acquired the mutated PT gene (*see* **Note 2**).

### 3.1.3. Production and Purification of Mutant PT

To perform ELISA or toxicity tests, *B. pertussis*-mutant strains are grown in small flasks. If larger amounts of proteins are required, strains are grown in fermentors. Here we describe a large-scale production and purification of PT.

1. Inoculate two BG agar plates with a loop of frozen stock of *B. pertussis* mutant strain containing the PT-9K/129G operon. Grow 72 h at 37°C. Collect the bacteria from the two plates and inoculate into 500 mL of modified SS medium in a 2-L flask.

2. Shake the flask at 250 rpm for 24 h at 37°C, and then use this culture to inoculate a 20-L fermentor: Grow the bacteria for 24 h, centrifuge the culture, and recover the supernatant.

3. Dilute the supernatant with an equal volume of sterile distilled $H_2O$.

4. Adsorb the sample on an 80-mL hydroxylapatite column.

5. Wash with 6 column volumes of 70 m$M$ phosphate buffer, pH 7.0.

6. Elute with 250 m$M$ phosphate buffer, pH 7.0.

7. Dilute the eluate with water until the concentration of phosphate is 0.2 $M$.

8. Apply the solution to a fetuin Sepharose affinity column (5 × 20 cm).

9. Wash the column with 6 column volumes of 50 m$M$ Tris-HCl, pH 7.4. This step will remove nonadsorbed proteins.

10. Wash the column with 50 m$M$ Tris-HCl, pH 7.4, 1 $M$ NaCl. This step allows the release of the FHA protein, and should be continued until no more proteins are released from the column.

11. Elute PT with 50 m$M$ Tris-HCl, pH 7.4, 3 $M$ MgCl$_2$.

12. Dialyze against 50 m$M$ Tris-HCl, pH 7.4, 0.5 $M$ NaCl.

13. Dialyze against PBS.

## 3.2. Heat-Labile Enterotoxin

### 3.2.1. Site-Directed Mutagenesis to Generate LT/K63-Mutated Operon

1. Generate the 1.3-kb *Sma*I-*Eco*RI fragment suitable for the mutagenesis experiment (**Fig. 2B**) from the plasmid pEWD299 *(20)*.

2. Subclone the 1.3-kb fragment containing the gene coding for the A subunit of LT along with its natural promoter into Bluescript KS vector (*see* **Fig. 2B**) and mutagenize using the oligonucleotide primer -(5')GTTTCCACTA**AAG**CTTA GTTTG(3')- where the codon TCT of Ser63 is substituted with the codon AAG (*in bold*) of Lys.

3. Digest the pEWD299 plasmid with *Eco*RI and *Hin*dIII restriction enzymes to obtain the 580-bp DNA fragment encoding for the B subunit of LT.

4. Gel-purify the 580-bp *Eco*RI-*Hin*dIII fragment and the *Sma*I-*Eco*RI fragment encoding for the A subunit containing the 63K (Ser63 → Lys) mutation and clone into Bluescript KS digested with *Sma*I-*Hin*dIII to generate a plasmid containing the mutated LT-K63 operon.

5. Transform the Bluescript-KS/LTK63 into the *E. coli* TG1 strain. The LT/K63 mutant protein is secreted into the periplasm of the host *E. coli* strain from which it can be purified.

### 3.2.2. Production and Purification of LT Mutant in E. coli

The purification of LT is performed according to a previously described protocol *(31)* with few modifications.

1. Streak the *E. coli* LT-mutant strain on an LB agar plate supplemented with 100 µg/mL ampicillin and incubate overnight at 37°C. Replate the strain and incubate at 37°C for 8 h. Collect bacteria from this plate and inoculate into 500 mL of LB medium containing 100 µg/mL of ampicillin in a 2-L flask.
2. Incubate at 37°C overnight and use the contents of the flask to inoculate a 20-L fermentor. Grow the bacteria in the fermentor for 12 h, centrifuge the culture, and recover the cells.
3. Weigh the cellular pellet and resuspend in 50 m*M* Tris-HCl, pH 8.0, at 10 mL/g pellet. Add EDTA, pH 8.0, to final concentration of 2 m*M*. Sonicate at 45 W for 6 min using a refrigerated vessel set at –15°C to maintain a low temperature.
4. Dilute the sonicated material with 2 vol of water and 3 vol of TEAN, pH 9.7.
5. Add 4 g of CPG resin/g of pellet and stir gently at 4°C overnight.
6. Pack the column and wash with 6 vol of TEAN, pH 9.7.
7. Elute proteins with 3 column volumes of TEAN, pH 9.7, 1 *M* NaCl.
8. Pool fractions containing the bulk proteins and concentrate 10-fold by using PM 10 Amicon filters.
9. Apply the concentrated proteins to an ASM agarose column (1.6 × 70 cm).
10. Let the proteins adsorb on the column and add 0.5 column volumes of TEAN, pH 9.7.
11. Elute LT with about 1 column volume of TEAN, pH 9.7, 0.2 *M* galactose.
12. Apply the eluate to a Sephacryl S-200 column (1.6 × 140 cm).
13. Elute the protein with at least 2 column volumes of TEAN, pH 7.4.

### 3.3. Cholera Toxin

### 3.3.1. Site-Directed Mutagenesis to Generate CT/K63 Mutated Operon

1. Generate by PCR-amplification the fragment of 1.1 kb *Xba*I-*Hin*dIII containing the CT(AB)-encoding genes suitable for the mutagenesis experiment from the plasmid pJM17 *(32)* (**Fig. 2C**).
2. Subclone the amplified *Xba*I-*Hin*dIII fragment into pEMBL19 vector *(33)* and mutagenize using the oligonucleotide (5')-GTTTCCACC**AAG**ATTAGTTTG-(3') where the codon TCA of Ser63 is changed with the codon AAG (in bold) to introduce a Lys.
3. Digest the pJM17 plasmid with *Pst*I and *Xba*I to obtain the 2.7-kb DNA fragment containing the CT promoter region.
4. Blunt-end the mutagenized *Xba*I-*Hin*dIII fragment containing the 63 K (Ser63 → Lys) mutation at the *Hin*dIII site.
5. Gel purify the 2.7-kb *Pst*I-*Xba*I fragment from pJM17 containing the CT promoter region and clone this fragment, together with the 1.1-kb *Xba*I-*Hin*dIII/filled fragment, into the pGEM3 vector digested with *Eco*RI, blunt-ended with Klenow enzyme, and then digested with *Pst*I. The resulting pGEM/CT-K63 plasmid, contains the mutated CT-K63 operon.
6. Electroporate the plasmid pGEM/CT-K63 into the *V. cholerae* strain 0395-NT *(19)* that contains a chromosomal deletion of the entire CT operon. The CT mutant protein is secreted in the supernatant of the host *V. cholerae* strain from which it can be purified.

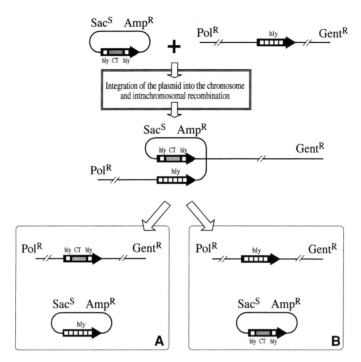

Fig. 5. Schematic representation of the events of recombination after conjugation of *V. cholerae* with *E. coli* to construct a strain stably expressing CTK63 mutant. Symbols: Sac, sucrose; Amp, ampicillin; Pol, polymixin; Gent, gentamycin; hly, hemolysin; CT, CTK63 mutant.

### 3.3.2. Transfer of the Mutated CT Gene into the V. cholerae Chromosome

To generate a *V. cholerae* strain that is able to express in a stable way the detoxified CTK63 mutant of cholera toxin, the procedure used **(Fig. 5)** resembles the one previously described for the transfer of the mutated PT gene into the *B. pertussis* chromosome. In this case, the gene used as locus for the homologous recombination is the hemolysin gene (*Hly*) *(34)*. The plasmid most commonly used for homologous recombination in *V. cholerae* is the CVD 442, a suicide vector that is unable to replicate in *V. cholerae (35)*. It contains the *ori*T for conjugative transfer from R6K plasmid, a vegetative origin of replication from ColE1, the β-lactamase gene that confers ampicillin resistance, and the *SacB* gene from *Bacillus subtilis*, coding for the levano-sucrase, that confers sucrose susceptibility to Gram-negative bacteria. These two genes are useful markers for homologous recombination. The recombinant CVD442 plasmid is transformed into *E. coli* SM10λpir donor strain *(26)*, containing the genes required for DNA transfer, and transferred to the *V. cholerae* recipient strain by conjugation.

The use of the hemolysin as genetic locus allows the selection of the recombinant strains on the basis of their hemolytic phenotype.

Briefly, the pCVD-*hly*::CTK63::*hly* plasmid, derived from the conjugative plasmid CVD442 and containing the CTK63 gene flanked by sequences of the *hly* gene, is introduced in *V. cholerae* by conjugation. Following a single recombination event, the plasmid is integrated into the *Vibrio* chromosome, and the recombinant *Vibrio* strain (gentamycin and polymixin-resistant strain) will acquire the genetic markers carried by the plasmid, becoming ampicillin-resistant and sucrose-sensitive. The second event of homologous recombination can be selected by growing bacteria in medium containing sucrose. The growing bacteria that are sucrose-resistant, have lost the plasmid sequences. By plating them on LB agar containing 20% sheep blood, it is possible to differentiate the colonies on the basis of the halo of hemolysis. The absence of hemolysis indicates the disruption of the *Hly* gene and the integration of the CTK63 gene into the chromosome.

### 3.3.2.1. CONSTRUCTION OF THE *V. CHOLERAE* RECOMBINANT STRAIN EXPRESSING CTK63 MUTANT

1. Digest the p*hly*3 plasmid with *Nru*I and *Hin*dIII. Following digestion, two fragments of 5 Kb and 1.5 Kb, respectively, are generated. The 1.5-Kb fragment contains the core region of the *hly* gene, whereas the 5-Kb fragment contains the vector sequences, 1.2 Kb of the 5' end and 0.8 Kb of the 3' end of the *hly* gene.
2. Digest the plasmid p*ct*K63 with *Eco*RI, fill with Klenow fragment of DNA polymerase I, and digest with *Hin*dIII. Following digestion a fragment of 1.3 Kb is generated.
3. Clone the 1.3-Kb *Eco*RI/blunt-ended-*Hin*dIII fragment into the 5-Kb NruI-*Hin*dIII fragment of p*hly*3, to generate p*hly*-*ct*K63 plasmid.
4. Digest the plasmid p*hly*-*ct*K63 with *Sac*I and *Sal*I, and clone the 3.3-Kb fragments obtained into CVD422 digested with *Sac*I and *Sal*I, generating the pCVD*hly*::*ct*K63::*hly* plasmid. This plasmid is used to transform the conjugative strain *E. coli* SM10λ*pir*.
5. Spread the *V. cholerae*-recipient strain and the SM10λ*pir* (pCVD*hly*::*ct*K63::*hly*) donor strain on LB agar plates and incubate for 16–18 h at 37°C.
6. Collect *V. cholerae* cells from the plate with a Dacron swab and spread uniformly on LB agar plate. Rotate the plate by 90°C and spread the SM10λ*pir* (pCVD*hly*::*ct*K63::*hly*) cells. The two strains must be present in a 1:5 ratio. Incubate the plates for 6 h at 37°C.
7. Collect all bacteria with a swab and plate them on LB agar supplemented with gentamycin, polymixin, and ampicillin to select for the first recombination event (integration of the plasmid into the chromosome). Incubate the plate for 16–18 h at 37°C.
8. Spread each single colony on selective medium and incubate at 37°C for 16–18 h. To confirm that the selected bacteria are *V. cholerae*, test a small amount of cells for agglutination using a polyclonal rabbit serum obtained by immunizing with *Vibrio* cells. The agglutination test is performed as follows: drop 50 µL of the LB medium on a glass, resuspend the bacteria in the drop, add 20 µL of anti-*Vibrio* serum. After 5 min, the agglutination of bacteria is detected.
9. To select for the second recombination event identifying the colonies that have lost the plasmid sequences, a single colony is inoculated in 10 mL of TYS medium containing 10% sucrose and incubated for 16–18 h at 28°C in a shaking bath.
10. To identify the non-hemolytic bacteria (which will have the disruption of the chromosomal hemolysin gene by insertion of CTK63 sequences), a dilution of the liquid culture (a $10^{-5}$ dilution is generally used) is plated on LB agar-blood and the plates are incubated at 37°C for 16–18 h.

11. Isolate the ampicillin-sensitive and sucrose-resistant nonhemolytic colonies, spread and store at −80°C.

### 3.3.3. Production and Purification of CT Mutant in V. cholerae

The protocol used for production and purification of CT from *V. cholerae* has been described previously *(36)*.

1. Spread *V. cholerae* strain 0395-CTK63 on LB agar plates supplemented with 200 µg/mL of ampicillin and incubate overnight at 37°C.
2. Inoculate a single colony in 250 mL of Syncase-modified medium in a 2-L flask.
3. Incubate the bacteria overnight at 37°C, then inoculate a 5-L fermentor by diluting bacteria to an OD of 0.05 at 590 nm. Grow the bacteria for 24 h at 30°C, maintaining the pH at 7.0, and filter the bacterial suspension by tangential microfiltration using a Sartocon minimodule.
4. Add 2.5 g/L of sodium hexametaphosphate to precipitate the CT, adjust the pH to 4.5 with concentrated HC1, and stir the mixture for 2.5 h at room temperature.
5. Collect the precipitate by centrifugation at 12,000*g* for 20 min and resuspend the pellet in 0.1 *M* sodium phosphate, pH 8.0.
6. Dialyze three times against 10 m*M* sodium phosphate, pH 7.0, and remove the insoluble material by centrifugation at 25,000*g* for 20 min.
7. Apply the solution to a 30–40-mL carboxy-methyl Sepharose CL-6B column and wash with 6 column volumes of 10 m*M* sodium phosphate, pH 7.0.
8. Elute the CT holotoxin with 1 column volume of 20 m*M* sodium phosphate buffer, pH 7.5, and the B pentamer (not assembled to the A subunit) with 1 column volume of 40 m*M* sodium phosphate buffer, pH 7.5.

### 3.4. Toxicity Testing and Immunological Testing

Wild-type CT, LT, and PT are able to induce morphological changes on tissue-culture cells. This property is useful to evaluate the toxic activity of mutant molecules. This assay is very sensitive, and toxicity can be detected using a few picograms of active toxins. The activity of CT and LT can be clearly detected using Y1 adrenal cells. The toxins are able to induce a rounding of monolayer growing cells *(28)*. In the case of PT, the toxicity can be evaluated by the induction of clustering activity of CHO cells *(29)*. These assays can also be used to evaluate the ability of the antibodies to neutralize the toxic activity of LT, CT, and PT.

### 3.4.1. Toxicity Test

1. Add 25 µL of the assay medium to each well of the microtiter plate.
2. Add the wild-type toxin and/or the mutants in the first well and then make 1:2 serial dilutions.
3. Add 50,000 cells in each well (200-µL volume).
4. Incubate at 37°C in a humidified atmosphere of 95% air, 5% $CO_2$.
5. Record the results after 48 h by visual inspection of the microtiter wells using an inverted microscope.

Under these conditions, 5 pg/well of LT and CT or PT can induce a morphological change of Y1 and CHO cells, respectively.

### 3.4.2. Neutralization Test

1. Add undeleted sera to the first well and then make 1:2 serial dilutions.
2. Add 80 pg of CT, LT, or PT to the sera and incubate the plate for 3 h at 37°C.
3. Add 50,000 cells in each well (200-μL volume).
4. Record the results after 48 h by visual inspection of the microtiter wells using an inverted microscope.

### 3.4.3. Immunogenicity

To test the ability of the mutant molecules to induce an immune response, mice and rabbits can be immunized systemically.

#### 3.4.3.1. MOUSE IMMUNIZATION

1. Immunize mice with 3 μg of toxoid in saline buffer at d 0, 15, 30, and 45. (No adjuvant is needed.)
2. Collect the sample bleed at d 0, 15, and 30.
3. Bleed out at d 60.

#### 3.4.3.2. RABBIT IMMUNIZATION

1. Immunize rabbits with 25 μg of mutant protein in saline buffer at d 0, 14, 28, and 56. (No adjuvant is needed.)
2. Collect sample bleed at d 0, 14, 28, and 56.
3. Bleed out at d 70.

The sera are analyzed by Western blots and ELISA tests.

#### 3.4.3.3. WESTERN BLOTTING

1. Load 3 μg of each toxin, treated with SDS loading buffer and boiled for 5 min, on a 15% polyacrylamide gel.
2. After electrophoresis, transfer the proteins from the gel onto a BA-85 nitrocellulose filter (Schleicher & Schuell) for 45 min at 200 mA in the transfer buffer.
3. Saturate the filter with PBMT.
4. Incubate the filter with the sera diluted 1:500 in PBMT.
5. Wash 3× for 10 min in PBMT.
6. Depending on whether antibodies have been raised in mice or rabbits, incubate with the antimouse or antirabbit γ-globulins conjugated to peroxidase (Sigma).
7. Wash 3× in PBMT.
8. Develop using a solution of 0.5 mL 0.3% (w/v) 4-chloro-1-naphthol, 16 μL $H_2O_2$, and 20 mL 0.175 $M$ Tris-HCl, pH 6.8, as the peroxidase substrate.

#### 3.4.3.4. ELISA ASSAY

1. Coat the microtiter plate with 100 μL/well of 1.5 μg/mL GM1 ganglioside (Sigma) for CT and LT ELISA, or with 200 μL of 2.5 μg/mL fetuin in PBS for PT ELISA.
2. Wash the plates 3× with PBS, 0.05% Tween 20 (PBS/T).
3. Add 200 μL/well of 1% (w/v) BSA and incubate for 1 h at 37°C.
4. Add 100 μL/well of 0.5 μg/mL LT, CT, or PT and incubate overnight at 4°C.
5. Add the sera to each well starting from a dilution of 1:50 and make 1:2 dilutions.
6. Wash 3× with PBS/T.

7. Add the anti-mouse or anti-rabbit immunoglobulin G conjugated to alkaline phosphatase.
8. Wash 3× with PBS/T.
9. Add 10 μL pNPP, the substrate for alkaline phosphatase, per well.
10. Read the absorbances at 450 nm.

## 4. Notes

1. This strain carries mobilizing genes of the broad host-range IncP-type plasmid RP4 integrated into the chromosome. A fresh, transformed colony of SMI0(pSS1129/ PT::Kan::PT) is then used for bacterial conjugation with a *B. pertussis* strain that is resistant to streptomycin and nalidixic acid. Therefore, exconjugants are selected on plates containing nalidixic acid, gentamycin, and kanamycin. Nalidixic acid is used to counter select *E. coli*, whereas gentamycin and kanamycin are used to select acquisition of the plasmid by *B. pertussis*. Since the vector cannot replicate into *B. pertussis*, growing colonies are exconjugants that have integrated the plasmid into the chromosome by homologous recombination. A second event of intrachromosomal recombination is selected by growing the exconjugants on BG plates containing streptomycin. (*see* **Fig. 3**).
2. To confirm this substitution, it is always recommended to perform Southern blot analyses on chromosomal DNA extracted from the kanamycin-sensitive isolates. These isolates should be negative in respect to the kanamycin cassette.

## References

1. Rappuoli, R. and Pizza, M. (1991) Structure and evolutionary aspects of ADP-ribosylating toxins, in *Sourcebook of Bacterial Protein Toxins* (Alouf, J. and Freer, J., eds.), Academic Press, New York, pp. 1–20.
2. Telford, J. L., Ghiara, P., Dell'Orco, M., Comanducci, M., Burroni, D., Bugnoli M., et al. (1994) Gene structure of the *Helicobacter pylori* cytotoxin and evidence of its key role in gastric disease. *J. Exp. Med.* **179,** 1653–1658.
3. Ramon, G. (1924) Sur la toxine et sur l'anatoxine diphtheriques. *Ann. Inst. Pasteur* **38,** 1–10.
4. Rappuoli, R. (1997) New and improved vaccines against diphtheria and tetanus, in *New Generation Vaccines* (Levine, M. M., Woodrow, G. C., Kaper, J. B., and Cobon, G. S., eds.), Marcel Dekker, New York, pp. 251–268.
5. Rappuoli, R. (1994) Toxin inactivation and antigen stabilization: two different uses of formaldehyde-short review. *Vaccine* **12,** 579–581.
6. Pizza, M., Covacci, A., Bartoloni, A., Perugini, M., Nencioni, L., De Magistris. M. T., et al. (1989) Mutants of pertussis toxin suitable for vaccine development. *Science* **246,** 497–500.
7. Rappuoli, R., Podda, A., Pizza, M., Covacci, A., Bartoloni, A., De Magistris, M. T., et al. (1992) Progress towards the development of new vaccines against whooping cough. *Vaccine* **10,** 1027–1032.
8. Podda, A., Deluca, E. C., Contu, B., Furlan, R., Maida, A., Moiraghi, A., et al. (1994) Comparative study of a whole-cell pertussis vaccine and a recombinant acellular pertussis vaccine. *J. Pediatr.* **124,** 921–926.
9. Pizza, M., Domenighini, M., Hol, W., Giannelli, V., Fontana, M. R., Giuliani, M. M., et al. (1994) Probing the structure-activity relationship of Escherichia coli LT-A by site-directed mutagenesis. *Mol. Microbiol.* **14,** 51–60.
10. Pizza, M., Fontana, M. R., Giuliani, M. M., Domenighini, M., Magagnoli, C., Giannelli, V., et al. (1994) A genetically detoxified derivative of heat-labile *E. coli* enterotoxin induces neutralizing antibodies against the A subunit. *J. Exp. Med.* **6,** 2147–2153.

11. Pizza, M., Giuliani, M. M., Fontana, M. R., Monaci, E., Douce, G., Dougan, G., et al. (2001) Mucosal vaccines: non toxic derivatives of LT and CT as mucosal adjuvants. *Vaccine* **19**, 2534–2541.

12. Tamura, M., Nogimori, K., Katada, T., Ui, M., and Ishii, S. (1982) Subunit structure of islet-activating protein, pertussis toxin, in conformity with the A-B model. *Biochemistry* **21**, 5516–5520.

13. Sixma, T. K., Pronk, S. E., Kalk, K. H., Wartna, E. S., van Zanten, B. A. M., Witholt, B., et al. (1991) Crystal structure of a cholera toxin-related heat-labile enterotoxin from *E. coli. Nature* **351**, 371–377.

14. Stein, P. E., Boodhoo, A., Armstrong, G. D., Cockle, S. A., Klein, M. H., and Read, R. J. (1994) The crystal structure of pertussis toxin. *Structure* **2**, 45–57.

15. Domenighini, M., Montecucco, C., Ripka, W. C., and Rappuoli, R. (1991) Computer modeling of the NAD binding site of ADP-ribosylating toxins: active site structure and mechanism of NAD binding. *Mol. Microbiol.* **5**, 23–3 1.

16. Domenighini, M., Magagnoli, C., Pizza, M., and Rappuoli, R. (1994) Common features of the NAD-binding and catalytic site of ADP-ribosylating toxins. *Mol. Microbiol.* **14**, 41–50.

17. Nicosia, A., Perugini, M., Franzini, C., Casagli, M. C., Borri, M. G., Antoni, G., et al. (1986) Cloning and sequencing of the pertussis toxin genes: operon structure and gene duplication. *Proc. Natl. Acad. Sci. USA* **83**, 4631–4635.

18. Locht, C. and Keith, J. M. (1986) Pertussis toxin gene: nucleotide sequence and genetic organization. *Science* **232**, 1258–1264.

19. Mekalanos, J. J., Swartz D. J., Pearson, G. D., Harford, N., Groyne, F., and de Wilde, M. (1983) Cholera toxin genes: nucleotide sequence, deletion analysis and vaccine development. *Nature* **306**, 551–557.

20. Dallas, W. S. and Falkow, S. (1980) Amino acid homology between cholera toxin and *Escherichia coli* heat labile toxin. *Nature* **288**, 499–501.

21. Zoller, M. J. and Smith, M. (1982) Oligonucleotide-directed mutagenesis using M13-derived vectors: an efficient and general procedure for the production of point mutations in any fragment of DNA. *Nucleic Acids Res.* **10**, 6487–6500.

22. Sambrook, J., Fritsch, E. F., and Maniatis, T. (1989) *Molecular Cloning. A Laboratory Manual.* Cold Spring Harbor Laboratory, Cold Spring Harbor, NY, pp. 68–73.

23. Pittman, M. (1984) *Genus Bordetella, in Bergey's Manual of Systemic Bacteriology* (Krief, N. R. and Holt, J. G., eds.), William and Wilkins, Baltimore, MD, pp. 338.

24. Stainer, D. W. and Scholte, M. J. (1971) A simple chemically defined medium for the production of phase I *Bordetella pertussis. J. Gen. Microbiol.* **63**, 211–220.

25. Stibitz, S. and Yang, M. S. (1991) Subcellular localization and immunological detection of proteins encoded by the *vir* locus of *Bordetella pertussis. J. Bacteriol.* **173**, 4288–4291.

26. Simon, R., Priefer, U., and Puhler, A. (1983) A broad host range mobilization system for in vivo genetic engineering: transposon mutagenesis in gram-negative bacteria. *BioTechnology* **1**, 784–791.

27. Lebens, M., Johansson, S., Osek, J., Lindblad, M., and Holmgren, J. (1993) Large- scale production of *Vibrio-cholerae* toxin-B subunit for use in oral vaccines. *BioTechnology* **11**, 1574–1578.

28. Donta, S. T., Moon, H. W., and Whipp, S. C. (1973) Detection and use of heat-labile *Escherichia coli* enterotoxin with the use of adrenal cells in tissue culture. *Science* **183**, 334–335.

29. Hewlett, E. L., Sauer, K. T., Myers, G. A., Cowell, J. L., and Guerrant, R. (1983) Induction of a novel morphological response in Chinese hamster ovary cells by pertussis toxin. *Infect. Immun.* **40**, 1198–1203.

30. Stibitz, S., Black, W., and Falkow, S. (1986) The construction of a cloning vector designed for gene replacement in *Bordetella pertussis*. *Gene* **50**, 133–140.

31. Pronk, S. E., Hofstra, H., Groendijk, H., Kingma, J., Swarte, M. B. A., Dorner, F., et al. (1985) Heat-labile enterotoxin of *Escherichia coli*: characterization of different crystal forms. *J. Biol. Chem.* **260**, 13,580–13,584.

32. Pearson, G. D. N. and Mekalanos, J. J. (1982) Molecular cloning of *Vibrio cholerae* enterotoxin genes in *Escherichia coli* K-12. *Proc. Natl. Acad. Sci. USA* **79**, 2976–2980.

33. Dente, L., Cesarini, G., and Cortese, R. (1983) pEMBL: a new family of single stranded plasmids. *Nucleic Acids Res.* **11**, 1645–1655.

34. Fontana, M.R., Monaci, E., Liu, YQ., Qi, GM., Guangcai, D., Rappuoli, R., Pizza, M. (2001) IEM101, a naturally attenuated *Vibrio cholera* strani as carrier for genetically detoxified derivatives of cholera toxin. *Vaccine* **19**, 75–85.

35. Donnenberg, M. S. and Kaper, J. K. (1991) Construction of an eae deletion mutant of enteropathogenic *Escherichia coli* by using a positive-selection suicide vector. *Infect. Immun.* **59**, 4310–4317.

36. Mekalanos, J. (1988) Production and purification of cholera toxin. *Meth. Enzymol.* **165**, 169–175.

# 10

## Preparation of Polysaccharide-Conjugate Vaccines

**Carla C. A. M. Peeters, Patrick R. Lagerman,
Odo de Weers, Lukas A. Oomen, Peter Hoogerhout,
Michel Beurret, and Jan T. Poolman**

**Revised by Karen M. Reddin**

### 1. Introduction

It was recognized early last century that small molecules, known as haptens, can be made immunogenic after conjugation to carrier proteins *(1)*. This principle has since been applied successfully to improve the immunogenicity of (poly)saccharides *(2,3)*. We now know that the carrier proteins ensure the involvement of T-helper lymphocytes in the activation of the hapten- or polysaccharide-specific antibody-producing B lymphocytes (**Fig. 1**). In contrast to small molecules or haptens, polysaccharides (or other macromolecules with a repeating structure) are able to induce an immune response, most likely by directly activating B-lymphocytes. Antigens that are able to induce an immune response without the involvement of T-helper lymphocytes are referred to as TI (thymus-independent) antigens *(4)* (**Table 1**). TI-2 antigens, such as plain polysaccharides, are not able to activate relatively immature B-cells. This is in contrast to TI-l antigens, which can activate immature B-cells because of their mitogenic activity. Lipopolysaccharides (LPS) are examples of TI-l antigens. Conventional T-cells recognize peptide sequences in association with the major histocompatibility complex (MHC). Recently, unconventional T-cells were found to recognize (glyco) lipids in a CD1-restricted way, γδT-cells were shown to respond to non-proteinaceous microbial ligands (that may include carbohydrates) in a virtually MHC-unrestricted way *(5)*. The findings of T-cell regulation of the immune response against polysaccharides *(6–8)* without biochemical demonstration of the specificity of the molecular interactions can best be explained by assuming a role for anti-idiotypic antibodies and T-cells specific for the idiotopes (carbohydrate mimotopes) or via the newly discovered unconventional T-cells.

From: *Methods in Molecular Medicine, Vol. 87: Vaccine Protocols, 2nd ed.*
Edited by: A. Robinson, M. J. Hudson, and M. P. Cranage © Humana Press Inc., Totowa, NJ

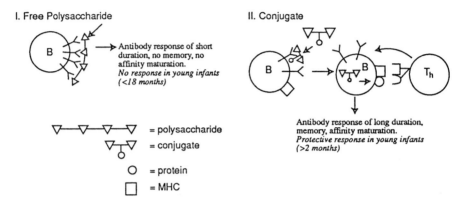

Fig. 1. Polysaccharides are poor in activating B-cells to the production of antibodies in children younger than 2 yr of age. If antibodies are formed, they are of short duration. For conjugate vaccines T-cells are involved in the activation of B-cells. Presumably, the conjugate is taken up by polysaccharide-specific B-cells, processed, and presented to carrier-specific T-cells. The involvement of T-cells results in the activation of B-cells to production of antibodies and induction of memory in children younger than 2 yr of age.

The characteristics of polysaccharides described here are reflected in the antibody responses found in humans. Plain polysaccharides induce a poor response in infants, and at later ages of life the responses are of short duration and cannot be boosted (*9–11*), and the affinity does not mature.

To overcome these problems, polysaccharides must be conjugated to carrier proteins in order to create effective vaccines.

The *Haemophilus influenzae* type b capsular polysaccharide conjugate vaccine has been successfully introduced in many national childhood vaccination programs (*12–15*). *N. meningitidis* serogroup C polysaccharide conjugate vaccines have now been developed. Clinical trials for these vaccines proved successful (*16*) and, as a result, a number of these vaccines were introduced into the UK vaccination schedules in 1999. These conjugate vaccines have already had a significant impact on the incidence of meningococcal serogroup C disease in immunized groups (*17,18*). This has led to a better definition of important criteria needed for potent conjugate vaccines (*see* **Subheading 1.1.**). Finally, in recent clinical trials, pneumococcal conjugate vaccines have been shown to be effective at preventing pneumococcal disease in children (*19*).

In this chapter, we describe details of the preparation of a pneumococcal type 19F polysaccharide-protein conjugate vaccine (*20*).

## 1.1. Development of Saccharide–Protein Conjugate Vaccines—Relation of Structure to Immunogenicity

### 1.1.1. Saccharide Chain Length

Both large-mol-wt polysaccharides and small, otherwise non-immunogenic oligosaccharides can be converted to thymus-dependent (TD) antigens by conjugation to a carrier protein (*21–27*). Bacterial saccharide antigens generally belong to the follow-

**Table 1**
**Characteristics of T-Cell Independent Antigens**

Type 1

        Bacterial cell-wall components

        Mitogenic or polyclonal B-cell activator

        Stimulate antibody responses in neonates

        Stimulate antibody responses in CBA/N mice

        Examples: lipopolysaccharide and hapten derivatives;
            *Brucella abortus*

Type 2

        Polysaccharides, polypeptides, polynucleotides

        High mol wt, multiple repeating antigenic determinants

        Slowly metabolized

        Tolerogenic in large doses or soluble form

        Activate alternative complement pathway (some)

        Generate few (if any) memory B-cells

        Restriction of isotypes induced

        Lack of affinity maturation

        Lack of T-cell memory

        Fail to stimulate antibody responses in neonates

        Fail to stimulate antibody responses in CBA/N mice

        Examples: Pneumococcal polysaccharides;
            *Haemophilus influenzae* type b polysaccharide;
            meningococcal polysaccharides

ing main categories: capsular polysaccharides (CPS), lipopolysaccharides (LPS), or lipo-oligosaccharides (LOS).

Their chemical structures have been extensively investigated, and several reviews present the current state of knowledge in this field *(28–34)*. Thus, the antigen may be an oligomer or a polymer, in which case depolymerization, if needed, can be accomplished by various means.

For a polysaccharide, it is theorized that a minimal number of unmodified repeat units (RU) must be present in a continuous chain to allow for sufficient immunogenicity. Numerous studies have shown the correlation between length of saccharide chain and antigenicity and immunogenicity *(35–41)*. Very short oligosaccharides of one or two RU may not always raise antibodies that are specific for the polysaccharide, as it exists on the bacterial surface, essentially for two reasons. First, one of the main epitopes present is a terminal non-reducing sugar that represents only a very low proportion of the natural polysaccharide. Second, antibodies directed at the internal part of a short saccharide chain may not bind strongly to the native polysaccharide, because of the absence in the former of secondary structures that are present only when a minimal number of RU is available *(42,44)*.

Most important is the need to retain antigenicity, and to retain or improve immunogenicity of the saccharide after conjugation. Small saccharides can have much reduced antigenicity in comparison with the corresponding native polysaccharides, but this is not necessarily a drawback in immunogenicity if the saccharide is conjugated to protein. In most cases, a minimal chain length of two RU is necessary to raise antibodies that bind polysaccharides with corresponding epitope patterns *(35,45)*. In some instances, protective antibodies have been generated with conjugate vaccines bearing only one RU from a bacterial polysaccharide *(46,47)*. However, this was only shown for adult animals. Other studies have shown that conjugate vaccines that are immunogenic in adult animals are not always able to induce an antibody response in neonatal animals. This might be explained by the fact that for primed B-cells, the binding on only a few receptors seems necessary, whereas for unprimed B-cells, more Ig receptors must be crosslinked by the saccharide antigen before the cell is activated.

In their native, high-mol-wt form, bacterial polysaccharides (CPS or LPS) are TI antigens and may retain some of these characteristics once conjugated to a TD carrier protein *(48)*. However, conjugated oligosaccharides of low mol wt may achieve the best T-dependent antigen recognition, and may be able to maximize carrier help function and allow easier preparation of conjugates. Therefore, polysaccharides are often depolymerized before coupling. A number of chemical and enzymatic methods are available for the specific degradation of polysaccharides *(49–53)*. These include mainly hydrolyses (acid-, alkali-, or glycanase-mediated), oxidations, and eliminations (alkali- or lyase-mediated β-elimination). Physical methods, such as sonication *(54,55)* and mechanical shearing *(56)* can also provoke stress-induced depolymerization of polysaccharides. Such methods can have the disadvantage of causing random cuts of glycosidic linkages, which in turn will lower the yield of coupling if a specific end group is needed for activation of the saccharide. However, it is also worth noting that chemically induced depolymerization methods are rarely specific for a given linkage, and can therefore promote loss of important side groups common in bacterial antigens, such as *O*-acetyls, pyruvates, or saccharide side-chains. When possible, specific bacterial or viral enzymes have the clear advantage of causing highly specific cuts without the need for potentially toxic reagents *(57–61)*. The purification of depolymerized saccharides and the selection of a defined range of mol wts can be accomplished by several techniques, such as ultrafiltration, liquid chromatography (e.g. gel permeation, ion exchange, or hydrophobic interaction), or electrophoresis. Finally, oligosaccharides of defined chain length can be obtained by chemical synthesis (*see* **Subheading 1.2.**), sometimes with the incorporation of a spacer to facilitate conjugation.

### 1.1.2. Carrier Protein

A variety of proteins, including bacterial pili, outer membrane proteins (OMPs), and excreted toxins of pathogenic bacteria, preferably in toxoid form, have been employed as carriers for carbohydrate antigens. Most popular as carrier proteins are tetanus and diphtheria toxoids, which are readily available and accepted for human use. However, the use of detoxified bacterial toxins as carrier proteins has some disadvantages. The process of chemically detoxifying produces lot-to-lot variations. Thus, physical and chemical properties of the toxin can be substantially modified, which can affect the conjugation efficiency. Conjugation of these proteins with large amounts of saccharide may further affect protein conformational features and inactivate T- and/or B-cell epitopes. This might limit the amount of saccharide to be coupled to the protein, since a precondition of the conjugation is to maintain the T-cell activating properties of the carrier protein. Bacterial toxins offer advantages over their corresponding toxoids if cytotoxic effects can be reduced by the conjugation itself. Alternative carrier proteins have been developed, such as $CRM_{197}$, a nontoxic analog of diphtheria toxoid *(62,63)*. These proteins have the same advantages as native toxins—light or heavy loading of saccharide is possible without influencing the carrier characteristics. Although diphtheria and tetanus toxin-derivatized proteins have proven to be successful carrier proteins, both in animal and human studies, such problems as hypersensitivity or suppression of anti-carbohydrate response caused by the pre-existence of anti-carrier antibodies may still be a matter of concern, especially when a broad range of saccharides is analyzed *(64–68)*. These negative effects could become more evident when conjugated carrier proteins are tested in polyvalent or combination vaccine formulations.

The use of a carrier protein derived from the homologous bacterial species from which the polysaccharide was obtained would avoid possible problems. Furthermore, a homologous carrier protein may afford protection by itself that would enhance the protective action of the anti-polysaccharide immunity through synergistic action. In addition, homologous T help will be boosted on infection. It may be necessary to develop and use multiple carrier proteins as an approach to reduce interference when more than one conjugate vaccine is used; alternative carrier proteins, such as *Bordetella pertussis* fimbriae, have been used experimentally *(69,70)*. Alternatively, the use of synthetic peptides corresponding to T-cell of proteins may be a viable approach to circumvent the phenomena described previously *(71–73)*. However, to be able to induce an immune response across HLA barriers in the human population, synthetic polypeptides containing multiple epitopes from proteins would have to be used.

### 1.1.3. Coupling Chemistry (Linkage)

To confer a TD character to a saccharide, it must be coupled to a carrier protein through a covalent bond. Other strong, noncovalent couplings or associations with proteins have not proven to be as effective in reaching that goal.

There are numerous existing or potential techniques available for the conjugation of bio-organic molecules, including saccharides and proteins *(74–81)*. A large variety of these, often derived from pioneering research in affinity chromatography, have been used for the preparation of conjugate vaccines *(24)*, including mainly reductive amination, amidation, and etherification reactions, but also the formation of disulfide, thiocarbamoyl, *O*-alkylisourea, or diazo couplings, among others. Conjugates obtained by reductive amination *(82–84)*, amidation *(85)*, the formation of a thioether bond *(21,86–88)*, or a combination of these *(89,90)* have been shown to be highly stable. However, at present, it is uncertain whether some other types of linkage (e.g. disulfide bonds) have enough stability in vivo. New techniques, sometimes adapted from other areas of biochemical research, constantly broaden the choice already available *(91–99)*. Because of the lability of some saccharide components, coupling conditions should be as mild as possible. Accordingly, reaction parameters (pH, temperature, reaction time, and chemical reagents), should be chosen with the goal of avoiding the denaturation of protein or unwanted hydrolysis of saccharides. The stability of the linkage formed by conjugation is also of paramount importance. Significant decoupling during storage could lead to loss of immunogenicity or of the TD character of the conjugate.

The choice of a coupling chemistry is also largely driven by the model of conjugate that is needed, namely a well-defined neoglycoprotein or a crosslinked lattice *(24,25)*. The former is obtained by activation of a single end of the saccharide, and is generally more efficient for the coupling of oligosaccharides or short polysaccharides *(100,101)*. The latter is obtained by random activation at several points on the saccharide chain, and is the more practical approach for the coupling of large polysaccharides. This model appears also to be the most appropriate for reducing the TI character of a polysaccharide, by controlling the length of continuous chains of intact RU in the conjugate. It should be noted that, in some rare instances, a well-defined crosslinked lattice can be obtained when a saccharide is amenable to specific activation of both ends of the chain—e.g. by periodate-induced depolymerization *(82,83)*.

When conjugating oligosaccharides, it is often desirable to use a spacer arm (e.g., adipic acid dihydrazide, diaminobutane, or 6-aminohexanoic acid) as a linker between the saccharide and the protein in order to avoid the shielding of important saccharide epitopes by the secondary structure of the carrier protein. A spacer can also provide greater efficiency of coupling with polysaccharides by reducing steric hindrance of activated moieties *(86,102–104)*. In turn, a spacer can create a neo-antigenic structure that may be either harmless or toxic (e.g. aromatic spacer), or may lead to the unnecessary production of large amounts of nonprotective antibodies on immunization with the conjugate. Other considerations that influence the choice of a coupling chemistry include the availability of active groups on both the saccharide and the carrier protein, or the practical feasibility of introducing new ones by chemical or enzymatic modifications. Moreover, unrelated groups must be deactivated after conjugation, to avoid uncontrolled reactions within the conjugate itself and with body tissues after immunization.

### 1.1.4. Saccharide-to-Protein Ratio

The spacing and density of the saccharide on the protein are likely to have major impacts on the ability of the conjugate to induce an immune response. Once the saccharide antigen is coupled to the carrier protein, measuring the relative ratio of those two moieties will provide some information about the conjugate structure. To obtain accurate data, it is essential that all free (uncoupled) material is removed from the final reaction mixture. This can be accomplished by ultrafiltration, liquid chromatography, electrophoresis, or differential precipitation. In some instances, it may be difficult to separate native polysaccharides from conjugates, since both components have high mol wts that are not always amenable to chromatographic separation. If a conjugate contains appreciable amounts of free polysaccharide, dose calculations for animal experiments become unreliable. In addition, the presence of a comparatively large amount of the TI form of the saccharide antigen, together with its coupled TD form, can have adverse effects on the immune response *(105–107)*. Long-term storage of a conjugate can equally lead to partial depolymerization or decoupling of the saccharide antigen, which in turn will affect the saccharide-to-protein ratio.

For a neo-glycoprotein model, the saccharide-to-protein ratio provides valuable information about the number of attachment points on the carrier. It then becomes possible to compare several conjugates with different ratios *(25,41,108)*, and to evaluate the importance of the shielding of protein epitopes. With high saccharide-to-protein ratios, essential carrier epitopes may be hidden from the immune system, preventing recognition of the conjugate as a TD antigen *(24–26,102)*. For a lattice model, since activation points are randomly distributed on the saccharide, information about linkage points to the protein is not readily available. Additional tests are needed, such as the titration of remaining activated groups on the carrier. Attachment points can also be measured when amino acids become covalently modified in such a way that physical (e.g., NMR) or chemical analysis is able to detect a change in their structure *(86,109)*. It is equally difficult to measure the extent of crosslinking or the length of intact saccharide chains between attachment points. Other characteristics, such as the actual mol wt of the conjugate, particularly if physical aggregation has taken place, certainly play a role in the way the conjugate is processed by the immune system. Finally, it should be emphasized that an optimal conjugation scheme must be determined for each particular saccharide and protein combination *(25)*.

## 1.2. Development of Synthetic Saccharide–Protein Conjugate Vaccines

Like natural saccharides, synthetic carbohydrates may be coupled to proteins by direct reductive amination *(110)*. However, groups with specific reactivity can also be introduced into synthetic carbohydrates *(42,111)*. Usually, a spacer arm with a reactive group is coupled to the anomeric center. Examples are the use of allyl *(112)*, 4-aminophenyl *(113,114)*, 8-methoxycarbonyloctyl *(115–117)*, and 3-aminopropyl glycosides *(118,119)*, all of which can be modified further for conjugation purposes.

During synthesis of carbohydrates containing repeating phosphodiester units, it is more convenient to modify a terminal phosphodiester with a spacer arm. In this way, phosphorylation was used to couple *N*-benzyloxycarbonyl-protected derivatives of 3-aminopropanol and glycine-*N*-(3-hydroxypropyl)-amide to oligosaccharides derived from capsular polysaccharides occurring in *Haemophilus pleuropneumoniae (120)* and *H. influenzae* type b *(121,122)* respectively. During deprotection of the oligosaccharides, the spacer amino group was liberated by catalytic hydrogenation.

Spacer-containing oligosaccharides of *H. influenzae* type b were directly conjugated to tetanus toxoid with glutaric dialdehyde *(123)*. Furthermore, the spacer amino group was modified with *S*-acetylthioglycolic acid N-hydroxysuccinimide ester (SATA). The SATA-functionalized oligosaccharides were coupled with 3-(2-pyridyldithio)-propionylated tetanus toxoid or *H. influenzae* outer membrane protein to give disulfide conjugates *(123)* and with bromoacetylated tetanus toxoid or diphtheria toxin to furnish thioether conjugates *(40)*. In immunization experiments, the most promising results were obtained with the thioether conjugates. Therefore, conjugation of carbohydrates (as well as peptides) via thioether linkages has become the method of choice. The method was used successfully to prepare conjugates of meningococcal LOS and proteins *(124)* or synthetic peptides *(125)*, and is currently also being used in pneumococcal vaccine development.

## *1.3. Development of a Pneumococcus Serotype 19F Saccharide–Protein Conjugate Vaccine*

The development of pneumococcal serotype 19F saccharide–protein (Pn19FTTd) conjugates was initiated by using a saccharide with a mean mol wt of approx 350 kDa, a spacer coupling via a thioether linkage, and tetanus toxoid as a carrier protein. Conjugates were prepared with either a high or low molar saccharide-to-protein ratio, aiming for theoretical value of 2.5:1 and 0.25:1, respectively. Furthermore, the influence of adding $AlPO_4$ as an adjuvant on the immunogenicity of the prepared conjugates was studied. The method for preparing and characterizing these conjugates is described in detail in the following section.

## 2. Materials

1. Native 19F polysaccharide from *Streptococcus pneumoniae*, mol wt 1250 kDa (American Type Culture Collection, Rockville, MD).
2. 0.01 $M$ sodium phosphate buffer, pH 7.2 (phosphate buffer).
3. GPC-HPLC (gel-permeation chromatography) columns Oltpak KB-805 and KB804, 8 × 300 mm (Shodex, Tokyo, Japan), connected in series.
4. Phosphate buffer, 0.9% (w/v) NaCl (phosphate-buffered saline [PBS]).
5. PBS containing 0.05% (v/v) Tween 80 (PBS-Tween).
6. Pullulan mol-wt standards (Shodex).
7. Pneumococcal cell-wall polysaccharide, provided by U. Sorensen, Statens Serum Institut, Copenhagen, Denmark.
8. High-titer rabbit anti-Pn19F PS IgG serum.
9. Tetanus toxoid (TTd), similar properties to that for vaccine production, provided by Laboratory for Vaccine Production, RIVM (Bilthoven, The Netherlands).
10. 1 $M$ sodium hydroxide.
11. *N,N*-dimethylformamide (DMFA) (890 µL) containing 22.2 mg cyanogen bromide (0.21 mmol).
12. 4.63 mL distilled water containing 185 mg diaminobutane (2.1 mmol).
13. Centriflo® CF25 (Amazon, Beverly, MA).
14. 0.1 $M$ ethylmorpholine buffer, pH 8.5.
15. 400 µL *N,N*-dimethylacetamide containing 60 mg (0.26 mmol) SATA (Sigma, St. Louis, MO).
16. 70 µL *N,N*-dimethylacetamide containing 9.9 mg (0.04 mol) N-succinimidyl bromoacetate (Sigma, St. Louis, MO).
17. 1.2 mL of 0.1 $M$ phosphate buffer, pH8.0 containing 17.5 mg TTd.
18. 0.1 $M$ phosphate buffer containing 5 m$M$ EDTA, pH 7.5.
19. 2 $M$ hydroxylamine in 0.1 $M$ phosphate buffer, pH 7.5, containing 5 m$M$ EDTA.
20. 2-aminoethanethiol (50 mg/mL) in 0.1 $M$ phosphate buffer, pH 7.5, containing 5 m$M$ EDTA.
21. PolySorp(tm) microtiter plates (Nunc, Roskilde, Denmark).
22. 0.04 $M$ carbonate buffer, pH 9.6.
23. Water containing 0.03% (w/v) Tween 80 (Water-Tween).
24. Horseradish peroxidase-labeled goat anti-mouse antibodies.
25. Tetramethylbenzidine (0.1 mg/mL) and 0.01% (v/v) $H_2O_2$ in 0.11 $M$ sodium acetate buffer, pH 5.5 (Sigma).
26. 2 $M$ $H_2SO_4$.

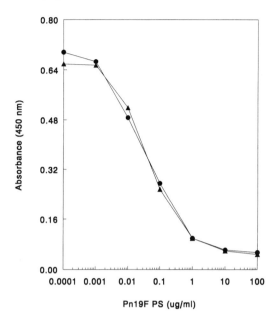

Fig. 2. Inhibition profiles of native polysaccharide, mol wt 1250 kDa (●) and sonicated polysaccharide, mol wt 350 kDa (▲). The antigenicity of the polysaccharides was found to be similar.

27. ELISA Titretek Multiscan spectrophotometer.
28. Swiss Webster mice (Harlan, Zeist, The Netherlands).
29. AlPO$_4$ (Superfos-Biosector, Denmark).

## 3. Methods
### 3.1. S. pneumoniae *Serotype 19F Saccharide*

1. To decrease the size of the native Pnl9F PS, mol wt 1250 kDa, sonicate a solution of polysaccharide (10 mg/mL in 0.01 *M* phosphate buffer, pH 7.2) for a total of 1.5 min on ice.
2. Monitor the decrease of the mol wt by GPC-HPLC (gel permeation chromatography) using PBS as eluent (1 mL/min), and pullulan fractions as standards (Shodex).
3. Compare the antigenicity of the sonicated polysaccharide to that of the native Pnl9FPS in a competition ELISA by pre-incubating a high-titer rabbit anti-Pnl9F PS IgG serum, preadsorbed for 30 min at 37°C with 100 µg/mL CPs (cell wall polysaccharide), with varying amounts of sonicated and native Pnl9F PS (**Fig. 2**). Then transfer these samples to a native Pnl9F PS-coated ELISA plate (*see* **Subheading 3.4.**). Process the ELISA further as described for polysaccharide and tetanus toxoid antibody determinations (*see* **Subheading 3.4.**). This will determine whether important epitopes have been affected by the breakdown of the polysaccharide.

### 3.2. Coupling of Saccharides to Protein

1. Cool 35 mg of sonicated polysaccharide (mol wt 350 kDa) at a concentration of 5 mg/mL in 0.005 *M* phosphate buffer, pH 7.2, to a temperature of 2.5°C.

2. Adjust the pH of this solution to 10.5 using 1 *M* sodium hydroxide.

3. Add a solution of cyanogen bromide (22.2 mg; 0.21 mmol) in 890 μL of *N*,*N*-DMFA while mixing.

4. Keep the solution at pH 10.5 for 6 min, then lower the pH to 7.2 using 1 *M* HCl

5. Add a solution of diaminobutane (185 mg; 2.1 mmol) in 4.63 mL distilled water while keeping the pH at 7.2.

6. After 45 min incubation at room temperature, dialyze the reaction mixture against distilled water.

7. Concentrate the dialysate by ultrafiltration (Centriflo CF-25, Amicon) and dry *in vacuo*.

8. Mix a solution of 22.4 mg modified polysaccharide in 1.1 mL 0.1 *M* ethylmorpholine buffer, pH 8.5, with 60 mg (0.26 mmol) SATA in 400 μL *N*,*N*-dimethylacetamide.

9. After 1 h incubation at room temperature, stop the reaction by addition of 100 μL of acetic acid.

10. Precipate the SATA-modified polysaccharide (Pnl9F-SATA) with acetone and dry *in vacuo*.

11. Dissolve the dried precipitate in water and further purify by ultrafiltration.

12. Mix a solution of *N*-succinimidyl bromoacetate (9.9 mg; 0.04 mol) in 70 μL *N*,*N* dimethylacetamide with a solution of TTd (17.5 mg) in 1.2 mL of 0.1 *M* phosphate buffer, pH 8.0.

13. After 1.5 h reaction at room temperature, subject the mixture to ultrafiltration and equilibrate in 1 mL of 0.1 *M* phosphate buffer containing 5 m*M* EDTA, pH 7.5.

14. Add the solution of bromoacetylated TTd thus obtained to the SATA-modified carbohydrate. For the preparation of conjugates with a theoretical saccharide-to-protein molar ratio of 0.25:1, mix 6.5 mg of Pnl9F-SATA in distilled water (410 μL) with 11 mg of bromoacetylated TTd (765 μL) in 0.1 *M* phosphate buffer, pH 7.5, containing 5 m*M* EDTA, and incubate with 27.5 μL of 2 *M* hydroxylamine (in 0.1 *M* phosphate buffer, pH 7.5, containing 5 m*M* EDTA). For the preparation of conjugates with a theoretical molar ratio of 2.5:1, mix 6.5 mg of Pnl9F-SATA in distilled water (410 μL) with 1.1 mg of bromoacetylated TTd (765 μL) in 0.1 *M* phosphate buffer, pH 7.5, containing 5 m*M* EDTA, and incubate with 27.5 μL of 2 *M* hydroxylamine (in 0.1 *M* phosphate buffer, pH 7.5, containing 5 m*M* EDTA). Follow the conjugation over time by GPC-HPLC.

15. After 43 h incubation at room temperature, block the remaining bromoacetyl groups by the addition of 2-aminoethanethiol (50 mg/mL) in 0.1 *M* phosphate buffer, pH 7.5, containing 5 m*M* EDTA. For the conjugate with a saccharide-to-protein ratio of 0.25:1, add 101 μL 2-aminoethanethiol; for a saccharide-to-protein ratio of 2.5:1, add 10.1 μL 2-aminoethanethiol.

16. After an additional period of 6 h, purify the conjugate and equilibrate in PBS by ultrafiltration.

17. Fractionate the conjugates by GPC-HPLC.

### 3.3. Characterization of Pn19F-TTd Saccharide–Protein Conjugates

1. After the reaction has been stopped, confirm the presence of conjugate by a sandwich ELISA detecting both polysaccharide and protein.

2. Isolate the conjugate by GPC-HPLC, monitoring the elution profile by both UV absorbance at 280 nm (for the presence of protein) and refractive index (**Fig. 3**).

3. Analyze all fractions for the presence of sugar *(126)* and protein *(127)* to estimate for the presence of covalent conjugates. In our experience, a low initial saccharide-to-protein ratio yields conjugates with a molar ratio ranging from 0.08:1 to 0.65:1, whereas a high initial saccharide-to-protein ratio yields a molar ratio ranging from 2.4:1 to 3.9:1.

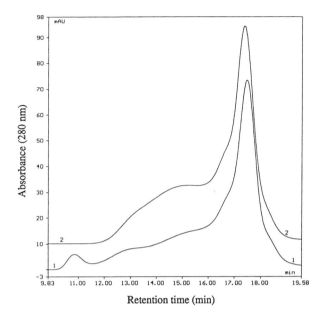

Retention time (min)

Fig. 3. Conjugation of modified Pnl9F PS to TTd was followed by GPC-HPLC. After a conjugation period of 15 h, at a retention time of 12–16 min, an increase in the absorbance at 280 nm was observed. This indicates the formation of conjugate. 1. Conjugation at $t = 0$. 2. Conjugation at $t = 15$ h.

4. Compare the antigenicity of the Pnl9FTTd conjugates with that of the native capsular polysaccharide in a competition ELISA.
5. Determine the level of unbound polysaccharide and protein by rocket immuno-electro-phoresis.
6. Select the conjugates with the lowest percentage of free polysaccharide and free protein for immunogenicity studies.

## 3.4. Determinations of Antibodies by ELISA

1. Coat PolySorp microtiter plates (Nunc) with TTd (2 mg/mL in 0.04 $M$ carbonate buffer, pH 9.6) for 2 h at room temperature and use to determine antibodies to TTd.
2. Coat similar plates for 5 h at 37°C followed by an overnight incubation at 4°C with Pnl9F PS (10 µg/mL in PBS) for the determination of antiPnl9F PS antibodies.
3. Wash the coated plates with water-Tween and incubate for 2 h at 37°C with three- or fivefold serial dilutions in PBS-Tween of serum samples that have been pre-incubated for 30 min at 37°C with 100 µg/mL CPs.
4. Wash the plates with water-Tween and incubate for 2 h at 37°C with horseradish peroxi-dase-labeled goat anti-mouse antibodies in PBS-Tween containing 0.5% (w/v) BSA.
5. Wash the plates again with water-Tween and incubate at room temperature with the per-oxidase substrate tetramethylbenzidine (0.1 mg/mL; Sigma)–0.01% (v/v) $H_2O_2$ in 0.11 $M$ sodium acetate buffer, pH 5.5.
6. After 10–30 min of incubation, stop the reaction by adding 100 µL of 2 $M$ $H_2SO_4$.
7. Read the $A_{450}$ on an ELISA Titertek Multiscan spectrophotometer.

## Table 2
## Immunogenicity of Pn19FTTd Conjugates in Adult Mice

| Group | Conjugate | Doses, μg | AntiPn19F antibody titers (geometric mean [+/−] SEM after the following immunization) | | | | | |
|---|---|---|---|---|---|---|---|---|
| | | | Primary | | Secondary | | Tertiary | |
| | | | Titer | Resp. | Titer | Resp. | Titer | Resp. |
| IgM | | | | | | | | |
| 1 | Pn19FTTd (0.65:1) | 1 | 22 (+/−) 2 | 0/6 | 39 (+/−) 1 | 5/6 | 42 (+/−) 2 | 6/6 |
| 2 | Pn19FTTd (0.65:1)[a] | 1 | 41 (+/−) 2 | 5/5 | 70 (+/−) 3 | 4/5 | 116 (+/−) 3 | 5/5 |
| 3 | Pn19FTTd (3.7:1) | 1 | 28 (+/−) 2 | 0/6 | 43 (+/−) 2 | 5/6 | 42 (+/−) 2 | 6/6 |
| 4 | Pn19FTTd (3.7:1)[a] | 1 | 24 (+/−) 2 | 0/5 | 34 (+/−) 2 | 2/5 | 43 (+/−) 3 | 4/5 |
| 5 | Saline | 1 | 11 (+/−) 4 | 0/6 | 10 (+/−) 3 | 0/5 | 6 (+/−) 1 | 0/5 |
| 6 | Saline[a] | — | 12 (+/−) 1 | 0/6 | 16 (+/−) 1 | 0/6 | 6 (+/−) 1 | 0/6 |
| IgG | | | | | | | | |
| 1 | Pn19FTTd (0.65:1) | 1 | 8 (+/−) 13 | 3/6 | 51 (+/−) 14 | 3/6 | 67 (+/−) 8 | 4/6 |
| 2 | Pn19FTTd (0.65:1)[a] | 1 | 15 (+/−) 6 | 3/5 | 446 (+/−) 5 | 5/5 | 1792 (+/−) 8 | 5/5 |
| 3 | Pn19FTTd (3.7:1) | 1 | 4 (+/−) 2 | 1/6 | 15 (+/−) 5 | 4/6 | 15 (+/−) 5 | 4/6 |
| 4 | Pn19FTTd (3.7:1)[a] | 1 | 3 (+/−) 4 | 1/5 | 7 (+/−) 4 | 2/5 | 27 (+/−) 6 | 4/5 |
| 5 | Saline | 1 | 1 (+/−) 1 | 0/6 | 2 (+/−) 7 | 0/5 | 2 (+/−) 1 | 0/5 |
| 6 | Saline[a] | — | 1 (+/−) 1 | 0/6 | 2 (+/−) 6 | 0/6 | 2 (+/−) 2 | 0/6 |

[a]Administered in the presence of 0.1% AlPO$_4$.

### 3.5. Immunogenicity of Saccharide–Protein Conjugate Vaccines

1. Immunize groups of six 8–12-wk-old female random outbred (Swiss Webster/Harlan) mice subcutaneously 3× with a 4-wk interval with 0.25 mL 0.9% NaCl solutions of conjugate containing 1 µg of saccharide. The conjugates can be administered in the presence or absence of 0.1% (w/v) $AlPO_4$.
2. Collect blood samples before each immunization and at d 14 after the third immunization.

Analysis of individual sera of mice immunized in our laboratory with either Pnl9FTTd (0.65:1) or Pnl9FTTd (3.7:1) on d 28 after first immunization showed that the highest percentage of mice responded to the Pnl9FTTd (0.65:1) conjugate (**Table 2**). Both antiPn19F IgM and IgG antibody responses could be observed. Booster injections with the homologous Pn 19FTTd conjugates showed a small increase of Pnl9F IgM antibodies, whereas a remarkable increase in the level of Pnl9F PS IgG antibodies was observed. A tertiary immunization further increased antiPnl9F PS antibody responses in mice immunized with Pnl9FTTd (0.65:1) adsorbed to $AlPO_4$, whereas for the other groups only minor increases were observed. The highest increase resulting from $AlPO_4$ was observed with the anti-Pnl9F PS antibody response of the Pnl9FTTd (0.65:1) conjugate.

Analysis of antiTTd antibody responses in individual sera demonstrated that each of the immunized mice could form anti-TTd antibodies (data not shown).

## 4. Conclusion

The application of conjugate vaccines has been shown to be successful for the prevention of infectious diseases caused by *H. influenzae* type b and pneumococci in infants and by serogroup C *N. meningitidis* in infants and young adults *(18)*. This approach is therefore also favoured for other encapsulated bacteria, such as pneumococci. In recent clinical trials, pneumococcal conjugate vaccines have been shown to be effective at preventing pneumococcal disease in children *(19)*.

Since there are large differences in the design of the conjugates shown to be protective in human infants, there is still no general formulation available for the development of optimal immunogenic conjugate vaccines with high potency. However, there is some evidence to suggest that the use of the same carrier can lead to epitopic suppression; therefore, clinical trials with multivalent pneumococcal and meningococcal conjugate vaccines, in which the same carrier protein is used, will be helpful to understand the important aspects of using combined vaccine formulations. Also, results obtained from these trials will improve the understanding of the immunological mechanisms of saccharide protein conjugate vaccines. Until now, no adjuvants other than alum are needed for generating high immune responses in infants with conjugate vaccines.

## References

1. Landsteiner, K. and Van der Scheer, J. (1929) Serological differentiation of steric isomers (antigens containing tartaric acids). *J. Exp. Med.* **50,** 407–417.
2. Avery, O. T. and Goebel, W. F. (1931) Chemo-immunological studies on conjugated carbohydrate-proteins. V. The immunological specificity of an antigen pre-pared by combining the capsular polysaccharide of type III Pneumococcus with foreign protein. *J. Exp. Med.* **54,** 437–447.

3.  Goebel, W. F. and Avery, O. T. (1931) Chemo-immunological studies on conjugated carbohydrate-proteins. IV. The synthesis of the *p*-aminobenzyl ether of the soluble specific substance of type III *Pneumococcus* and its coupling with protein. *J. Exp. Med.* **54,** 431–436.
4.  Mosier, D. E., Zaldivar, N. M., Goldings, E., Mond, J., Scher, I., and Paul, W. E. (1977) Formation of antibody in the newborn mouse: study of T-cell-independent antibody response. *J. Infect. Dis.* **136,** S14–S19.
5.  Kaufmann, S. H. E. and Reimann, J. (1999) Immunology of infection, in: *Methods in Microbiology* (Perlmann, P. and Wigzell, H., eds.), Springer, New York, pp. 21–42.
6.  Baker, P. J., Stashak, P. W., Amsbaugh, D. F., Prescott, B., and Barth, R. F. ( 1970) Evidence for the existence of two functionally distinct types of cells which regulate the antibody response to type 3 pneumococcal polysaccharide. *J. Immunol.* **105,** 1581–1583.
7.  Baker, P. J., Reed, N. D., Stashak, P. W., Amsbaugh, D. F., and Prescott, B. (1973) Regulation of the antibody response to type 3 pneumococcal polysaccharide. I. Nature of regulatory cells. *J. Exp. Med.* **137,** 1431–1441.
8.  Braley-Mullen, H. (1974) Regulatory role of T-cells in IgG antibody formation and immune memory to type III pneumococcal polysaccharide. *J. Immunol.* **113,** 1909–1920.
9.  Kayhty, H., Karanko, V., Peltola, H., and Makela, P. H. (1984) Serum antibodies after vaccination with *Haemophilus influenzae* type b capsular polysaccharide and responses to reimmunization: no evidence of immunologic tolerance or memory. *Pediatrics* **74,** 857–865.
10. Peltola, H., Kayhty, H., Sivonen, A., and Makela, P. H. (1977) *Haemophilus influenzae* type b capsular polysaccharide vaccine in children: a double-blind field study of 100,000 vaccinees 3 months to 5 years of age in Finland. *Pediatrics* **60,** 730–737.
11. Baker, P. J., Amsbaugh, D. F., Stashak, P. W., Calder, G., and Prescott, B. (1981) Regulation of the antibody response to pneumococcal polysaccharide by thymus-derived cells. *Rev. Infect. Dis.* **3,** 332–341.
12. Eskola, J., Kayhty, H., Takala, A. K., Peltola, H., Ronnberg, P.-R., Kela, E., et al. (1990) A randomized, prospective field trial of a conjugate vaccine in the protection of infants and young children against invasive *Haemophilus influenzae* type b disease. *N. Engl. J. Med.* **323,** 1381–1387.
13. Santosham, M., Wolff, M., Reid, R., Hohenboken, M., Bateman, M., Goepp, J., et al. (1991) The efficacy in Navajo infants of a conjugate vaccine consisting of *Haemophilus influelizae* type b polysaccharide and *Neisseria meningitidis* outer-membrane protein complex. *N. Engl. J. Med.* **324,** 1767–1772.
14. Black, S. B., Shinefield, H. R., Fireman, B., Hiatt, R., Polen, M., Vittinghoff, E., and The Northern California Kaiser Permanente Vaccine Study Center Pediatrics Group (1991) Efficacy in infancy of oligosaccharide conjugate *Haemophilus influenzae* type b (HbOC) vaccine in a United States population of 61,080 children. *Pediatr. Infect. Dis. J.* **10,** 97–104.
15. Wenger J. D., Heath, P. T., Moxon, R., and Booy, R. (1997) Epidemiological impact of conjugate vaccines against invasive disease caused by *H. influenzae* type b, in *New Generation Vaccines* 2nd ed. (Levine, M. M., Woodrow, G. C., Kaper, J. B., and Cobon, G. S., eds.), Marcel Dekker, NY, pp. 489–502.
16. Maclennan, J. M., Shackley, F., Heath, P. T., Deeks, J. J., Flamark, C., Herbert, M., et al. (2000) Safety, immunogenicity and induction of immunological memory by a serogroup C meningococcal conjugate vaccine in infants; a randomised controlled trial. *J. Am. Med. Assoc.* **283,** 2795–2801.

17. Ramsey, M. E., Andrews, N., Kaczmarski, E. B., and Miller, E. (2001) Efficacy of meningococcal serogroup C conjugate vaccine in teenagers and toddlers in England. *Lancet* **357,** 195–196.

18. Miller, E., Salisbury, D., and Ramsey, R. (2001) Planning, registration and implementation of an immunisation campaign against meningococcal serogroup C disease in the UK: a success story. *Vaccine* **20,** S58–S67.

19. Black S., Shinefield, H., Fireman B., Lewis, E., Ray, P., Hansen, J.R., and the Northern California Kaiser Permanents Vaccine Study Center Group. (2000) Efficacy, safety and immunogenicity of heptavalent pneumococcal conjugate vaccine in children. *Pediatr. Infect. Dis. J.* **19,** 187–195.

20. de Weers, O, Beurret M., van Buren L., Oomen L. A., Poolman J. T., and Hoogerhout P. (1998). Application of cystamine and *N,N'*-bis(glycyl)cystamine as linkers in polysaccharide-protein conjugation. *Bioconjugate Chem.* **9,** 309–315.

21. Alonso de Velasco, E., Verheul, A. F. M., Veeneman, G. H., Gomes, L. J. F., van Boom, J, H., et al. (1993) Protein-conjugated synthetic disaccharide and trisaccharide of pneumococcal type 17F exhibit a different immunogenicity and antigenicity than tetrasaccharide. *Vaccine* **11,** 1429–1436.

22. Anderson, P. W. and Insel, R. A. (1988) Prospects for overcoming maturational and genetic barriers to the human antibody response to the capsular polysaccharide of *Haemophilus influenzae* type b. *Vaccine* **6,** 188–191.

23. Bundle, D. R. (1979) Antibody to an artificial disaccharide antigen cross-reactive with *Neisseria gonorrhoeae* lipopolysaccharide. *Can. J. Biochem.* **57,** 367–371.

24. Dick, W. E., Jr. and Beurret, M. (1989) Glycoconjugates of bacterial carbohydrate antigens. A survey and consideration of design and preparation factors, in *Contributions to Microbiology and Immunology, vol. I0. Conjugate Vaccines* (Cruse, J. M. and Lewis, R. E., Jr., eds.), Kruger, Basel, pp. 48–114.

25. Stein, K. E. (1994) Glycoconjugate vaccines. What next? *Int. J. Technic. Assess. Health Care* **10,** 167–176.

26. Szu, S. C., Bystricky, S., Hinojosa-Ahumada, M., Egan, W., and Robbins, J. B. (1994) Synthesis and some immunologic properties of an *O-acetyl* pectin [poly $(1\rightarrow4)$-α-D-GalpA]-protein conjugate as a vaccine for typhoid fever. *Infect. Immun.* **62,** 5545–5549.

27. Verheul, A. F. M., Braat, A. K., Leenhouts, J. M., Hoogerhout, P., Poolman, J. T., Snippe, H., et al. (1991) Preparation, characterization, and immunogenicity of meningococcal immunotype L2 and L3,7,9 phosphoethanolamine group-containing oligosaccharide-protein conjugates. *Infect. Immun.* **59,** 843–851.

28. Jann, K. and Westphal, O. (1975) Microbial polysaccharides, in *The Antigens,* vol. 3. (Sela, M., ed.), Academic Press, New York, pp. 1–125.

29. Jennings, H. J. (1983) Capsular polysaccharides as human vaccines. *Adv. Carbohydr. Chem. Biochem.* **41,** 155–208.

30. Kenne, L. and Lindberg, B. (1983) Bacterial polysaccharides, in *The Polysaccharides,* vol. 2. (Aspinall, G. O., ed.), Academic Press, Orlando, FL, pp. 287–363.

31. Jennings, H. J. (1990) Capsular polysaccharides as vaccine candidates, in *Current Topics in Microbiology and Immunology, vol. 150. Bacterial Capsules* (Jann, K. and Jann, B., eds.), Springer-Verlag, Berlin, pp. 97–127.

32. Knirel', Y. A. and Kochetkov, N. K. (1993) The structure of lipopolysaccharides of gramnegative bacteria. II. The structure of the core region (a review). *Biokhimiya* **58,** 84–99.

33. Lee, C.-J. (1987) Bacterial capsular polysaccharides-biochemistry, immunity and vaccine. *Mol. Immunol.* **24,** 1005–1019.

34. Luderitz, O., Freudenberg, M. A., Galanos, C:, Lehmann, V., Rietschel, E. T., and Shaw, D. H. (1982) Lipopolysaccharides of gram-negative bacteria. *Curr. Top. Membranes Transp.* **17,** 79–151.

35. Geyer, H., Stirm, S., and Himmelspach, K. (1979) Immunochemical properties of oligosaccharide-protein conjugates with *Klebsiella*-K2 specificity. I. Specificity and crossreactivity of anti-conjugate versus anti-bacterial antibodies. *Med. Microbial. Immunol. (Berl.)* **165,** 271–288.

36. Jaton, J. C., Huser, H., Braun, D. G., Givol, D., Pecht, I., and Schlessinger, J. (1975) Conformational changes induced in a homogeneous anti-type III pneumococcal antibody by oligosaccharides of increasing size. *Biochemistry* **14,** 5312–5315.

37. Kabat, E. A. and Bezer, A. E. (1958) The effect of variation in molecular weight on the antigenicity of dextran in man. *Arch. Biochem. Biophys.* **78,** 306–318.

38. Maeda, H., Schmidt, K. A., Engel, J., and Jaton, J. C. (1977) Kinetics of binding of oligosaccharides to a homogeneous pneumococcal antibody: dependence on antigen chain length suggests a labile intermediate complex. *Biochemistry* **16,** 4086–4089.

39. Makela, O., Peterfy, F., Outschoorn, I. G., Richter, A. W., and Seppala, I. (1984) Immunogenic properties of α(1→6) dextran, its protein conjugates, and conjugates of its breakdown products in mice. *Scand. J. Immunol.* **19,** 541–550.

40. Peeters, C. C. A. M., Evenberg, D., Hoogerhout, P., Kayhty, H., Saarinen, L., van Boeckel, C. A. A., et al. (1992) Synthetic trimer and tetramer of 3-β-D-ribose-(1-1)-D-ribitol-5-phosphate conjugated to protein induce antibody responses to *Haemophilus influenzae* type b capsular polysaccharide in mice and monkeys. *Infect. Immun.* **60,** 1826–1833.

41. Seppala, I. and Makela, O. (1989) Antigenicity of dextran-protein conjugates in mice. Effect of molecular weight of the carbohydrate and comparison of two modes of coupling. *J. Immunol.* **143,** 1259–1264.

42. Pozsgay, V. (2000) Oligosaccharide-protein conjugates as vaccine candidates against bacteria. *Advances in Carbohydrate Chemistry and Biochemistry* **56,** 153–199.

43. Jennings, H. J., Roy, R., and Michon, F. (1985) Determinant specificities of the group B and C polysaccharides of *Neisseria meningitidis. J. Immunol.* **134,** 2651–2657.

44. Lifely, M. R., Mareno, C., and Lindon, J. C. (1987) An integrated molecular and immunological approach towards a meningococcal group B vaccine. *Vaccine* **5,** 11–26.

45. Richter, A. W. and Eby, R. (1985) Studies on artificial oligosaccharide-protein antigens: induction of precipitating antibodies to defined epitopes on natural and synthetic dextrans and mannans. *Mol. Immunol.* **22,** 29–36.

46. Goebel, W. F. (1939) Studies on antibacterial immunity induced by artificial antigens. I. Immunity to experimental pneumococcal infection with an antigen containing cellobiuronic acid. *J. Exp. Med.* **69,** 353–364.

47. Goebel, W. F. (1940) Studies on antibacterial immunity induced by artificial antigens. II. Immunity to experimental pneumococcal infection with antigens containing saccharides of synthetic origin. *J. Exp. Med.* **72,** 33–48.

48. Makela, O., Mattila, P., Rautonen, N., Seppala, I., Eskola, J., and Kayhty, H. (1987) Isotype concentrations of human antibodies to *Haemophilus influenzae* type b polysaccharide (Hib) in young adults immunized with the polysaccharide as such or conjugated to a protein (diphtheria toxoid). *J. Immunol.* **139,** 1999–2004.

49. Lindberg, B., Lönngren, J., and Svensson, S. (1975) Specific degradation of polysaccharides. *Adv. Carbohydr. Chem. Biochem.* **31,** 185–240.

50. Pigman, W. W. and Wolfram, M. L., eds. (1945–1968) *Advances in Carbohydrate Chemistry*, vol. 1–23, Academic, Orlando, FL.

51. Whistler, R. L., Wolfram, M. L., Shafizadeh, F., and BeMiller, J. N., eds. (1962–1980) *Methods in Carbohydrate Chemistry*, vol. 1–8. Academic Press, Orlando, FL.

52. Wolfram, M. L., Tipson, R. S., and Horton, D., eds. (1969–1994) *Advances in Carbohydrate Chemistry and Biochemistry*, vol. 24–50. Academic Press, Orlando, FL.

53. Yalpani, M. (1985) A survey of recent advances in selective chemical and enzymic polysaccharide modifications. *Tetrahedron* **41**, 2957–3020.

54. Kubo, K., Nakamura, T., Takagaki, K., Yoshida, Y., and Endo, M. (1993) Depolymerization of hyaluronanby sonication. *Glycoconjugate J.* **10**, 435–439.

55. Szu, S. C., Zon, G., Schneerson, R., and Robbins, J. B. (1986) Ultrasonic irradiation of bacterial polysaccharides. Characterization of the depolymerized products and some applications of the process. *Carbohydr. Res.* **182**, 7–20.

56. Kniskern, P. J., Ip, C. C., Hagopian, A., Hennessey, J. P., Jr., Miller, W. J., Kubek, D. J., et al. (1992) Pneumococcal polysaccharide conjugate vaccine. *Eur. Pat. Appl.* 0 497 525 A2. Merck and Co., Inc., Rahway, N.J.

57. Baker, E. E. and Whiteside, R. E. (1965) Preparation and properties of a Vi antigen-degrading enzyme. *J. Bacteriol.* **89**, 1217–1224.

58. Dutton, G. G. S., Di Fabio, J. L., Leek, D. M., Merrifield, E. H., Nunn, J. R., and Stephen, A. M. (1981) Preparation of oligosaccharides by the action of bacteriophage-borne enzymic on Klebsiella capsular polysaccharides. *Carbohydr. Res.* **97**, 127–138.

59. Geyer, H., Himmelspach, K., Kwiatkowski, B., Schlecht, S., and Stirm, S. (1983) Degradation of bacterial surface carbohydrates by virus-associated enzymes. *Pure Appl. Chem.* **55**, 637–653.

60. Kwiatkowski, B., Boschek, B., Thiele, H., and Stirm, S. (1983) Substrate specificity of two bacteriophage associated endo-N-acetylneuraminidases. *J. Virol.* **45**, 367–374.

61. Tomlinson, S. and Taylor, P. W. (1985) Neuraminidase associated with coliphage E that specifically depolymerizes the *Escherichia coli* KI capsular polysaccharide. *J. Virol.* **55**, 374–378.

62. Uchida, T., Pappenheimer, A. M., Jr., and Harper, A. A. (1972) Reconstitution of diphtheria toxin from two nontoxic cross-reacting mutant proteins. *Science* **175**, 901–903.

63. Pappenheimer, A. M., Jr., Uchida, T., and Harper, A. A. (1972) An immunological study of the diphtheria toxin molecule. *Immunochemistry* **9**, 891–906.

64. Barington, T., Skettrup, M., Juul, L., and Heilmann, C. (1993) Non—specific suppression of the antibody response to *Haemophilus influenzae* type b conjugate vaccines by preimmunization with vaccine components. *Infect. Immun.* **61**, 432–438.

65. Barington, T., Gyhrs, A., Kristensen, K., and Heilmann, C. (1994) Opposite effects of actively and passively acquired immunity to the carrier on responses of human infants to a *Haemophilus influenzae* type b conjugate vaccine. *Infect. Immun.* **62**, 9–14.

66. Peeters, C. C. A. M., Tenbergen-Meekes, A.-M., Poolman, J. T., Beurret, M., Zegers, B. J. M., and Rijkers, G. T. (1991) Effect of carrier priming on immunogenicity of saccharide-protein conjugate vaccines. *Infect. Immun.* **59**, 3504–35 10.

67. Dintzis, H. M. and Dintzis, R. Z. (1992) Profound specific suppression by antigen of persistent IgM, IgG, and IgE antibody production. *Proc. Natl. Acad. Sci. USA* **89**, 1113–1117.

68. Fattom, A., Hee Cho, Y., Chu, C., Fuller, S., Fries, L., and Naso, R. (1991). Epitopic overload at the site of injection may result in supression of the immune response to combined capsular polysaccharide conjugate vaccines. *Vaccine* **17**, 126–133.

69. Crowley-Luke, A., Reddin, K. M., Gorringe, A. R., Hudson, M. J., and Robinson, A. (2001) Formulation and characterisation of *Bordetella pertussis* fimbriae as novel carrier proteins for Hib conjugate vaccines. *Vaccine* **19**, 3399–3407.

70. Reddin, K. M., Crowley-Luke, A., Clark, S. O., Vincent, P. J., Gorringe, A. R., Hudson, M. J., et al. *Bordetella pertussis* fimbriae are effective carrier proteins in *Neisseria meningitidis* serogroup C conjugate vaccines. *FEMS Immunol. Med. Micro.* **31,** 153–162.

71. Paradiso, P. R., Dermody, K., and Pillai, S. (1993) Novel approaches to the development of glycoconjugate vaccines with synthetic peptides as carriers. *Vacc. Res.* **2,** 239–248.

72. Bixler, G. S., Jr., Eby, R., Dermody, K. M., Woods, R. M., Seid, R. C., Jr., and Pillai, S. (1989) Synthetic peptide representing a T-cell epitope of CRM197 substitutes as carrier molecule in a *Haemophilus influenzae* type B (Hib) conjugate vaccine. *Adv. Exp. Med. Biol.* **251,** 175–180.

73. Lett, E., Gangloff, S., Zimmermann, M., Wachsmann, D., and Klein, J.-P. (1994) Immunogenicity of polysaccharides conjugated to peptides containing T- and B-cell epitopes. *Infect. Immun.* **62,** 785–792.

74. Aplin, J. D. and Wriston, J. C., Jr. (1981) Preparation, properties, and applications of carbohydrate conjugates of proteins and lipids. *CRC Crit. Rev. Biochem.* **10,** 259–306.

75. Pazur, J. H. (1981) Affinity chromatography of macromolecular substances on adsorbents bearing carbohydrate ligands. *Adv. Carbohydr. Chem. Biochem.* **39,** 405–447.

76. Porath, J. (1974) General methods and coupling procedures. *Meth. Enzymol.* **34B,** 13–30.

77. Stowell, C. P. and Lee, Y. C. (1980) Neoglycoproteins. The preparation and application of synthetic glycoproteins. *Adv. Carbohydr. Chem. Biochem.* **37,** 225–281.

78. Wilchek, M., Miron, T., and Kohn, J. (1984) Affinity chromatography. *Meth. Enzymol.* **104C,** 3–55.

79. Hermanson, G.T. (1996). *Bioconjugate Techniques.* Academic Press, San Diego, CA.

80. Jennings, H.J. and Sood, R.K. 1994. Synthetic glycoconjugates as human vaccines. In Lee, Y.C. and Lee, R.T. (eds.), *Neoglycoconjugates: Preparation and Applications* (pp. 325–371). San Diego: Academic Press, Inc.

81. Kohn, J. and Wilchek, M. (1986) The use of cyanogen bromide and other novel cyanylating reagents for the activation of polysaccharide resins. *Appl. Biochem. Biotechnol.* **9,** 285–305.

82. Anderson, P. W., Pichichero, M. E., Insel, R. A., Betts, R., Eby, R., and Smith, D. H. (1986) Vaccines consisting of periodate-cleaved oligosaccharides from the capsule of *Haemophilus influenzae* type b coupled to a protein carrier: structural and temporal requirements for priming in the human infant. *J. Immunol.* **137,** 1181–1186.

83. Beuvery, E. C., Roy, R., Kanhai, V., and Jennings, H. J. (1986) Characteristics of two types of meningococcal group C polysaccharide conjugates using tetanus toxoid as carrierprotein. *Dev. Biol. Stand.* **65,** 197–204.

84. Jennings, H. J. and Lugowski, C. (1981) Immunochemistry of groups A, B, and C meningococcal polysaccharide-tetanus toxoid conjugates. *J. Immunol.* **127,** 1011–1018.

85. Beuvery, E. C., Miedema, F., van Delft, R., and Haverkamp, J. (1983) Preparation and immunochemical characterization of meningococcal group C polysaccharide-tetanus toxoid conjugates as a new generation of vaccines. *Infect. Immun.* **40,** 39–45.

86. Marburg, S., Jorn, D., Tolman, R. L., Arison, B., McCauley, J., Kniskem, P. J., et al. (1986) Bimolecular chemistry of macromolecules: synthesis of bacterial polysaccharide conjugates with *Neisseria meningitidis* membrane protein. *J. Am. Chem. Soc.* **108,** 5282–5287.

87. Shafer, D. E., Toll, B., Schuman, R. F., Nelson, B. L., Mond, J. J., and Lees, A. (2000) Activation of soluble polysaccharide with 1-cyano-4-dimethylaminopyridium tetrafluoroborate (CDAP) for use in protein-polysaccharide conjugate vaccines and immunological

reagents. II Selective cross-linking of proteins to CDAP-activated polysaccharides. *Vaccine* **18**, 1273–1281.

88. Schneller, M. and Geiger, R.E. (1992) An effective method for the synthesis of neoglycoproteins and neogangliosideproteins by use of reductively aminated sulfhydryl-containing carbohydrate conjugates. *Biol. Chem. Hoppe-Seyler* **373**, 1095–1104.

89. Costantino, P., Viti, S., Vannozzi, F., Serafini G., Marsili, I., and Valeri, A. (1986) Immunochemistry of some bacterial oligosaccharide protein conjugates. *Ann. Sclavo Collana Monogr.* **3**, 359–366.

90. Cryz, S. J., Jr., Furer, E. P., Cross, A. S., Wegmann, A., Germanier R., and Sadoff, J. C. (1987) Safety and immunogenicity of a *Pseudomonas aeruginosa* O-polysaccharide toxin A conjugate vaccine in humans. *J. Clin. Investig.* **80**, 51–56.

91. Akerblom, E., Dohlsten, M., Bryno, C., Mastej, M., Steringer, I., Hedlund, G., et al. (1993) Preparation and characterization of conjugates of monoclonal antibodies and staphylococcus enterotoxin A using a new hydrophilic cross-linker. *Bioconjugate Chem.* **4**, 455–466.

92. Andersson, M., Oscarson, S., and Ohberg, L. (1993) Synthesis of oligosaccharides with oligoethylene glycol spacers and their conversion into glycoconjugates using $N,N,N^1,N^1$-tetramethyl(succinimido)uronium tetrafluoroborate as coupling reagent. *Glycoconjugate J.* **10**, 461–465.

93. Collioud, A., Clemence, J. F., Sanger, M., and Sigrist, H. (1993) Oriented and covalent immobilization of target molecules to solid supports: synthesis and application of a light-activatable and thiol-reactive cross-linking reagent. *Bioconjugate Chem.* **4**, 528–536.

94. Jennings, H. J. (1992) Further approaches for optimizing polysaccharide-protein conjugate vaccines for prevention of invasive bacterial disease. *J. Infect. Dis.* **165**, S156–S159.

95. Pozsgay, V. (1993) A method for glycoconjugate synthesis. *Glycoconjugate J.* **10**, 133–141.

96. Romanowska, A., Meunier, S. J., Tropper, F. D., Laferriere, C. A., and Roy, R. (1994) Michael additions for syntheses of neoglycoproteins. *Meth. Enzymol.* **242A**, 90–101.

97. Vilaseca, L. A., Rose, K., Werlen, R., Meunier, A., Offord, R. E., Nichols, C. L., et al. (1993) Protein conjugates of defined structure: synthesis and use of a new carrier molecule. *Bioconjugate Chem.* **4**, 515–520.

98. Yoshida, T. and Lee, Y. C. (1994) Glycamine formation via reductive amination of oligosaccharides with benzylamine: efficient coupling of oligosaccharides to protein. *Carbohydr. Res.* **251**, 175–186.

99. Zara, J. J., Wood, R. D., Boon, P., Kim, C.-H., Pomato, N., Bredehorst, R., et al. (1991) A carbohydrate-directed heterobifunctional cross-linking reagent for the synthesis of immunoconjugates. *Anal. Biochem.* **194**, 156–162.

100. Pawlowski, A., Källenius, G., and Svenson, S.B. (1999) A new method of non-cross-linking conjugation of polysaccharides to proteins via thioether bonds for the preparation of saccharide-protein conjugate vaccines. *Vaccine* **17**, 1474–1483.

101. Pawlowski, A., Källenius, G., and Svenson, S.B. (2000) Preparation of pneumococcal capsular polysaccharide-protein conjugate vaccines utilizing new fragmentation and conjugation technologies. *Vaccine* **18**, 1873–1885.

102. Beuvery, E. C., Van de Kaaden, A., Kanhai, V., and Leussink, A. B. (1983) Physico-chemical and immunological characterization of meningococcal group A polysaccharide-tetanus toxoid conjugates prepared by two methods. *Vaccine* **1**, 31–36.

103. Lepow, M. L., Samuelson, J. S., and Gordon, L. K. (1984) Safety and immunogenicity of *Haemophilus influenzae* type b polysaccharide-diphtheria toxoid conjugate vaccine in adults. *J. Infect. Dis.* **150**, 402–406.

104. Schneerson, R., Robbins, J. E., Chu, C. Y., Sutton, A., Schiffman, G., and Vann, W. F. (1983) Semi-synthetic vaccines composed of capsular polysaccharides of pathogenic bacteria covalently bound to proteins for the prevention of invasive diseases. *Prog. Allergy* **33**, 144–158.

105. Braley-Mullen, H. (1980) Antigen requirements for priming of IgG producing B memory cells specific for Type III pneumococcal polysaccharide. *Immunology* **40**, 521–527.

106. Peeters, C. C. A. M., Tenbergen-Meekes, A.-M. J., Poolman, J. T., Zegers, B. J. M., and Rijkers, G T. (1992) Immunogenicity of a *Streptococcus pneumoniae* type 4 polysaccharide-protein conjugate vaccine is decreased by admixture of high doses of free saccharide. *Vaccine* **10**, 833–840.

107. Wilson, D. and Braley-Mullen, H. (1981) Antigen requirements for priming of type III pneumococcal polysaccharide-specific IgG memory responses: suppression of memory with the T-independent form of antigen. *Cell. Immunol.* **64**, 177–186.

108. Peeters, C. C. A. M., Tenbergen-Meekes, A.-M., Evenberg, D. E., Poolman, J. T., Zegers, B. J. M., and Rijkers, G. T. (1991) A comparative study of the immunogenicity of pneumococcal type 4 polysaccharide and oligosaccharide tetanus toxoid conjugates in adult mice. *J. Immunol.* **146**, 4308–43 14.

109. Seid, R. C., Jr., Boykins, R. A., Liu, D.-F., Kimbrough, K. W., Hsieh, C.-L., and Eby, R. (1989) Chemical evidence for covalent linkages of a semi-synthetic glycoconjugate vaccine for *Haemophilus influenzae* type b disease. *Glycoconjugate J.* **6**, 489–498.

110. Brett, S. J., Payne, S. N., Gigg, I., Burgess, P., and Gigg, R. (1986) Use of synthetic glycoconjugates containing the *Mycobacterium leprae* specific and immunodominant epitope of phenolic glycolipid I in the serology of leprosy. *Clin. Exp. Immunol.* **64**, 476–483.

111. Pozsgay, V. (1998) Synthesis of glycoconjugate vaccines against *Shigella dysenteriae* type 1. *J. Org. Chem.* **63**, 5983–5999.

112. Nashed, M. A. (1983) Glycosidic derivatives of 2-acetamido-2-deoxy-D-galactopyranose suitable for use as ligands in affinity chromatography. *Carbohydr. Res.* **123**, 241–246.

113. Ekborg, G., Eklind, K., Garegg, P. J., Gotthammar, B., Carlsson, H. E., Lindberg, A. A., et al. (1977) Artificial disaccharide-protein conjugates as immunogens for the preparation of specific anti-Salmonella O-antisera. *Immunochemistry* **14**, 153–157.

114. Roy, R., Andersson, F. O., Harms, G., Kelm, S., and Schauer, R. (1992) Synthesis of esterase-resistant 9-0-acetylated polysialoside as inhibitor of influenza C virus haemagglutinin. *Angew. Chem. Int. Ed. Eng.* **31**, 1478–1481.

115. Bock, K. and Meldal, M. (1984) Synthesis of the branchpoint tetrasaccharide of the O-specific determinant of *Salmonella* serogroup B. *Acta Chem. Scand. B.* **38**, 71–77.

116. Lee, H.-H., Schwartz, D. A., Harris, J. F., Carver, J. P., and Krepinsky, J. J. (1986) Syntheses of model oligosaccharides of biological significance. 7. Synthesis of a fucosylated $N,N^I$-diacetylchitobioside linked to bovine serum albumin and immunochemical characterization of rabbit antisera to this structure. *Can. J. Chem.* **64**, 1912–1918.

117. Tahir, S. H. and Hindsgaul, O. (1986) Substrates for the differentiation of the *N*-acetylglucosaminyltransferases. Synthesis of βDGlcNAc-(1,2)-αDMan-(1,6)-βDMan and βDGLcNAc-(1,2)-αDMan-(1,6)-[αLDMan-(1,3)]-βDMan glycosides. *Can. J. Chem.* **64**, 1771–1780.

118. Boons, G. J. P. H., van der Marel, G. A., Poolman, J. T., and van Boom, J. H. (1989) Synthesis of L-*glycero*-α-D-*manno*-heptopyranose-containing disaccharide derivatives

of the *Nesseria meningitidis* dephosphorylated inner-core region. *Recl. Trav. Chim. Pays-Bas.* **108,** 339–343.

119. Veeneman, G. H., Notermans, S., Hoogerhout, P., and van Boom, J. H. (1989) Synthesis of an immunologically active component of the extra cellular polysaccharide produced by *Aspergillus* and *Penicillium* species. *Recl. Trav. Chim. Pays-Bas.* **108,** 344–350.

120. Veeneman, G. H., Brugghe, H. F., Hoogerhout, P., van der Marel, G. A., and van Boom, J. H. (1988) Synthesis of a cell wall component of *Haemophilus (Actinobacillus) pleuropneu-moniae* type 2. *Recl. Tray. Chim. Pays-Bas.* **107,** 610–612.

121. Hoogerhout, P., Evenberg, D., van Boeckel, C. A. A., Poolman, J. T., Beuvery, E. C., van der Marel, G. A., et al. (1987) Synthesis of fragments of the capsular polysaccharide of *Haemophilus influenzae* type b, comprising two and three repeating units. *Tetrahedron Lett.* **28,** 1553–1556.

122. Hoogerhout, P., Funke, C. W., Mellema, J.-R., Wagenaars, G. N., van Boeckel, C. A. A., Evenberg, D., et al. (1988) Synthesis of fragments of the capsular polysaccharide of *Haemophilus influenzae* type b. Part II. Preparation and structural analysis of fragments comprising two and three repeating units. *J. Carbohyd. Chem* **7,** 399–416; erratum, *ibid.* (1989) **8,** 167.

123. Evenberg, D., Hoogerhout, P., van Boeckel, C. A. A., Rijkers, G. T., Beuvery, E.C., van Boom, J. H., et al. (1992) Preparation, antigenicity, and immunogenicity of synthetic ribosylribitol phosphate oligomer-protein conjugates and their potential use for vaccination against *Haemophilus influenzae* type b disease. *J. Infect. Dis.* **165,** S152–S155.

124. Verheul, A. F. M., Boons, G. J. P. H., van der Marel, G. A., van Boom, J. H,, Jennings, H. J., Snippe, H., et al. (1991) Minimal oligosaccharide structures required for induction of immune responses against meningococcal immunotype L1, L2, and L3,7,9 lipopolysaccharides determined by using synthetic oligosaccharide-protein conjugates. *Infect. Immun.* **59,** 3566–3573.

125. Boons, G. J. P. H., Hoogerhout, P., Poolman, J. T., van der Marel, G. A., and van Boom, J. H. (1991) Preparation of a well-defined sugar-peptide conjugate. A possible approach to a synthetic vaccine against *Neisseria meningitidis. Bioorg. Medicinal. Chem. Lett.* **1,** 303–308.

126. Dubois, M., Gilles, K. A., Hamilton, J. K., Rebers, P. A., and Smith, F. (1956) Calorimetric method for determination of sugars and related substances. *Anal. Chem.* **28,** 350–356.

127. Lowry, O. H., Rosebrough, N. J., Farr, A. L., and Randall, R. J. (1951) Protein measurement with the Folin phenol reagent. *J. Biol. Chem.* **193,** 265–275.

# 11

## Adjuvant Formulations for Experimental Vaccines

### Duncan E. S. Stewart-Tull

### 1. Introduction

An adjuvant (immunopotentiator), when added to a vaccine, will enhance the immunogenicity of the antigen with the stimulation of an elevated humoral immune response. Some adjuvants may also stimulate a cell-mediated response against the antigen. One advantage of including an adjuvant in the vaccine mixture is that smaller quantities of the antigen are usually required to stimulate a good response. New synthetic experimental vaccines may require the presence of an adjuvant to achieve an immunogenic response. There is no single universal adjuvant, but numerous adjuvants are available alone (e.g., muramyl dipeptide and Quil A derivatives), or conjugated to the antigen (e.g., Immune-stimulating complexes [ISCOMs]), or in mixtures (e.g., Montanides, Guildhay or MF-59 adjuvants). The adjuvant selected will be based on experimental data produced with a variety of antigen preparations, taking into consideration the nature and dose to be administered, the route of vaccine administration, and any contraindications. For human vaccines, it should be remembered that aluminum salt adjuvants have been the only licensed preparations for the past sixty yr.

One difficulty in the selection of a suitable adjuvant has been that, until recently, they have been ignored in standard texts on immunology. Thus, it was necessary to search through original research papers in the hope that sufficient guidance on the use and preparation of adjuvanted experimental vaccines was described. There are now a number of texts that will assist in the choice of a suitable adjuvant (*1–5*), and a compendium of 100 different preparations was published in 1994 (*4*). There was agreement in 1988 for adjuvant standards: aluminum hydroxide and Freund's complete adjuvant were selected; the former as a licensed adjuvant for veterinary and human use and the latter as the best-documented adjuvant. In addition, two standard antigens were designated for use in experimental research—namely, ovalbumin and influenza hemagglutinin (*6*).

From: *Methods in Molecular Medicine, Vol. 87: Vaccine Protocols, 2nd ed.*
Edited by: A. Robinson, M. J. Hudson, and M. P. Cranage © Humana Press Inc., Totowa, NJ

## 1.1. Aluminum Hydroxide Gels

There has been a general belief that alum-precipitated antigens, made by mixing the protein with potassium alum [$KAl(SO_4)_2 \cdot 12H_2O$], are retained at the site of injection, "the depot effect," with the slow release of the antigen over a prolonged period and the nonspecific irritation of the immune system. Subsequently, the importance of protein antigen adsorption to aluminum hydroxide [$Al(OH)_3$] or aluminum phosphate [$AlPO_4$] was stressed *(7)*. It is possible to prepare the latter as gels in the laboratory, but it is less time-consuming and more profitable to obtain the well-defined and standardized commercial preparations, such as Alhydrogel (Brenntag Biosector, Denmark). The ability of aluminum hydroxide gel [$Al_2O_3 \cdot H_2O$] to adsorb protein antigens depends on a number of physicochemical characteristics of the gel, namely particle-size distribution, internal surface, degree of hydration, and charge of the particles. Hem and White *(8)* reported that the charge was positive below pH 9.0. The adsorption capacity of an aluminum hydroxide gel varies *(9,10)*, even among those proteins that are related phylogenetically, for example, bovine and human serum albumins.

The main use for aluminum hydroxide gels is in vaccines where a Th2 humoral immune response against a protein antigen is required, especially for the stimulation of IgG and IgE; however, they are not particularly useful with peptide antigens. In addition, it is doubtful whether a Th1-cell-mediated response can be elicited with aluminum-adsorbed antigen. Before the selection of an adjuvant for a particular vaccine is made, it would be useful to refer to articles by Mossmann and Sad *(11)* and Cox and Cooper *(12)*. The use of cytokines to potentiate immune responses will not be considered here for the following reason: in 1979, a letter to the *Journal of Immunology*, signed by thirty-nine leading immunologists, reduced the confusion about a wide range of cytokines with similar activities by collating them all under the name Interleukins, IL-1 or IL-2. Since this time and at regular intervals, new interleukins have been reported, and it is apparent that they have important functions in the intricate steady-state system of the immune response. Until such time as doubts about the activity of an as yet unidentified cytokine being adversely affected by the presence of an interleukin in a vaccine, it may be wise to caution their use, and they will not be considered further in this chapter.

## 1.2. Freund-Type and Oil-Emulsion Formulations

Freund's complete adjuvant (FCA), the standard adjuvant, has been used extensively in experimental vaccines in animals because of its strong adjuvant effect *(6)*. The combination of mineral oil and heat-killed *Mycobacterium tuberculosis* cells, together with an emulsifier such as mannide monooleate, produced a specific cellular reaction in experimental animals. FCA stimulated active humoral and cell-mediated immune responses, but there may be concomitant contraindications because of the reactogenicity of some types of mineral oil, particularly those causing the formation of an epithelioid macrophage granuloma and local ulceration at the site of injection when the injection was administered subcutaneously. Pyrogenicity, stimulation of experimental autoimmune diseases, and adjuvant arthritis were also recorded (reviewed in detail by Stewart-Tull **refs.** *13,14*).

Since the 1970s, new procedures have been used in the manufacture of white oils, and today the use of the term FCA is a misnomer. At best, the average laboratory can only produce a "Freund-type" emulsion *(3)*, and reputable journals should disallow the use of the term FCA in research articles for laboratory preparations without some evidence of the source of the components. The general use of FCA for the routine production of antisera is both unnecessary and ethically unwarranted because other adjuvants usually achieve an acceptable result. Similarly, it is surprising that experimenters continue to inject animals intra-footpad despite very clear contrary recommendations *(15–18)*. Indeed, it is doubtful if any pharmaceutical company would market a veterinary vaccine with such a recommended route of injection! Vaccine development laboratory workers must be aware of the licensing requirements for a human vaccine and devise realistic dose levels and injection protocols such as the route and number of injections, *(16)*.

The conclusion from a workshop on the escape from the use of FCA (at the 1999 conference on "*Alternatives and Animal Use in the Life Sciences*") was that the use of the standard FCA may be justifiable in "*special cases where less potent adjuvants would fail to elicit an adequate response, or in which adjuvants are used as tools to investigate parameters of the immune system itself*" *(19)*. As stated by Salk: "*If I thought it would cure the patient, I should have no doubts about including Freund Complete Adjuvant in an HIV vaccine*" (Salk J, personal communication, 1990).

Consideration should be given to new oil formulations that are less reactogenic and have fewer contraindications than products marketed before 1970, partly because of changes in the oils *(3)* and improved methods to measure the hydrocarbon content *(14)*. In this respect, Montanide 80, a highly refined mannide oleate, was used in Phase I *(20)* and Phase II *(21)*, Montanide ISA 51 in Phase I *(22–24)* and Phase II *(25)*, ISA 720 in Phase I *(26)*, and ISA 724 in Phase I *(27,28)* clinical trials of human immunodeficiency virus (HIV)-1 vaccine. ISA 51 was used in Phase I/II trials with a cancer vaccine *(29,30)* and ISA 720 alone *(31)* or with *Plasmodium falciparum* vaccine *(32–34)*. In the melanoma cancer trials with ISA 51, in which a more aggressive immunotherapeutic response was required, the volume of emulsion used varied from 0.5 mL to 2.0 mL with as many as eight repetitive injections. The adverse reactions after subcutaneous (sc) injection were local and mild to moderate; the benefit:risk ratio must be carefully gauged when considering the injection dose with a prophylactic vaccine! For the malaria trials, volumes of the ISA 720 emulsion were in the order of 0.36–1.8 mL injected intramuscularly with 1–3 injections at different sites. In my opinion, for a prophylactic vaccine, the intramuscular (im) route would be the most suitable for an injection volume of 250 µL. For veterinary vaccines, Montanides ISA 50, 57, and 206 were tested in a FMDV vaccine for calves, and ISA 57 proved to be the most useful *(35)*.

Synthetic oligodeoxynucleotides (ODN) containing immunostimulatory cytosine-phosphorothioate-guanine (CpG ODN) possessed adjuvant activity for protein antigen after either im injection or intranasal (in) inhalation *(36,37)*. Subsequently, CpG ODN was tested with purified hepatitis B surface antigen by the oral route and both the Th1 and Th2 responses were stimulated in Balb/c mice *(38)*, with IgA in lung, vaginal, and gut washes. It was concluded that after im, in, or sc injection that the Th2 stimulation was associated with the phosphorothioate ODN backbone, and that the presence of CpG motifs shifted this toward a Th1 response *(39)*. Manders and Thomas *(40)* reviewed the role of CpG motifs as adjuvants for DNA vaccines. With a gp120-depleted whole-killed HIV antigen (HIV-1) in combination with synthetic CpG ODN in a Freund's incomplete adjuvant (FIA), both CD4+ and CD8 + T-cell HIV-specific responses were stimulated in rats *(41,42)*. These studies indicate a cirumvention of the increasing resistance to the use of mycobacterial *(43)* or toxin *(44)* derivatives in Freund-type complete adjuvant mixtures; although many whole-cell bacterial vaccines do contain peptidoglycan or lipopolysaccharide (LPS), respectively *(45)*. It is also worth noting that intranasal administration of radiolabeled cholera toxin (CT) or CT-B subunit targeted the olfactory nerves/epithelium and olfactory bulbs via a GM1 monosialoganglioside, and doubts were raised about the role of such GM1-binding molecules as mucosal adjuvants *(46)*. However, intracerebral injection of CT-B containing 0.2% CT at the 10-$\mu$g dose/mouse caused death within 7 d, but <3.0 $\mu$g did not. Intranasal (in) administration of 0.1 $\mu$g CT-B thirty times caused no effect on the brain but some slight effect on the nasal mucosa and the associated lymphoid tissue *(47)*. With the background knowledge that CpG ODN possesses adjuvant activity, it would be interesting to combine this with ISA 51 or 720—tailor-made for human application, as shown by the clinical trials mentioned previously—and show whether microbial adjuvants could be eliminated from the equivalent of FCA.

## 1.3. Immune-Stimulatory Complexes (ISCOMS)

In the first edition of this book, the indication was that the main focus of research on the use of ISCOMs was with viral antigens and veterinary vaccines *(48)*. In the ISCOM matrix, the Quil A is bound with cholesterol and phosphatidylcholine to form a stable, cage-like structure (similar in shape to a plastic practice golf ball) that binds the hydrophobic moiety of the antigen and presents the hydrophilic moiety to the immune cells. Human volunteers have now been injected with influenza ISCOM vaccines and compared with a group that received the non-adjuvanted, inactivated, split-virion vaccine in a double-blind trial. The ISCOM vaccines induced Th2 responses in the test and control groups, but the incidence of Th1 responses was higher in the ISCOM group *(49)*. It was apparent that a hydrophobic anchor on hydrophilic proteins assisted in the production of an active influenza ISCOM *(50)*. Initially, it seemed that this technology was confined to viral vaccines, but some studies with other infective agents are now appearing. In addition, mice injected with ISCOMs containing synthetic peptides of the erythrocyte surface antigen of *P. falciparum* produced antibodies that inhibited the parasite *(51)*; such studies may also renew interest in peptide vaccines.

The delays in the development of such vaccines were caused by the difficulties workers found in the preparation of ISCOMs; however, a commercial preparation of the ISCOM-matrix is available from Iscotec AB (Uppsala, Sweden) in the form of the matrix without antigen incorporated into the stucture; thus, further use will be made of this technology. There is still a requirement for careful monitoring of the balance of Quil A and antigen in the complex. The latter should be hydrophobic or amphipathic in nature *(52)*, but one would expect to see more human ISCOM vaccines developed in future years.

## 1.4. Liposomes

The use of artificial lipid bilayers in the form of vesicles is an efficient means of antigen presentation *(53,54)*. A large variety of natural phospholipids or other polar amphiphiles can be used in an aqueous solution of an antigen to form either unilamellar or multilamellar spherules. The antigen(s) may either be lipid-soluble and insert into the artificial lipid bilayer, or bind to the bilayer, or become entrapped inside the spherule. In multilamellar liposomes, the antigen(s) may also be trapped in the aqueous compartments between the lipid bilayers. The surface of the liposome may also be positively or negatively charged by the addition of suitable charged amphiphiles. Many of the natural adjuvant substances are amphiphilic, and may insert into the liposome through hydrophobic groups *(55,56)*. The purity of the phospholipid will affect the stability of the final preparation of liposomes and their leakiness. For instance, Gregoriadis *(53)* points out that high-density plasma lipoproteins will remove low-melting phospholipids from liposomes and cause leakiness. With high-melting phospholipids or with an excess of cholesterol, the lipid bilayers become rigid at 37°C, and the result is a slower release of the antigen. Space does not permit the author to record the many combinations that could be used; the preparation of a pure sample of phosphatidylcholine (ovo-lecithin) and positively and negatively charged liposomes are described as examples.

Current research and improved preparation and stability of liposomes *(57,58)* has enabled their use in liposome-mediated DNA transfer. Such work has culminated in a licensed hepatitis A virosome vaccine *(59)*; thus, further advances may be expected in the future with such technology. For example, the mumps virus hemagglutinin was engineered into a plasmid vector and combined with an influenza virosome, a liposome containing influenza hemagglutinin and neuraminidase, and both Th1 and Th2 responses were elicited *(60)*.

Seventy-five years have passed since studies began on the use of alum as an adjuvant. Despite the vast effort to produce suitable adjuvant formulations for use in human vaccines we still have few licensed adjuvanted vaccines. At the ECPI World Vaccine Congress *(61)*, it was stated that "*it would be incorrect of WHO or any other health authority to attempt to paint vaccines as being totally safe. As with any medicine or health intervention, there will always be some risk. Severe complications as a result of the interaction between the individual and the vaccine can occur after even the best known of childhood vaccines*" *(62)*.

Nevertheless, strenuous attempts will continue to be made to ensure that no adjuvanted vaccine is licensed without the most rigorous toxicity testing *(63,64)*, and the U.S. Center for Biologics Evaluation and Research will expect to review the toxicity profile of both the adjuvant alone, as well as the adjuvant-antigen combination *(65)*. Mankind will continue to face new challenges with emergence of new diseases and re-emergence of old diseases with migration of peoples and climatic changes. Modern travel *(66)* leads to the transfer of diseases to new environments; in the United

Kingdom we have no safeguards against Ebola virus or against West Nile Fever, which has emerged as a problem in the United States and Canada.

In this chapter, prominence has been given to a comparatively small area of adjuvant research with the associated human clinical trials, but it is hoped that this and studies on the 100 adjuvants and delivery systems *(4)* will soon achieve success in the development of efficacious vaccines for human use.

## 2. Materials

### 2.1. Aluminum Preparations

1. The standard antigen solution: (e.g., ovalbumin) 1.0 mg/mL in sterile distilled water. A small amount of the ovalbumin should be placed in a clean glass container in a desiccator for 24–48 h to remove residual water; this can account for some 50% of the weight of protein.
2. Alhydrogel available as 2.0% (w/v) and 3.0% (w/v) aluminum hydroxide, a white gelatinous precipitate in aqueous suspension, from Brenntag Biosector, Elsenbakkien 23, 3600 Frederikssund, Denmark.
3. Sodium diethylbarbiturate buffer, 0.07 $M$ at pH 8.6. The formulation of an effective buffer is 2.76 g diethyl barbituric acid and 15.4 g sodium diethyl barbiturate dissolved in sterile distilled water, to a final volume of 1.0 L. Prolonged storage of buffer solution is not recommended, especially if the solution is not sterile. Ideally, buffer should be prepared daily and kept refrigerated until use.
4. Gel medium: Dissolve 2.0 g purified agar in 100 mL diethylbarbiturate buffer, pH 8.6, by heating in a steamer. Add 1.0 mL thiomersal as a preservative. Dispense into glass, wide-necked bottles in 7.0-mL quantities.
5. Polyclonal rabbit anti-ovalbumin anti-serum or the specific anti-serum against the candidate vaccine antigen.
6. Amido-black stain, 0.1% (w/v) solution. Prepared by dissolving 100 mg in methanol: water: acetic acid solution (5:5:1, v/v/v).
7. Methanol-acetic acid (9: 1, v/v) washing solution.
8. Rotating mixer (e.g., Matburn-blood-cell suspension mixer).

### 2.2. Standard Freund's Complete and Incomplete Adjuvants

1. Freund's complete adjuvant (FCA), produced by the Statens Seruminstitut and available from Brenntag Biosector, Elsenbakkien 23, 3600 Frederikssund, Denmark, consists of a mixture of 85% mineral oil (Marcol 52) and 15% emulsifier (Arlacel A-mannide monooleate) with 500 μg heat-killed, dried *Mycobacterium tuberculosis* per mL. The mixture is used in a 1:1 ratio with the antigen-containing aqueous phase (*see* **Note 1**).
2. FIA: as in above **item 1**, but without the *M. tuberculosis*.

### 2.3. Montanide Incomplete Seppic Adjuvants (ISA)

1. This is a series of ready-to-use preparations for animal and human vaccines produced by Seppic, Siege Social, 75 Quai D'Orsay, 75321 Paris, Cedex 07, France.
2. Montanide ISA 51 is a mixture of Montanide 80, a highly refined mannide oleate, in Drakeol 6VR as a ready-to-use preparation at a ratio of 50:50 v/v, with the aqueous phase containing the antigen (*see* **Note 2**).
3. Montanide ISA 720 contains the highly refined emulsifier in natural metabolizable oil designed for the production of water-in-oil emulsions. This ready-to-use preparation is mixed with the aqueous antigen preparation in the ratio 70:30 v/v (*see* **Note 2**).

## 2.4. Non-Ulcerative Freund's Adjuvant (NUFA)

A commercial preparation of Freund-type adjuvant has been introduced by Morris of Guildhay Ltd. (Guildford, Surrey, UK), which can be administered by im, sc, and intradermal (id) routes in small doses at multiple sites. The im sites create a longer depot stimulus and fewer adverse reactions than the other routes. The main difference between this product and others relies on the use of Evans Medical Bacillus Calmette-Guérin (BCG) vaccine to provide the *M. tuberculosis* for FCA. The BCG vaccine is formulated for id use (BCG vaccine BP, BNF [id] supplied by John Bell and Croydon, 52-54 Wigmore Street, London, W1H 0AU, UK). After reconstitution, 0.1 mL is added to 0.9 mL of the aqueous antigen solution and 2.0 mL of the FIA containing highly refined base oil that conforms to US and EU Pharmacopoeia requirements and complies with FDA regulations 21 CFR 172.878 and 178.3620(a). The dose varies from one animal to another, between 0.25 and 0.5 mL.

## 2.5. Liposomes

1. Cholesterol (Sigma).
2. Spectroscopic-grade chloroform (Uvasol; Merck, Rahway, NJ).
3. Dicetyl phosphate (Dihexadecyl phosphate; Sigma) for negatively charged liposomes.
4. Octadecylamine (Stearylamine; Sigma) for positively charged liposomes.
5. Phosphatidylcholine, or purified from fresh newly-laid eggs as ovolecithin *(67)*.
6. Antigen: A preparation of a suitable amphipathic antigen in distilled water or 20 m*M* phosphate-buffered saline (PBS) (*see* **Note 3**).
7. Newly laid eggs, <24-h-old.
8. Chloroform, spectroscopic grade (Uvasol).
9. Acetone.
10. Ethanol.
11. Petroleum ether.
12. Cadmium chloride.
13. Silver nitrate.
14. Rhodamine 6G: 0.012% w/v aqueous solution (Sigma).
15. 0.145 *M* potassium and sodium chloride: 1.08 g KC1 and 0.847 g NaC1/100 mL.

## 3. Methods

All procedures should be carried out in accordance with appropriate safety regulations.

## 3.1. Preparation of Antigen Adsorbed to Aluminum Hydroxide

1. Prepare a stock solution of the vaccine candidate protein antigen in sterile, nonpyrogenic, glass-distilled water.
2. Sterilize a sample of aluminum hydroxide gel (*see* **Note 4**): For small amounts, it is acceptable to autoclave at 121°C and a pressure of 103.4 kPa (15 lb/in$^2$) for 1 h. With larger quantities, a stirring mechanism may be required because of the low heat conductivity of the aluminum hydroxide. Alhydrogel is nonpyrogenic, noncarcinogenic, and nonteratogenic, and it is assumed that the antigen preparation will also have been tested and shown to be free of these properties.
3. Mix aliquots of the stock protein solution aseptically with the aluminum hydroxide gel, e.g., 0.5–1.0 mL with 0.5 mL sterile Alhydrogel. Incubate the mixture for a minimum of 1 h at 37°C (a maximum period of 18 h); stir slowly or rotate on a mixer.

4. Repeat the adsorption process at different pH values; start at pH 6.0 and increase at 0.5 pH intervals to pH 9.0 (*see* **Notes 5–7**). If the antigen mixture is complex, there may be preferential binding at a particular pH value.

5. Place the mixtures at 0–1°C for 1 h; centrifuge at 1000$g$ for 10 min. Separate the clear supernates and measure the unadsorbed antigen(s) by a quantitative radial immunodiffusion test *(68)* (*see* **Subheading 3.2.**; **Note 8**).

## 3.2. Radial Immunodiffusion Test to Measure Antigen Unadsorbed to AL (OH)$_3$

1. Note that antibodies are not damaged by exposure to 50°C, and agar solidifies at temperatures below 38°C. Place a 5-cm-diameter Petri dish on a leveling table. Warm the specific anti-serum by placing in a water bath at 50°C for 5 min and add 0.75 mL to the 7.0-mL molten diethylbarbiturate agar. Mix anti-serum and gel thoroughly and pour into the Petri dish; ensure that the gel mixture is distributed evenly over the surface and leave to set at room temperature. Repeat with different anti-sera if a complex antigen mixture is being used.

2. Prepare standard twofold dilutions of antigens in sodium diethylbarbiturate buffer (e.g., 0.5–3.0 µg/mL antigen). These standard antigen solutions will depend on the original protein estimations of the candidate antigen.

3. Cut out basins in the anti-serum-agar layer with a sterile stainless-steel cutter. It should be possible to suck out the small agar plug at the same time as the basin is cut. Cut out 12 basins in a ring and mark their positions. Transfer 5.0 µL of the standard antigen dilutions or the test supernates to fill each of the basins. Some care is required to avoid spilling the antigen over the surface of the agar. Use a micropipet, automatic pipetter, or Hamilton syringe.

4. Leave the plate in a moist chamber at room temperature for 24 h. Measure the diameters of the circular immunoprecipitates around the basins with a graduated mono-ocular magnifier, or place the plate over a centimeter scale and measure with a hand lens.

5. Plot the $d^2$ values (squares of the diameters; square millimeters) minus the square millimeters of the basin itself from each of the antigen dilutions against the concentration of the standard antigen. A straight-line standard antigen curve should be obtained, but note that the origin on the $y$-axis will be at the point (diameter of basin)$^2$. Read the corresponding protein concentration of each test $d^2$ value from this standard curve and calculate the amount of protein in the total volume of each respective supernate.

6. If the precipitates are difficult to measure, it is possible to stain them. Wash the plate in physiological saline for 2 d to remove non-precipitated protein. Stain for 5–10 min with Amido black solution and wash with methanol-acetic acid mixture.

7. Calculate the amount of protein bound to the aluminum hydroxide and select the most appropriate combination of aluminum hydroxide to antigen. Make allowance for a slight excess of antigen to ensure that there is a small amount of free antigen in the final vaccine mixture (*see* **Notes 9–11**).

## 3.3. Preparation of a Complete Freund-Type Adjuvant

1. Dissolve the dried antigen (e.g., crystallized ovalbumin) in an appropriate volume of sterile distilled water. (Water-soluble equivalents of the mycobacterial adjuvant are dissolved in the saline component.)

2. Add the aqueous immunogen to the Guildhay NUFA incomplete adjuvant (1:2 v/v) or Montanide ISA 720 (3:7 v/v), *see* **Note 2**, or the FIA from Statens Seruminstitut at 1:1 v/v.

3. Add the aqueous phase to the oil phase and mix thoroughly until a creamy white emulsion is produced (*see* **Note 12**). This can be achieved by either drawing up into a 1.0-mL glass Luer syringe fitted with a medium-bore needle, passing from syringe to syringe through a sterile adapter, or by mild ultrasonication.
4. The nature of the resulting emulsion should be tested to ensure that a water-in-mineral oil emulsion has been prepared. Expel a drop of the emulsion onto the surface of water in a shallow dish. An oil-in-water emulsion will immediately disperse over the surface, whereas a water-in-oil emulsion will retain the integrity of the drop.
5. Store the final mixture at 4°C or at room temperature, depending on the nature of the antigen, but do not freeze because this will break the emulsion.

## 3.4. Preparation of an Incomplete Oil Adjuvant

The procedure is as described in **Subheading 3.3.**, but the mycobacterial component or its equivalent is omitted from the mixture.

## 3.5. Immunization Procedure (see Notes 12–14)

1. Warm the experimental vaccine to 37°C before injection. This avoids shock to the small animal, and helps the flow of the vaccine from the syringe. For large-scale use in the field this may not always be possible, but it is not recommended to use vaccine immediately from the refrigerator.
2. The size of the injection dose will depend on the animal and the route of injection. For example, 0.2 mL of a water-in-oil emulsion containing 2.0 mg of ovalbumin and 200 µg *M. tuberculosis* im into the left hindlimb of the guinea pig is suitable. However, 200 µg *M. tuberculosis* in the vaccine dose will completely suppress the humoral response in a mouse; 25–50 µg is the optimal dose. Different regimens may be required for larger animals; those for rabbits and sheep have been described where it may be advisable to use multiple injection sites (*69*).

## 3.6. Preparation of Pure Ovolecithin (Phosphatidylcholine; see Note 15)

This method is based on that described by Pangborn (*67*), as follows:
1. Separate the yolks from 12 <24-h-old eggs and blend in a suitable mixer.
2. Add acetone (400-mL aliquots) and blend the mixture for a further 30 s. Allow to separate and decant the acetone extract. Repeat until the yolk powder is creamy white when the final acetone extract is removed by filtering the mixture through a Buchner funnel.
3. Transfer the yolk filter cake to a stoppered flask, add 800 mL ethanol, and shake the mixture intermittently by hand for 30 min. Filter off the alcoholic extract by suction through a Buchner funnel, precipitate with approx 15.0 mL of 50% (w/v) aqueous cadmium chloride, and leave at 4°C for 1 h. Filter the precipitate through the Buchner funnel and wash with acetone on the filter.
4. Dissolve the washed precipitate in 100 mL chloroform, pour into a mixture of 700 mL alcohol + 10 mL 50% (w/v) aqueous cadmium chloride with constant stirring, and leave at room temperature for 10 min. Separate the cadmium-precipitated floccules by filtration, and redissolve in 100 mL chloroform. Re-precipitate the cadmium salt twice in the alcohol-cadmium chloride mixture, suspend in 150 mL petroleum ether, and place in a stoppered separating funnel.
5. Add 500 mL of 80% (v/v) ethanol (saturated with petroleum ether and containing 0.1% (w/v) cadmium chloride) to the suspended cadmium salt. Vigorously shake the mixture

by hand until the lecithin-cadmium chloride salt has dissolved, draw off, and retain the alcohol layer. Re-extract the petroleum ether layer once with 300 mL and once with 100 mL of the 80% (v/v) alcohol mixture.

6. Pool and concentrate the alcoholic extracts *in vacuo* in a rotary evaporator to a vol of 600 mL. Leave the concentrate at 4°C overnight to precipitate the lecithin-cadmium chloride.
7. Collect the precipitate by filtration through a Buchner funnel, dissolve in 150 mL chloroform, and mix with 150 mL 30% (v/v) ethanol in a separating funnel. After mixing, draw off the dilute alcohol layer and test for the presence of chloride with 5% (w/v) silver nitrate solution. Repeat this alcohol extraction until the chloride test is negative.
8. Evaporate the cadmium-free chloroform solution to dryness in a rotary evaporator, wash the residue with acetone to remove residual alcohol and chloroform, and finally dry *in vacuo*. Dissolve the lecithin in 100 mL anhydrous ether and add 20 mL acetone. Leave the mixture at 4°C overnight and remove the precipitate by filtration on a Buchner funnel. Evaporate the clear ether-acetone filtrate to dryness *in vacuo*, weigh the purified lecithin, and dissolve in spectroscopic-grade chloroform (Uvasol). Store in brown glass bottles in 25-mL aliquots at –70°C.

## *3.7. Preparation of Liposomes (Lipid Spherules)*

1. To obtain liposomes containing antigen, place 4.75 mL of the stock solution containing 14.75 mg pure lecithin/mL chloroform (1.75 μmol/ mL), 0.4 mL stock solution containing 241.66 mg cholesterol/25 mL chloroform (25.0 μmol/mL), and either 2.0 mL stock solution containing 136.7 mg dicetyl phosphate/25.0 mL chloroform (10 μmol/mL) for negatively charged liposomes or 2.0 mL stock solution containing 67.38 mg octadecylamine/25.0 mL chloroform (10 μmol/mL) for positively charged liposomes, in a 100-mL long-necked, round-bottomed flask. For best results, all solutions are prepared in spectroscopic-grade chloroform (Uvasol). Dry down the mixture *in vacuo* on a rotary evaporator and flush the flask with nitrogen to remove any residual solvent from the dry lipid film.
2. Vigorously resuspend the 100 μmol of lipid (70 μmol lecithin: 10 μmol cholesterol: 20 μmol dicetyl phosphate or octadecylamine) in 6.0 mL of the antigen in aqueous solution or 20 m*M* phosphate-buffered saline, at a temperature above the gel-liquid crystalline transition temperature of the phospholipid, before the liposomes are used as a vaccine. Further dispersion of the lipids may be achieved by mild ultrasonication. Allow the liposome:antigen mixture to equilibrate for 1 h before im injection. In some cases, it may be desirable to leave some free antigen in the final mixture, but this can be removed as indicated in **Subheading 3.8.** (*see* **Note 16**).

## *3.8. Calculation of Liposomal Antigen Entrapment Levels*

1. Liposomes containing antigen may be separated from free antigen on a Sephadex GSO column (20 × 2 cm) equilibrated with 0.145 *M* potassium and sodium chloride. It is common to collect 12–16 mL of the milky suspension of liposomes from the column.
2. Determine the amount of free antigen eluted from the column and thus calculate the amount of antigen entrapped in or linked to the liposomes. An alternative is to centrifuge the mixture at 10,000*g* for 30 min to remove free antigen.

## *3.9. Long-Term Storage of Liposomal Vaccines*

The use of a two-container system—with dried lipid in one and antigen solution in another, which requires mixing just prior to injection—is satisfactory for experimental purposes, but would not seem to be commercially viable. However, it is possible to

**Table 1**
**The Grades of Montanide ISA Which May Be Used**
**to Produce a Water-in-Oil Emulsion**

| | Type of oil | | |
|---|---|---|---|
| Emulsion type | Mineral adjuvant /antigen v/v | Nonmineral adjuvant /antigen v/v | Mineral/nonmineral adjuvant/antigen v/v |
| Water in oil | ISA 51 (50/50) | ISA 720 (70/30) | ISA 740 (70/30) |
| | ISA 50 (50/50) | ISA 708 (70/30) | ISA 773 (70/30) |
| | ISA 70 (70/30) | ISA 763A (70/30) | |
| Oil in water | ISA 25 (25/75) | ISA 27 (25/75) | ISA 28 (25/75) |
| | | ISA 35 (25/75) | |

freeze-dry the preformed liposomes *(70,71)* and resuspend prior to intraperitoneal (ip), sc, or im injection.

## 4. Notes

1. The use of poorly defined oils in Freund-type mixtures may give rise to severe toxic reactions *(6,43)* with accompanying ulceration. For this reason, it is recommended that the manufacturer supply evidence of quality-control tests on the oil—for example, GLC mass spectrometric analyses and systemic toxicity and pyrogenicity test results for a production batch. GLC analyses are carried out with a 2.77-m column packed with 3% OV-17 coated on Gas Chrom Q (Phase Separations Ltd.).
   Samples are dissolved in ether (ca. 5 mg/mL) and injected (1–2 µL) via a self-sealing septum into the apparatus. Analyses are carried out initially at 100°C for 16 min, followed by temperature programming at 8°C/min to 275°C. Standard hydrocarbons $nC_{11}H_{22}$, $nC_{18}H_{38}$, and $nC_{20}H_{42}$ are used as the reference compounds. The optimum hydrocarbon chain length is between $C_{18}$ and $C_{24}$ *(15)*.

2. Montanide ISA 720 and ISA 51 preparations should not be stored below 4°C after they have been included in a water-in-oil emulsion, otherwise there is separation into the two phases. The emulsion has a viscosity of 1500 mPa and is a fine emulsion with a droplet size of 1.0 µ (determined by laser scattering). Storage in an airtight container under nitrogen is recommended, as it can be damaged by oxidation. The shelf-life of ISA 720 is 2 yr. **Table 1** shows a selection of the Montanide ISA types available for the water-in-oil emulsions; there are also types for oil-in-water and water-in-oil-in-water, but these release the antigen more rapidly. The detailed manufacturing process is available on request from Seppic.

3. It must not be assumed that liposomes can be used for the presentation of all antigens, but a wide range of viral, bacterial, and mammalian amphipathic preparations have been used *(71)*.

4. It is essential to start with a sterile preparation; microbial contamination of the aluminum hydroxide gel may lead to unexpected antigens being added to the experimental vaccine. Furthermore, bacterial cell-wall (peptidoglycan) may modify the adjuvanticity or possibly induce pyrogenicity. Contaminating protein may also interfere with the adsorption capacity of the aluminum hydroxide.

5. At a pH of 6.0–6.5 some proteins may be labile, so it may be necessary to use a slightly higher pH value.

**Table 2**
**The Dose and Sites Injection for Oil-Adjuvanted Vaccines**

| Species | Maximum volume per injection site | Injection sites | |
| --- | --- | --- | --- |
| | | Primary response | Secondary response |
| Mice or hamsters | 50 µL | sc; im | sc; im |
| | 200 µL | | oral |
| Guinea-pigs or rats | 200 µL | sc; im into one hindlimb | sc; im into one hindlimb |
| | 300 µL | | oral |
| Rabbit | 250 µL (if in multiple sites <25 µL /site*) | sc; im into one thigh muscle; id* | sc; im into one thigh muscle; id* |
| Large animal | 500 µL (if in multiples sites <250 µL/site*) | sc; im into one hindlimb; id* | sc; im into one hindlimb; id* |
| Chicken | 250 µL | sc; im | sc; im |
| Human | 250 µL* | im | im |

*But note the increased volumes used in aggressive human cancer immunotherapy.

6. An aluminum adjuvant will dissociate if frozen. This is easily detected, as an upper, clear layer is formed.

7. Multiple negatively charged ions—such as phosphate, sulfate, and borate—may interfere with the adsorption to aluminum salts of negatively charged proteins, so buffer systems with these should be used with caution.

8. An alternative to the radial immunodiffusion assay for protein has recently been suggested—namely, a modified bicinchoninic acid assay (Dr. E.E. Lindblad, Brenntag Biosector; personal communication). In addition, one manufacturer was requested to calculate the amount of residual unconjugated aluminum salt in a vaccine mixture. This value could be determined from an aliquot of the supernate in an analytical laboratory by atomic absorption spectroscopy.

9. The injection dose of aluminum hydroxide in an aluminum-adjuvanted vaccine should be carefully calculated because too much may be toxic—e.g., a 25-g mouse will tolerate 1.0 mg aluminum hydroxide, whereas for human vaccines 1.25 mg aluminum hydroxide is acceptable.

10. Aluminum adjuvants have been shown to be ineffective with influenza, typhoid, or peptide vaccines. In addition, aluminum hydroxide is more useful for the stimulation of the primary immune response. There is no evidence that it acts as an immunogen or hapten by itself.

11. Contraindications: Aluminum adjuvants may cause the formation of small local granulomas of 5.0–10.0 mm in diameter, or transient erythema at the site of injection. These have been described with the DTP vaccine, but they usually regress after a few weeks.

12. The ratio of the oil phase to the aqueous phase may be altered, depending on the product used (**Table 1**). For example, the Montanide ISA 720 from Seppic is used at a 70:30 ratio to yield stable emulsions; if economies are made and this ratio is altered, the emulsion may separate into two phases and reduce the stability during storage.

There are also grades for water-in-oil-in-water formulations, and these can be obtained

**Table 3**
**Oil-Adjuvanted Vaccines: Local Reactions in Humans**

| Vaccine investigator | Year | Country | Group size | Adverse reactions | Frequency (%) |
|---|---|---|---|---|---|
| INFLUENZA: | | | | | |
| Salk (79) | 1951 | US | 18,000 | | <10 |
| Bell (80) | 1951–55 | US | 10,864 | 24 | 0.2 |
| MRC (81) | 1953–55 | UK | 7,547 | 9 | 0.1 |
| Heggie (82) | 1958 | US | 85 | 0 | – |
| Himmelweit (83) | 1958 | US | 224 | 0 | – |
| MRC (84) | 1960 | UK | 6123 | 2 | 0.03 |
| Meiklejohn (85) | 1960 | US | 2694 | 0 | – |
| Seal (86) | 1955 | US | 8000 | 3 | 0.04 |
| POLIO: | | | | | |
| Salk (87) | 1951 | US | 90 | 0 | – |
| Cutler (88) | 1960 | US | 23,917 | 93 | 1.1 |
| | | | | 14 nodules | 0.2 |
| TRACHOMA: | | | | | |
| Snyder (89) | 1966 | US | 1393 | 0 | – |
| TYPHOID: | | | | | |
| Snyder (89) | 1966 | US | 1189 | 87 | 7.3 |
| TETANUS: | | | | | |
| McLennan (90) | 1965 | US | Purified  39 | 9 (minor) | 23.0 |
| | | | Crude  327 | 193 | 59.0 |
| CHOLERA: | | | | | |
| Ogonuki et al. (91) | 1964 | US | Adjuvanted* | | |
| | | | 143,600 | 2844 | 1.95 |
| | | | | Abcess 1018 | 0.71 |
| | | | Aqueous | 75 | |
| | | | 440,000 | Abcess 21 | 0.005 |

*Note that this vaccine was injected subcutaneously and not by the recommended im route for oil formulations.

from Seppic. In general, it is not recommended to inject these adjuvants intradermally, because of the local reactivity and ulceration. There may also be species differences found after ip injection; for example, the ip route caused ascites production in Balb/c mice, but booster injections in rabbits or sheep did not cause adverse effects (72). The recommended injection volumes for oil emulsions are shown in **Table 2**. It is doubtful that human patients would be willing to accept intravenous (iv) or ip vaccine injections as a routine procedure, so these routes are not recommended for oil emulsions in research leading to the development of human vaccines. In addition, there may be risks involved in repeated oral (73) or in administration (74) of adjuvanted preparations.

13. Care must be exercised to ensure that the operator does not accidentally inject his/her or the assisting person's hand with a Freund-type complete adjuvant emulsion; a veterinary surgeon required amputation of part of a finger because of restriction of the blood supply

caused by local granuloma formation *(75)*. If self-inoculation does occur, it is advisable to seek medical attention at the earliest opportunity.

14. With consideration of the foregoing comments, it is worth noting that the Committee on Clinical Trials concluded that the adjuvant effect of emulsified influenza vaccines was clearly demonstrated, and therefore the economy in the amount of antigen needed was obvious *(3)*. An oil-adjuvanted influenza vaccine was administered to American servicemen in the 1940s, and the long-term surveillance for 35 yr has not shown a greater incidence of hypersensitivity states, autoimmune diseases, or cancers in these vaccinees than found in a contemporaneous control group *(76–78)* (*see also* **Table 3**).

15. Phospholipid purity is essential to maintain stable liposomes. For this reason, phosphatidylcholine was routinely prepared by the method described above, **Subheading 3.6** . Commercial preparations should be examined by thin-layer chromatography prior to their use to check for levels of impurities. Polygram Sil G plates are developed to the 15-cm mark with undiluted spectroscopic-grade chloroform or di-isobutyl-ketone ($C_9H_{18}O$). Spots are visualized either by charring with a spray of 50% (v/v) sulfuric acid or with 0.012% (w/v) rhodamine.

16. The phospholipid:antigen ratio may be important. Gregoriadis and colleagues *(70)* noted with liposomes of equimolar phosphatidylcholine and cholesterol plus 0.2 µg tetanus toxoid that a ratio of phospholipid: antigen of 346:1 stimulated significantly higher levels of antitoxin than a ratio of 17,804:1. It is necessary to prepare a range of experimental vaccines with different compositions before concluding that liposomes are ineffective.

One advantage is the ability to formulate the lipid bilayer to mimic the mammalian-cell membrane so that it is seen as "self," and thus, anti-phospholipid antibodies are not stimulated and the antigen stimulus survives for a longer period until the liposomes slowly degrade.

## References

1. Jollès, P. and Paraf, A. (1973) Chemical and biological basis of adjuvants (Kleinzeller, A., Springer G. F., and Wittman, H. G., eds.) in *Molecular Biology and Biophysics* Springer, New York **13**, 1–53.
2. Adam, A. (1985) Synthetic adjuvants in *Modern Concepts in Immunology* (Bona C., ed.). Wiley, Chichester, UK, **1**, 1–239.
3. Stewart-Tull, D. E. S., ed. (1994) *The Theory and Practical Application of Adjuvants*. Wiley, Chichester and New York, pp. 1–380.
4. Vogel, F. R. and Powell, M. F. (1994) A compendium of vaccine adjuvants and excipients, in *Vaccine Design* (Powell, M. F. and Newman, M. J., eds.), Plenum, New York, pp. 141–229.
5. O'Hagan, D.T., ed. (2000) *Vaccine Adjuvants: Preparation Methods and Research Protocols*. Humana Press Inc., Totowa, NJ, pp. 1–342.
6. Stewart-Tull, D. E. S. (1988) Recommendations for the assessment of adjuvants (immunopotentiators), in *Immunological Adjuvants and Vaccines*, NATO ASI Series A: Life Sciences, vol. 179 (Gregoriadis, G., Allison, A. C., and Poste, G., eds.), Plenum, New York, pp. 213–226.
7. Lindblad, E. B. (1994) Aluminium adjuvants, in *The Theory and Practical Application of Adjuvants* (Stewart-Tull, D. E. S., ed.), Wiley, Chichester and New York, pp, 21–35.
8. Hem, S. L. and White, J. L. (1984) Characterization of aluminium hydroxide for use as an adjuvant in parenteral vaccines. *J. Parenter. Sci. Technol.* **38**, 2–11.
9. Weeke, B., Weeke, W., and Lowenstein, H. (1975) The adsorption of serum proteins to

aluminium hydroxide gel examined by means of quantitative immuno-electrophoresis, in *Quantitative Immuno-electrophoresis: New Developments and Applications* (Axelsen, N. H., ed.), Universitetsforlaget, Denmark, pp. 149–154.

10. Seeber, S. J., White, J. L., and Hem, S. L. (1991) Predicting the adsorption of proteins by aluminium-containing adjuvants. *Vaccine* **9,** 201–203.
11. Mosmann, T. R. and Sad, S. (1996) The expanding universe of T-cell subsets: Th1, Th2 and more. *Immunol. Today* **17,** 138–146.
12. Cox, J.C., and Coulter, A.R. (1997) Adjuvants—a classification and review of their modes of action. *Vaccine* **15,** 248–256.
13. Stewart-Tull, D. E. S. (1983) Immunologically important constituents of mycobacteria, in *The Biology of the Mycobacteria*, vol. 2 (Ratledge, C. and Stanford, J., eds.), Academic Press, London, pp. 3–84.
14. Stewart-Tull, D. E. S. (1985) Immunopotentiating activity of peptidoglycan and surface polymers, in *Immunology of the Bacterial Cell Envelope* (Stewart-Tull, D. E. S. and Davies, M., eds.), Wiley, Chichester and New York, pp. 47–89.
15. Stewart-Tull, D. E. S., Shimono, T., Kotani, S., and Knights, B. A. (1976) Immunosuppressive effect in mycobacterial adjuvant emulsions of mineral oils containing low molecular weight hydrocarbons. *Int. Arch. Allergy Appl. Immunol.* **52,** 118–128.
16. Stewart-Tull, D. E. S. (2000) Harmful and Beneficial Activities of Immunological Adjuvants in *Vaccine Adjuvants: Preparation Methods and Research Protocols* (O'Hagan D. T., ed.), Humana Press, Totowa, NJ, pp. 29–48.
17. Lindblad, E. B. (2000) Freund's adjuvants in *Vaccine Adjuvants: Preparation Methods and Research Protocols* (O'Hagan D. T., ed.), Humana Press, Totowa, NJ, pp. 49–63.
18. Leenaars, P. P. A. M., Hendriksen, C. F. M., de Leeuw, W. A., Carat, F., Delahaut, P., Fischer, R., et al. (1999) The production of polyclonal antibodies in laboratory animals. The Report and Recommendations of ECVAM/FELASA Workshop 35. *ATLA* **27,** 70–102.
19. Lindblad, E. B. (2000) Escaping from the use of Freund's complete adjuvant, in *Progress in the Reduction, Refinement and Replacement of Animal Experimentation* (Balls, M., van Zeller, A. M. and Halder, M. E., eds.), Elsevier, Amsterdam, pp. 1681–1685.
20. Turner, J. L., Trauger, R. J., Daigle, A. E., and Carlo, D. J. (1994) HIV-1 immunogen induction of HIV-1 specific delayed-type hypersensitivity: results of a double-blind, adjuvant-controlled dose-ranging trial. *AIDS* **8,** 1429–1435.
21. Trauger, R. J., Giermakowska, W., Wormsley, S., Turner, J. L., Jensen, F. C., and Carlo, D. J. (1995) Autoproliferation in HIV-1 infected patients undergoing active HIV-1-specific immunotherapy. *Clin. Exp. Immunol.* **100,** 7–12.
22. Gringeri, A., Santagostino, E., Muca-Perja, M., Mannucci, P. M., Zagury, J. F., Bizzini, B., et al. (1998) Safety and immunogenicity of HIV-1 Tat toxoid in immunocompromised HIV-1-infected patients. *J. Hum. Virol.* **1,** 293–298.
23. Gringeri, A., Musico, M., Hermans, P., Bentwich, Z., Cusini, M., Bergamasco, A., et al. (1999) Active anti-interferon-a immunisation: A European-Israeli, randomised, double-blind, placebo-controlled clinical trial in 242 HIV-infected patients (The Euris Study). *J. Acquir. Immune Defic. Syndr. Hum. Retrovirol.* **20,** 358–370.
24. Pinto, L. A., Berzofsky, J. A., Fowke, K. R., Little, R. F., Merced-Galindez, F., Humphrey, R., et al. (1999) HIV-specific immunity following immunization with HIV synthetic envelope peptides in asymptomatic HIV-1 infected patients. *AIDS* **22,** 2003–2012.
25. van Driel, W. J., Ressing, M. E., Kenter, G. G., Brandt, R. M., Krul, E. L., van Rossum, A. B., et al. (1999) Vaccination with HPV16 peptides of patients with advanced cervical carcinoma clinical evaluation of a Phase I-II trial. *Eur. J. Cancer* **35,** 946–952.
26. Duarte Cano, C.A. (1999) The multi-epitope polypeptide approach in HIV-1 vaccine development. *Genet. Anal: Biomol. Eng.* **15,** 149–153.

27. Picard, O., Achour, A., Bernard, J., Halbreich Bizzini, B., Boyer, V., Desgranges, C., et al. (1992) A 2-year follow up of an anti-HIV immune reaction in HIV-1 gp160 immunized healthy sero-negative humans, evidence for persistent cell-mediated immunity. *J. Acquir. Immune Defic. Syndr.* **5,** 539–546.

28. Gringeri, A., Santagostino, E., Mannucci, P. M., Tradati, F., Cultraro, D., Buzzi, A., et al.(1994) A randomised placebo-controlled blind anti-AIDS clinical trial. Safety and immunogenicity of a specific anti-IFNα immunization. *J. Acquir. Immune Defic. Syndr.* **7,** 978–979.

29. Rosenberg, S. A., Yang, J. C., Schwartzentruber, D. J., Hwu, P., Marincola, F. M., Topalian, S. L., et al. (1998) Immunologic and therapeutic evaluation of a synthetic peptide vaccine for a treatment of patients with metastatic melanoma. *Nat. Med.* **4,** 321–327.

30. Yamshchikov, G. V., Barnd, D. L., Eastham, S., Galavotti, H., Patterson, J. W., Deacon, D. H., et al. (2001) Evaluation of peptide vaccine immunogenicity in draining lymph nodes and peripheral blood of melanoma patients. *Int. J. Cancer* **92,** 703–711.

31. Lawrence G. W., Saul, A., Giddy, A. J., Kemp, R., and Pye, D. (1967) Phase I trial in humans of an oil-based adjuvant SEPPIC Montanide ISA 720. *Vaccine* **15,** 176–178.

32. Saul, A., Lawrence, G., Simillie, A., Rzepezyk, C., Reed, C., Taylor, D., et al. (1999) Human phase I vaccine trial of 3 recombinant asexual stage malaria antigens with Montanide ISA 720 adjuvant. *Vaccine* **17,** 3145–3159.

33. Lawrence, G., Cheng, Q. Q., Reed, C., Taylor, S., Stowers, A., Cloonan, N., et al. (2000) Effect of vaccination with 3 recombinant asexual-stage malaria antigens on initial growth rates of *Plasmodium falciparum* in non-immune volunteers. *Vaccine* **17,** 1925–1931.

34. Genton, B., Al-Yaman, F., Anders, R., Saul, A., Brown, G. T., Rare, L., et al. (2000) Safety and immunogenicity of a three-component blood stage malaria vaccine in adults living in an endemic area of Papua New Guinea. *Vaccine* **22,** 2504–2511.

35. Iyer, A.V., Ghosh, S., Singh, S.N., and Deshmukh, R.A. (2000) Evaluation of three 'ready to formulate' oil adjuvants for foot and mouth disease vaccine production. *Vaccine* **19,** 1097–1105.

36. McCluskie, M. J. and Davis, H. L. (1998) CpG DNA is a potent enhancer of systemic and mucosal immune responses against hepatitis B surface antigen with intranasal administration to mice. *J. Immunol.* **161,** 4463–4466.

37. McCluskie, M. J., Weeratna, R. D., Payette, P. J., and Davis, H. L. The potential of CpG oligodeoxynucleotides as mucosal adjuvants. (2001) *Crit. Rev. Immunol.* **21,** 103–120.

38. McCluskie, M. J. and Davis, H. L. (2000) Oral, intrarectal and intranasal immunizations using CpG and non-CpG oligodeoxynucleotides as adjuvants. *Vaccine* **19,** 413–422.

39. McCluskie, M. J., Weeratna, R. D., Krieg, A. M., and Davis, H. L. (2000) CpG DNA is an effective oral adjuvant to protein antigens in mice. *Vaccine* **19,** 950–957.

40. Manders, P. and Thomas, R. (2000) Immunology of DNA vaccines: CpG motifs and antigen presentation. *Inflamm. Res.* **49,** 199–205.

41. Moss, R. B., Diveley, J., Jensen, F. C., Gouveia, E., Savary, J., and Carlo, D. J. (2000) HIV-specific CD4 (+) and CD8 (+) immune responses are generated with a gp-depleted, whole-killed HIV-1 immunogen with CpG immunostimulatory sequences of DNA. *J. Interferon and Cytosine Res.* **20,** 1131–1137.

42. Moss, R. B., Diveley, J., Jensen, F. C., Gouveia, E., and Carlo, D. J. (2001) Human immunodeficiency virus (HIV)-specific immune responses are generated with the simultaneous vaccination of a gp120-depleted, whole-killed HIV-1 immunogen with cytosine-phosphorothioate-guanine dinucleotide immunostimulatory sequences of DNA. *J. Hum. Virol.* **4,** 39–43.

43. Leenaars, P. P. A. M., Koedam, M. A., Wester, P. W., Baumans, V., Claassen, E., and Hendriksen, C. F. M. (1998) Assessment of side-effects induced by injection of different adjuvant/antigen combinations in rabbits and mice. *Lab. Anim.* **32,** 387–406

44. Tamura, S. I. and Kurata (2000) A proposal for safety standards for human use of cholera toxin (or *Escherichia coli* heat-labile enterotoxin derivatives as an adjuvant of nasal inactivated influenza vaccine. *Jpn. J. Inf. Dis.* **53,** 98–106.

45. Stewart-Tull, D. E. S. (1985) Immunopotentiating activity of peptidoglycan and surface polymers, in *Immunology of the Bacterial Cell Envelope* (Stewart-Tull, D. E. S. and Davies, M., eds.), Wiley, Chichester, UK, pp. 47–89.

46. Van Ginkel, F. W., Jackson, R. J., Yuki, Y., and McGhee, J. R. (2000) Cutting edge: the mucosal adjuvant cholera toxin redirects vaccine proteins into olfactory tissues. *J. Immunol.* **165,** 4778–4782.

47. Hagiwara, Y., Iwasaki, T., Asanuma, H., Sato, Y., Sata, T., Aizawa, C., et al. (2000) Effects of intranasal administration of cholera toxin (or *Escherichia coli* heat-labile toxin) B subunits supplemented with a trace amount of the holotoxin on the brain. *Vaccine* **19,** 1652–1660.

48. Stewart-Tull, D. E. S. (1996) The use of adjuvants in experimental vaccines IV ISCOMS, in *Methods in Molecular Medicine: Vaccine Protocols* (Robinson, A., Farrar, G. and Wiblin, C., eds.), Humana Press, Inc., Totowa, NJ, pp. 153–155.

49. Rimmelzwaan, G. F., Nieuwkoop, N., Brandenburg, A., Sutter, G. Bayer, W. E., Maher, D., et al. (2000) A randomised double blind study in young healthy adults comparing cell-mediated and humoral immune responses induced by influenza ISCOM vaccines and conventional vaccines. *Vaccine* **19,** 1180–1187.

50. Voeten, J. T., Rimmelzwaan, G. F., Nieuwkoop, N. J., Lövgren-Bengtsson, K., and Osterhaus, A. D. (2000) Introduction of the hemagglutinin transmembrane region in the influenza virus matrix protein facilitates its incorporation into ISCOM and activation of specific CD8 (+) cytotoxic T lymphocytes. *Vaccine* **19,** 514–522.

51. Chopra, N., Biswas, S., Thomas, B., Sabhani, L., and Rao, D.N. (2000) Inducing protective antibodies against ring-infected erythrocyte surface peptide antigen of *Plasmodium falciparum* using immunostimulating complex (ISCOMs) delivery. *Med. Microbiol. Immunol.* **189,** 75–83.

52. Lövgren-Bengtsson, K. and Morein, B. (2000) The ISCOM(tm) technology, in *Vaccine Adjuvants: Preparation Methods and Research Protocols* (O'Hagan, D. T., ed.), Humana Press, Totowa, NJ, pp. 239–258.

53. Gregoriadis, G. (1988) Fate of injected liposomes: observations on entrapped solute retention, vesicle clearance and tissue distribution *in vivo,* in *Liposomes as Drug Carriers: Recent Trends and Progress* (Gregoriadis, G., ed.), Wiley, Chichester and New York, pp. 3–18.

54. van Rooijen, N. and Su, D. (1989) Immunoadjuvant action of liposomes: mechanisms, in *Immunological Adjuvants and Vaccines* (Gregoriadis, G., Allison, A. C. and Poste, G., eds.), Plenum, New York, pp. 95–106.

55. Stewart-Tull, D. E. S., Davies, M., and Jackson, D. M. (1978) The binding of adjuvant-active mycobacterial peptidoglycolipids and glycopeptides to mammalian membranes and their effect on artificial lipid bilayers. *Immunology* **34,** 57–67.

56. Davies, M., Stewart-Tull, D. E. S., and Jackson, D. M. (1978) The binding of lipopolysaccharide from *Escherichia coli* to mammalian cell membranes and its effect on liposomes. *Biochim. Biophys. Acta* **508,** 260–276.

57. Stewart-Tull, D. E. S. (1996) The use of adjuvants in experimental vaccines III Lipo-

somes, in *Methods in Molecular Medicine: Vaccine Protocols* (Robinson, A., Farrar, G. and Wiblin, C., eds.), Humana Press, Inc., Totowa, NJ, pp. 147–151.

58. Gregoriadis, G., McCormack, B., Obrenovic, M., Perrie, Y., and Saffie, R (2000) Liposomes as immunological adjuvants and vaccine carriers, in *Vaccine Adjuvants: Preparation Methods and Research Protocols* (O'Hagan, D. T., ed.), Humana Press, Totowa, NJ, pp. 137–150.

59. Loutan, L., Bovier, P., Althaus, B., and Gluck, R. (1994) Inactivated virosome hepatitis a vaccine. *Lancet* **343**, 322–324.

60. Cusi, M. G., Zurbriggen, R., Valassina, M., Bianchi, S., Durrer, P., Valensin, P. E., et al. (2000) Intranasal immunization with mumps virus DNA vaccine delivered by influenza virosomes elicits mucosal and systemic immunity. *Virology* **277**, 111–118.

61. ECPI World Vaccine Congress 1999. (2001) Collected papers. *Vaccine* **19**, 1559–1615.

62. Jodar, L., Duclos, P., Milstein, J. B., Griffiths, E., Aguado, M. Y., and Clements, C. J. (2001) Ensuring vaccine safety in immunization programmes. *Vaccine* **19**, 1594–1605.

63. Seibert, H., Balls, M., Fentem, J. H., Bianchi, V., Clothier, R. H., Dierickx, P. J., et al. (1996) Acute toxicity testing in vitro and the classification and labelling of chemicals. The Report and Recommendations of ECVAM Workshop 16. *ATLA* **24**, 499–510.

64. Cooper, J. F. (2001) The bacterial endotoxins test: past, present and future. *Eur. J. Parenteral Sci.* **6**, 89–93.

65. Falk, L. A. and Ball, L. K. (2001) Current status and future trends in vaccine regulation. *Vaccine* **19**, 1567–1572.

66. Masterton, R. G. and Green, A. D. (1991) Dissemination of human pathogens by airline travel. *J. Appl. Bacteriol.* **70**, 31S–38S.

67. Pangborn, M. C. (1951) A simplified purification of lecithin. *J. Biol. Chem.* **188**, 471–476.

68. Mancini, G., Carbonara, A. O., and Heremans, J. F. (1965) Immunochemical quantitation of antigens by single radial immunodiffusion. *Immunochemistry* **2**, 235–255.

69. Stewart-Tull, D. E. S. (1991) The assessment and use of adjuvants, in *Vaccines* (Gregoriadis, G., Allison, A., and Poste, G., eds.), Plenum, New York, pp. 85–92.

70. Gregoriadis, G., Davis, D., and Davies, A. (1987) Liposomes as immunological adjuvants in vaccines: antigen incorporation studies. *Vaccine* **5**, 145–151.

71. Gregoriadis, G., Tan, L., and Xiao, Q. (1989) The immunoadjuvant action of liposomes: role of structural characteristics, in *Immunological Adjuvants and Vaccines* (Gregoriadis, G., Allison, A. C., and Poste, G., eds.), Plenum, New York, pp. 79–94.

72. Stewart-Tull, D. E. S., and Rowe, R. E. C. (1975) Procedures for large-scale antiserum production in sheep. *J. Immunol. Methods* **8**, 37–46.

73. Stewart-Tull, D. E. S. and Jones, A. C. (1992) Adjuvanted vaccines should not induce allergic responses to dietary antigens. *FEMS Microbiol. Lett.* **100**, 489–496.

74. Tamura, S. I. and Kurata, T. (2000) A proposal for safety standards for human use of cholera toxin (or *Escherichia coli* heat-labile enterotoxin) derivatives as an adjuvant of nasal inactivated influenza vaccine. *Jap. J. Inf. Dis.* **53**, 98–106.

75. Stones, P. B. (1979) Self injection of veterinary oil-emulsion vaccines. *Br. Med. J.* **I**, 1627.

76. Davenport, F. M., Hennessy, A. V., Houser, H. B., and Cryns W. F. (1956) Evaluation of adjuvant influenza virus vaccine tested against influenza B, 1954-1955. *Am. J. Hyg.* **64**, 304–313.

77. Davenport, F. M. and Hennessy, A. V. (1956) Serologic recapitulation of past experiences with influenza A: antibody response to monovalent vaccine. *J. Exp. Med.* **104**, 85–97.

78. Davenport, F. M. (1968) Seventeen years experience with mineral oil adjuvant influenza virus vaccines. *Ann. Allergy* **26**, 288–292.

79. Salk, J. E., Contakos, A.B., and Laurent, A.M. (1953) Use of adjuvants in studies on influ-

enza immunization III Degree of persistence of antibody in human subjects two years after vaccination. *JAMA* **151**, 1169–1175.

80. Bell, J. A., Philip, R. N., Davis, D. J., Beem, M. O., Beigelman, P. M., Engler, J. I., et al. (1961) Epidemiologic studies on influenza in familial and general populations, 1951–1956: IV vaccine reactions. *Am. J. Hyg.* **73**, 148–163.

81. Medical Research Council (1955) Report of the Committee on Clinical Trials of Influenza Vaccine. *Br. Med. J.* **2**, 1229–1232.

82. Heggie, A. D., Crawford, Y. E., and Miller, L. F. (1960) Failure to demonstrate increased hypersensitivity to egg protein after immunization with an influenza vaccine of the oil-adjuvanted type. *N. Engl. J. Med.* **263**, 959–962.

83. Himmelweit, F. (1960) Serological responses and clinical reactions to influenza virus vaccines. *Br. Med. J.* **2**, 1690–1694.

84. Medical Research Council (1964) Clinical trials of oil-adjuvant influenza vaccines 1960-63. Report of the Medical Research Council by its Committee on Influenza and other respiratory virus vaccines. *Br. Med. J.* **i**, 267–271.

85. Meiklejohn, G. (1960) Observations on live influenza vaccine. *J. Am. Med. Assn.* **172**, 1354–1356.

86. Seal, J. R. (1955) Reactions to influenza vaccine. *US Armed Forces Med. J.* **6**, 1559–1563.

87. Salk, J. and Salk, D. (1977) Control of influenza and poliomyelitis with killed virus vaccines. *Science* **195**, 834–847

88. Cutler, J. C., Lesesne, L., and Vaughn, I. (1960) Use of poliomyelitis virus vaccine in light mineral oil adjuvant in a community immunization program and report of reactions encountered. *J. Allergy* **33**, 193–209.

89. Snyder, J. C., Bell, S. D., and Murray E. S. (1966) Reactions among infants immunized intramuscularly with typhoid vaccine in adjuvant. *J. Bacteriol.* **91**, 902

90. MacLennan, R., Schofield, F. D., Pittmann, M., Hardegree, M. C., and Barile, M. F. (1965) Immunization against neonatal tetanus in New Guinea: antitoxin response of pregnant women to adjuvant and plain toxoids. *Bull. WHO* **32**, 683–697

91. Ogonuki, H., Hashizume, S., and Abe, H (1967) Histopathological tests of tissues in the sites of local reactions caused by the injection of oil-adjuvant cholera vaccine: international symposium on adjuvants of immunity. *Symp. Ser. Immunobiol. Stand.* **6**, Karger, New York, pp. 125–128.

# 12

## Incorporation of Immunomodulators into Plasmid DNA Vaccines

### Linda S. Klavinskis, Philip Hobson, and Andrew Woods

### 1. Introduction

The success of candidate vaccines against infectious disease depends on their ability to activate components of the immune response (innate, cellular, and/or humoral) appropriate to the correlates of protection identified for the particular pathogen. Recombinant DNA technology has provided the opportunity to rationally design vaccines based upon the identified protective antigens, and also to modulate the type and magnitude of the immune response by the incorporation of genetic adjuvants. These may include cytokines, chemokines, costimulatory molecules, or hemopoietic growth factors (*see* **ref. *1***). The choice of immunomodulatory molecule reflects the polarization of the immune response (Th1 and cell-mediated or Th2 and antibody) selected to eliminate the particular pathogen by the vaccine candidate. The presence of IL-12, IL-15, IL-18, or interferon-gamma (IFN-$\gamma$) are critical in the development of Th1 responses that are directed toward cell-mediated immunity *(2)*, and the presence of IL-4, IL-5, and IL-10 are critical in the development of Th2 responses that are directed toward antibody production *(2)*. For weakly immunogenic antigens, the incorporation of genes that code for pro-inflammatory cytokines (e.g., IL-1$\alpha$, TNF-$\alpha$, or TGF-$\beta$) or costimulatory molecules (CD80, CD86, and CD40-ligand) may provide maturation signals to antigen-presenting cells (APC) to enhance their ability to present vaccine antigens, and result in an increased adaptive immune response *(3,4)*. More recently, cytokines and chemokines, including granulocyte-macrophage colony-stimulating factor (GM-CSF), monocyte chemotactic proteins (MCPs) and macrophage inflammatory proteins (MIPs), have been incorporated into vaccines in lieu of their potential to increase recruitment of blood-borne dendritic cells and monocytes to interstitial sites of vaccine delivery *(5)*.

With increasing emphasis to achieve vaccine delivery by noninvasive, patient-compliant routes, nasal or oral vaccine delivery has become an attractive alternative to needle injection. The approach has the added advantage of stimulating both systemic

From: *Methods in Molecular Medicine, Vol. 87: Vaccine Protocols, 2nd ed.*
Edited by: A. Robinson, M. J. Hudson, and M. P. Cranage © Humana Press Inc., Totowa, NJ

and mucosal immune responses *(6)*. However, nonreplicating antigens are generally nonimmunogenic at mucosal inductive sites, and thus can induce tolerance when delivered *(6)*. The incorporation of immunomodulators into DNA vaccines has thus raised new possibilities for the design of effective mucosal vaccines. Numerous cytokines and chemokines have been successfully cloned into DNA expression vectors and have been co-administered with DNA coding immunogens by the intranasal (in) route *(5,7,8)*.

The incorporation of the IL-12 gene into a DNA vaccine is used here to illustrate the methods utilized for cloning into a bicistronic expression vector, in vitro verification of immunomodulator expression from an expression vector, and in delivery of cytokine- and immunogen-coding plasmid DNA.

## 2. Materials

1. pCRscript kit (Stratagene).
2. PFU DNA polymerase (Stratagene).
3. Taq DNA polymerase (Promega).
4. Reverse-transcription kit (ProStar, Stratagene).
5. pBluscript II SK+ (Stratagene).
6. pCI mammalian expression plasmid (Promega).
7. pIRES (Clontech).
8. Gene clean gel purification kit (Bio 101).
9. *Escherichia coli* XL-1 Blue (Stratagene).
10. RNAzol (Bio101).
11. Oligonucleotides (MWG).
12. Restriction enzymes (New England Biolabs).
13. Agarose (Invitrogen).
14. 2× TY media (Difco, Becton and Dickinson).
15. IPTG (isopropyl-β-D-thio-galactopyraoside, Sigma Aldrich).
16. X-gal (Sigma Aldrich).
17. LB medium (Pharmacia).
18. LBA (Pharmacia).
19. Miniprep kit (Qiagen).
20. Midiprep kit (Qiagen).
21. Nova blot buffer.
22. Sodium dodecyl sulfate polyacrylamide gel electrophoresis (SDS-PAGE) Running buffer.
23. 100-bp DNA ladder (Promega).
24. 1K-bp DNA ladder (Promega).
25. Polymerase chain reaction (PCR) mastermix 1.1 m$M$ MgCl$_2$ (Abgene).
26. Acrylamide; *bis*-acrylamide (39:1) (Biorad).
27. TEMED (Sigma Aldrich).
28. Ammonium persulfate (Sigma Aldrich).
29. Shrimp alkaline phosphatase (Promega).
30. PCR Mastermix 1.1 m$M$ MgCl$_2$ (Abgene).
31. PfuTurbo® DNA Polymerase (Stratagene).
32. *EcoR I* (New England Biolabs).
33. *Nhe I* (New England Biolabs).
34. *Not I* (New England Biolabs).
35. *Hind III* (New England Biolabs).

36. *Sal I* (New England Biolabs).
37. Cell-transfection medium: Dulbecco's Modified Eagle's Medium (DMEM) (D-5796), penicillin/streptomycin, L-glutamine (Life Technologies).
38. FuGENE 6 transfection reagent (Roche).
39. Detection of p40 (goat polyclonal anti-mouse p40 IL-12 **α-M-20** sc-1283 Santa Cruz Biotechnology).
40. Detection of p35 (goat polyclonal anti-mouse p35 IL-12 **α-M-19** sc-9350 Santa Cruz Biotechnology).
41. Rabbit anti-goat IgG biotin (**RαGt**, Dako).
42. Strepatavidin-horesradish peroxidase conjugate (**S-HRP**, Southern Biotechnology).
43. Recombinant IL-12 (R and D Systems).
44. Hybond-C nitrocellulose membrane (AP Bioscience).
45. Enzyme chemiluminescence amplification kit (AP Bioscience).
46. OptEIA™ mouse IL-12 p40 ELISA, Cat No: 551116 (Becton and Dickinson).
47. OptEIA™ mouse IL-12 p70 ELISA Cat No: 559528 (Becton and Dickinson).
48. Recombinant mouse IFN-γ (R and D Systems).
49. RNase-free DNase (Stratagene).
50. DMRIE-C (Life Technologies cat. No.10459-014).

## 3. Methods

### 3.1. Expression Plasmid

The details of the construction of a modified plasmid, for simultaneous expression of the murine interleukin 12 (mIL-12) p35 and p40 chains, which are modified to contain conservative mutations and unique restriction sites, are detailed in **Subheadings 3.1.1.** to **3.1.4.** This includes a description of the pCI-IRES expression plasmid and details of its generation. The method described can be applied to expression of an immunogen and single-chain immunomodulatory molecule from the same plasmid or the co-expression of a second immunomodulator 3' from the IRES. Also described are the isolation, cloning, and introduction of conservative mutations into the IL-12 p35 (mut-p35) and p40 (mut-p40) subunits of the murine IL-12 p35 and p40 cDNAs, to differentiate endogenous from transgenic expressed IL-12. The final section describes the subcloning of mut-p35 and mut-p40 into the pCI-IRES expression plasmid.

### 3.1.1. Cloning of an Immunomodulatory Gene

1. Stimulate a subconfluent culture of WEHI-3B cells (European Collection of Animal Cell Cultures, ECACC, CAMR (Salisbury, UK), accession number 86013003) overnight with LPS at 1 µg/mL.
2. Wash stimulated cells 2× in PBS and isolate total RNA with RNAzol.
3. Reverse-transcribe 1 µg of total RNA with either mIL-12 p35- or mIL-12 p40-specific primers and a Stratagene reverse-transcription kit (*see* **Table 1**; **Note 1**).
4. PCR 10 ng of IL-12 p35 or p40 cDNA with PFUtubo® DNA polymerase and p35- or p40-specific primers (Stratagene) (*see* **Table 2**; **Note 2**). Analyze 10 µL of each reaction by gel electrophoresis using a 1.2% agarose gel (according to standard methods, *see* **ref. 9**).
5. Purify the p35 and p40 PCR products using Geneclean (Bio101).
6. Individually clone PCR products into PCRscript (Stratagene) according to the manufacturer's instructions. These products are thereafter designated PCRscript-35 and PCRscript-40, respectively.

**Table 1**
**mIL-12 Reverse-Transcription Primers**

| Primer name | Primer sequence | Tm (°C) (specific) |
|---|---|---|
| mIL-12p35 rev | 5' AGTCCGCCTCGAGTCTAT 3' | Tm = 52 |
| mIL-12p40 rev | 5' CTAGGATCGGACCCTGC 3' | Tm = 53 |

rev = reverse.

**Table 2**
**mIL-12p35 and p40 Cloning Primers**

| Primer name | Primer sequence | Tm (°C) (specific) | Tm (°C) (total) | Product size (bp) |
|---|---|---|---|---|
| mIL-12 p35 for | 5' ATGTGTCAATCACGCTACCT 3' | 53 | 51 | |
| mIL-12 p35 rev | 5' AGTCCGCCTCGAGTCTAT 3' | 52 | 52 | 672 |
| mIL-12 p40 for | 5' ATGTGTCCTCAGAAGCTAAC 3' | 48 | 48 | |
| mIL-12 p40 rev | 5' CTAGGATCGGACCCTGC 3' | 53 | 53 | 1032 |

for = forward.

7. DNA sequence PCRscript-35 and PCRscript-40 inserts using T3 and T7 primers (Stratagene) with an ABI PCR dye terminator sequencing kit (Perkin-Elmer) and analyse reactions with an ABI 377 sequencer (according to the instructions of the manufacturer) (*see* **Note 3**).

### 3.1.2. Generation of mut-p35 and mut-p40

Primers for mutation can be designed using the pDRAW32 software to incorporate a novel restriction-enzyme site and generate a specific PCR primer site by the introduction of conservative mutations into the mIL-12 p35 and p40 cDNA sequences (**Tables 3**, **4** respectively, *see* **Notes 4, 5**).

1. Linearize 1 μg of PCRscript-35 and PCRscript-40 by digestion with 10 U of Not I for 1 h at 37°C. Heat to 65°C for 10 min (to inactivate the restriction enzyme) and place on ice for 10 min.
2. To 100 μL of PCR mastermix add 10 ng of linearized PCRscript-35 plasmid DNA and 1 μL of the p35 5' primers or the p35 3' primers (**Table 3**) and cycle (*see* **Note 6**). Repeat as above with the PCRscript 40 and p40 5' or 3' primers (**Table 4**, *see* **Note 6**).
3. Purify the PCR products with Geneclean (Bio101) according to the manufacturer's instructions, mix and anneal by PCR with PFUtubo® DNA polymerase (*see* **Note 2**).
4. Analyze the products on a 1.2% agarose gel, purify with Geneclean and clone using the PCRscript kit as previously.

**Table 3**
**mIL-12 p35 Mutation Primers**

| Primer name | Primer sequence | Tm (°C) (specific) | Tm (°C) (total) | Restriction site | Product size (bp) |
|---|---|---|---|---|---|
| mIL-12 p35 for | 5' **CTGATGGCTAGC**ATGTGTCAATCACGCTACCT 3' | 53 | 70 | *Nhe I* | 597 |
| mut p35 5' rev | 5' CAATAATATACAAAGCTTCATCTTCACTCTGTAAGGGTCTGCTT 3' | 51 | 69 | *Hind III* | |
| mut p35 3' for | 5' AAGATGAAGCTTTGTATATTATTGCACGCCTTCAGCACCC 3' | 56 | 73 | *Hind III* | |
| mIL-12 p35 rev | 5' AGTCCGCCTCGAGTCTATC**TCTTAAGTCAACTCA** 3' | 52 | 68 | *EcoR I* | 99 |

**Table 4**
**mIL-12 p40 Mutation Primers**

| Primer name | Primer sequence | Tm (°C) (specific) | Tm (°C) (total) | Restriction site | Product size (bp) |
|---|---|---|---|---|---|
| mIL-12 p40 for | 5' **CGATAAGTCGAC**ATGTGTCCTCAGAAGCTAAC 3' | 48 | 68 | *Sal I* | 699 |
| mut p40 5' rev | 5' ATCACGAATAAAGAAGCTTGTCGAGTAGTTCTCATATTTAT TCTGC 3' | 51 | 69 | *Hind III* | |
| mut p40 3' for | 5' TCGACAAGCTTCTTTATTCGTGATATCATCAAACCAGACCCG 3' | 56 | 73 | *Hind III* | 357 |
| mIL-12 p40 rev | 5' CTAGGATCGGACCCTGC**CGCGGCGTATTAG** 3' | 53 | 78 | *Not I* | |

5. Prepare plasmid minipreps (*see* **Subheading 3.1.1.**) and check for inserts by restriction digestion and agarose gel electrophoresis.
6. DNA-sequence inserts with T3 and T7 plasmid primers and analyze sequence (*see* **Subheading 3.1.1.**).
7. Products are now referred to as PCRscript-35mut and PCRscript-40mut.

### 3.1.3. Generation of pCI-IRES

1. PCR the IRES sequence from pIRES, for primers (*see* **Table 5**; **Note 3**).
2. Digest the PCR products with *EcoR I* and *Sal I* and purify with Geneclean.
3. Digest pCI neo with *EcoR I* and *Sal I* and gel-purify with Geneclean.
4. Ligate the PCR product into PCI using Ligafast (Promega), transfect into *E. coli*. XL-1 blue (Stratagene) and select on LBA-ampicillin plates overnight at 37°C.
5. Select single colonies, inoculate LB media (containing ampicillin), culture overnight, and isolate plasmid DNA using a Midi prep isolation kit. Check the size and orientation of the insert by restriction digestion and agarose gel electrophoresis (*see* **Note 5**).

### 3.1.4. Generation of the pCI-IRES p35mut-p40mut Expression Plasmid

1. Excise the p35mut from the PCRscript-35mut multiple cloning site with EcoR I and Nhe I.
2. Isolate the p35mut insert by agarose gel electrophoresis and purify with Geneclean (Bio 101).
3. Cut the pCI-IRES vector with Nhe I and EcoR I and phosphatase the digestion products with shrimp alkaline phosphatase (*see* **Note 6**) and heat-inactivate the enzyme at 65°C for 10 min. Check the products by agarose gel electrophoresis (1%).
4. Ligate the p35mut cassette into the 5' of the IRES sequence of pCI-IRES with Ligafast, transfect into *E. coli* XL-1 blue (*see* **Subheading 3.1.3.**) and select on ampicillin plates overnight at 37°C.
5. Generate plasmid DNA minipreps from single colonies (Qiagen, miniprep kit) according to the manufacturer's instructions and check isolated plasmid DNA for inserts and their orientation by restriction digestion. Repeat the above process to insert the p40mut cassette into pCI-IRES 3' of the IRES sequence using the restriction enzymes *Sal I* and *Not I*.
6. Sequence the entire multiple cloning site (*see* **Note 7**).

## 3.2. In Vitro Characterization of Immunomodulator Expression

Described in this section are methods, to i) verify expression of the immunomodulator from the IRES construct by in vitro transfection, ii) quantitate levels of the expressed protein, iii) verify correct conformational folding, and iv) verify biological activity. The latter will depend entirely upon the immunomodulator being examined (for example, migration, or calcium-flux assay for chemokines or proliferation of responsive cell lines to specific cytokines). The general principles are illustrated with the expression of murine IL-12.

### 3.2.1. In Vitro Transfection

Numerous cell lines and transfection protocols are available. The cell line of choice in our laboratory is 293T (a human embryonic kidney-cell line), which can be obtained from the European Collection of Animal Cell Cultures, CAMR (Salisbury, UK), (ECACC no: 85120602). This cell line is easy to grow in standard media and transfects with high efficiency. Although many transfection reagents are available com-

**Table 5**
**IRES Cloning Primers**

| Primer name | Primer sequence | Tm (°C) (specific) | Tm (°C) (total) | Restriction site | Product size (bp) |
|---|---|---|---|---|---|
| IRES for | 5' **TGATATGAATT**CCACGCGTCGAGCATGCAT 3' | 61 | 73 | *EcoR I* | 634 |
| IRES rev | 5' AATAGTAGCACAAAAGTTTCC**CAGCTGC**CGATAA 3' | 49 | 68 | *Sal I* | |

mercially to increase gene delivery, it is widely reported that different cationic lipids (cytofectins) and cationic polymers show enhanced transgene expression for specific, but not all, cell lines *(10)*. In our laboratory, the commercial cytofectin of choice for use with 293T cells is FUGENE (Roche) and the proprietary formulation is DMRIE/ DOPE (Vical Inc.).

1. Expand 293T cells in DMEM medium (D5796, Life Technologies), supplemented with 10% fetal calf serum (FCS), 1X L-glutamine and penicillin-streptomycin (Life Technologies), referred to as complete medium and maintain in log phase (*see* **Note 8**). Passage at 1:10 split ratio every 2–3 d.
2. Wash monolayer carefully with sterile PBS. Remove cells from the flask by repeated gentle pipetting (trypsin/ethylenediaminetetraacetic acid [EDTA] is not required, since 293T are semi-adherent). Transfer the cells to an appropriate tube, sediment by centrifugation at 100*g*, wash once with complete medium, sediment (as before), aspirate the supernatant, and count with Trypan Blue (Sigma) using a hemocytometer.
3. Resuspend cells in complete DMEM. Add 1.0 mL cells at $1 \times 10^5$/mL per well of a 24-well plate (*see* **Note 9**). Ensure that cells are evenly distributed by tapping the plate.
4. Add FUGENE 6 transfection reagent (Roche) to plasmid DNA at a 3:1 ratio (µL and µg, respectively) according to the manufacturer's instructions, using a starting mass of 0.5 µg plasmid DNA per well of 24-well plate (*see* **Notes 10, 11**).
5. Add the complexed plasmid DNA dropwise to the recently plated 293T cells (which should still be in suspension). Swirl the wells to ensure even dispersal.
6. Harvest supernatants and/or cell lysates at 72 h for functional and immunochemical analysis (*see* **Subheadings 3.2.2., 3.2.3.**).

## *3.2.2. Immunochemical Analysis of IL-12 Expression by Western Blot*

### 3.2.2.1. GENERATION OF CELL LYSATES

1. Dissociate 293T cells from the culture plate by repeated pipetting. Transfer the cells to an appropriate tube, sediment by centrifugation at 100*g*. Aspirate the supernatant and store aliquots at –80°C.
2. Wash the cells once more in complete medium and an additional 2× in phosphate-buffered saline (PBS) and count.
3. Lyse the cells at $2 \times 10^6$ per mL in ice-cold lysis buffer (1× PBS, NP40 0.5% v/v) containing 1× complete™ protease inhibitors (Roche).
4. Homogenize lysate by passing through a fine-tipped 1-mL automatic pipet, vortex, and place on ice. Vortex every 5 min for 30 min.
5. Aliquot into 1.5-mL microcentrifuge tubes, and spin at 13,000*g* in a refrigerated benchtop microcentrifuge at 4°C for 10 min. Aspirate the supernatant and store as 100-µL aliquots at –80°C.

### 3.2.2.2. WESTERN BLOTTING

1. Cast and run duplicate 12% polyacrylamide gels (*see* **Table 6**) on an SDS-PAGE minigel system according to the protocols outlined by Laemmli *(11)*.
2. Transfer protein bands from gels onto Hybond-C nitrocellulose membranes (AP Biosciences) with a Biorad semi-dry electrophoretic transfer apparatus.
3. Block nonspecific protein binding by incubation of blots in PBST (PBS + 0.05% v/v Tween-20) containing 5% (w/v) powdered milk for one h at 37°C.

**Table 6**
**SDS-PAGE Layout**

| Lane | Sample | Anti-p35 banding pattern | Anti-p40 banding pattern | Volume /quantity |
|------|--------|--------------------------|--------------------------|------------------|
| 1 | Pre stained High MW markers | N/A | N/A | 1 μL |
| 2 | Medium | None | None | 5 μL |
| 3 | Non transfected tissue-culture supernatant | None | None | 5 μL |
| 4 | Non transfected cell lysate | None | None | 5 μL |
| 5 | Control transfected tissue-culture supernatant | None | None | 5 μL |
| 6 | Control transfected-cell lysate | None | None | 5 μL |
| 7 | pIRES p35mut transfected tissue-culture supernatant | None | None | 5 μL |
| 8 | pIRES p35mut cell lysate | 35 kDa | None | 5 μL |
| 9 | pIRES p40mut transfected tissue-culture supernatant | None | 40kDa | 5 μL |
| 10 | pIRES p40mut cell lysate | None | 40 kDa | 5 μL |
| 11 | pIRES p35mut p40mut transfected tissue-culture supernatant | 70 kDa | 40, 70kDa | 5 μL |
| 12 | pIRES p35mut p40mut transfected-cell lysate | 35, 70 kDa | 40, 70 kDa | 5 μL |
| 13 | Recombinant murine IL-12 | 70 kDa | 70 kDa | 200 ng |

N/A = not applicable.

4. Sequentially apply antibody layers in PBST for 1 h with rotation at room temperature, followed by washing each blot 5× for 5 min with 10 mL of PBST between layers.
5. For detection of IL-12 subunits, use anti-p35 or anti-p40 antibodies (1:500) followed by a biotinylated rabbit anti-goat IgG (1:2000) and strepatavidin-horseradish peroxidase conjugate (1:6000).
6. Finally, detect bound antibody complexes by enzyme chemiluminescence according to the manufacturer's instructions and record-banding pattern on ECL Hyperfilm (AP Biosciences).

### 3.2.3. Functional Expression: IL2 Bioassay

The assay of choice for testing transfected supernatants is entirely dependent upon the immunomodulator. A migration or calcium flux assay can be used for chemokines *(12)*, although several cytokines (e.g., IL-2, IL-4, IL-5, IL-6, IL-10, TNFα, and TGFβ) can be detected via their ability to stimulate the proliferation of selected cell lines *(12)*. For IL-12, a bioassay based upon the ability of IL-12 to induce IFN-γ production by resting splenocytes can be used (*see* **Note 12**). For convenience, commercial cytokine- and chemokine-specific ELISAs are available to demonstrate expression, although they do not reflect functional activity.

1. 72 h following transfection of 293T (*see* **Subheading 3.2.1.**), harvest the supernatant.
2. Seed 96-well U-bottomed plates (Costar) with 100 μL of naïve mouse spleen cells (at 2 × $10^6$/mL) in RPMI-1640 medium containing 10% fetal calf serum (FCS), 1× penicillin- streptomycin (Life Technologies), and 100U/mL recombinant mouse IL-2 (R and D Systems).
3. To separate wells, add 100 μL of supernatant (from either pCI-IRES p35mut-p40mut or the empty vector-transfected cells) diluted 1/2, 1/4, and 1/8 in RPMI-1640 (Life Technologies), medium alone, or serial dilutions of recombinant mouse IL-12.
4. Incubate for 48 h at 37°C and 5% $CO_2$. Harvest the supernatants and test for the presence of IFN-γ, using an OptEIA™ mouse IFNγ ELISA kit (Becton and Dickinson, Cat. no. 550582).

## 3.3. Characterization of Immunomodulator Expression In Vivo

Prior to initiating immunogenicity studies, it is essential to first demonstrate that the immunomodulator is actually expressed from the plasmid in vivo, and then, to determine the duration of expression (since to achieve the desired modulation or enhancement of the immune response may require repeated administration). Consideration should also be given to the timing when the immunomodulator is administered relative to the antigen coding plasmid DNA (*see* **Note 13**).

### 3.3.1. mRNA Localization

Numerous strategies exist for the in vivo detection of recombinant IL-12 mRNA and include *in situ* hybridization, *in situ* PCR, and semi-quantitative reverse transcriptase-polymerase chain reaction (RT-PCR). This chapter focuses on the latter, since the other methods are beyond the scope of this chapter. Detection of recombinant vs endogenous IL-12 mRNA relies upon specific amplification of the recombinant mRNA sequences. The inclusion of an amplification control primer set is of paramount importance to control for differences in the efficiency of RNA recovery, reverse transcription, and amplification efficiency between RNA preparations and PCR reactions. Several primer design strategies are available to achieve this, and are detailed in **Note 14**).

1. Administer 50 μg of either pCI-IRES mut35 mut 40 or pCI-IRES plasmid DNA condensed with cytofectins (*see* **Subheading 3.4.1.**) by topical delivery to the nares of 6–8-wk-old mice (*see* **Subheading 3.4.2.**). Include a further control group, which receive the cytofectin formulation alone.
2. Euthanize mice (according to nationally approved licensed procedures) at d 0, 1, 3, 5, 7, and 14. Harvest tissues (nasal, lung, draining cervical lymph node, spleen, and peripheral [noninvolved] lymph nodes) for immediate storage in liquid nitrogen. Additional tissues (liver, kidney, thymus, and large and small intestine) may be collected for complete investigation of immunomodulator dissemination.
3. Extract RNA with RNAzol according to the manufacturer's instructions from a pre-weighed mass of each tissue (previously ground over liquid nitrogen). Incubate the isolated RNA with 50 U of RNase-free DNase per μg of RNA for 1.5 h at 37°C (*see* **Note 15**). Reverse-transcribe 5 μg total RNA with random hexamers and a Stratagene ProStar reverse-transcription kit.

**Table 7**
**G3PDH Control Primers**

| Primer name | Primer sequence | Tm (°C) (specific) | Product size (bp) |
|---|---|---|---|
| G3PDH For | 5' TCA'TGA'CCACAGTCCATGC CATCAC 3' | 65 | |
| | | | 436 |
| G3PDH Rev | 5' GACCATACTGTTACTTATG CCGATG 3' | 57 | |

4. Perform PCR reactions in duplicate with 10 ng of cDNA template from each tissue sample at three log dilution using junctional plasmid and recombinant-specific primers (*see* **Note 14**) and include internal amplification control primers (*see* **Table 7**; **Note 16**).
5. Analyze PCR products by agarose gel electrophoresis and record band intensity by UV transillumination (UV Products).

## *3.4. Intranasal Vaccination Protocol*

All in vivo procedures must comply with national and institutionally approved regulations. The upper concentration of immunogen and immunomodulator plasmid DNA-cytofectin complex administered is governed by the maximum approved volume, which can be applied to the nares of mice. In our own laboratory, the UK Home Office specifies a maximum administered volume of 60 µL over a period of 6 h to the nares of 20-g mice.

### *3.4.1. DNA:Cytofectin Formulation for In Vivo Delivery*

Commercial cytofectins available for in vivo plasmid DNA delivery are restricted. DMRIE-C is available from Life Technologies (cat. No. 10459-014). The proprietary cytofectin of choice in our laboratory for intranasal (in) delivery is DMRIE/DOPE (Vical Inc.).

1. Condense plasmid DNA (coding for the immunomodulator and/or immunogen) with DMRIE/DOPE at a molar DNA-to-cytofectin ratio of 8:1. Assume that DNA concentration at 1 mg/mL is 3 m$M$ and cytofectin concentration is 1.5 m$M$. Aim to administer 50 µg pCI-IRES mut35 mut40 or pCI-IRES plasmid DNA combined with 50 µg of plasmid DNA that codes an immunogen.
2. Add an equal volume of diluted stock plasmid DNA (in endotoxin-free PBS) dropwise to DMRIE/DOPE (in water) to achieve a final 8:1 DNA to DMRIE/DOPE ratio.
3. Vortex on a low level and incubate 30 min at room temperature.

### *3.4.2. Intranasal Administration*

1. For 6–8-wk-old mice, administer dropwise (using a fine plastic tip) a maximum dose of 5 µL plasmid DNA-cytofectin complex to one nostril. Allow the mouse to recover for at least 25 min.

2. Add further plasmid DNA-complex (5 µL per application) in a round robin fashion, to the alternate nostril until the full dose has been applied.
3. Re-administer plasmid DNA at 14 d and 28 d.
4. Analyze enhancement of the cellular and or humoral immune response at 7 d following the final immunization, using standard assays for immunogen-specific CD8$^+$ and CD4$^+$ T-cell responses and antibody-secreting cells (ASC) by ELIspot assay *(13)*.

## 4. Notes

1. For reverse transcription of specific genes an anealing temperature of 42°C should be used. When numerous reactions are to be performed using multiple primers, transcripts should be reverse-transcribed with random heaxmers at 25°C. Large-scale reactions are preferable (up to 5 µg of total RNA) to provide a pool of cDNA which can be used in numerous experiments.
2. It is preferable to add nonproof-reading enzyme for the addition of 3' and 5' nonhomologous sequences to PCR products (for example, restriction-enzyme digestion sites). PCRturbo from Stratagene is a mixture of pfu (proof-reading) and Taq DNA polymerase (nonproof-reading) in a compatible buffer. It is possible to use this buffer to add Taq initially to the first four cycles of a PCR, and then add PFU with its proof-reading activity to the last 25 cycles of the reaction.
3. All primers are used at 100 p*M* per µL. All PCR reactions are based around the information that typically Taq DNA polymerase extends a template on average by 1000 bp every min at 72°C. Primer annealing temperatures are obtained from the appropriate table and are typically 2.5°C lower than the lowest melting temperature given for any primer pair. When primers include nonspecific regions of sequence the first four cycles are performed using the specific melting temperature to gain the initial annealing temperature and the subsequent 25 cycles are performed using the melting temperature of the entire primer. By raising the melting annealing temperature after four PCR cycles, the specificity of the reaction is enhanced and driven toward the formation of specific product.
4. cDNA-specific primers: The introduction of conservative mutations into the recombinant protein cDNA sequence allows primers that are specific to the recombinant protein to be generated. Bases at the 3' end of the primer sequence should be mutated, as hybridization of this region of the primer is required for extension by polymerase. Whenever possible mutations should be from adenine and thymidine to guanine and cytosine residues respectively, as this allows the annealing temperature of the mutant primer to be raised in the PCR reaction and introduces a further degree of specificity. Preferential amino acids for mutation include arginine, leucine, and serine and these show the greatest redundancy in their codon usage. Primers should be analyzed by blast search, against the murine cDNA database at the NCBI website for homology to endogenous murine cDNAs. They should be altered to show the minimum level of hybridization at the 3' end.
5. Using the pDRAW32 software, it is possible to produce a restriction map of the vector and insert under construction. To check for the presence and orientation of the insert, a restriction enzyme must be selected that is present in the multiple cloning site once and in an asymmetric position within the insert. The size of the resulting fragments, as determined by agarose gel electrophoresis, will allow the determination of the presence and orientation of the insert.
6. The enzyme shrimp alkaline phosphatase removes the 5' phosphate from both strands of a DNA molecule. The 5' phosphate moiety is required for the ligation of DNA fragments by the enzyme T4 DNA ligase. Its removal prevents religation of vector in the absence of

insert. The 5' phosphate group for the ligation reaction may be provided by another DNA molecule, such as the insert to be cloned. However, the presence of phosphatase activity will inhibit ligation reactions. The activity of shrimp alkaline phosphatase can be completely ablated by heating reactions to 65°C for 10 min. This is a distinct advantage over Calf Intestinal Alkaline Phosphatase, which requires removal by purification of DNA from protein (Geneclean).

7. For DNA sequencing, follow the procedures detailed in the sequencing kit. DNA for sequencing must be of high quality, and therefore it is recommended that a Qiagen miniprep kit be used to generate templates for sequencing.

8. Optimal transfection efficiency is achieved with cells in log phase, which have been passaged over several weeks at a consistent cell density. Do not allow cells to reach greater than 70–80% confluency prior to passage, otherwise transfection efficiency is much reduced.

9. In some cell types, transfection efficiency is improved in reduced or serum-free conditions. For 293Tcells, we recommend including serum. However, if problems arise, try transfecting for 2–4 h in 0.5 mL serum-free media, then add 0.5 mL media containing 20% FCS. Alternatively, transfection efficiency of some cells may be improved by transfecting a semi-confluent monolayer.

10. Ensure that FuGENE 6 transfection reagent and plasmid DNA are at room temperature (30 min) before complexing. Always add plasmid DNA (at a concentration of 0.2–2 mg/mL) dropwise to the prediluted FuGENE 6 transfection reagent, and incubate for a minimum of 30 min at room temperature, before addition to cells.

11. Highly purified nucleic acid (e.g., caesium chloride gradient or Quiagen column purified) is critical for successful cell transfection. Traces of residual caesium chloride, phenol, or chloroform are cytotoxic.

12. IL-12 p35 and p40 subunits are assembled through processing to produce a p70 secreted product. However, p40 is also secreted, which is an IL-12-receptor antagonist. If low levels of IL-12 are detected from transfected cell supernatants by functional bioassay, quantitate the levels of p70 and p40 in the media by enzyme-linked immunosorbent assay (ELISA) (OptEIA™ mouse IL-12 p40 ELISA, Cat No: 551116 and mouse IL-12 p70 ELISA Cat. No. 559528, Becton and Dickinson).

13. Consideration should be given to the timing when the immunomodulator is administered relative to the immunogen coding plasmid DNA. When immunomodulatory molecules are designed to increase hematopoiesis and/or enhance recruitment of antigen-presenting cells (APCs) to the site of vaccine delivery—e.g., through GM-CSF, MCPs, MIPs, or FLT-3L, optimal efficacy has been achieved by delivering the immunomodulator 1–5 d prior to administration of the antigen coding plasmid from the vaccine *(14)*. When the goal is to enhance antigen presentation (particularly for weakly immunogenic proteins), co-delivery of genes that encode pro-inflammatory cytokines or modulators of dendritic-cell maturation (e.g., IL-1α, TNF- α, CD80, CD86, CD40ligand) has generally proven successful *(15)*. Polarization of the ensuing immune response toward antibody or Th2 immunity can be achieved by co-delivery of antigen and cytokine encoding plasmid DNA—e.g., IL-4, IL-5, or IL-10 *(15)*. Similarly, redirection of the immune response toward CD8 T cell or Th1 immunity can be achieved by co-delivery of antigen and cytokine (e.g., IL-12, IL-15, and IL-18) *(15)*. However, cytokines such as IL-2 (selected to increase the number of responding T-cells that enter the long-term memory pool) generally need to be administered 2 d following administration of the plasmid-encoded antigen *(16)*.

14. Junctional primers: These primers incorporate plasmid-derived sequence and immunomodulatory protein-specific sequence. The PCR product amplified is thus derived from the recombinant plasmid. A further degree of specificity may be obtained by designing the forward primers to plasmid sequence and performing 4–5 asymmetric PCR cycles (including the forward primer only) to specifically amplify the recombinant cDNA, after which the reverse primer may be added to further amplify this sequence. Construct specific primers: The combination of plasmid junctional and cDNA-specific primers provides the highest stringency for the amplification of recombinant cDNA. This is because none of this primer sequence should exist in vivo.

15. RNA preps should be treated with RNase-free DNase (2 U/10 µg RNA) to remove recombinant plasmid. Reactions must be stopped by the addition of EDTA as heating to 65°C in the presence of $Mg^{2+}$ ions destroys RNA. After reverse trancription (with random hexamers) the reverse reaction should be stopped by heating to 65°C for 10 min to destroy enzymic activity and endogenous RNA.

16. A prerequisite is that pooled cDNA preps are used for titration experiments and an internal amplification control, such as G3PDH specific primers (**Table 7**) must be included to compare samples within and between tissues. This is to compensate for variation between efficiency of cDNA preparation PCR amplification.

17. p32Draw v5.0 beta DNA analysis software reference (web page http://www.geocities.com/acaclone/) Kjeld Olesen, Ph.D (ACACLONE software) Department of Chemistry, Carlsberg Laboratory, Copenhagen Valby, Denmark.

## Acknowledgments

We would like to thank the MRC and the Charitable Foundation of Guys and St. Thomas' Hospital for supporting HIV vaccine studies and to the Arthritis and Rheumatism Council for supporting gene therapy studies in the Klavinskis laboratory. P. Hobson was supported by a PhD training studentship from the BBSRC. We are grateful to the EU Programme EVA for providing invaluable reagents.

## References

1. Ryan, E. J., Daly, L. M., and Mills, H. G. (2001) Immunomodulators and delivery systems for vaccination by mucosal routes. *TRENDS Biotechnol.* **19**, 293–304.
2. O'Garra, A. (1998) Cytokines induce the development of functionally heterogeneous T helper cell subsets. *Immunity* **8**, 275–283.
3. Kim, J. J., Nottingham, L. K., Wilson, D. M., Bagarazzi, M. L., Tsai, A., Morrison, L. D., et al. (1998) Engineering DNA vaccines via co-delivery of co-stimulatory molecule genes. *Vaccine* **16**, 1828–1835.
4. Kim, J. J., Yang, J. S., Dentchev, T., Dang, K., and Weiner, D. B. (2000) Chemokine gene adjuvants can modulate immune responses induced by DNA vaccines. *J. Interferon Cytokine Res.* **20**, 487–498.
5. Novelli, P., Hobson, P., Barnes, A., and Klavinskis, L. S. (2000) Enhancing immunity induced by a plasmid DNA encoded antigen by co-immunisation with a MIP-3α expression vector. *Immunology* **101 (Suppl. 1)**, 12–21.
6. Czerkinsky, C., Anjuere, F., McGhee, J. R., George-Chandy, A., Holmgren, J., Kieny, M. P., Fujiyashi, K., Mestecky, J. F., Pierrefite-Carle, V., Rask, C., and Sun, J. B. (1999) Mucosal immunity and tolerance: relevance to vaccine development. *Immunol. Rev.* **170**, 197–222.

7. Eo, S. K., Lee, S., Chun, S., and Rouse, B. T. (2001) Modulation of immunity against herpes simplex virus infection via mucosal genetic transfer of plasmid DNA encoding chemokines. *J. Virol.* **75**, 569–578.

8. Chun, S., Daheshia, M., Lee, S., Eo, S. K., and Rouse B. T. (1999) Distribution fate and mechanism of immune modulation following mucosal delivery of plasmid DNA encoding IL-10. *J. Immunol.* **163**, 2393–2402.

9. Sambrook, J., Fritsch, E. F., and Maniatis, T. (1989) *Molecular Cloning: A Laboratory Manual,* 2nd ed., Cold Spring Harbor Laboratory Press, Cold Spring Harbor, New York.

10. Haines, A. M., Irvine, A. S., Mountain, A., Charlesworth, J., Farrow, N. A., Hussain, R. D., et al. (2001) CL22 - a novel cationic peptide for eficient transfection of mammalian cells. *Gene Ther.* **8**, 99–110.

11. Laemmli, U. K. (1970) Cleavage of structural proteins during the assembly of the head of bacteriophage T4. *Nature* **227**, 680–685

12. Coligan, J. E., Kruisbecek, A. M., Margulies, D. H., Shevach, E. M., and Strober, W. (1992) *Current Protocols in Immunology.* John Wiley and Sons, Chapter 6.

13. Klavinskis, L. S., Barnfield, C., Gao, L., and Parker, S. (1999) Intranasal immunization with plasmid DNA-lipid complexes elicits mucosal immunity in the female genital and rectal tracts. *J. Immunol.* **162**, 254–262.

14. He, Y., Pimenov, A. A., Nayak, J. V., Plowey, J., Faldo, L. D., and Huang, L. (2000) Intravenous injection of naked DNA encoding secreted flt3 ligand dramatically increases the number of dendritic cells and natural killer cells *in vivo. Hum. Gene Ther.* **11**, 547–554.

15. Kim, J. J., Trivedi, N. N., Nottingham, L. K., Morrison, L., Tsai, A., Hu, Y., et al. (1998) Modulation of amplitude and direction of in vivo immune responses by co-administration of cytokine gene expression cassettes with DNA immunogens. *Eur. J. Immunol.* **28**, 1089–1103.

16. Barouch, D. H., Santra, S., Steenbeke, T. D., Zheng, X. X., Perry, H. C., Davies, M., et al. (1998) Augmentation and suppression of immune responses to an HIV-1 DNA vaccine by plasmid cytokine/Ig administration. *J. Immunol.* **161**, 1875–1882.

# 13

## Microencapsulation of Vaccine Antigens

### David H. Jones

## 1. Introduction

Despite obvious successes in controlling most serious childhood infections, there is a need to develop cheaper and more effective programs in infant vaccination. However, with the knowledge that adults are susceptible to diseases once believed to be only relevant to children, these criteria are equally applicable to adult vaccination programs. Furthermore, with the emphasis on safety, the vaccine industry is slowly replacing existing vaccines with recombinant alternatives that are safer and less reactogenic than their nonrecombinant counterparts, yet also less immunogenic. Thus, any improvements to vaccines in the foreseeable future are likely to arise through the introduction of better adjuvants and delivery systems. For example, a single injection comprising primary and booster doses of vaccine would improve compliance in a cost-effective manner by reducing the number of visits to clinics or medical centers. Equally, administering existing vaccines orally would remove the trauma of injection and the reliance on medical staff to perform the injections. Many vaccines are dependent on a cold chain; improving the stability of vaccines would thus help to reduce the cost of vaccination. To tackle such issues, researchers have borrowed ideas from other areas of the pharmaceutical industry in an attempt to improve the performance of vaccines and reduce the cost of these important health-care interventions.

It is recognized that the sustained release of subunit antigens from depots by their formulation with adjuvants, such as alum and oil-based adjuvants, is a prerequisite for the generation of potent immune responses (*see* Chapter 11). However, the release of antigens from these systems is short-lived compared to the escape of some microencapsulated drugs used for contraception or cancer therapy, which are microencapsulated in biodegradable matrices *(1,2)*. Use of biodegradable matrices for the encapsulation of antigens may provide an extra degree of control in the delivery of vaccines *(3–5)*.

Of the many biodegradable polymers that have been used experimentally for the delivery of vaccines, homo- or co-polymers of glycolidic and lactidic acids have

From: *Methods in Molecular Medicine, Vol. 87: Vaccine Protocols, 2nd ed.*
Edited by: A. Robinson, M. J. Hudson, and M. P. Cranage © Humana Press Inc., Totowa, NJ

proven to be the most promising candidates. Poly(lactide-co-glycolide) (PLG) has been used for resorbable sutures and implants for over 30 yr (6,7), and has a history of biosafety and biocompatibility as both a medical and veterinary product (8). The copolymer can be made to a reproducibly high standard, and decays in vivo by non-enzymic hydrolysis to the natural metabolites, lactic and glycolic acids (9,10).

The rate of decay is dependent on—among other things—the size of the micro-particles, the mol wt of the polymer, and the ratio of lactidic:glycolidic acids in the polymer (10,11). Thus, by encapsulating a vaccine in separate polymers of two or three different compositions and/or sizes, and administering the different encapsu-lated formulations simultaneously, it should be possible to release vaccine over an extended period, thereby delivering primary and booster doses in a single administra-tion (12). Studies have shown that this is possible—for example, injection of mice with antigen encapsulated in microspheres of 1–10 μm and 20–50 μm in diameter resulted in both primary and secondary antigen-specific antibody responses (13). It was suggested that the adjuvanting effects observed by injection of PLG-entrapped antigens were dependent on the microparticles being smaller than 10 μm, allowing phagocytosis of large amounts of antigen by macrophages and other accessory cells followed by migration of these cells to draining lymph nodes at the injection site (14).

Microencapsulation of antigens offers more tangible advantages than conventional adjuvants and delivery systems, including the potential for mucosal delivery. When formulated in microparticles, antigens can pass through the stomach unaffected (15,16) allowing their use for oral administration. Orally administered particulate materials of diameter <10 μm are selectively taken up by the specialized M cells, which overlie the immune-inductive tissues (the Peyer's patches) in the gastrointestinal tract (GIT), (17,18). It is the function of these cells to transport phagocytosed particles across the epithelium and present them to professional antigen-presenting cells (APCs) in the germinal core of the Peyer's patches. Thus, the formulation of antigens into micron-sized microparticles should facilitate their uptake into the Peyer's patches, and initiate the generation of potent immune responses. Several studies have confirmed this: the controlled release of antigens from PLG microparticles of diameter <10 μm but not from particles >10 μm, given orally to animals, elicited high levels of antigen-specific serum (systemic) antibodies, but perhaps more importantly, also induced antigen-spe-cific mucosal immune responses (13,15,16,19,20). With the realization that the major-ity (>95%) of human pathogens gain access to their host cells across a mucosal surface, the induction of immune responses at these mucosal surfaces—which may inhibit or even abrogate trans-mucosal passage of pathogens—has taken on additional signifi-cance. Over the last few years, major efforts have been devoted to the development of mucosal vaccines (21–23). Many studies now document the successful induction of mucosal immunity and protection against challenge with live pathogens, following immunization of animals with PLG-microencapsulated vaccines (24).

However, despite the promise of delivering "single shot" vaccines by mucosal routes, very few human studies or clinical trials of PLG-encapsulated vaccines have been performed, principally because of concerns about the integrity of the entrapped antigens. In our experience (see Note 1), we observed no gross loss of conformational or biologically important epitopes in either encapsulated *Bordetella pertussis* fimbriae *(25)* or the highly labile human immunodeficiency virus HIV-1 gp120 *(26)*. However, other studies with the important pediatric vaccines, diphtheria and tetanus toxoids, have suggested that the encapsulation process itself can cause degradation of antigens *(27)*, or that, as microparticles degrade to lactic and glycolic acids, the resulting drop in pH can cause antigen denaturation, fragmentation, and/or aggregation *(28,29)*. Whether some antigens are more susceptible to loss of integrity than others has not been determined, but in the meantime, various strategies have been used in attempts to overcome these issues. This topic is discussed further in **Note 2**.

Strategies used to combat the loss of protein integrity include the addition of excipients and stabilizers to antigens during the encapsulation process *(30–33; see* **Note 3**), chemical stabilization of antigens prior to encapsulation *(34)*, PLG-entrapment of antigens under polarity-reducing conditions *(35; see* **Note 3**), adsorption of antigens to PLG substrates *(36; see* **Note 4**), and adsorption of DNA to cationized microparticles *(37; see* **Note 4**). Although strictly not encapsulation, the latter two examples comprise preformed lamellae or empty, derivatized micro-particles, both used as supports, and they are made essentially as described in **Subheading 3.2.** (*see* **Note 4**). Once made, they are simply mixed with antigens. Antigens adsorbed onto surfaces of these substrates are thus not exposed to potentially denaturing solvents or shear during encapsulation, and are not exposed to detrimental pH changes during bulk polymer degradation. These biodegradable supports are believed to act as immunopotentiators by slowly releasing adsorbed antigens in a depot effect.

The issue of loss of antigenic integrity may hinder progress toward clinical trials of PLG-encapsulated vaccines. Nevertheless, numerous animal studies have shown that even with antigens that are potentially denatured, PLG-formulated vaccines are highly immunogenic, and are capable of eliciting humoral and cell-mediated immune responses. Here we provide a description of the methods used for the efficient microencapsulation of a model protein, bovine serum albumin (BSA), into PLG microparticles in a form that is suitable for administration to experimental animals.

## 2. Materials

1. A standard Silverson Laboratory mixer with a three-quarter-inch probe, fitted with an emulsor screen (Silverson Machines Ltd., Chesham, Bucks, UK).
2. Poly(lactide-co-glycolide) (PLG):e.g., Resomer RG506, 50:50 ratio of lactide:glycolide, mol wt 22,000 kDa (Boehringer Ingelheim KG, D-6507 Ingelheim, Germany or Alfa Chemicals Ltd., Bracknell, Berks, UK) (*see* **Note 5**).
3. Polyvinyl alcohol (PVA):87–89% hydrolyzed, 13,000–23,000 mol wt (Aldrich Chemical Company, Gillingham, Dorset, UK).
4. Latex beads:10% aqueous suspension of polystyrene beads; range of diameters available from 0.1 μm–26 μm (Sigma Chemicals Ltd., Poole, Dorset, UK). An accurate diameter for each batch of beads is provided.
5. Protein estimation kit:e.g., Pierce BCA Protein Assay Reagent (Pierce & Warriner, Chester, Cheshire, UK).
6. Dichloromethane: high-performance liquid chromatography (HPLC) grade (Aldrich Chemical Company, Gillingham, Dorset, UK).

7. BSA (Sigma Chemicals Ltd., Poole, Dorset, UK).
8. NaOH/sodium dodecyl sulfate (SDS):0.1 *M* NaOH containing 1% (w/v) SDS.

## 3. Methods
### 3.1. Principle of Using PLG

The principle of encapsulating subunit vaccines is straightforward. However, every antigen behaves differently, and thus the general method outlined here may need to be modified for each different application. Essentially, the methods described here and in the Notes were adopted and/or developed by the author with colleagues when he was employed at the Centre for Applied Microbiology and Research, UK.

A primary (water-in-oil) emulsion is prepared by mixing the antigen solution (internal aqueous phase) with a solution of PLG in dichloromethane (oil phase). The emulsion is then stabilized by addition of polyvinyl alcohol (external aqueous phase) and mixing, forming a double, (water-in-oil)-in-water emulsion. Removal of the organic solvent, by extraction in a large volume of water, results in the formation of microparticles containing the antigen. Microparticles are harvested by centrifugation, repeatedly washed in water, and lyophilized.

The procedure provided here, developed from two published procedures *(38,39)*, describes the microencapsulation of a model protein (BSA–*see* **Note 6**) in micro particles, and how the resulting microparticles are characterized.

The conditions described have been used to microencapsulate well-characterized proteins in microparticles of a defined size range. It is appreciated that readers with their own applications will have different requirements. The reader is therefore referred to the literature (*see* **ref. 38**), in which the effects on the final microparticle preparations when varying the concentrations, volumes, and ratios of the oil—as well as the internal and external aqueous phases—are described.

### 3.2. Encapsulation of Protein Antigens

1. Weigh 600 mg of PLG into a screw-topped glass container fitted with a rubber or teflon seal, and dissolve in 3.6 mL of dichloromethane.
2. Prepare a solution of BSA in distilled or deionized water to a final concentration of 1–30 mg/mL. (*see* **Note 7**).
3. Weigh 8 g of PVA into a beaker and dissolve in 80 mL of boiling, distilled, or deionized water. When dissolved, allow to cool. Make up to 100 mL with distilled or deionized water and transfer to a screw-topped container.
4. Measure 60 mL of 8% (w/v) PVA solution (**step 3**) into a 150-mL beaker.
5. Measure 1 L of distilled water into a 2-L beaker, add a magnetic follower, and place on a magnetic stirrer.
6. Using a glass pipet, aliquot 3 mL of PLG solution into a 10-mL beaker.
7. Immerse the probe of the Silverson laboratory mixer into the PLG solution and run the mixer at full speed (8000–9000 rpm).
8. Add 0.3 mL of BSA solution and mix for 2.5 min.
9. Switch off the mixer and wait until the shaft has completely stopped revolving before withdrawing it from the PLG/BSA emulsion to avoid damaging the probe.

10. Immerse the probe into the PVA solution and run the mixer at full speed.
11. Using a glass Pasteur pipet, quickly add the PLG/BSA primary emulsion to the PVA and emulsify for 2.5 min.
12. Add the double emulsion to the 1 L of water and stir rapidly to disperse the emulsion.
13. Divide the suspension of microparticles into six 250-mL centrifuge bottles and centrifuge at $10,000g_{av}$ for 20 min.
14. Gently decant the liquid from the bottles without disturbing the pellets and add 10 mL of water to each bottle.
15. Resuspend the pellets (*see* **Note 8**), pool, and divide equally between two bottles. Fill the bottles with water, invert several times to mix, and recentrifuge at $10,000g_{av}$ for 20 min.
16. Repeat **steps 14** and **15**, twice.
17. Repeat **step 14**. Resuspend the pellets, pool and transfer the suspension to a container suitable for freeze-drying the microparticles.
18. Shell freeze the suspension in solid carbon dioxide and freeze-dry.
19. Transfer the freeze-dried microparticles to a glass screw-topped tube and store at –20°C over desiccant.
20. Microparticles containing no protein ("empty microparticles") are made in the same way, adding water instead of albumin solution to the PLG solution in the initial emulsification stage (**step 8**).

### 3.3. Determination of Protein Loading and Entrapment Efficiency

1. Dissolve BSA in NaOH/SDS to 1 mg/mL in a screw-top Eppendorf tube.
2. Accurately weigh out samples of microparticles containing BSA, and empty micro-particles (*see* **Note 9**) into screw-top Eppendorf tubes.
3. Resuspend the weighed samples of microparticles in NaOH/SDS to a 25% (w/v) suspension (*see* **Note 10**).
4. Place the tubes containing microparticle samples and BSA solution in a heating block set at 100°C, and incubate for 15 min.
5. Allow to cool and centrifuge the samples in a benchtop centrifuge at $250g_{max}$ for 15 min.
6. Prepare protein standards by pipetting 0, 2, 4, 6, 8, and 10 µL of NaOH/SDS and 10, 8, 6, 4, 2, and 0 µL of treated BSA in duplicate, into wells of a microtiter plate, to make a volume of 10 µL in each well.
7. Pipet 10 µL of supernatants from the microparticle suspensions into adjacent wells.
8. Make up the protein assay reagent as directed in the manufacturer's instructions and add 190 µL to each well containing sample or BSA standard.
9. Incubate the plate for 30 min at 37°C.
10. Allow the plate to cool and read in an ELISA plate reader at 560 nm.
11. Construct a curve of absorbance vs protein concentration for the albumin and from it, determine the protein content of the supernatants from the microparticle suspensions (*see* **Note 11**).
12. From these figures, establish the protein loading per unit weight of microparticles (X µg BSA per mg of PLG microparticles).
13. The microencapsulation process began with 500 mg of PLG, allowing the overall incorporation of BSA to be estimated ($500 \times X = Y\mu g$).
14. Since the amount of BSA initially added to the PLG is known (Z µg), the efficiency of entrapment is described by the ratio of the (actual entrapment [Y]/theoretical entrapment [Z]) × 100%).

### *3.4. Determination of Microparticle Diameter*

1. The sizing of microparticle preparations can be performed with a Coulter Counter model ZM fitted with a Channelyzer 256 (Coulter Electronics Ltd, Luton, Beds, UK). The instrument, fitted with a 30-µm orifice tube, is set up and standardized according to the manufacturer's instructions.
2. Add 10 µL of the latex suspension to 100 mL of phosphate-buffered saline (PBS) previously filtered through a disposable 0.22-µm plastic filter unit. Calibrate the channelyzer by drawing the suspension into the orifice tube until a peak is visible on the channelyzer. Adjust the cursor to reveal the window containing the maximum number of particles, type in the diameter of the beads (given in the documentation accompanying the beads) and press the *calibrate* button.
3. Weigh out 0.5 mg of microparticles and resuspend in 100 mL of filtered PBS and draw the suspension into the orifice tube until a peak is visible on the channelyzer. Adjust the cursor to reveal the window containing the maximum number of particles and read the corresponding diameter (*see* **Note 12**).

### *3.5. Determination of the Rate of Protein Release From Microparticles*

1. Make a stock solution of 1 mg/ mL BSA in PBS containing 0.05% (w/v) sodium azide. Aliquot and freeze all but one of the aliquots.
2. Weigh out seven 10-mg samples of microparticles in screw-top Eppendorf tubes and add 30 µL of PBS containing 0.1% (w/v) sodium azide, to each tube. Ensure that the contents of the tubes are mixed and that the tops are tightly screwed on.
3. Place six of the seven tubes containing microparticle suspensions on a rotating wheel in a 37°C incubator.
4. Centrifuge the seventh tube at $250g_{max}$ in a benchtop centrifuge for 15 min.
5. Remove the supernatant, and assay for protein as detailed in **Subheading 3.3.**
6. At weekly intervals (or more frequently), remove a tube containing a suspension of microparticles from the rotating wheel, centrifuge as in **step 4**, and assay for protein in the supernatant as detailed in **Subheading 3.3.**
7. The protein released into the supernatant can be expressed as a percentage of the total load of the microparticle sample (determined in **Subheading 3.3.**), and can be plotted against time. In this way the half-life of release of BSA from microparticles can be determined.
8. The released protein can also be analyzed to evaluate the extent of protein denaturation as a result of microencapsulation (*see* **Note 1**).

## 4. Notes

1. One of the major issues concerning the microencapsulation of proteins is whether the microencapsulation process denatures the protein, and if so, to what degree. Attempts have been made to address this issue by comparing electrophoretic or isoelectric profiles of a model protein (ovalbumin) before and after microencapsulation—no significant differences between the profiles were observed *(38)*. Western blotting was also used to demonstrate that ovalbumin retained antigenicity following encapsulation.
   Dissolution of microparticles with organic solvents has been used to recover entrapped tetanus toxoid, which was then analyzed by HPLC, sodium dodecyl sulfate-polyacryla-

mide gel electrophoresis (SDS-PAGE), and immunodiffusion *(40)*. The authors of this study demonstrated partial aggregation of the toxoid with a concomitant loss of antigenicity that may have been the result of prolonged exposure to organic solvents and/or the final freeze-drying stage of the microencapsulation process.

We have evaluated the detrimental effects of microencapsulation on *Bordetella pertussis* fimbriae by enzyme-linked immunosorbent assay (ELISA) using a panel of monoclonal antibodies (MAbs) binding to linear or nonlinear (conformational) fimbrial epitopes *(25)*. Their binding to fimbriae recovered from microparticles was compared with their binding to native or chemically denatured fimbriae, and showed that encapsulation did not result in any gross denaturation *(25)*. A similar study using a panel of nine MAbs that bound to linear or nonlinear epitopes on the highly labile HIV-1 envelope recombinant glycoprotein, HIV-1 gp120, showed that this protein was not subject to any gross denaturation as a result of encapsulation *(26)*.

Another approach we have used is to compare the biological activity of proteins recovered from microparticles with the native protein when a well-characterized biological activity can be assayed (e.g., the binding of HIV-1 gp120 to CD4). The similarity in the CD4-binding affinities of native and recovered gp120 again demonstrated the lack of gross denaturation during encapsulation *(26)*.

Using a variety of techniques such as size-exclusion chromatography, ELISAs using mapped MAbs, CD4 binding, and circular dichroism, similar results on this labile glycoprotein were obtained elsewhere *(41)*.

2. In limited studies, we were able to show that as a result of encapsulation, i) unique conformational epitopes were not lost and linear epitopes were not gained *(25,26)*, and ii) epitopes responsible for an exquisite biological activity (CD4 binding) were not damaged *(26)*. Using essentially the same encapsulation procedures, we were also able to encapsulate plasmid DNA (pDNA), which was transcribed following administration to animals, leading to expression of the encoded protein and induction of immune responses against it *(42–46)*. A significant amount of pDNA must have remained in circular form (e.g., transcribable), and was not irrevocably damaged by the encapsulation process. Thus, the processes described here appear to cause remarkably little denaturation of entrapped antigens or pDNA-encoding antigens, in contrast to other studies with tetanus and diphtheria toxoids that suggested otherwise *(27–35)*. There may be several possible explanations for these apparently contradictory results.

   Apart from process differences (emulsifying, washing, freeze-drying, or storage), there may be fundamental physicochemical differences between the different antigens used in the studies mentioned previously. It may be that these toxoid antigens are more susceptible to denaturation during encapsulation than other antigens (although pDNA is highly susceptible to shear and significant amounts appeared to survive the process relatively intact, which would indicate the benign nature of our process). Another explanation may be that our studies were performed in vitro on antigens released from freshly prepared microparticles, immediately after preparation, and that the microparticles had not had time to degrade, thereby sparing entrapped antigens from the acid conditions that would prevail if the microparticles had time to degrade. These explanations are speculation—clearly, considerably more work must be done to get to the core of the issues and resolve them.

3. Attempts to improve the stability of entrapped proteins have involved the inclusion of excipients and stabilizers in the encapsulation process, and entrapment of antigens under polarity-reducing conditions *(30–33,35)*. Interested readers are encouraged to refer to the articles cited to obtain details of the procedures used.

4. Attempts to circumvent problems over antigen integrity have involved adsorbing antigens to the surfaces of preformed PLG lamellae or particles. Lamellae are made by adding water to a stirred solution of PLG in solvent, allowing the solvent to evaporate, and finally washing the resulting lamellar particles *(47)*. Antigens are adsorbed by simple mixing of a suspension of lamellae with an aqueous solution of antigen followed by washing.

   Cationic microparticles are prepared by substituting PBS for protein at **step 8** in **Subheading 3.2.** This primary emulsion is then emulsified with an aqueous solution of cetyltrimethylammonium bromide (CTAB) instead of PVA at **steps 10** and **11** in **Subheading 3.2.**, and solvent allowed to evaporate by stirring the (water-in-oil)-in-water emulsion overnight at ambient temperature *(37)*. pDNA was adsorbed by simply mixing cationized microparticles with DNA solutions and washing.

   Although neither protocol is strictly an encapsulation, they are included for the sake of completeness, and because they offer a simple alternative to encapsulation proper, if the reader has concerns about maintaining the integrity of his or her antigen. The reader is encouraged to refer to the cited articles for more details of these processes.

5. Poly(lactide-co-glycolide) (PLG) polymers degrade by non-enzymic hydrolysis to lactic and glycolic acids. It is thus imperative to maintain the polymer under dry conditions as much as possible. Store the dry polymer or microencapsulated protein at $-20°C$ over desiccant and allow the polymer or microparticles to reach ambient temperature before exposing to air.

6. BSA has been used in this example merely for convenience. We have encapsulated a range of proteins from 10mer peptides to large proteins of 250-kDa size. The basic principles remain the same, although it has been our experience that some proteins encapsulate with high efficiency and others encapsulate with very poor efficiency. However, most proteins fall into an "average" category, and typically encapsulate with efficiencies of approx 50%.

7. The protein load of microparticles (% protein per unit weight) is important in determining the distribution of the protein, and thus its release profile from the microparticles. At protein loads greater than about 10% (>100 µg of protein per mg of microparticles), most of the protein tends to adsorb to the external surface of the microparticles. In these cases, release of protein is largely independent of the decay of the matrix, and protein is consequently "released" in a burst over the first 1–2 d in an aqueous environment. At less than 5% protein load (<50 µg of protein per mg of microparticles), most of the protein is entrapped homogeneously within the matrix of the microparticles; thus, the release profile is slower and is highly dependent on the rate of decay of the microparticle matrix.

   The requirement for a rapid or a slow but sustained release of protein will therefore determine the amount and concentration of protein added to the PLG solution in the initial phase of the microencapsulation process (preparation of the primary emulsion). These figures must be calculated in advance with a target protein load in mind (assuming that 50% of the protein will be entrapped). A protein loading of 0.5–1.0%, which should be suitable for most studies can be routinely achieved.

8. Washing of the microparticles is necessary to remove both the PVA and dichloromethane (although some microparticle preparation methods *(38)* simply allow the dichloromethane to evaporate during overnight stirring of the double emulsion made in **Subheading 3.2.**, **step 2**). Complete removal of PVA (and dichloromethane) is important for performing animal experiments with microparticles, and imperative for human studies.

   The pellets resulting from the first centrifugation are difficult to completely disperse, and therefore it is necessary to wash the microparticles thoroughly. The pellets are resuspended, and carefully and gently dispersed in a hand-held homogenizer with a large clearance (0.2 mm) between the plunger and tube. The pellets from subsequent centrifugation steps are much easier to disperse as a result. It can be beneficial to heat the 1L of water used in **Subheading 3.2.**, **step 12**, to 37°C to facilitate the rapid removal of the volatile dichloromethane.

9. The procedure given to determine protein loading and entrapment (*see* **Subheading 3.3.**) releases all the protein from the microparticles, although in a denatured state. On the assumption that entrapment efficiency is about 50%, half the protein added in the initial emulsification stage will be recovered in 500 mg of microparticles. Thus, the weight of microparticles containing sufficient protein to fall within the range of the BSA standard (1–10 μg) can be estimated.

10. The volume of NaOH/SDS solution that should be used to resuspend the microparticles will depend on their estimated protein loading (*see* **Note 5**). In our laboratory, we would recommend the use of a minimum of 30 μL of NaOH/SDS solution per 10 mg of microparticles.

11. Supernatants resulting from treating "empty" microparticles with NaOH/SDS at 100°C as described in **Subheading 3.3.**, contain compounds that undergo a colorimetric reaction with the protein assay reagents. The supernatant will appear to contain protein and by extrapolation from the standard curve, an apparent protein concentration can be derived for empty microparticles. This figure must be subtracted from the equivalent figure for microparticles containing protein to provide a true figure for protein entrapment.

12. Depending on the orifice tube attached, the diameter of particles within the range of 1–100 μm can be accurately measured by use of a Coulter Counter. For accurate determination of the diameter of submicron microparticles, Photon Correlation Spectroscopy or Laser Diffractometry should be used to estimate particle diameters. For such micro-particles, a Brookhaven BI-90 Particle Size Analyzer (Brookhaven Instruments Corporation, Holtsville, NY) can be used, and the author can highly recommend the more modern BI-90 plus instrument. Both the BI-90 and BI-90 plus will accurately determine particle sizes within a range of 1–1000 nm, and the BI-90 plus instrument can also measure the zeta potential (surface charge) of the microparticles.

Alternatively, Scanning Electron Microscopy can be used. Knowing the magnification at which images are viewed, diameters of a range of microparticles can be determined. This technique offers the added bonus of allowing their surfaces to be viewed. Microparticles with smooth surfaces will release their contents at a constant rate as the outer shell of the microparticle hydrolyzes. Pitted microparticles will release their contents erratically and more rapidly, as water will be able to randomly penetrate the core of the microparticles, allowing more rapid diffusion of the contents from the center.

# References

1. Beck, L. E., Pope, V. Z., Flowers, C. E., Cowsar, D. R., Tice, T. R., Lewis, D. H., et al. (1983) Poly(DL-lactide-co-glycolide)/norethisterone microparticles: an injectable biodegradable contraceptive. *Biol. Reprod.* **28**, 186–195.

2. Verrijk, R., Smolders, I. J. H., Bosnie, N., and Begg, A. C. (1992) Reduction of systemic exposure and toxicity of cisplatin by encapsulation in poly-lactide-co-glycolide. *Cancer Res.* **52**, 6653–6656.

3. Kohn, J., Niemi, S. M., Albert, E. C., Murphy, J. C., Langer, R., and Fox, J. (1986) Single-step immunization using controlled release biodegradable polymer with sustained adjuvant activity. *J. Immunol. Methods* **95**, 31–38.

4. Morris, W., Steinhoff, M. C., and Russell, P. K. (1994) Potential of polymer microencapsulation technology for vaccine innovation. *Vaccine* **12,** 5–11.
5. Walker, R. I. (1994) New strategies for using mucosal vaccination to achieve more effective immunization. *Vaccine* **12,** 387–400.
6. Reul, G. J. (1977) Use of vicryl (polyglactin 910) sutures in general surgery and cardiothoracic procedures. *Am. J. Surg.* **134,** 297–299.
7. Vert, M., Christel, P., Chabot, F., and Leray, L.F. (1984) Bioresorbable plastic materials for bone surgery, in *Macromolecular Biomaterials* (Hastings, H. W. and Ducheyne, P., eds.), CRC Press, Boca Raton, FL, pp. 119–142.
8. Visscher, G. E., Robinson, R. L., Maulding, H. V., Fong, J. W., Pearson, J. E., and Argentieri, G. J. (1985) Biodegradation and tissue reaction to 50:50 poly(D,L-lactide-co-glycolide) microparticles. *J. Biomed. Mater. Res.* **19,** 349–365.
9. Wise, D. L., Fellman, T. D., Sanderson, J. E., and Wentworth, R. L. (1979) Lactic/glycolic acid polymers, in *Drug Carriers in Biology and Medicine* (Gregoriadis, G., ed.), Academic Press, London, pp. 237–270.
10. Vert, M., Li, S., and Garreau, H. (1991) More about the degradation of LA/GA-derived matrices in aqueous media. *J. Control. Rel.* **16,** 15–26.
11. Cohen, S., Yoshioka, T., Lucarelli, M., Hwang, L. H., and Langer, R. (1991) Controlled delivery systems for proteins based on poly(lactic/glycolic acid) microspheres. *Pharm. Res.* **8,** 713–720.
12. Aguado, M. T. and Lambert, P.-H. (1992) Controlled release vaccines—biodegradable polylactide/polyglycolide (PL/PG) microspheres as antigen vehicles. *Immunobiology* **184,** 113–125.
13. Eldridge, J. H., Staas, J. K., Meulbroek, J. A., McGhee, J. R., Tice, T. R., and Gilley, R.M. (1991) Biodegradable microspheres as a vaccine delivery system. *Mol. Immunol.* **28,** 287–294.
14. Eldridge, J. H., Staas, J. K., Meulbroek, J. A., Tice, T. R., and Gilley, R.M. (1991) Biodegradable and biocompatible poly(DL-lactide-co-glycolide) microspheres as an adjuvant for staphylococcal enterotoxin B toxoid which enhances the level of toxin-neutralizing antibodies. *Infect. Immun.* **59,** 2978–2986.
15. Eldridge, J. H., Hammond, C. J., Meulbroek, J. A., Staas, J. K., Gilley, R. M., and Tice, T. M. (1990) Controlled vaccine release in the gut-associated lymphoid tissues. 1. Orally administered biodegradable microspheres target the Peyer's patches. *J. Control. Rel.* **11,** 205–214.
16. Mestecky, J., Moldoveanu, Z., Novak, M., Huang, W-Q., Gilley, R. M., Staas, J. K., et al. (1994) Biodegradable microspheres for the delivery of oral vaccines. *J. Control. Rel.* **28,** 131–141.
17. Bockman, D. E. and Cooper, M. D. (1973) Pinocytosis by epithelium associated with lymphoid follicles in the bursa of Fabricius, appendix and Peyer's patches. An electron microscope study. *Am. J. Anat.* **136,** 455–477.
18. O'Hagan, D. T. (1990) Intestinal translocation of particulates—implications for drug and antigen delivery. *Adv. Drug Delivery Rev.* **5,** 265–285.
19. Challacombe, S. J., Rahman, D., Jeffery, H., Davis, S. S., and O'Hagan, D. T. (1992) Enhanced secretory IgA and systemic IgG antibody responses after oral immunisation with biodegradable microparticles containing antigen. *Immunology* **76,** 164–168.
20. Maloy, K. J., Donachie, A. M., O'Hagan, D. T., and Mowat, A. McI. (1994) Induction of mucosal and systemic immune responses by immunisation with ovalbumin entrapped in poly(lactide-co-glycolide) microparticles. *Immunology* **81,** 661–667.

21. Corthesy, B. and Spertini, F. (1999) Secretory immunoglobulin A: from mucosal protection to vaccine development. *Biol. Chem.* **380**, 1251–1262.
22. Chen, H. (2000) Recent advances in mucosal vaccine development. *J. Control. Release* **67**, 117–128.
23. van Ginkel, F. W., Nguyen, H. H., and McGhee, J. R. (2000) Vaccines for mucosal immunity to combat emerging infectious diseases. *Emerg. Infect. Dis.* **6**, 123–132.
24. Gupta, R. K., Singh, M., and O'Hagan, D. T. (1998) Poly(lactide-co-glycolide) microparticles for the development of single-dose controlled-release vaccines. *Adv. Drug Deliv. Rev.* **6**, 225–246.
25. Jones, D. H., McBride, B. W., Jeffery, H., O'Hagan, D. T., Robinson, A., and Farrar, G. H. (1995) Protection of mice from *Bordetella pertussis* respiratory infection using microencapsulated pertussis fimbriae. *Vaccine* **13**, 675–681.
26. Jones, D. H., Partidos, C. D., Steward, M. W., and Farrar, G. H. (1997) Oral administration of poly(lactide-co-glycolide) encapsulated vaccines. *Behring Inst. Mitt.* **98**, 220–228.
27. Raghuvanshi, R. S., Goyal, S., Singh, O., and Panda, A. K. (1998) Stabilization of dichloromethane-induced protein denaturation during microencapsulation. *Pharm. Dev. Tech.* **3**, 269–276.
28. Xing, D. K.-L., Crane, D. T., Bolgiano, B., Corbel, M. J., Jones, C., and Sesardic, D. (1996) Physicochemical and immunological studies on the stability of free and microsphere-encapsulated tetanus toxoid in vitro. *Vaccine* **14**, 1205–1213.
29. Takahata, H., Lavelle, E. C., Coombes, A. G. A., and Davis, S. S. (1998) The distribution of protein associated with poly(DL-lactide-co-glycolide) microparticles and its degradation in simulated body fluids. *J. Control. Rel.* **50**, 237–248.
30. Chang, A. C. and Gupta, R. K. (1996) Stabilization of tetanus toxoid in poly(DL-lactide-co-glycolide) microspheres for the controlled release of antigen. *J. Pharm. Sci.* **85**, 129–132.
31. Johansen, P., Men, Y., Audran, R., Corradin, G., Merkle, H. P., and Gander, B. (1998) Improved stability and release kinetics of microencapsulated tetanus toxoid by co-encapsulation of additives. *Pharm. Res.* **15**, 1103–1110.
32. Audran, R., Men, Y., Johansen, P., Gander, B., and Corradin, G. (1998) Enhanced immunogenicity of microencapsulated tetanus toxoid with stabilizing agents. *Pharm. Res.* **15**, 1111–1116.
33. Schwendeman, S. P., Tobio, M., Joworowicz, M., Alonso, M. J., and Langer, R. (1998) New strategies for the microencapsulation of tetanus vaccine. *J. Microencapsul.* **15**, 299–318.
34. Schwendeman, S. P., Constantino, H. R., Gupta, R. K., Siber, G. R., Klibanov, A. M., and Langer, R. Stabilization of tetanus and diphtheria toxoids against moisture-induced aggregation. *Proc. Natl. Acad. Sci. USA* **92**, 11,234–11,238.
35. Lavelle, E. C., Yeh, M. -K., Coombes, A. G. A., and Davis, S. S. (1999) The stability and immunogenicity of a protein antigen encapsulated in biodegradable microparticles based on blends of lactide polymers and polyethylene glycol. *Vaccine* **17**, 512–529.
36. Jabbal-Gill, I., Lin, W., Jenkins, P., Watts, P., Jimenez, M., Illum, L., et al. (2000) Potential of polymeric lamellar substrate particles (PLSP) as adjuvants for vaccines. *Vaccine* **18**, 238–250.
37. Singh, M., Briones, M., Ott, G., and O'Hagan, D. (2000) Cationic microparticles: a potent delivery system for DNA vaccines. *Proc. Natl. Acad. Sci. USA* **97**, 811–816.
38. Jeffery, H., Davis, S. S., and O'Hagan, D. T. (1993) The preparation and characterisation of poly(lactide-co-glycolide) microparticles. II. The entrapment of a model protein using a (water-in-oil)-in-water emulsion solvent evaporation technique. *Pharm. Res.* **10**, 362–368.

39. Eldridge, J. H., Staas, J. K., Meulbroek, J. A., Tice, T. R., and Gilley, R. M. (1991) Biodegradable and biocompatible poly(DL-lactide-co-glycolide) microspheres as an adjuvant for staphylococcal enterotoxin B toxoid which enhances the level of toxin-neutralizing antibodies. *Infect. Immun.* **59,** 2978–2986.
40. Alonso, M. J., Gupta, R. K., Min, C., Siber, G. R., and Langer, R. (1994) Biodegradable microspheres as controlled-release tetanus toxoid delivery systems. *Vaccine* **12,** 299–306.
41. Cleland, J. L., Powell, M. F., Lim, A., Barron, L., Berman, P. W., Eastman, D. J., et al. (1994) Development of a single-shot subunit vaccine for HIV-1. *AIDS Res. Hum. Retrovir.* **10,** S21–S26.
42. Jones, D. H., Corris, S., McDonald, S., Clegg, J. C. S., and Farrar, G. H. (1997) Poly(DL-lactide-co-glycolide) encapsulated plasmid DNA elicits systemic and mucosal antibody responses to encoded protein after oral administration. *Vaccine* **15,** 814–817.
43. Jones, D. H., Clegg, J. C. S., and Farrar, G. H. (1998) Oral delivery of microencapsulated DNA vaccines. *Dev. Biol. Stand.* **92,** 149–155.
44. Chen, S. C., Jones, D. H., Fynan, E. F., Clegg, J. C. S., Farrar, G. H., Greenberg, H. B., et al. (1998) Mucosal immunity induced by oral immunization with a rotavirus VP6 DNA vaccine encapsulated in microparticles. *J. Virol.* **72,** 5757–5761.
45. Jones, T. (1998) Mucosal Immunity elicited by DNA Vaccines. *IDrugs* **1,** 103–108.
46. Herrmann, J. E., Chen, S. C., Jones, D. H., Tinsley-Bown, A., Fynan, E. F., Greenberg, H. B., et al. (1999) Immune responses and protection obtained by oral immunization with rotavirus VP4 and VP7 DNA Vaccines encapsulated in microparticles. *Virology* **259,** 148–153.
47. Coombes, A. G. A., Lavelle, E. C., and Davis, S. S. (1999) Biodegradable lamellar particles of poly(lactide) induce sustained immune responses to a single dose of adsorbed protein. *Vaccine* **17,** 2410–2422.

# 14

## Lyophilization of Vaccines

*Current Trends*

### Gerald D. J. Adams

### 1. Introduction

Regardless of how effective a vaccine may be in the laboratory, unless the suspension can be stabilized for storage and distribution, its commercial potential will be limited. Lyophilization (freeze-drying) is a well-established technique used in the pharmaceutical industry for stabilizing high-cost, labile bioproducts, such as vaccines. Alternative techniques that require the establishment of a cold chain can present problems, including the potential loss of vaccine stocks resulting from freezer failure and difficulties and costs when distributing frozen materials.

Methods of stabilizing biomaterials by desiccation can be traced back to prehistoric times. One of the earliest recorded vaccine applications was by Jenner, who prepared dried vaccinia impregnated threads to protect against smallpox. By the end of the 19th century, Altman and Shackell described lyophilization on a scientific basis, and in 1913, Vansteenberg used the method to dry rabies virus *(1)*. Since the 1930s, lyophilization has become firmly established as an industrial process for manufacturing pharmaceuticals and foods *(2)*.

Since the publication of the first volume of *Vaccine Protocols*, there has been progress in lyophilization technology, particularly in the area of validation and process control, the adoption of topical, oral, or inhalation administration techniques, the need to replace human or bovine excipients in pharmaceutical formulations, and advances in the fundamental understanding of vaccine technology.

### 2. Principles of the Lyophilization Process

The individual stages in freeze-drying a vaccine may be summarized as:

1. Preparation and purification of the vaccine;
2. Formulation of the suspension to stabilize the vaccine and satisfy marketing demands;
3. Sample freezing;

From: *Methods in Molecular Medicine, Vol. 87: Vaccine Protocols, 2nd ed.*
Edited by: A. Robinson, M. J. Hudson, and M. P. Cranage © Humana Press Inc., Totowa, NJ

4. Main or primary drying (sublimation);
5. Final or secondary drying (desorption);
6. Chamber gas back-filling, product stoppering, vacuum release, and product removal;
7. Post-drying operations, packaging, and storage;
8. Product quality assessment; and
9. Vaccine distribution, reconstitution, and administration to the patient.

## 2.1. Sample Preparation

The salient features of vaccines, including their method of preparation and purification, are discussed more fully elsewhere in this volume. For the purposes of this chapter, vaccines are regarded as: live, attenuated organisms, including carrier bacteria containing introduced genes; whole killed microorganisms; purified subunit and DNA vaccines; and microencapsulated vaccines, in which the antigenic component is contained in a polymer carrier to prevent proteolytic or aerosol denaturation for oral or respiratory delivery *(3)*.

Alternative methods of preparing an apparently identical bioproduct can influence the response of the product to freeze-drying, and this aspect should be considered when vaccines are prepared and purified *(4)*.

## 2.2. Formulation

Lyophilization is often regarded as a bland method of drying materials, although in practice the individual stages in the process are a series of interrelated stresses that may damage labile bioproducts *(5)*. In this context, it is important to appreciate that a molecule may sustain damage during an early stage in the process, which becomes more extensive as the cycle progresses. Formulation aspects will be discussed more fully in **Subheading 5**.

## 2.3. Product Dispensing

It is probable that there will be a significant difference in dispensing times when development trials are compared with Good Manufacturing Process (GMP) manufacturing. For this reason, the dispensing operation should be validated to ensure, for example, that denaturation by protease activity is minimized. For pharmaceutical applications, the dispensing reservoir is typically maintained at 5°C.

## 2.4. Alternative Dose Formats

Until recently lyophilization dose formats for pharmaceutical application have focused predominantly on products filled into trays, ampoules (all glass sealed containers) or rubber-stoppered vials. However, there has recently been a move to alternative dose formats including double-chambered syringes, containing both lyophilized product and diluent, topical delivery systems, and aerosol packs for powder delivery by inhalation. Each of these formats is presently undergoing trials for the delivery of attenuated or subunit vaccines.

## 2.5. Freezing the Product

It is important to differentiate between cooling and freezing. Strictly speaking, cooling refers to a reduction in temperature of the lyophilizer shelves, container, and sample, without implying a phase change in the suspension. The shelves are also cooled during drying to process the product at a low temperature to minimize sample inactivation or collapse (*6*).

Considered the first step in the process, freezing will reduce thermal inactivation of the sample and immobilize the components in the suspension to prevent product foaming when the chamber is evacuated. Freezing is a two-step process during which water initially nucleates around microscopic particle impurities within the suspension. This is followed by growth and proliferation of ice crystals into the solute phase (*7,8*). In practice, ice nucleates heterogeneously around microscopic particles within the suspension, and is facilitated by reducing temperature and agitating the sample. In contrast, ice proliferation is encouraged by warming the sample to reduce viscosity.

Ice nucleation is inhibited at temperatures below the glass transition temperature (Tg'), and ice will melt at temperatures above the melt point (Tm). The relationships between these temperatures are important factors when developing a product formulation or developing a drying cycle.

Essentially, a slow freezing rate of 0.1°C–1.0°C/min is advocated to promote large, contiguous ice crystals, orientated within the frozen mass to provide an open structure that is conducive to vapor migration. Lyophilizers are typically designed to operate with shelf-cooling rates of 0.25–2°C/min (*9,10*). More rapid cooling induces an ice matrix in which smaller crystals are distributed in a convoluted geometry which impedes drying. Freezing behavior is complex, and is dependent on the sample formulation, cleanliness, fill depth, and the extent of supercooling. Samples should be cooled below their freezing point and left for a consolidation period to ensure that the entire batch has been completely frozen. The biological consequences of freezing are discussed in the following section.

## 2.6. Primary Drying

### 2.6.1. Condenser Temperature

The driving force of the system represents the difference in vapor pressure, rather than a difference in temperature between the condenser and the sample. Since temperature and water vapor pressures are interrelated, the condenser must be operated at a lower temperature than that of the shelf.

### 2.6.2. Primary Drying Conditions

The primary drying stage is also referred to as sublimation or main drying. The triple-point diagram, which summarizes the interrelationships between temperature, pressure, and water physical state, indicates that at sub-atmospheric pressures ice will convert directly into water vapor (*10*). This is known as sublimation, and forms the basis of the lyophilization process. In practice, a vacuum of 0.5 mBar is required to reduce the system pressure enough to promote efficient sublimation. Reducing pressure further has little effect on drying rate. At very low pressures (high vacuum conditions), the sublimation rate decreases because the number of gas or vapor molecules capable of conducting heat into the product is reduced (*11*).

### 2.6.3. Warming the Product

Sublimation cooling will lower the sample temperature appreciably, and the sample must be warmed to compensate for sublimation cooling to complete drying. Heat enters the product by conduction from the shelf through the container base and frozen mass to the to the sublimation front, molecular conduction through vapor or gas molecules in the chamber, radiation, and convection at high chamber pressures. Under high-pressure conditions (poor vacuum), product warming is facilitated by vapor and gas molecular conduction. In contrast, when the system is operated at low pressures (high vacuum), radiation (a relatively inefficient heat-transfer mechanism) becomes more significant. These contrasting conditions have significant influences on drying rates and cycle times as discussed in the following section *(11)*.

### 2.6.4. The Sublimation Interface

Variously described as the drying front or freeze-drying front, the sublimation interface, where ice is converted into vapor, is macroscopically a discrete boundary which progresses through the frozen matrix producing an increasing layer of dried sample. The sublimation interface represents a zone of maximal change of sample temperature and moisture content from frozen to dried product, and is the region in which structural collapse is often observed.

As the dry layer increases in depth, vapor migration through the matrix is progressively impeded, and the sublimation rate consequently falls. To control cycle conditions, it is therefore important to monitor interface temperature during drying *(6)*.

### 2.6.5. Heat and Mass Transfer

The essence of the freeze-drying process depends on warming the sample sufficiently to compensate for sublimation cooling while ensuring that the sample does not melt or collapse. Heat is extracted from the sample as water vapor and it is essential to maintain the heat input and vapor extraction equilibrium, termed heat and mass transfer equation, during the cycle. This equilibrium is simple to maintain during the early stages of drying, when impedance to vapor flow by the dry layer is minimal, but becomes progressively more difficult to control as the dry layer thickens and vapor impedance increases. The dry structure represents the major source of vapor impedance during lyophilization.

### 2.6.6. Primary Drying Conditions

Conditions that encourage primary drying include the use of relatively low shelf temperatures and high chamber pressures to facilitate sample warming by molecular conduction, although these conditions should not compromise product quality or induce collapse.

### 2.6.7. Secondary Drying (Final Drying) Conditions

At the end of sublimation, the sample could be removed without the risk of ice melt. However, moisture contents of the dried samples are usually too high (approx 10%) for optimal stability, and consequently the drying cycle is extended to remove additional moisture. The extended drying stage has been defined as secondary, desorption or final drying. Desorption is less efficient than sublimation and may represent 40% of the total process time. In contrast to processing conditions for primary drying, which should avoid product melt or collapse, desorption is completed by reducing chamber pressure and using high shelf temperatures, although live organisms may be damaged and proteins may be aggregated by exposure to high processing temperatures *(12)*.

### 2.6.8. Stoppering the Product

Exposing the hygroscopic dried matrix to moist air may result in degradative changes in the sample and reduced shelf stability. The rubber-stoppered vial is a convenient format for freeze-drying, since samples can be sealed within the dryer at the end of a cycle without exposure to air *(13)*. Stoppering under a full vacuum provides ideal conditions for product stability. However, when reconstitution fluid is injected into an evacuated vial, sample foaming may be induced. To prevent foaming, an inert gas such as argon or nitrogen is introduced into the chamber prior to stoppering. Samples should be back-filled to a negative pressure to ensure that the stopper is retained within the vial. Rubber-stoppered vials are susceptible to leakage during storage, particularly at sub-zero temperatures, which may cause the stopper to lose elasticity *(14)*. Glass-sealed ampoules overcome these problems, but the ampoule must be removed from the dryer prior to sealing.

## 3. Equipment Design and Operations

### 3.1. Design

Essentially all lyophilizers conform to a common design comprising a sample chamber connected to a vacuum pump. Industrial units are fitted with a refrigerated vapor trap (the process condenser), interposed between the chamber and pump *(6)*. Process condensers may be sited within the drying chamber (internal condenser) or in a separate sub-chamber (external condenser). The internal condenser offers advantages of compact size, economy of manufacture, and improved access for topical cleaning. The external condenser can be isolated from the drying chamber for independent defrost at the end of the cycle and verifying the end of primary drying. Either design will satisfy processing requirements *(9)*.

Samples can be cooled on shelves fitted into the chamber. Both the shelves and process condenser may be cooled by conventional or liquid nitrogen refrigeration. The process condenser is typically cooled by direct expansion, and this method can be used for shelf cooling on small lyophilizers. For industrial units, where GMP practice necessitates maintaining the shelf at +/1°C, a diatherm fluid (invariably silicone oil), which can be alternately heated or cooled in a heat exchanger, is circulated through the shelves to maintain a precise temperature control.

For pharmaceutical applications, for which cleanliness is essential, lyophilizers are fabricated from stainless steel and fitted with moveable shelves to facilitate cleaning and steam sterilization. Stainless steel is chemically inert, and can be decontaminated or topically cleaned using a wide range of sanitizing agents. Technical difficulties when using or validating vaporized hydrogen peroxide as a sterilant, have limited its application for lyophilization *(15)*. Cleaning-in-place (CIP) mechanisms may be incorporated into lyophilizers. Because of mechanical complexities, CIP systems are expensive to install, and require extensive validation *(16)*.

Considerable attention has been paid to reducing in-leaks into the dryer, and industrial standards are applied to assess this parameter *(17,18)*.

To eliminate any risk of pump oil back-migrating to the product, oil-free vacuum pumps may be fitted to pharmaceutical lyophilizers. Potentially it is also possible that the product could be contaminated with hydraulic fluid from the ram mechanism included in the chamber for vial stoppering, and devices such as flexible bellows are now fitted around the ram to eliminate fluid leak.

## 3.2. Ablation

The high velocities of vapor water migrating from containers during sublimation can result in the loss of contents from the vial *(19,20)*, resulting in contamination of the lyophilizer interior, condenser, and vacuum pump, and ultimately the dispensing area *(18)*. This problem has been termed ablation and has been reviewed by Adams *(21)*. Potential hazards resulting from ablation should be considered whenever attenuated vaccines are freeze-dried. Ablation can be prevented by incorporating protective devices such as filters into the lyophilizer *(19,22)*.

## 3.3. Validation

Fail-safe operation and validation have received considerable attention during the past decade. Devices for determining endpoints in the process and monitoring product response may be incorporated into the lyophilizer for automatic cycle control and in-process validation purposes *(6,10)*.

## 4. Formulation Development for Lyophilization

Products should be formulated to ensure batch uniformity using a cycle that is economically practical and reproducible. The purpose of the formulation exercise is to establish the factors that influence the impact of the suspending medium on the bioproduct and to optimize the freeze-drying cycle. All of the factors related to the process should be considered, since seemingly insignificant changes in the procedure—for example, the use of a moulded rather than a tube-drawn vial—may influence the acceptability of the vaccine. Formulating exercises should be completed on a rational basis rather than relying on a pragmatic approach. It is important to consider freeze-drying formulation at an early stage of the vaccine-development program, since attempts to modify formulations later in the program will inevitably reflect a compromise when optimizing freeze-drying conditions.

## 4.1. Impact of Freezing on Biological Activity

Ice proliferation throughout the suspension results in a concentration of medium solutes. Biopolymers or live cells generally tolerate chilling (a reduction in temperature in the absence of ice formation), although there have been reports that complex biomolecules may be damaged by reducing temperature *(23)*. Biopolymers are more likely to be damaged during freezing as a result of exposure to increasing solute concentration as ice forms *(24–26)*. These damaging effects include the concentration of biopolymers that will be encouraged to aggregate; alterations in the suspension ionic composition leading to "salting out" effects; variations in the suspension pH caused by crystallization of individual buffer salts *(27)*; freeze concentration of impurities above a toxic limit; and precipitation of sparingly soluble salts.

In addition to damage to individual polymers within the cell, microorganisms may also be damaged by plasmolytic effects that compromise the selective permeability characteristics of membranes. Concentration effects may be appreciable—for example, an aqueous solution of 1% (w/w) sodium chloride will concentrate to 30% (w/w) prior to complete sample freezing. Under freezing conditions, microorganisms tolerate plasmolysis to approx 60% without suffering irreversible damage, although more extensive plasmolysis will result in injury *(28)*. Damage will be exacerbated by prolonging exposure to media concentration, and cells should be cooled rapidly to minimize concentrate exposure *(26,29–33)*. However, at very rapid cooling rates, water is unable to diffuse freely from the cell and freezes intracellularly, causing internal structural damage. For optimal survival, cells should be cooled at a rate that minimizes solution effects while preventing intracellular ice formation *(34)*.

## 4.2. Heat Annealing

We have noted that a slow rate of cooling provides a physical matrix that is conducive to sublimation. However, slow cooling may compromise the product physiologically, and may also concentrate solutes at the sample surface, which can develop into an impervious surface skin that impedes vapor flow *(35)*.

An ice structure that is conducive to drying but minimizes biomolecule damage can be achieved by introducing a heat-annealing step at the freezing stage. Heat annealing is completed by cooling the suspension rapidly to minimize skin formation and sample inactivation. The sample is then warmed before re-cooling prior to sublimation *(24)*. Warming encourages small ice crystals that are formed by rapid cooling to re-crystallize into larger crystals that are conducive to efficient sublimation. Heat annealing also encourages crystallization of solutes, which do not readily crystallize when cooled.

When selecting the upper limit for sample warming, it is important to ensure that the formulation does not melt or undergo an eutectic transition, since biomolecules may be inactivated when exposed to hypertonic conditions during heat annealing.

## 4.3. Solution Responses to Cooling and Freezing

Eutectic freezing, leading to the separation of ice and solute crystals, represents the simplest formulation, in which sublimation of ice from the eutectic will produce a dry solute cake that exhibits low moisture content. The typical solutions presented for freeze-drying do not describe eutectic behavior *(35)*. Labile biomolecules, including proteins and microorganisms, which are damaged when freeze-dried in eutectic media, require protection by including excipients in the formulation that persist in an amorphous (glassy) state *(36–39)*. Attempts to freeze-dry amorphous formulations often present problems, since the sample may collapse as drying progresses. When suspensions are frozen, although a portion of the water will convert to ice, solutes—

including the active component—respond to cooling in one of several ways, depending on the nature and concentration of individual solutes, interactions between these *solutes*, and cooling or drying conditions.

The ways solutes respond to cooling are *(37)*:

1. Solute crystallizes readily during freezing to produce a mixture of ice and solute crystals (= eutectic behavior).
2. Solute crystallizes only when a slow cooling rate is used.
3. Solute crystallizes only when the cooled mass is warmed—for example, during the earlier stages of freeze-drying or when a heat-annealing step is introduced into the cycle.
4. Solute fails to crystallize during freezing, regardless of the cooling conditions used, and remains associated with a proportion of unfrozen water as an amorphous concentrate or glass.

Regardless of the precise freezing behavior of a solution, ice formation will result in an increase in solute concentration. Although individual solutes may crystallize as cooling progresses, a proportion, including vaccine components and stabilizers, will persist as a non-crystalline, amorphous concentrate. At low temperatures, this concentrate will exhibit high viscosity and behave as a brittle solid. Warming the concentrate, perhaps when heat is applied during freeze-drying, will result in a viscosity decrease. At temperatures above the glass transition temperature (Tg'), the concentrate may soften and collapse as drying progresses to form a structureless, sticky residue within the vial. The temperature at which collapse is observed is termed the collapse temperature (Tc) *(37,40–42)*. As well as being cosmetically unacceptable, a collapsed product often exhibits reduced activity or stability, displays an unacceptably high moisture content, and is poorly soluble *(43,44)*.

Collapse can be avoided by formulating the product with additives that exhibit high Tg' or Tc values (*see* **Table 1**) or by freeze-drying the product below Tc throughout the drying cycle. One result of reducing the shelf temperature to avoid collapse is that the drying cycle will be prolonged.

It is important to determine both Tg' or Tc when formulating a freeze-dried product, and techniques used to measure these parameters include:

1. Determination of electrical resistance: Developed by Greaves *(45)*, the principal of this method depends on measuring the electrical conductivity of a suspension as it freezes or thaws. A suspension will exhibit high conductivity (low resistance). In contrast, the conductivity of the frozen or dried sample will be low (high resistance).
2. Differential thermal analysis (DTA): Tg' can also be determined by relating solution temperature (T) to exothermic or endothermic changes as the sample freezes, melts, or softens *(45–47)*. In this laboratory, we also use Differential Scanning Calorimetry (DSC), a commercial instrument which operates on a similar principle to DTA.
3. Freeze-drying microscopy: Based on an original design by Mackenzie *(48)*, the freeze-drying microscope used in this laboratory consists of a small freeze-drying chamber fitted with optical windows through which the behavior of a sample during freeze-drying can be observed. Collapse temperatures are determined by varying the sample temperature over the range of –120 to 30°C to induce drying with collapse or structure. Collapse temperatures are markedly depressed by the addition of low mol-wt solutes, for example

**Table 1**
**Relationship Between Tc Determined by Freeze-Drying Microscopy and Tg' Determined by DSC for Common Excipients Used in Lyophilization**

| Excipient | Tc (°C) | Tg' (°C) |
|---|---|---|
| Fructose | −46 | −48 |
| Lactose plus sodium chloride (ratio 10:3) | −43 | −46 |
| Glucose | −41 | −42 |
| Sucrose | −31 | −32 |
| Lactose | −28 | −28 |
| Trehalose | −28 | −28 |
| Polyvinyl pyrrolidone (MW 70,000) | −21 | −24 |
| Dextran (MW 120,000) | −11 | −11 |
| Mannitol (eutectic) | −1.4 | −3.0 |
| Mannitol (amorphous) | −42 | −40 |

the collapse temperature of lactose is depressed from −28°C to 50°C by adding sodium chloride (*see* **Table 1**).

All of these techniques can be used to determine eutectic, collapse, or glass transition temperatures in crystalline or amorphous matrices.

### 4.4. Eutectic and Collapse "Zones"

The term "eutectic zone" has been used to define a range of temperatures encompassing all eutectic temperatures within a system. When a single eutectic is observed, the eutectic point represents a discrete, definable temperature. In contrast, multi-crystallising systems exhibit a zone in which the minimum eutectic temperature will be lower than that of any individual eutectic temperature within the system.

We have also suggested the concept of a collapse zone based on the extent of sample collapse, by defining Tg' as a temperature at which a viscosity change is observed but the extent of collapse is minimal. At a higher temperature, collapse may be sufficient to compromise product quality. The region between these values may be defined as a collapse zone.

### 5. Biological Consequence of Formulation

An understanding of the physical behavior of a formulation during the freezing and drying process provides only part of the information necessary to develop a successful product *(49)*. Damage should be anticipated at any stage in the cycle, and a vaccine bioassay is recommended at each stage. The bioassay should be sufficiently sensitive to determine losses in vaccine titer with precision. For this reason, data from this laboratory describing the stability of freeze-dried influenza virus was derived by using a chick-cell assay *(50)* rather than the less precise egg assay used by Grieff and Rightsel *(51)*.

## 5.1. Nonspecific Adsorption

Significant amounts of a biopolymer may irreversibly adsorb to the surfaces of filling lines, or vials, and this is known as "nonspecific adsorption." When low concentrations of active component are freeze-dried, adsorption can reduce the dose to an unacceptable level. Adsorption can be prevented by adding an inert bulking protein to the formulation. Since adsorption is a result of the surface topography of the vial, bulking agents should closely resemble the active component. Serum proteins or degraded gelatines were favored to prevent adsorption, although their ethical acceptability for inclusion into vaccines is now questionable because of the risks of contamination with infectious agents.

Cammack and Adams reported that individual batches of serum stabilizers varied markedly in their efficiency and required co-stabilizing with calcium lactobionate for consistent response *(52)*.

## 5.2. The Role of Excipients

Excipients are not universal protectants, but may protect a biomolecule or whole cell only during individual stages of the drying cycle. Although a wide range of additives—including amino acids, sugars, and polymers—protect against freezing damage (cryoprotectants), excipients that protect against dehydration (desicco-protectants) appear to act by specific interactions between excipient and biomolecule, including interactions between sugar molecules and polar residues in cell membranes and stabilization of hydrophobic bonds *(53)*.

The choice of additives that can be included in formulations for human parenteral use is limited *(54,55)*, and most present problems when included in freeze-drying formulations. Sugars are widely used as freeze-drying protectants, either individually or in combination with other solutes *(56)*. Although Adams has used a mixture of glucose and mannitol for freeze-drying pharmaceuticals, including *Mycobacterium* vaccines, the formulation was developed to satisfy commercial rather than freeze-drying criteria. Glucose exhibits a low Tg' and typically dries with collapse, forming a dried cake with a low Tg' that is consequently not shelf-stable. Disaccharides are effective freeze-drying protectants, and are preferred to monosaccharides because they display higher Tc in suspension and solid (*see* **Tables 1** and **3**). The possibility that reducing sugars may induce damage by Maillard reactions should be considered, and non-reducing disaccharides *(57)*, such as sucrose or trehalose *(58)*, should be used in preference to reducing sugars, such as lactose. (We have also observed poor shelf-stability with formulations containing trehalose compared to similar formulations containing sucrose).

Because the inclusion of salts in formulations containing sugars will markedly depress Tg', suspensions based on mixtures of sugars and salts may require the addition of a polymer, such as dextran, to increase Tg' and ensure successful freeze-drying.

A complicating factor in the development of a suitable formulation is the need to use excipients that are compatible with the freeze-drying process and are ethically acceptable. These constraints in formulation development have resulted in the evolution of complex media, which often include excipients added to augment deficiencies in a previously developed formulation *(59)*.

The possibility that excipients derived from human or bovine sources, such as human serum albumin, lactose, or gelatins, may be contaminated by infectious agents such as human immunodeficiency virus (HIV) or transmissible spongiform encephalopathy (TSE), has detracted from their inclusion in vaccine formulations. The composition of the dried cake can induce free-radical activity *(60)*, and attenuators such as threonine or cysteine may be added to formulations to minimize such damage *(35)*.

Dried material exhibiting a high solid content may exhibit poor solubility, which can be improved by including surfactants such as Tweens in the formulation. Flavorings may be incorporated into oral vaccines to improve palatability, although their impact on freeze-drying behavior should be validated prior to use.

Azides were added to vaccine preparations to inhibit the growth of contaminants. The hazards in lyophilization associated with ablation of azides from samples resulting in the formation of explosive compounds have been described *(52)*. Merthyolate has been substituted for azide in vaccine formulation, although the toxicity of this additive should be evaluated before use.

The impact of any excipient included in a vaccine should be validated carefully, particularly when additives such as surfactants and merthyolate, which are present in low concentration in the suspension, can freeze-concentrate to a toxic or damaging level when the sample is cooled. To avoid such problems, it may be preferable to include these additives in the reconstitution fluid.

When attempting to incorporate adjuvants such as alhydrogel into the freeze-drying formulation, we have noted that the gel structure that is responsible for improving the antigenic response of the vaccine is physically disrupted by freezing and drying.

## 6. Microorganism Sensitivity to Lyophilization

Microorganisms vary markedly in their sensitivity to lyophilization. In general, bacteria can be successfully freeze-dried, although as genera become physiologically more complex, they often become more sensitive to freeze-drying damage. Gram-positive bacteria and spores can be freeze-dried, with high survival in a wide range of formulations. In contrast, Gram-negative genera exhibit poor survival when dried under similar conditions *(35)*. Growth conditions will also influence survival, and cells harvested from the logarithmic phase of growth are typically more sensitive to freeze-drying than cells harvested from the stationary phase *(35)*.

Although physiologically the simplest of living organisms, viruses vary markedly in their responses to freeze-drying, reflecting both their type-sensitivity to the process and their inability to repair drying damage. Greiff and Rightsel have categorized viruses into groups, depending on their sensitivity to freeze-drying *(61)*. Members of Group VI, which includes poliovirus, are particularly sensitive to freeze-drying *(62)*.

It is possible that microorganisms that survive freeze-drying may be damaged by the process, and induced to mutate during post-drying repair *(35)*. To prevent mutation by freeze-drying, formulations may require the inclusion of sulfhydryl-rich compounds, such as cysteine, into the drying medium.

## 7. Damage in the Dried State

Freeze-dried products should be: active, shelf stable, dry, clean, and sterile (for pharmaceutical applications), as well as ethically acceptable, pharmaceutically elegant, readily soluble, and simple to reconstitute *(52,63)*.

Lyophilized products are not immune to storage decay, and vaccines may lose activity in the dried state through mechanisms that include inactivation by residual gases (such as oxygen or carbon dioxide) in the sealing environment, Maillard reactions, free-radical activity, light, temperature (when thermal inactivation may be direct or indirect as a result of softening the cake structure), and background irradiation *(35)*.

### 7.1. Collapse in the Solid State

A dry sample resulting from an amorphous formulation will persist as a glass within the vial. These cakes will soften and distort when stored above the solid-state Tg' or Tc (solid) *(42)*. Collapsing products decay at a faster rate than predicted by the Arrhenius equation because viscosity changes will influence the diffusion and interactions of solute molecules in the amorphous mass. In collapsing structures, it is necessary to use a more complex equation, such as the William-Land-Ferry (WLF) equation to determine sample stability *(42)*.

Collapse in the dried sample is dependent on the formulation, residual moisture, and storage temperature, and these factors should be determined as part of the development program. In this laboratory, Tg' and Tc (solid) are determined by DSC and by the Tsouroflouris technique *(64)*, in parallel with moisture content determinations described by Adams *(65)* (*see* **Table 2**). **Table 3** illustrates the impact of moisture content on solid-state collapse.

## 8. Product Stability

### 8.1. Residual Moisture Content

It is a mandatory requirement to specify the water content of vaccines distributed for clinical use. Premature removal of samples displaying high moisture contents from the lyophilizer can result in poor stability, since sufficient free water may remain in the sample to permit conformational changes in a biomolecule *(72,73)*. To reduce sample moisture content, the drying cycle is extended by secondary drying.

Greiff and Rightsel demonstrated that overdrying influenza virus could compromise stability by removing a protective molecular film of "ordered" water surrounding the virus particle, thereby exposing sensitive hydrophilic sites to inactivation by gases, including oxygen or carbon dioxide *(72)*. The authors concluded that influenza preparations, suspended in a serum albumin/saline formulation, should be dried to 1.8% moisture content for optimal stability. Underdrying and overdrying (to 4.0% and 0.6%, respectively) markedly reduced stability, especially when the dried cake collapsed. We have confirmed their findings, although different water content optima were observed for alternative suspending media (*see* **Table 4**).

Partly on the basis Greiff's data, the Center for Biologics Evaluation and Control, has recognised the importance of drying vaccines to an optimal value *(74)*. Definitions that specify water existing as "bound," or "structured" *(75,76)* should be treated with caution. From analysis of data derived from a number of techniques used to estimate

**Table 2**
**Summary of Methods Used to Estimate Moisture Content
of Lyophilized Samples**

| Method | Description/reference |
|---|---|
| Heating method | Dried sample heated and weight loss equated with loss of moisture *(66)*. |
| Heating method (Baker technique) | Dried sample heated and weight loss equated with loss of moisture. Weight loss extrapolated to zero time to compensate for moisture adsorption during assay *(67)*. |
| Karl Fischer | Chemical technique which relies on reaction between free iodine in reagent and moisture in sample ($2I+H_2 \rightarrow 2HI$) *(68,69)*. |
| Thermogravimetric technique | Precise heating technique using Thermal Analysis combined with gas chromatography *(70)*. |
| Gas chromatography | Relies on phase separation of water from solvent/sample extract *(71)*. |

**Table 3**
**Relationship Between Solid-State Collapse Temperatures Determined
by Tsourouflis Technique *(64)* and Dried Sample Moisture Content
Determined by Karl Fischer Technique for Glucose, Sucrose, Lactose,
or Trehalose**

| Excipient (formulation before drying) | Moisture content % w/w | Solid-state collapse temperature (°C) |
|---|---|---|
| 1% w/w trehalose | 1.0 | 110 |
| | 2.0 | 96 |
| | 5.0 | 64 |
| 1% w/w lactose | 1.0 | 105 |
| | 2.0 | 94 |
| | 5.0 | 58 |
| 1% w/w sucrose | 1.0 | 66 |
| | 2.0 | 55 |
| | 5.0 | 21 |
| 1% w/w glucose | 2.5 | 34 |
| | 3.5 | 15 |

water content, Beale has suggested that it is more appropriate to use the concept of diffusional correlation times for water molecules in dried samples *(77)*.

## 8.2. Shelf Stability Assessment

An important aspect of the formulation exercise is to produce a vaccine that is shelf-stable.

**Table 4**
**Stability of Influenza A Virus (Strain WSN) Lyophilized to**
**Various Residual Moisture Contents and Stored**
**Under 0.5-Bar Helium or Nitrogen**

| Fill gas | Moisture content (% w/w) | Time (d) to lose 1.0 log virus infectivity when stored at −20°C |
|----------|--------------------------|------------------------------------------------------------------|
| Helium   | 3.6 | 670 |
|          | 1.8 | 2,600 |
|          | 0.6 | 540 |
| Nitrogen | 3.8 | 475 |
|          | 1.7 | 930 |
|          | 0.6 | 525 |

Data Derived by Real Time-Assay. Moisture Contents Determined by Baker Technique *(67)*. Drying medium ~ 1:5 diluted allantoic fluid plus 1.0% human serum albumin plus 1.0% calcium lactobionate plus 0.9% sodium chloride (pH 7.0).

### 8.2.1. Accelerated Storage Testing

These tests are used during development trials and manufacturing to monitor batch variations by providing early data to predict the rate of sample decay *(78–80)*. When stored vaccines are to be used clinically, accelerated storage test data must be confirmed by real-time assay to assess the potency of the vaccine. Based on data by Greiff and Rightsel, we have used a logarithmic form of the Arrhenius equation to calculate inactivation rates (K) for influenza vaccines dried to different moisture contents or stored under different sealing gases. The method consists of determining K values for dried, live virus samples stored at 45°C, 32°C, and 20°C, and predicting storage times at lower temperature such as 4°C. It is important to establish that a linear relationship exists between virus titers at the higher and lower storage temperatures. Deviations from a straight-line relationship indicate either a different mechanism of damage at the two temperatures or changes in the cake structure, both of which would invalidate the use of the Arrhenius equation.

### 8.2.2. Sealing Atmosphere

Sealing vaccines in the presence of reactive gases, such as oxygen (air), may markedly reduce product stability. Studies by Greiff and his colleagues *(72)*, suggest that chemically inert gases such as argon provide enhanced stability compared to nitrogen.

### 8.2.3. Seal Integrity Testing

Leaking of moist air into the vial may reduce shelf life, and may contaminate clinical material. For these reasons, the integrity of the seal should be confirmed on all batches of vaccines issued for clinical use. Samples sealed under vacuum can be tested using a high-voltage tester *(81)*. We have experimentally confirmed that this test, known as glow-discharge, does not significantly inactivate freeze-dried organisms

*(30)*. The test is only applicable to vaccines sealed under vacuum, and is not applicable for testing containers which are back-filled with gas. Sealed ampoules may be tested by immersion in a solution of methylene blue. Dye penetration into a leaking container is encouraged by applying pressure/vacuum pulses to the test system *(35)*. Collapse of the dried cake and the presence of dye in the sample indicates container leak. The test is not suitable for vaccines in gas-filled vials.

### 8.2.4. Light

Experimental evidence suggests that samples are damaged only by prolonged exposure to direct sunlight *(82)*, and thus it is doubtful whether light is a damaging factor when vaccines are boxed and stored in darkened refrigerators.

### 8.2.5. Temperature (see **Subheading 7.1.**)

Although freeze-dried preparations are much more thermostable than suspension, dried vaccines are not immune to thermal inactivation, and storage at low temperatures will improve stability. In a well-formulated sample, storage at 4°C should be adequate for long-term stability, and short excursions to higher temperatures—for example, during distribution—should not effect biostability.

### 8.2.6. Gamma, Background Irradiation, and Free-Radical Induction

Desiccated live organisms will be inactivated by ionizing radiation, particularly by secondary effects such as the induction of ozone or free radicals.

### 8.2.7. Maillard Reactions

These are specific reactions between free amino groups on protein molecules and reducing sugars, leading to the formation of unstable Amadori compounds and ultimately protein inactivation by aggregation. Maillard reactions have been associated only with sample storage at high temperatures, although Cox has reported that biopolymers may be inactivated by these reactions, even at ambient temperatures.

## 9. Changes in the Characteristics of a Lyophilized Vaccine

Lyophilization can induce genetic changes in an inoculum, and this potential should be considered when attenuated vaccines are stabilized. Although Calcott and Gargett *(83)* have reported that freezing may induce genetic reversion, most authors suggest that mutation is restricted to the drying stages of freeze-drying. All desiccation processes induce mutation, including spray or air-drying. It is probable that under dry-state conditions, mutation is caused by free-radical activity.

## 10. Reconstitution

After lyophilization, attenuated vaccines comprise of mixture of killed, live, and damaged cells, and the damaged population can progress to killed or live depending on the method of rehydration. The consequences of sample reconstitution in vivo have not been extensively reviewed. Typically microorganisms rehydrated in water display a reduced viability or protracted lag phase, compared to similar samples reconstituted in saline or culture media. Wilson et al. *(84)* have developed specific selective membrane systems that improve the efficacy of pharmaceuticals, including vaccines, intended for injection or oral administration. Vapor-phase rehydration remains controversial.

The pharmacological efficacy of attenuated *Salmonella* vaccines may be improved by reconstitution in sodium bicarbonate solution.

## 11. Safety Considerations

Biohazards associated with the lyophilization process should always be considered whenever live or antigenic materials are processed. Biohazards associated with freeze-drying have been reviewed by Adams *(19)*. When Genetically Manipulated Organisms (GMO) are lyophilized to Good Manufacturing Practice (GMP) standards, operational procedures required to satisfy FDA, Medicines Control Agency, UK (MCA), or Health and Safety legislation may restrict the operational procedures. These restrictions may have a significant impact on the vaccine lyophilization program, since the design and operation of dispensing and lyophilization areas may require extensive modification and manufacturers may be prohibited from lyophilizing vaccines derived from GMO sources in facilities used to manufacture orthodox pharmaceuticals.

## 12. Cycle Development
### 12.1. Conventional Cycles

Conventional cycles, based on the presumption that a processing defect such as collapse has occurred early in the cycle, often use low shelf temperatures during the initial stages of primary drying, increasing shelf temperature as the cycle progresses. An air bleed into the chamber may also be applied to facilitate heat conduction into the drying sample.

As a result of sublimation cooling, the drying front temperature may be appreciably below the glass transition or collapse temperature. Although these conditions will ensure that the sample remains below the collapse temperature, they may result in unnecessarily protracted processing times. If the shelf temperature is maintained at a constant value or raised later in main drying (when the cake depth increases and impedance to vapor flow rises), the sublimation interface temperature may exceed Tg' or Tc, resulting in sample collapse. Collapse may be exacerbated when heat transfer is encouraged by the continual use of pressure control *(85)*.

### 12.2. Optimized Cycles (85)

Adams and Ramsey have described how shelf temperatures can be raised early in main drying, when the dry layer is thin and impedance to vapor flow is minimal, but should be reduced later in the cycle as the dry cake develops, so that the sublimation front is maintained at approx 4 to 5°C below Tg' or Tc throughout primary drying *(85)*. Pressure control should also be activated strategically in order to precisely control the sample temperature. In this way, it is possible to optimize process cycles to ensure a minimum processing time combined with a satisfactory dried cake. For final drying, higher shelf temperatures and low chamber-pressure conditions can be used to facilitate desorption.

Cycles optimized with this principle require a detailed analysis of the sample to determine Tg' and Tc or the impact of processing defects, such as surface skin formation. The product should also be carefully monitored during drying, using techniques such as thermometry, thermal or gas analysis, or humidity control.

## References

1. Vansteenberge, M. P. (1903) Precede de conservation a l'etat sec. *Cr. Seanc. Soc. Biol.* **55,** 1646–1647.
2. Flosdorf, E. W. and Mudd, S. (1935) Procedure and apparatus for preservation in the lyophile form of serum and other biological substances. *J. Immunol.* **29,** 389–425.
3. Wong, J. P., Yang, H., Nagata, L., Kende, M., Levy., H., Schnell, G., et al. (1999) Liposome-mediated immunotherapy against respiratory influenza virus infection using double-stranded RNA poly ICLC. *Vaccine* 1999 1788–1795.
4. Jameson, P., Greiff, D., and Grossberg, S. E. (1979) Thermal stability of freeze-dried mammalian interferons. *Cryobiology* **16,** 301–314.
5. Adams, G. D. J. (1991) Freeze-drying of biological rnaterials. *Drying Technol.* **9,** 891–925.
6. Oetjen, G. (1999) Industrial freeze-drying For pharmaceutical applications, in *Freeze-Drying/Lyophilization of Pharmaceutical and Biological Products* (Rey, L. and May, J. C., eds.), Marcel Dekker, New York, pp. 267–335.
7. Mackenzie, A. P. (1966) Basic principles of freeze-drying for pharmaceuticals. *Bull. Parenter. Drug Assoc.* **26,** 101–129.
8. Mackenzie, A. P. (1977) The physico-chemical basis for the freeze-drying process, in *Developments in Biological Standards*, Vol. 36. Karger, Basel, pp. 51–57.
9. Rowe, T. W. G. (1971) Machinery and methods in freeze-drying. *Cryobiology* **8,** 153–172.
10. Cameron, P. (1997) Good Pharmaceutical Freeze-Drying Practice, Interpharm Press, Buffalo Grove, IL.
11. Adams, G.D.J. (1995) Freeze-Drying—The Integrated Approach. *Pharmaceutical Manufacturing International*, pp. 177–180.
12. Pikal, M. J. (1999) Mechanisms of protein stabilization during freeze-drying and storage: the relative importance of thermostabilization and glassy state relaxation dynamics, in *Freeze-Drying/Lyophilization of Pharmaceutical and Biological Products* (Rey, L. and May, J. C., eds.), Marcel Dekker, New York, pp. 161–198.
13. Willemer, H. (1999) Experimental freeze-drying: procedures and equipment, in *Freeze-Drying/Lyophilization of Pharmaceutical and Biological Products* (Rey, L. and May, J. C., eds.), Marcel Dekker, New York, pp. 79–121.
14. Barbaree, J. M. and Smith, S. J. (1981) Loss of vacuum in rubber stoppered vials stored in a liquid nitrogen phase freezer. *Cryobiology* **18,** 528–531.
15. Klapes, N. A. and Vesley, D. (1990) Vapor-phase hydrogen peroxide as a surface decontaminant and sterilant. *Appl. Environ. Microbiol.* **56,** 503–506.
16. Beurel, G.A. (1999) Technical procedures for operation of cleaning-in-place and sterilization-in-place process for production freeze-drying equipment, in *Freeze-Drying/Lyophilization of Pharmaceutical and Biological Products* (Rey, L. and May, J. C., eds.), Marcel Dekker, New York, pp. 423 –432.
17. Bindschaedler, C. (1999) Lyophilization process validation, in *Freeze-Drying/Lyophilization of Pharmaceutical and Biological Products* (Rey, L. and May, J. C., eds.), Marcel Dekker, New York, pp. 373–408.
18. Jennings, T.A. (1986) Validation of the lyophilzation process, in *Validation of Aseptic Pharmaceutical Processes* (Carleton, F. J. and Agalloco, J. P., eds.), Marcel Dekker, New York, pp. 595–633.

19. Adams, G. D. J. (1994) Freeze-drying of biohazardous products, in *Biosafety in Industrial Biotechnology* (Hambleton, P., Melling, J. and Salusbury, T. T., eds.), Blackie Academic and Professional, London, pp. 178–212.

20. Thorne, A. L. C. (1953) Recovery of caprinized and lapinized rinderpest viruses from condensed water vapor removed during desiccation. *Nature* **171**, 605.

21. Adams, G. D. J. (1991) The loss of substrate from a vial during freeze-drying using *Escherichia coli* as a trace organism. *J. Chem. Technol. Biotechnol.* **52**, 511–518.

22. Parker, J. and Smith, H. M. (1972) Design and construction of a freeze-drier incorporating improved standards of biological safety. *J. Appl. Chem. Biotech.* **22**, 925–932.

23. Franks, F. (1985) *Biophysics and Biochemistry at Low Temperatures.* Cambridge University Press, Cambridge, UK.

24. Pikal, M. J. (1991) Freeze-drying of proteins I: process design. *Pharm. Technol. Intern.* **3**, 37–43.

25. Franks, F. (1990) Freeze-drying: from empiricism to predictability. *Cryoletters* **11**, 93–110.

26. Mazur. P. (1970) Cryobiology: the freezing of biological systems. *Science* **168**, 939–949.

27. Taylor, M. J. (1981) The meaning of pH at low temperature. *Cryobiology* **2**, 231–239.

28. Meryman, H. I., Williams, R. J., and St. J. Douglas, M. (1977) Freezing injury from solution effects and its prevention by natural or artificial cryoprotection. *Cryobiology* **14**, 287–302.

29. Grout, B. W. W. and Morris G. J. (1987) *The Effects of Low Temperatures on Biological Systems.* Edward Arnold, London.

30. Arakawa, T., Carpenter, I. F., Kita, Y. A., and Crowe, 1. H. (1990) The basis for toxicity of certain cryoprotectants: a hypothesis. *Cryobiology* **27**, 401–415.

31. Ashwood-Smith, M. I. and Farrant, J. (1980) *Low Temperature Preservation in Medicine and Biology.* Pitman Medical, Tonbridge Wells, UK.

32. Grout, B., Morris, I., and McLellan, M. (1990) Cryopreservation and the maintenance of cell lines. *Tibtech* **8**, 293–297.

33. Farrant, J. (1980) General observations on cell preservation, in *Low Temperature Preservation in Medicine and Biology* (Ashwood-Smith, M. I. and Farrant, J., eds.), Pitman Medical, Tonbridge Wells, UK, pp. 1–18.

34. Mazur, P., Leibo, S. P., and Chu, C. H. Y. (1972) A two factor hypothesis of freezing injury. Evidence from Chinese Hamster tissue cells. *Exp. Cell Res.* **71**, 345–355.

35. Adams, G. D. J. (1995) The preservation of inocula, in *Microbiological Quality Assurance: A Guide Towards Relevance and Reproducibility of Inocula* (Brown, M. R. W. and Gilbert, P., eds.), CRC Press, 89–119.

36. Pikal, M. J. (1991) Freeze-drying of proteins II: formulation selection. *Pharm. Technol. Intern.* **3**, 40–43.

37. Mackenzie, A. P. (1985) A current understanding of the freeze-drying of representative aqueous solutions, in *Refrigeration Science and Technology: Fundamentals and Applications of Freeze-Drying to Biological Materials, Drugs and Foodstuffs.* International Institute of Refrigeration, Paris, pp. 21–34.

38. Franks, F. (1989) Improved freeze-drying: an analysis of the basic scientific principles. *Process Biochem.* **24**, iii–vii.

39. Franks, F. (1992) Freeze-drying: from empiricism to predictability. The significance of glass transitions, in *Developments in Biological Standards.* Karger, Basel, pp. 9–19.

40. Bellows, R. J. and King, C. J. (1972) Freeze-drying aqueous solutions: maximal allowable operating temperatures. *Cryobiology* **9**, 559–561.

41. Franks, F., Hatley, R. H. M., and Mathias, S. F. (1991) Materials science and the production of shelf-stable biologicals. *Pharm. Technol. Intern.* **3**, 24–34.

42. Levine, H. and Slade, L. (1988) Water as plastizer: physico-chemical aspects of low moisture polymeric systems. *Water Sci. Rev.* **5,** 79–185.
43. Adams, G. D. J. and Irons, L. I. (1992) Practical aspects of formulation: the avoidance of product collapse. *Pharm. J.* **249,** 442–443.
44. Adams, G. D. J. and Irons, L. I. (1993) Some implications of structural collapse during freeze drying using *Erwinia caratovora* L-asparaginase as a model. *J. Chem. Technol. Biotechnol.* **58,** 71–76.
45. Greaves, R. I. N. (1954) Theoretical aspects of drying by vacuum sublimation, in *Biological Applications of Freezing and Drying* (Harris, R. J. C., ed.), Academic, New York, pp. 87–127.
46. Rey, L. R. (1999) Glimpses into the Realm of Freeze-Drying: Classic Issues and New Ventures, in *Freeze-Drying/Lyophilization of Pharmaceutical and Biological Products* (Rey, L. and May, J. C., eds.), Marcel Dekker, New York, pp. 1–30.
47. Mackenzie, A. P. (1985) Changes in electrical resistance during and their application to the control of the freeze-drying process, in *Fundamentals and Applications of Freeze-Drying to Biological Materials, Drugs and Foodstuffs.* International Institute of Refrigeration, Paris, pp. 155–163.
48. Mackenzie, A. P. (1964) Apparatus for microscopic observations during freeze-drying. *Biodynamica* **9,** 223–231.
49. Adebayo, A. A., Sim-Brandenburg, J. W., Emmel, H., Olaeye, D. O., and Niedrig. M. (1998) Stability of Yellow Fever Virus vaccine using different stabilisers. *Biologics* 309–316.
50. Appleyard, G. and Maber, H. B. (1974) Plaque formation by influenza viruses in the presence of trypsin. *J. Gen. Viral.* **25,** 351–357.
51. Greiff, D. and Rightsel, W. A. (1968) Stabilities of influenza virus dried to different contents of residual moisture by sublimation in vacuo. *Appl. Microbiol.* **16,** 835–840.
52. Cammack, K. A. and Adams, G. D. J. (1985) Formulation and storage, in *Animal Cell Biotechnology*, vol. 2 (Spiers, R. E. and Griffiths, J. B., eds.), Academic Press, London, pp. 251–288.
53. Carpenter, J. F., Izutsu, K., and Randolph, T. W. (1999) Freezing- and drying-induced perturbations of protein structure and mechanisms of protein protection by stabilizing additives, in *Freeze-Drying/Lyophilization of Pharmaceutical and Biological Products* (Rey, L. and May, J. C., eds.), Marcel Dekker, New York, pp. 123–161.
54. Fanget, B. and Francon, A. (1996) A Varicella vaccine stable at 5 degrees C. *Dev. Biol. Stand.* **87,** 167–171.
55. Gheorghiu, M., Lagranderie, M., and Balazuc, A. M. (1996) Stabilisation of BCG vaccines. *Dev. Biol. Stand.* **87,** 251–261.
56. Adams, G. D. J. (1996) Lyophilization of vaccines, in *Vaccine Protocols*, (Robinson, A., Farrar, G. H., and Wiblin, C. N., eds.), Humana Press, Totowa, NJ, pp. 167–185.
57. Cox, C. S. (1991) *Roles of Maillard Reactions in Disease.* HMSO Publications, London.
58. Gribbon, E. M., Sen, S. D., Roser, B. J., and Kampinga, J. (1996) Stabilisation of Vaccines using Trehalose (Q-T4) Technology. *Dev. Biol. Stand.* **87,** 193–199.
59. Jansen, D.L. and Meade, B.D (1996) Preparation and standardization of US standard pertussis vaccines lot No 11. *Biologicals* **24,** 263–270.
60. Heckly, R. J. and Quay, J. (1983) Adventitious chemistry at reduced water activities: free radicals and polyhydroxy compounds. *Cryobiology* **20,** 613–624.
61. Greiff, D. and Rightsel, W. A. (1965) Stabilities of suspensions of virus after vacuum sublimation and storage. *Cryobiology* **3,** 435–443.
62. Rightsel, W. A. and Grieff, D. (1967) Freezing and freeze-drying of viruses. *Cryobiology* **3,** 423–431.

63. Funk, J. M. and Knudsen, H. (1983) An introduction to freeze-drying. Handbook, by Heto Lab Equipment AIS, Birkerod, Denmark.

64. Tsourouflis, S., Funk, J. M., and Karel, M. (1976) Loss of structure in freeze-dried carbohydrate solutions: the effect of temperature, moisture content and composition. *J. Sci. Food Agricul.* **27,** 509–519.

65. Adams, G. D. J. (1990) Residual moisture and the freeze-dried product, in *Lyophilization Technology Handbook.* The Center for Professional Advancement, Academic Center, PO Box H, East Brunswick, NJ, pp. 581–604.

66. Pemberton, I. R. (1977) Critical factors of the vacuum oven technique which influence the estimation of moisture in veterinary biologics, in *International Symposium on Freeze-Drying of Biological Products, vol. 36: Developments in Biological Standards.* Karger, Basel, pp. 191–199.

67. Baker, P. R. W. (1955) The microdetermination of residual moisture in freeze-dried biological materials. *J. Hyg.* **53,** 426–435.

68. May, J. C., Grim, E., Wheeler, R. M., and West, J. (1982) Determination of residual moisture in freeze-dried viral vaccines: Karl Fischer, gravimetric and thermogravimetric methodologies. *J. Biol. Stand.* **10,** 249–259.

69. Hydranal Manual (1988) Eugen Scholz reagents. Handbook, by Reidel-de-Haan Aktiengeseuschaft, Wunstorfer Strasse, 40. D-30 16 Seelze, Germany.

70. May, I. C., Wheeler, R. M., and Grim, E. (1989) The gravimetric method for the determination of residual moisture in freeze-dried biological products. *Cryobiology* **26(3),** 277–284.

71. Robinson, L. C. (1972) A gas chromatography method of measuring residual moisture in freeze-dried smallpox vaccine. *Bull. WHO* **47,** 7–11.

72. Greiff, D. and Rightsel, W. A. (1969) Stabilities of freeze-dried suspensions of influenza virus sealed in vacuum or under different gases. *Appl. Microbiol.* **17,** 830–835.

73. Greiff, D. (1971) Protein structure and freeze-drying: the effects of residual moisture and gases. *Cryobiology* **8,** 145–152.

74. Center for Biologics Evaluation and Research (1990) Guidelines for the determination of residual moisture in dried biological products. Docket No. 89D-0 140 Docket Management Branch (HFA 305), Food and Drug Administration, Room 4–62, 5600 Fischers Lane, Rockville, MD.

75. Bellissent-Funel, M. and Teixera. J. (1999) Structural and dynamic properties of bulk and confined water additives, in *Freeze-Drying/Lyophilization of Pharmaceutical and Biological Products* (Rey, L. and May, J. C., eds.), Marcel Dekker, New York, pp. 53–77.

76. Phillips, G. O., Harrop, R., Wedlock, D. J., Srbova, H., Celba, V., and Drevo, M. (1981) A study of the water binding in lyophilised viral vaccine systems. *Cryobiology* **18,** 414–419.

77. Beale, P. T. (1983) Water in biological systems. *Cryobiology* **20,** 528–531.

78. Cowdery, S., Frey, M., Orlowski, S., and Gray, A. (1977) Stability characteristics of freeze-dried human live virus vaccines, in *International Symposium on Freeze-Drying of Biological Products, vol. 36: Developments in Biological Standards.* Karger, Basel, pp. 297–303.

79. Nicholson, A. E. (1977) Predicting stability of lyophilized products, in *International Symposium on Freeze-Drying of Biological Products, vol. 36: Developments in Biological Standards.* Karger, Basel, pp. 69–75.

80. Griffin, C. W., Cook, F. C., and Mehaffrey, M. A. (1981) Predicting the stability of freeze-dried *Fusobacterium montiferum.* Proficiency testing samples by accelerated storage tests. *Cryobiology* **18,** 420–425.

81. Rudge. R. H. (1984) Maintenance of bacteria by freeze-drying, in *Maintenance of Microorganisms* (Kirsop, B. F. and Snell, J. J. S., eds.), Academic Press, London, pp. 23–35.

82. de Rizzo, E., Pereira, C. A., Fang, F. L., Takata, C. S., Tenorio, E. C., Pral, M. M., et al. (1990) Photosensitivity and stability of freeze-dried and/or reconstituted measles vaccines. *Rev. Saude Publ.* **24,** 51–59.

83. Calcott, P. H. and Gargett, A. M. (1981) Mutagenicity of freezing and thawing. *FEMS Microbiol. Lett.* **10,** 151–155.

84. Wilson, M., Monro, P., and Cutting, W. A. (1993) Osmotic production of sterile oral rehydration solutions—an economic, low technology method. *Trop. Doct.* **23,** 69–72.

85. Adams, G. D. J and Ramsay, J. R. Optimising the lyophilization cycle and the consequences of collapse on the pharmaceutical acceptability of *Erwinia* L-asparaginase. *J. Pharm. Sci.* **8606,** 1301–1305.

# 15

## Stimulation of Mucosal Immunity

### David J. M. Lewis and Christopher M. M. Hayward

### 1. Introduction

The mucosal immune system is composed of distinct regional immune tissue (e.g., "GALT," gut-associated lymphoid tissue; "NALT," nasal-associated lymphoid tissue; "BALT," bronchus-associated lymphoid tissue; reproductive tract, and breast tissue) interconnected by trafficking of primed lymphocytes as a common "mucosa-associated lymphoid tissue" ("MALT") *(1)*. In addition, immune responses within MALT may occur independently of systemic immunity, with distinctive regulatory mechanisms and the induction of dimeric secretory IgA (SIgA) at the mucosal surface. As a result, traditional methods for inducing systemic immunity may not induce significant SIgA, and techniques have been developed to deliver antigen directly to a mucosal surface in such a way as to induce immunity rather than immunological tolerance. The trafficking of primed B- and T-cells between mucosal sites, regulated by specific adhesion molecules, such as α4β7 integrin on lymphocytes and MAdCAM-1 on mucosal blood vessels *(2)*, leads to dissemination of the mucosal immune response. One benefit of this is that immunization of an accessible mucosal surface may induce an immune response at less accessible mucosal sites (such as the genital tract). Furthermore, by characterizing mucosa-homing lymphocytes trafficking in the blood, it may be possible to indirectly study mucosal responses.

A major problem is that the majority of soluble protein antigens or peptides rarely induce a mucosal response when given orally, and may in fact induce oral tolerance (active suppression of response to subsequent parenteral challenge). Certain antigens, usually bacterial toxins, that have the ability to bind directly to mucosal surfaces may enter by alternative pathways, and result in high-level mucosal and even systemic responses, including memory. The prototype for these mucosal immunogens is cholera toxin, and its nontoxic B subunit (CTB) has been developed as a human vaccine against cholera *(3)* and as a safe and powerful tool to investigate mucosal responses in health *(4)* and human disease states, such as acquired immunodeficiency syndrome

From: *Methods in Molecular Medicine, Vol. 87: Vaccine Protocols, 2nd ed.*
Edited by: A. Robinson, M. J. Hudson, and M. P. Cranage © Humana Press Inc., Totowa, NJ

(AIDS) *(5,6)*. Cholera toxin is also a mucosal adjuvant capable of abrogating tolerance and inducing immunity to coadministered antigens *(7)*. This chapter explores methods of inducing and evaluating mucosal immune responses to CTB as a model human and murine mucosal immunogen. The techniques described can be used as a template for other antigens and animal models, for which cholera toxin and CTB may be used as controls. The references should be consulted for ways to exploit cholera and related toxins *(8)* as adjuvants for protein *(9,10)* or polysaccharide antigens *(11)*, and for descriptions of alternative strategies for inducing mucosal responses (including cell-mediated immunity), such as antigen-containing microparticles (*12* and *see* Chapter 13) or live attenuated pathogens such as *Salmonella typhi* (*13–15* and *see* Chapter 6).

The most intensively studied route for mucosal priming is oral immunization. However, nasal, genital/rectal *(13–15)*, and directly injected (e.g., intratonsilar *(16)*, Peyer's patch *(17)*, draining lymph node *(18)*, or intraperitoneal (ip) *(12,19)* routes can be exploited. This chapter will focus on oral and nasal immunization and the measurement of B-cell and humoral responses in mice and humans. Circulating mucosal T-cell responses may also be detected *(20,21)*, immunodominant epitopes determined *(21)*, and primed mucosal T-cells characterized by detecting cytokine secretion (*23,24*, and *see* Chapter 16). Nasal immunization with CTB subunit is extremely effective, and can induce responses in a wide range of mucosal sites, such as the genital tract in human *(25,26)* and murine *(27)* models. For other antigens, an adjuvant such as CTB may be required for optimal nasal responses, or the highly effective nasal delivery system chitosan—a bioadhesive polycationic polysaccharide, reviewed by Illum *(28)*. Chitosan acts to localize antigen within the nasal cavity, reduce cilia activity, and increase transepithelial penetration through tight junctions. We have successfully used it as a nasal adjuvant in humans *(28a)*.

## 2. Materials

### 2.1. Immunization of Mice

1. Immunogen: purified cholera toxin B subunit (CTB) (Sigma Aldrich, Poole, UK) (*see* **Note 1**).
2. Chitosan glutamate 213 ("Protasan G 213" from FMC Biopolymer, http://www.fmcbiopolymer.com) as 5 mg/mL solution in 10% sucrose, 10 m*M* phosphate buffer, pH 5.6 can be used as a nasal delivery system for other antigens *(21,28)*.
3. Animals: 6–8-wk-old mice (*see* **Note 2**).
4. Gavage needles (International Market Supply Ltd., Congleton, UK) (*see* **Note 3**).
5. 1- and 5-mL syringes.

### 2.2. Immunization of Humans

1. Immunogen: killed whole-cell/B subunit oral cholera vaccine (SBL Vaccin AB, Stockholm, Sweden) (*see* **Note 4**).
2. Others have used live *Salmonella typhi* orally or rectally (*see* **Note 4**), and we have used chitosan (*see* **Subheading 2.1., item 2**) 7 mg dry powder in humans to deliver diphtheria toxoid CRM197 (50 μg) nasally with success.

## 2.3. Immunoassays

1. 10- and 24-mL syringes.
2. 50-mL Falcon tubes.
3. Preservative-free heparin, 1000 IU/mL.
4. Ficoll-hypaque.
5. RPMI-1640 medium.
6. Square 25-well bacterial culture plates (Sterilin, Stone, UK), 96-well nitrocellulose bottom plates, or 96/24-well tissue-culture plates for ELIspot (*see* **Note 5**).
7. 96-well immunoassay plates and V-bottomed plates for enzyme-linked immunosorbent assay (ELISA).
8. 60-mm plastic Petri dishes.
9. 0.45-μm filters (Sartorius, Göttingen, Germany).
10. Dispase (Boehringer Mannheim, Mannheim, Germany).
11. Monosialoganglioside $GM_1$ (Sigma Aldrich).
12. Purified cholera holotoxin (Sigma Aldrich) (*see* **Note 6**).
13. Unlabeled antibodies: goat antihuman/mouse IgG, IgA, and IgM (Sigma Aldrich).
14. Antibody-alkaline phosphatase conjugates (*see* **Note 7**): rabbit antigoat IgG and goat antihuman/mouse IgG, IgA, and IgM (Sigma Aldrich).
15. 104 alkaline phosphatase substrate (Sigma Aldrich).
16. 5-Bromo-4-chloro-3-indolyl phosphate (BCIP, Sigma Aldrich).
17. AMP buffer (Sigma Aldrich) (*see* **Note 8**).
18. 2% w/v 37°C melting-point agarose.

## 2.4. Solutions and Buffers

1. Solution A: 40 g NaC1, 1 g KCl, 14.5 g $Na_2HPO_4.12H_2O$, 1 g $KH_2PO_4$, 5 L distilled water, pH 7.4.
2. Solution B: 2.93 g $NaHCO_3$, 1.59 g $Na_2CO_3$, 1 L distilled water, pH 9.6.
3. Solution C: solution A plus 0.05% v/v polyoxyethylene sorbitan monolaurate (Tween 20) (Sigma Aldrich).
4. Solution D: Hammarsten Casein (BDH, Poole, UK): 10 g boiled in 100 mL 75 m*M* NaOH until dissolved (*see* **Note 9**).
5. Solution E: solution B plus 10% (v/v) solution D.
6. Solution F: solution C plus 10% (v/v) solution D.
7. Solution G: 1% (v/v) diethanolamine (Sigma Aldrich).
8. Solution H: 25 mg BCIP in 20 mL AMP working buffer, pH 10.25 (*see* **Note 10**).
9. Solution I: Solution A with 50 m*M* EDTA, 0.1 mg/mL Soya trypsin inhibitor.

# 3. Methods
## 3.1. Oral and Nasal Immunization of Mice

1. Prebleed mice on arrival and then settle 5–7 d prior to immunization (*see* **Note 11**).
2. Allow blood to coagulate for 1 h at room temperature. Dislodge clot, then place at 4°C to allow clot retraction.
3. Centrifuge at 4000*g* for 10 min. Aliquot serum and store at –20°C.
4. Dilute 10–20 μg immunogen with 250 μL buffer A.
5. Immunize five mice orally using a gavage needle attached to a 1-mL syringe: pick up the mouse by the nape of the neck; introduce the gavage needle through the mouth into the stomach, hyperextending the neck during transit to facilitate smooth passage (*see* **Note 12**).

6. Immunize an additional five mice nasally with a 20-μL aliquot (10 μL per nostril) using a Gilson pipet, under light halothane anesthesia.

7. After 10 d, prepare a second batch of antigen and boost animals.

8. At d 7, 14, 21, and 28 take test bleeds from tail veins to determine numbers of mice responding and kinetics of the response for each antigen being evaluated (*see* **Note 13**).

9. Collect stool at similar time-points to evaluate coproantibody levels.

10. Nasal and vaginal washes can be collected by gently flushing the nasal passage or vaginal canal with sterile PBS—20 μL or 50 μL, respectively. Saliva can be obtained by ip injection of mice with 100 μL of 1 mg/mL pilocarpine (Sigma) to stimulate flow.

11. At an appropriate time-point (usually after 14–28 d), sacrifice animals and remove organs to be analyzed—e.g., spleen (*see* Chapter 16, **Subheading 3.2., step 1**) and Peyer's patches (*see* **Subheading 3.5.**). Excised lungs can be homogenized in RPMI containing 8% FCS and 0.1 m*M* of a protease inhibitor—e.g., phenylmethyl sulfonyl fluoride (Sigma), for the determination of lower respiratory tract antibody responses.

## 3.2. Oral Immunization of Humans

1. Subjects should fast for 1 h, then swallow resuspended antacid solution provided with vaccine in accordance with manufacturer's recommendations (*see* **Note 14**). Shake a single dose vial of vaccine to resuspend sediment, add to antacid solution, and swallow. Subjects then fast for an additional 1 h.

2. Booster immunizations may be given 1–6 wk later (*see* **Note 15**).

3. Draw blood 7 d after first immunization or 5 d after booster for peak circulating B-cell response. Allow 1 mL heparinized blood for each well in ELIspot assay (*see* **Note 16**). Use at once in an ELIspot assay.

4. Draw 5 mL blood 10–14 d after immunization for serum IgG and IgA, and allow to clot. Separate serum by centrifugation and store aliquots at –20°C. Measure specific antibody by ELISA.

5. Collect saliva 5–14 d after immunization by free drooling into Falcon tubes (*see* **Note 17**). Aliquot and store immediately at –20° to –70°C (*see* **Note 18**). Measure specific antibody by ELISA.

## 3.3. Estimation of Specific Coproantibody Levels

1. Collect measured weight of stool in 1 mL solution I (*see* **Note 19**).

2. Sonicate and then pellet samples by centrifugation.

3. Harvest supernatant and store at –20°C.

4. Measure specific antibody by ELISA (*see* **Note 20**).

## 3.4. Estimation of Specific IgG and IgA in Serum, Mucosal Secretions, or Stool by ELISA

1. Incubate 96-well ELISA plates with 100 μL/well of 5 μg/mL cholera holotoxin in solution B at 37°C for 1 h or 4°C overnight (*see* **Note 21**).

2. Empty plates and block wells for 1 h at 37°C with 200 μL solution E.

3. Wash with solution C.

4. In an uncoated 96-well V-bottomed plate, prepare serial twofold dilutions of test samples (starting at 1 in 4) diluted with solution F (*see* **Note 22**).

5. Transfer 100 μL reference and test samples to an immunoassay plate and incubate at 37°C for 2–3 h.

6. Wash then incubate for 1–2 h at 37°C with 100 μL goat antihuman/mouse IgG or IgA diluted in solution F (usually 1:250–1000).

7. Wash and add 100 µL freshly prepared Sigma 104 substrate dissolved in solution G.
8. Observe plates for color reaction and read at 405 nm.

## 3.5. Isolating Antibody-Secreting Cells From Peyer's Patches

1. Carefully excise Peyer's patches (*see* **Note 23**) from the intestinal wall and place in a 60-mm Petri dish containing 5 mL RPMI-1640 and 1.5 mg/mL dispase.
2. Gently disassociate nodules with blunt dissection and tease apart.
3. Place cell suspension in a Falcon tube and incubate with shaking for 45 min at 37°C.
4. Allow tube to stand for 5 min; collect and save cells in suspension.
5. Add fresh media to the tissue debris and repeat **step 3**.
6. Discard remaining tissue debris and pool cell suspensions in a fresh tube.
7. Pellet mononuclear cells by centrifuging at 1200 rpm for 5 min.
8. Resuspend cells in 1 mL RPMI-1640.
9. Determine viability and adjust cell count to $5 \times 10^6$ PBMCs/mL with RPMI-1640 (with gentamicin 20 µg/mL), then use immediately in an ELISpot assay.

## 3.6. Isolating Antibody-Secreting Cells From Blood

1. Separate mononuclear cells from heparinized blood by Ficoll-hypaque discontinuous centrifugation (*see* Chapter 16, **Subheading 3.2., step 3**).
2. Wash at least 3× in solution A.
3. Resuspend in 1 mL RPMI-1640.
4. Determine viability and adjust cell count to $5 \times 10^6$ PBMCs/mL with RPMI-1640 and use immediately in an ELISpot assay.

## 3.7. ELISPOT Assay for Specific Antibody-Secreting Cells

1. Precoat Sterilin 25-well plates with 500 µL of 1.5 µg/mL GM1 in solution B overnight at room temperature or 4°C (*see* **Note 24**).
2. Discard $GM_1$ and block wells with 1 mL solution E at 37°C for 30 min.
3. Wash wells with solution A (*see* **Note 25**), then incubate at 37°C for 1 h with 500 µL of 5 µg/mL cholera holotoxin in solution A.
4. Wash with solution A (*see* **Note 25**), then add 500 µL of cell suspensions. Aim for $2.5 \times 10^6$ cells/well (*see* **Note 26**). Record number of mononuclear cells/well.
5. Incubate in 5% $CO_2$ at 37°C in a leveled, vibration-free incubator (*see* **Note 27**). 3 h for humans; mice may require overnight incubation.
6. Discard cells and wash plates thoroughly with solution C to remove adherent cells.
7. Add goat anti-human/mouse IgG, IgA, or IgM (diluted 1:250–1000 in buffer F) and incubate at 37°C for 3 h, or overnight at 4°C (*see* **Note 28**).
8. Wash with solution C, then incubate with rabbit anti-goat IgG-alkaline phosphatase and conjugate 3 h at 37°C or overnight at 4°C.
9. Wash with solution C and leave wells full.
10. Heat solution H to approx 50°C in water bath or microwave. Add 1 mL melted agarose to 4 mL solution H and vortex well. Allow 1 mL/well.
11. Quickly draw up substrate/agarose solution into a syringe, then filter through a 0.45-µm membrane into wells until the bottom is completely covered (*see* **Note 29**).
12. Count spots under low magnification with an inverted microscope (*see* **Note 30**). Express the number of isotype and antigen-specific antibody-forming cells/$10^6$ mononuclear cells studied.

## 4. Notes

1. Cholera toxin and CTB are also obtainable from Calbiochem (San Diego, CA) and List Biologicals (San Diego, CA). Highly purified, recombinant Escherichia coli enterotoxin B subunit (rEtxB) may be used, but is not commercially available (29,30); an alternative is to use the Escherichia coli LT holotoxin available from Sigma.

2. Responses depend on the strain of mouse and the antigen. Humoral responses to oral CTB and rEtxB are H2 haplotype-dependent:- rEtxB: $H-2^d > H-2^b = H-2^q\ H-2^a > H-2^k$. CTB: $H-2^b > H-2^d$. For a complete review, *see* ref. *30*.

3. Use 15-gauge 4-cm-long steel needles with a blunt bulbous tip.

4. This vaccine, developed by Jan Holmgren and colleagues, has been pivotal in the study of human mucosal immune responses to protein antigens in health and disease, including immunodeficiency states. It contains $10^{11}$ killed whole cholera vibrios and 1 mg purified CTB in single-dose vials with two sachets of antacid buffer. Permission of the manufacturer and appropriate regulatory authorities will be required. The vaccine is licensed in Sweden and Norway. Further details from the SBL website (http://www.sblvaccin.se).
   An alternative is the live attenuated Salmonella typhi Ty 21a (Vivotif Berna, Berna Products Corporation, Coral Gables, FL) vaccine. This has been given orally, and immune responses characterized in humans in terms of mucosal homing and phenotype of response. Additionally, the vaccine can be given rectally to study genital-tract immunity. See references for details *(13–15)*. A drawback with this live vaccine is that immune-deficient or HIV-infected subjects should not be exposed.

5. Some workers use 96-well nitrocellulose-bottomed or tissue-culture plates. Agarose is omitted from the substrate solution and lower concentrations of coating antigens are required, but fewer cells are assayable per well ($10^5$), and false spots are more difficult to distinguish. These have the advantage that they can be automatically counted by ELIspot plate readers. This technique is well-established for cytokine assays. Reader-specific plates may be required.

6. Holotoxin (both CT and LT are available from Sigma) is less expensive than CTB, and CT crossreacts with rEtxB.

7. Horseradish peroxidase conjugates may be used with appropriate substrates, alone or in a two-color assay with alkaline phosphatase conjugates.

8. This can be purchased ready for use from Sigma ("2-amino-2-methyl-1-propanol Alkaline Buffer Solution 1.5M" with an unusual catalog number "221").

9. Store in aliquots at –20°C and keep working the solution at 4°C because this rapidly becomes contaminated.

10. This solution may be kept at 4°C for several months.

11. Because serial serum collection from an individual mouse facilitates monitoring of immune responses, facilities for blood collection by tail-vein snip are advantageous.

12. This procedure is generally well-tolerated by the mice, but in <1%, immunization leads to esophageal trauma and mediastinitis. These mice must be culled.

13. If a response is not detectable, give a third dose of antigen and repeat sampling as before.

14. Alternatively, stomach acid can be neutralized by swallowing 2 g sodium bicarbonate dissolved in 100 mL water. The vaccine can be administered 10–20 min later when the rise in pH will be at a maximum.

15. Maximum responses occur after the second or third immunization.

16. Cells appear in distal sites (gut, salivary glands) after the first week.

17. "Parafilm" (Sigma Aldrich) may be chewed to stimulate flow. Keep saliva cold during processing to minimize bacterial action. Pure parotid saliva can be collected through a suction cup placed over the opening of the parotid duct *(31)*.

18. Rapid freezing minimizes degradation of IgA by bacterial proteases. Some workers add protease inhibitors such as 0.1 mM phenylmethyl sulfonyl fluoride (*see* **Note 19**).
19. This procedure minimizes degradation of IgA (especially IgA1) by bacterial proteases during processing *(32)*.
20. *See* **ref. 33** for further details of measurement of coproantibody responses to CTB and other antigens given orally.
21. Prior coating with $GM_1$ ganglioside is not required if purified toxins are used on high-binding immunoassay plates. If the toxin source is impure (e.g., culture filtrate), then coat with $GM_1$ and block with casein as for ELIspot assay **steps 1** and **2**, before adding toxin.
22. To calibrate the assay, a reference serum of known activity can be used. This can be prepared by standard parenteral immunization with adjuvant.
23. These are 1–2-mm pale pearly nodules visible on the serosol surface.
24. This procedure significantly reduces background, although the mechanism is unclear.
25. Do not use solution C, because "Tween-20" will lyse cells!
26. Ideally have at least 50–100 spots/well. The cell numbers can be titrated because too many spots are hard to count. More than $10^7$ cells/well results in crowding and poor spot formation.
27. If cells move during the incubation, spot duplication may occur.
28. Mouse monoclonal antibodies (MAbs) may be used at this stage to determine subclass-specific responses. A lower dilution (1:100 is typical) is usually required. Appropriate anti-mouse conjugate should be substituted in the next step.
29. Do not allow the substrate to become too hot or the enzyme conjugate may be denatured. Fill wells quickly since agarose will begin to set in the syringe and block filter (which may be omitted if there are no problems with spots from BCIP crystals). Avoid returning to wells to add more substrate because this increases movement artifact. Allow the gel to set before moving the plate or the gel will shift, causing spot duplication. Some workers omit agarose and use BCIP/AMP only, discarding excess from wells when spots develop. We find that agarose increases spot intensity.
30. Spots develop overnight at room temperature, but may be visible after a few hours. Avoid heating plates since this increases background. Characteristic ELIspots appear granular with a darker center. Small, dense spots represent adherent cells or crystals of BCIP. A control well with cells but no antigen is useful to distinguish such artifacts.

## References

1. Czerkinsky, C. and Holmgren, J. (1994) Exploration of mucosal immunity in humans; relevance to vaccine development. *Cell. Mol. Biol.* **1,** 37–44.
2. Quiding, J. M., Lakew, M., Nordstrom, I., Banchereau, J., Butcher, E., Holmgren, J., et al. (1995) Human circulating specific antibody-forming cells after systemic and mucosal immunizations: differential homing commitments and cell surface differentiation markers. *Eur. J. Immunol.* **25,** 322–327.
3. Holmgren, J., Svennerholm, A. M., Jertborn, M., Clemens, J., Sack, D. A., Salenstedt, R., et al. (1992) An oral B subunit: whole cell vaccine against cholera. *Vaccine* **10,** 911–914.
4. Lewis, D. J., Novotny, P., Dougan, G., and Griffin, G. E. (1991) The early cellular and humoral immune response to primary and booster oral immunization with cholera toxin B subunit. *Eur. J. Immunol.* **21,** 2087–2094.
5. Lewis, D. J., Gilks, C. F., Ojoo, S., Castello, B. L., Doughy, G., Evans, M. R., et al. (1994) Immune response following oral administration of cholera toxin B subunit to HIV-1-infected UK and Kenyan subjects. *AIDS* **8,** 779–785.

6. Eriksson, K., Kilander, A., Hagberg, L., Norkrans, G., Holmgren, J., and Czerkinsky, C. (1993) Intestinal antibody responses to oral vaccination in HIV- infected individuals. *AIDS* **7,** 1087–1091.

7. Holmgren, J., Lycke, N., and Czerkinsky, C. (1993) Cholera toxin and cholera B subunit as oral-mucosal adjuvant and antigen vector systems. *Vaccine* **11,** 1179–1184.

8. Pizza, M., Giuliani, M. M., Fontana, M. R., Monaci, E., Douce, G., Dougan, G., et al. (2001) Mucosal vaccines: non toxic derivatives of LT and CT as mucosal adjuvants. *Vaccine* **19,** 2534–2541.

9. Roberts, M., Bacon, A., Rappuoli, R., Pizza, M., Cropley, I., Douce, G., et al. (1995) A mutant pertussis toxin molecule that lacks ADP-ribosyltransferase activity, PT-9K/129G, is an effective mucosal adjuvant for intranasally delivered proteins. *Infect. Immun.* **63,** 2100–2108.

10. Douce, G., Turcotte, C., Cropley, I., Roberts, M., Pizza, M., Domenghini, M., et al. (1995) Mutants of Escherichia coli heat-labile toxin lacking ADP-ribosyltransferase activity act as nontoxic, mucosal adjuvants. *Proc. Natl. Acad. Sci. USA* **92,** 1644–1648.

11. Bergquist, C., Lagergard, T., Lindblad, M., and Holmgren, J. (1995) Local and systemic antibody responses to dextran-cholera toxin B subunit conjugates. *Infect. Immun.* **63,** 2021–2025.

12. O' Hagan, D. T., McGee, J. P., Holmgren, J., Mowat, A. M., Donachie, A. M., Mills, K. H., et al. (1993) Biodegradable microparticles for oral immunization. *Vaccine* **11,** 149–154.

13. Kutteh, W. H., Kantele, A., Moldoveanu, Z., Crowley-Nowick, P. A., and Mestecky, J. (2001) Induction of specific immune responses in the genital tract of women after oral or rectal immunization and rectal boosting with Salmonella typhi Ty 21a vaccine. *J. Reprod. Immunol.* **52(1–2),** 61–75.

14. Kantele, A., Westerholm, M., Kantele, J. M., Makela, P. H., and Savilahti, E. (1999) Homing potentials of circulating antibody-secreting cells after administration of oral or parenteral protein or polysaccharide vaccine in humans. *Vaccine* **17(3),** 229–236.

15. Kantele, A., Hakkinen, M., Moldoveanu, Z., Lu, A., Savilahti, E., Alvarez, R. D., et al. (1998) Differences in immune responses induced by oral and rectal immunizations with Salmonella typhi Ty21a: evidence for compartmentalization within the common mucosal immune system in humans. *Infect. Immun.* **66(12),** 5630–5635.

16. Quiding, J. M., Granstrom, G., Nordstrom, I., Holmgren, J., and Czerkinsky, C. (1995) Induction of compartmentalized B-cell responses in human tonsils. *Infect. Immun.* **63,** 853–857.

17. Cripps, A. W., Dunkley, M. L., and Clancy, R. L. (1994) Mucosal and systemic immunizations with killed Pseudomonas aeruginosa protect against acute respiratory infection in rats. *Infect. Immun.* **62,** 1427–1436.

18. Lehner, T., Bergmeier, L. A., Tao, L., Panagiotidi, C., Klavinskis, L. S., Hussain, L., et al. (1994) Targeted lymph node immunization with simian immunodeficiency virus p27 antigen to elicit genital, rectal, and urinary immune responses in nonhuman primates. *J. Immunol.* **153,** 1858–1868.

19. Lue, C., van den Wall Bake, A. W., Prince, S. J., Julian, B. A., Tseng, M. L., Radl, J., et al. (1994) Intraperitoneal immunization of human subjects with tetanus toxoid induces specific antibody-secreting cells in the peritoneal cavity and in the circulation, but fails to elicit a secretory IgA response. *Clin. Exp. Immunol.* **96,** 356–363.

20. Castello-Branco, L. R. R., Griffin, G. E., Poulton, T. A., Dougan, G., and Lewis, D. J. M. (1994) Characterization of the circulating T cell response after oral immunisation of human volunteers with cholera toxin B subunit. *Vaccine* **12,** 65–72.

21. McNeela, E. A., O'Connor, D., Jabbal-Gill, I., Illum, L., Davis, S. S., Pizza, M., et al. (2000) A mucosal vaccine against diphtheria: formulation of cross reacting material (CRM(197)) of diphtheria toxin with chitosan enhances local and systemic antibody and Th2 responses following nasal delivery. *Vaccine* **19,** 1188–1198.

22. Castello-Branco, L. R. R., Griffin, G. E., Dougan, G., and Lewis, D. J. M. (1995) A method to screen T lymphocyte epitopes after oral immunisation of humans: application to cholera toxin B subunit. *Vaccine* **13,** 817–820.

23. Lagoo, A. S., Eldridge, J. H., Lagoo, D. S., Black, C. A., Ridwan, B. U., Hardy, K. J., et al. (1994) Peyer's patch CD8+ memory T cells secrete T helper type 1 and type 2 cytokines and provide help for immunoglobulin secretion. *Eur. J. Immunol.* **24,** 3087–3092.

24. Hiroi, T., Fujihashi, K., McGhee, J. R., and Kiyono, H. (1994) Characterization of cytokine-producing cells in mucosal effector sites: CD3+ T cells of Thl and Th2 type in salivary gland-associated tissues. *Eur. J. Immunol.* **24,** 2653–2658.

25. Rudin, A., Johansson, E. L., Bergquist, C., and Holmgren, J. (1998) Differential kinetics and distribution of antibodies in serum and nasal and vaginal secretions after nasal and oral vaccination of humans. *Infect. Immun.* **66,** 3390–3396.

26. Johansson, E. L., Wassen, L., Holmgren, J., Jertborn, M., and Rudin, A. (2001) Nasal and vaginal vaccinations have differential effects on antibody responses in vaginal and cervical secretions in humans. *Infect. Immun.* **69,** 7481–7486.

27. Isaka, M., Yasuda, Y., Kozuka, S., Taniguchi, T., Matano, K., Maeyama, J., et al. (1999) Induction of systemic and mucosal antibody responses in mice immunized intranasally with aluminium-non-adsorbed diphtheria toxoid together with recombinant cholera toxin B subunit as an adjuvant. *Vaccine* **18,** 743–751.

28. Illum, L., Jabbal-Gill, I., Hinchcliffe, M., Fisher, A. N., and Davis, S. S. (2001) Chitosan as a novel nasal delivery system for vaccines. *Adv. Drug Deliv. Rev.* **51,** 81–96.

28a. Mills, K., Cosgrove, C., McNeela, E. A., et al. (2003) Protective diptheria immunity induced in healthy volunteers by unilateral prime-boost intranasal immunization associated with ipsilateral mucusal secretory IgA. *Infect. Immun.* **71(2),** 726–732.

29. Marcello, A., Loregian, A., Palu, G., and Hirst, T. R. (1994) Efficient extracellular production of hybrid Escherichia coli heat-labile enterotoxin B subunits in a marine vibrio. *FEMS Microbiol. Lett.* **117,** 47–51.

30. Hashar, T. H. and Hirst, T. R. (1995) Immunoregulatory role of H-2 and intra-H-2 alleles on antibody responses to recombinant preparations of B-subunits of Escherichia coli heat labile enterotoxin (rEtxB) and cholera toxin (rCtxB). *Vaccine* **13,** 803–810.

31. Schaefer, M. E., Rhodes, M., Prince, S. J., Michalek, S. M., and McGhee, J. R. (1977) A plastic intraoral device for the collection of human parotid saliva. *J. Dent. Res.* **56,** 728–733.

32. Gaspari, M. M., Brennan, P. T., Solomon, S. M., and Elson, C. O. (1988) A method of obtaining, processing, and analyzing human intestinal secretions for antibody content. *J. Immunol. Methods* **110,** 85–91.

33. de Vos, T. and Dick, T. A. (1991) A rapid method to determine the isotype and specificity of coproantibodies in mice infected with *Trichinella* or fed cholera toxin. *J. Immunol. Methods* **141,** 285–288.

# 16

# Induction and Detection of T-Cell Responses

## Kingston H. G. Mills

## 1. Introduction
### 1.1. Role of T-Cells in Immunity to Infectious Diseases

The fundamental basis of immunity to infectious diseases involves a complex interplay between humoral and cell-mediated immune responses against antigens on the foreign pathogen. Humoral immunity, either in the form of local IgA antibodies at the mucosal site of infection or neutralizing antibodies in the serum, provides the first line of defense against invading microorganisms. However, cellular immunity, mediated by T-cells, also plays a major role in protection against foreign pathogens. $CD8^+$ cytotoxic T-lymphocytes (CTLs) kill target cells infected with viruses or bacteria, whereas $CD4^+$ T-helper (Th) cells provide help for B-cells in antibody production and secrete a range of cytokines that are involved in a variety of immunoregulatory functions or have a direct effect on invading microorganisms (1–3). $CD4^+$ T-cells can be divided into subpopulations on the basis of their function and cytokine secretion (4). Th1 cells secrete interleukin 2 (IL-2), $\gamma$-interferon (IFN-$\gamma$), and tumor necrosis factor-$\beta$ (TNF-$\beta$) and are involved in delayed-type hypersensitivity and inflammatory responses, and display CTL activity in vitro. A key function of this $CD4^+$ Th1 population in the immunological defense mechanism in vivo appears to be the activation of macrophages, which are stimulated to take up and kill invading microorganisms. In contrast, Th2-cells, which secrete IL-4, lL-5, IL-6, and IL-10, are considered to be the true helper T-cells; their secreted cytokines play a crucial role in immunoglobulin (Ig) class switching and B-cell differentiation, in particular for IgE, IgA, and IgG1 antibody production (5). Thus, it has been concluded that Th1-cells and $CD8^+$ CTL mediate cellular immunity against intracellular pathogens, whereas Th2-cells stimulate humoral immunity against extracellular pathogens. However, Th1 cells have been shown to function as helper T-cells by promoting B-cell production of complement fixing and virus-neutralizing antibodies of the IgG2a subclass in the mouse (6). Furthermore, $CD4^+$ T-cells that secrete high levels of IL-10 or TGF-$\beta$—known as regula-

From: *Methods in Molecular Medicine, Vol. 87: Vaccine Protocols, 2nd ed.*
Edited by: A. Robinson, M. J. Hudson, and M. P. Cranage © Humana Press Inc., Totowa, NJ

tory T-cells—have recently been cloned, and have been shown to suppress Th1 responses and to play a role in the maintenance of self tolerance *(7–9)*.

## 1.2. Induction of T-Cell and Antibody Responses; The Basis of Vaccination

The repertoire of T- and B-lymphocytes in the immune system is vast, with an almost infinite capacity to respond to foreign antigens. In a naïve individual, the frequency of lymphocytes that are specific for an individual epitope on a foreign antigen is very low. However, following exposure to a microorganism or antigen expressing that epitope, clonal expansion of precommitted lymphocytes occurs, memory T- and B-cells are generated, and the precursor frequency is greatly increased. Therefore, primary infection with a microorganism—or vaccination by exposure to an attenuated or killed virus or bacteria, or to a purified native or recombinant antigen—results in the stimulation of a small but specific population of lymphocytes in vivo. In a subsequent encounter with the antigen, as through infection with the pathogen, the memory B- and T-cells proliferate rapidly and allow the immune system to deal effectively with the invading microorganism.

In contrast to B-cell recognition of a foreign pathogen, which involves direct binding of the antibody molecule to an epitope on the surface of a viral or bacterial antigen, T-cells only recognize antigenic peptides in association with major histocompatibility complex (MHC) molecules on the surface of an antigen-presenting cell (APC) *(10,11)*. The foreign microorganism or antigen is taken up by macrophages, dendritic cells (DCs), B-cells, or other APC, either by receptor-mediated endocytosis or by nonspecific mechanisms, such as phagocytosis or pinocytosis, and is then processed into fragments or peptides prior to association with MHC molecules *(12–14)*. The APCs process and present the antigen to CD4$^+$ and CD8$^+$ T-cells using distinct mechanisms *(15)*. In general, CD4$^+$ T-cells recognize exogenous antigen in association with MHC class II molecules; the internalized antigens are processed (denatured and degraded) in endosomes into short fragments or peptides that bind to the MHC molecules and, following expression on the APC's surface, the MHC/peptide complex is recognized and bound by the T-cell receptor of a CD4$^+$ T-cell that is specific for that T-cell epitope *(12,14)*. In contrast, CD8$^+$ cells recognize endogenous antigen in association with MHC class I molecules *(14,15)*. Therefore, CD4$^+$ T-cells are readily generated following immunization with killed bacteria, viruses, or soluble antigens, whereas the induction of CD8$^+$ normally requires the antigen to be synthesized within the APC—for example, a viral antigen in a virus-infected cell. However, it has also been demonstrated that live or killed bacteria or soluble antigens presented in adjuvant formulations based on particles, emulsions, or lipids can allow exogenous antigen to gain access to the endogenous route of processing for presentation to class I-restricted T-cells *(16)*. The demonstration of distinct mechanisms of antigen processing for class I- and class II-restricted T-cells is crucial in the design of vaccines for the induction of distinct T-cell responses required for effective immunity to different pathogens.

### 1.3. Factors Affecting the Induction of T-Cell Responses Following Immunization

The nature of the antigen, dose, choice of adjuvant, route of immunization, and number of inoculations are all known to affect the strength, duration, and repertoire of T-cell responses.

#### 1.3.1. Antigen

The choice of live or killed whole virus or bacteria, purified native or recombinant antigen, or naked DNA as the immunogen considerably influences the induction of T-cell responses in both qualitative and quantitative terms. In general, the more prolonged the exposure of antigen to the immune system—for example, following infection—the stronger and more persistent the T-cell response. This is reflected in the observation that the strongest T-cell responses and the highest level of immune protection against an infectious organism are usually provided by prior exposure to the pathogen in a self-limiting infection. This observation is exploited in vaccination, in which infection with attenuated viruses, such as poliovirus, measles, mumps and rubella, is highly effective at preventing disease. Although killed viruses (e.g., poliovirus or rabies), killed bacteria (e.g., *Bordetella pertussis*), bacterial subunit antigens (e.g., tetanus toxoid or diphtheria toxoid), or viral subunit antigens (e.g., hepatitis B surface antigen [HbsAg]), are also highly effective vaccines, the immune responses induced with these vaccines may not be as durable, and often require a greater number of booster inoculations.

Because of their relative safety and ease of production, considerable time and expense have been expended on the search for recombinant vaccines against a range of human pathogens. However, the use of purified recombinant proteins for the induction of a protective T-cell or antibody response against an infectious virus, bacteria, or parasite presents a range of problems.

First, it is necessary to identify the protective antigen(s)—i.e., the antigen(s) against which the appropriate T-cell or antibody responses are directed. Second, it is necessary to ensure that the recombinant antigen mimics the structure in its native form. Failure to mimic the conformation of the native antigen can preclude the induction of protective neutralizing antibody responses, which are predominantly directed against the three-dimensional (3D) structure of the antigen. In addition, the processing of T-cell epitopes can be affected by antigen conformation or amino acid substitutions in flanking regions or at distant sites in the primary structure *(17,18)*. Finally, the induction of CD8+ class I-restricted T-cell responses is more difficult with purified recombinant proteins *(16)*. The use of live attenuated microorganisms, such as vaccinia virus, attenuated salmonella, or bacillus Calmett-Guérin (BCG), as vectors for the expression of foreign antigens provides an alternative means of allowing the induction of CD8+ T-cell responses, but has added safety complications associated with the use of live vectors, and can result in poor takes owing to prior exposure to the parent organism.

### 1.3.2. Adjuvant, Vaccine Delivery, or Recombinant Expression Systems

Immunization with soluble proteins, including purified native or recombinant antigens, results in weak and transient T-cell responses, and when given by a mucosal route (e.g., oral or intranasal [in]) can result in a state of immunological tolerance, whereby subsequent exposure to the antigen can fail to elicit an immune response *(19)*. Experimental immunization protocols in animals have employed a variety of agents that boost the immune response to the injected antigen by maintaining the antigen at the site of inoculation for longer periods of time, by enhancing antigen uptake through particle formation, or by including immunomodulators, usually bacterial components, that activate cells of the innate immune system, which in turn directs the induction of T-cell responses *(20)*. Recent evidence from murine studies suggests that the components of bacteria or parasites can activate distinct populations of DCs, termed DC1 or DC2, that selectively stimulate the induction of Th1- and Th2-cells, respectively *(21,22)*. IL-12 and IL-4 production appears to play critical roles in the directing naïve T cells to Th1 or Th2 cells *(5,21)*, whereas DCs that secrete IL-10 appear to drive the induction of type 1 regulatory T cells (Tr1) cells *(9)*. The selective stimulation of T-cell subtypes is an important consideration in the induction of a protective immune response, and must be carefully considered for effective vaccine design.

A large number of experimental adjuvants and vaccine-delivery systems have recently been developed, and some of these are already in clinical trials in humans *(23)*. Particulate-delivery systems, including liposomes, immunostimulating complexes (ISCOMs), biocompatible microparticles, or metabolizable oil-in-water emulsions enhance uptake of soluble antigens by APC and facilitate the induction of CD4$^+$ and CD8$^+$ T-cell responses *(20,24–26)*. Other experimental antigen-presentation systems, such as yeast-derived Ty-virus-like particles, hepatitis B core particles, or lipid-linked peptide, have been reported to have varying degrees of success in the induction of T-cell responses to foreign antigens *(20,27)*. Furthermore, a number of immunomodulators, including nontoxic bacterial derivatives, such as mutants of *Escherichia coli* heat-labile toxin (LT) and cholera toxin (CT), muramyl dipeptide (MDP), or monophosphoyrl lipid A (MPL) *(28–30)*, function by activating DC maturation and cytokine production, leading to more potent induction of T-cell responses *(20)*. Adjuvants and immunomodulators are discussed more fully in Chapters 11 and 12.

### 1.3.3. Immunization Schedule

The dose of antigen used in experimental and routine human immunization has often been chosen on an empirical basis. The notion that the higher the dose, the stronger the immune response pervades the scientific literature on immunogenicity studies with protein antigens. Indeed, within a certain range, increasing the dose of antigen does increase the titer and persistence of the antibody response. However, this may not be the case for the induction of T-cell responses, especially for Th1 cells, for which relatively low doses of antigens are equally or more effective than high doses.

Injection of antigen by a systemic route (sc, ip, or im) is most commonly used, and generates the most potent circulating antibody and T-cell responses. However, the majority of infectious pathogens enter the body at mucosal sites, where local immune responses may be an important first line of defense. The role of secretory IgA in local immunity is well documented against a variety of human pathogens *(31)*. Although in theory IgA can be induced by immunization at any of the common sites of the mucosal system, a recent clinical study with a nasal diphtheria vaccine in adult human volunteers demonstrated that anti-toxin IgA was only induced in the vaccinated nostril *(32)*. There is also evidence that immunization at mucosal sites can induce systemic T-cell responses *(26,32)* and recent studies have suggested that mucosal immunization may favor the induction of Th2-cells *(32)*. Furthermore, we have demonstrated that immunization by the ip route favors the induction of Th1-cells, whereas the sc route favors Th2-cells *(26)*.

Vaccination with attenuated viruses and/or bacteria is an efficient means of eliciting T-cell responses *(6)*. However, because of the transient nature of the infection, booster inoculations are often required to raise and maintain the immune response to the level that would be achieved following more prolonged infection with the wild-type pathogen. Effective immunization with subunit vaccines, even when formulated with the majority of current adjuvants, requires repeated booster injections to maintain T-cell and antibody responses at detectable levels. Despite the wide range of reported studies, there is no clear indication of the optimum rest period between booster doses. However, it does appear that a rest period of 4 wk or greater does result in a more persistent T-cell response.

## 1.4. Techniques for the Detection of T-Cell Responses

Once a T-cell response is induced in vivo, the response can be detected in vitro using a variety of laboratory assays. One of the simplest and most routinely used techniques to detect T-cell responses is the lymphocyte proliferation assay. This assay is based on the principle that on exposure to antigen in the presence of autologous or MHC-matched APC, T-cells respond by dividing, and the proliferation can be readily quantified to provide a measure of the responding T-cell population. However, this technique is relatively crude, and in its simplest form, cannot discriminate between T-cells of different phenotype or function, or even between T-cells and B-cells, which can also proliferate in response to foreign antigen. More recently, the detection of T-cell responses has encompassed a sophisticated range of assays that can discriminate between the responding populations on the basis of their function or cytokine production.

Semipurified mononuclear leukocyte preparations can be used ex vivo for many of the assays used to detect T-cell responses. Since almost all assays involve T-cell recognition of antigen as the first step, a source of APC as well as T-cells is necessary. Unseparated spleen or lymph-node cells and peripheral-blood mononuclear cells (PBMC), separated by density-gradient centrifugation, are rich sources of lymphocytes, and also contain sufficient DCs or macrophages for antigen presentation, without additional APC. Although contaminated with relatively small numbers of polymorphs and red blood cells, spleen cells can be used for many of the T-cell assays without further separation. Where necessary, the contaminating cells can be removed by density-gradient centrifugation; 18% metrizamide, Ficoll 1.077, and Percoll 1.081 have been used in the author's laboratory to purify murine, human, and macaque mononuclear cells, respectively *(27,33)*.

Although these relatively crude mononuclear-cell preparations can be used for most assays, they do not allow definition of the responding T-cell subpopulation. Further-more, for the assays of T-cell function (e.g., helper or CTL assays), purified T-cells, CD4+ or CD8+ T-cell subpopulations, B-cells, or APCs are required. After the initial density-gradient purification of the mononuclear-cell population, which includes T-cells, B-cells, NK cells, monocytes, and DCs, the following methods can be used to enrich appropriate cells:

1. T-cells by passing the cells down a nylon wool column, rosetting with sheep red blood cells (human only), or depletion of B-cells on Ig-coated beads and monocytes by adher-ence to plastic (34,35);
2. B-cells by depletion of T-cells using anti-thy-l or anti-CD3 antibodies and complement;
3. Monocytes by recovery of plastic-adherent cells.

These techniques do not require sophisticated equipment, and are cheap and rela-tively simple to perform. However, they permit only enrichment rather than a purifica-tion of a particular cell population. The most definitive approach for high levels of purity involves labeling of the cell population with a specific monoclonal antibody (MAb) and separation on a fluorescence-activated cell sorter (FACS) (35). Apart from the limited access to FACS machines, this method is relatively slow, and is not practi-cal for the separation of large numbers of cells or cells from several samples on the same day, which would often be required for the routine evaluation of T-cell responses. An alternative approach that involves a similar principle involves the use of antibody-coated magnetic beads or glass beads on affinity columns (35). Cells are depleted by direct or indirect binding to antibody-coated beads immobilized on a column or by being placed in a magnetic field. These techniques, if performed carefully, can give high levels of purity and allow separation of relatively large numbers of cells (up to $10^9$/column), with several columns run simultaneously.

The most definitive technique for the analysis of the specificity and function of T-cells induced by immunization or infection involves the generation of antigen-specific T-cell lines and clones from immune animals or humans. This technique is more suit-able for detailed qualitative rather than for quantitative assessment of T-cell responses, and has been described in detail elsewhere (see Chapter 17; aslo ref. 33). Furthermore, limiting dilution analysis (36) and HLA-peptide tetrameric complexes (37) have been used to quantify the frequency of T-cells that are specific for individual antigens in naive or immune animals or humans. Although limiting dilution analysis is a very powerful tool, it is quite laborious, and is unsuitable for routine detection of T-cell responses. MHC class I tetramers allow direct visualization of antigen-specific T cells by flow cytometry and have proven very useful for quantifying human CD8+ CTL responses ex vivo. Although the synthesis of tetramers is now becoming more straight-forward, the technique is currently limited by the commercial availability of a wide range of HLA-peptide tetrameric complexes. MHC class II tetramers have also been used. Here, the application of this technology to routine analysis of T-cell responses following infection or vaccination is limited by the wide range of peptides recognized by T-cells in association with a single MHC haplotype (38).

Although the techniques described here mainly relate to the induction of T-cell responses and their detection in animals following experimental immunization or exposure to infectious organisms, similar methods can be used to detect T-cell responses in humans following routine vaccination, in clinical trials of candidate vaccines, or following infection with a foreign microorganism.

## 2. Materials

1. Ethanol 70% (v/v): 700 mL industrial alcohol added to 300 mL of distilled water.
2. Phosphate-buffered saline (PBS): 8.0 g/L NaCl, 0.2 g/L KCl, 1.15 g/L $Na_2HPO_4$ (anhydrous), 0.2 g/L $KH_2PO_4$.
3. Complete medium: Roslin Park Memorial Medium (RPMI)-1640 medium, supplemented with 10% (v/v) heat-inactivated fetal calf serum (FCS), 100 m$M$ L-glutamine, 100 U/mL penicillin, 100 µg/mL streptomycin, and 50 µ$M$ 2-mercaptoethanol.
4. RPMI-2: RPMI-1640 medium supplemented with 2% (v/v) FCS. Hank's Balanced Salt Solution (HBSS) supplemented with 2% (v/v) FCS or 1% (w/v) BSA, or 1% (w/v) gelatin can be substituted for RPMI-2 for cell washing.
5. Stock ethidium bromide (EB) and acridine orange (AO) solution for vital staining: 100 mg EB and 100 mg acridine orange in 100 mL PBS, stored at –20°C (working solution: 1/1000 dilution of stock in PBS). **Caution:** These compounds are carcinogenic, and should be handled with care and under local guidelines.
6. Metrizamide 18% (w/v): Prepare a stock solution of 35.3% (w/v) metrizamide (analytical grade) in distilled water. Filter-sterilize and store at 4°C, concealed from light. Before use, dilute 35% (w/v) metrizamide to 18% (w/v) as follows: 1.02 mL of stock, 0.94 mL PBS, and 0.04 mL of FCS. (The concentration and density can be checked by measuring the refractive index, which should be 1.3613).
7. Glycine-NaOH buffer 0.1 $M$, pH 8.6: Prepare 0.1 $M$ glycine in O.1 $M$ NaCl (7.51 g glycine + 5.84 g NaCl/L), and add 94.7 mL to 5.3 mL O.1 $M$ NaOH.
8. Enzyme-linked immunosorbent assay (ELISA) coating buffer: PBS, pH 7.2, or carbonate-bicarbonate buffer, pH 9.6 (1.59 g $NA_2CO_3$ anhydrous, 2.93 g $NaHCO_3$ in 1.0 L distilled water).
9. ELISA washing buffer: 0.5 mL Tween-20 in 1.0 L PBS.
10. ELISA blocking buffer: PBS with 1% (w/v) BSA or 5% (w/v) milk protein (dried milk powder).
11. Alkaline phosphatase substrate solution for immunoassays: *p*-nitrophenyl phosphate, disodium, hexahydrate (available from Sigma [Poole, Dorset, UK] as preweighed tablets), 1.0 mg/mL in 10% (w/v) di-ethanolamine buffer containing 0.54 m$M$ magnesium chloride, pH 9.8 (97 mL di-ethanolamine, 800 mL distilled water, 100 mg $MgCl_2$ 6 $H_2O$; adjust to pH 9.8 with 1 $M$ HCl; bring volume up to 1.0 L with distilled water. Store at 4°C in the dark; warm to 25°C before use.
12. Phosphatase substrate for ELISpot assays: Dissolve one 5-bromo-4-chloro-3-indolyl phosphate (BCIP) / nitro blue tetrazolium (NBT) tablet (Sigma Cat. no. B5655) in 10 mL deionized water; yields a ready-to-use buffered solution containing BCIP/NBT pH 9.5.
13. $^3$H-thymidine: [methyl-$^3$H] thymidine, 20 µCi/mL; specific activity 5 Ci/mmol.
14. $^{51}$Chromium: $^{51}$Cr, SA 350–600 µCi/µg chromium (because of the short half-life, $^{51}$Cr cannot be stored for more than 1–2 wk).

15. MAb: Antibodies against cell-surface antigens and cytokines can be obtained from a range of commercial suppliers as purified antibodies, either uncoupled or labeled with biotin, enzymes, or fluorescent compounds. Alternatively, hybridomas that secrete appropriate antibodies can be obtained from the American Tissue Culture Collection (ATCC).

## 3. Methods

### 3.1. Immunization of Mice

### 3.1.1. Preparation of Alum-Adsorbed Antigens (see Chapter 11)

Most commercially prepared alum-absorbed vaccines use alhydrogel (aluminum hydroxide), which is suitable for use in the laboratory. The antigen is simply mixed with the aluminum hydroxide (100 µg antigen/mg alum) and allowed to adsorb at 4°C overnight. Alternatively, the procedure described here uses potassium aluminum sulfate to form a complex protein-salt precipitate.

1. Prepare solutions of 0.2 $M$ potassium aluminum sulfate (can be stored at room temperature for several months) and 1.0 $M$ sodium bicarbonate.
2. Add 1 vol of 1.0 $M$ sodium bicarbonate and 2 vol of antigen in PBS or Tris buffer to a 10-mL glass beaker (e.g., if the stock antigen concentration is 0.5 mg/mL and 125 µg of alum-adsorbed antigen is required, take 250 µL of antigen and 125 µL of sodium bicarbonate).
3. Place beaker on a magnetic stirrer and, with constant stirring, slowly (dropwise) add 2 vol of 0.2 $M$ potassium aluminum sulfate.
4. After allowing to stand at 4°C for 1–2 h or overnight, transfer to a hard plastic centrifuge tube and pellet the precipitate by centrifugation at 1000$g$ for 10 min.
5. Resuspend the pellet in PBS. The final volume to be determined by the route of immunization (maximum volumes per mouse: 0.3 mL for intraperitoneal [ip], 0.2 mL for subcutaneous [sc], 0.05 mL for intramuscular [im] or interdermal [id] routes).

### 3.1.2. Immunization Procedure

Mice can be immunized systemically by the sc or ip routes with volumes up to 0.2 or 0.3 mL, respectively, without the use of an anesthetic (for precise details, *see* Dresser **ref. 39**).

For immunization by the intranasal (in) route, mice are anesthetized in an atmosphere saturated with metofane inhalation anesthetic (large glass beaker with lid containing a wad of cotton wool to which a few drops of the anesthetic has been added). Using a Gilson or Oxford pipet, drop 10 µL of antigen preparation into the nose (with the mouth occluded) of the anesthetized mouse, and allow it to inhale.

### 3.2. Preparation of Mononuclear Cells

Murine spleens provide the most convenient source of large numbers of responder T-cells and APC for T-cell assays. Lymph nodes (LN), although they do not provide as high a yield, have a greater proportion of T-cells (50%) compared with spleen (30%). Draining LN from the site of immunization (e.g., popliteal LN from the foot pad or inguinal and peraortic LN from the base of the tail) or from the source of infection (e.g., tracheobronchial LN from the lungs) provides a rich source of primed T-cells. For studies in humans, peripheral blood is usually the only source of lympho-cytes that is readily available (*see* **Note 1**).

### 3.2.1. Preparation of Murine Spleen and LN Cells (see **Note 2**)

1. Sacrifice mouse by cervical dislocation, and immerse in 70% (v/v) ethanol. Using sterile scissors and forceps, lift, cut, and pull back the skin on the left side of the abdomen. Spray exposed abdomen with 70% (v/v) ethanol and, using fresh sterile scissors and forceps, make an incision over the spleen, and remove spleen with forceps, carefully cutting away the connecting tissue. Transfer the organ to sterile medium.
2. Pour spleen(s) and medium onto sterile wire in a Petri dish or a nylon cell strainer (Becton Dickinson) over a 25-mL tube and, using the plunger of a 5-mL syringe, grind spleen until a fine suspension is obtained.
3. Transfer spleen-cell suspension to 15-mL centrifuge tube and allow debris/cell clumps to settle for 10 min or centrifuge at 100*g* for 30 s.
4. Pipet off cells in supernatant and add to a fresh 15-mL tube.
5. Centrifuge at 300*g* for 5 min, and resuspend the cell pellet in complete medium.
6. Perform a cell count (*see* **Subheading 3.2.4.**).

### 3.2.2. Purification of Viable Mononuclear Cells From Murine Spleen

1. Resuspend spleen cells (prepared as described in **Subheading 3.2.1.**) at $5 \times 10^7$ cells/mL in RPMI-2, and carefully layer 1 mL of cell suspension onto 2 mL of 18% (w/v) metrizamide in a 15-mL ($12 \times 75$ mm) centrifuge tube.
2. Centrifuge at 500*g* for 15 min in a benchtop centrifuge fitted with a swing-out rotor.
3. Recover the cells from the interface, wash twice with 8–10 mL of RPMI-2, and perform a cell count.

### 3.2.3. Preparation of Human PBMC

1. Dilute heparinized blood (10 U heparin/mL blood) 1/2 in RPMI medium or HBSS.
2. Carefully layer onto Ficoll density-gradient medium (density 1.077); 8 mL of diluted blood on 2 mL of Ficoll in 15-mL centrifuge tube or 15 mL diluted blood on 5-mL Ficoll in a 25-mL centrifuge tube.
3. Centrifuge at 400*g* for 30 min at room temperature (if using a refrigerated centrifuge, ensure that the temperature is set at 20°C).
4. Remove the cells from the interface of Ficoll and plasma with a Pasteur pipet and transfer to a fresh tube. Dilute the cell suspension at least fivefold with RPMI-2 medium or HBSS.
5. Centrifuge at 300*g* for 7–10 min, discard supernatant, and resuspend cells in 10 mL of RPMI-2.
6. Centrifuge at 200*g* for 5 min. (The slower spin is designed to allow separation of plate-lets from the mononuclear cells.)
7. Resuspend in complete medium at approx $5 \times 10^6$/mL and perform a cell count.

### 3.2.4. Viable Cell Count with Ethidium Bromide and Acridine Orange (see **Note 3**)

1. Prepare a working solution of EB/AO containing 0.1 mg of both EB and AO in 100 mL PBS.
2. Mix a measured volume (20–50 μL) of cell suspension with an appropriate volume (20 μL–1 mL) of EB/AO so that the estimated final cell concentration is in the range of $2 \times 10^5$–$2 \times 10^6$/mL.

3. Fill a hemocytometer, and count the number of viable (green) and nonviable (orange) cells using a fluorescence microscope with a combination of ultraviolet (UV) and visible light.

## 3.3. Purification of T-Cells, B-Cells, and T-Cell Subpopulations (see *Note 4*)

A number of methods, including complement-mediated lysis, affinity columns, immunomagnetic beads, rosetting, panning, or separation on the basis of MAb labeling on an FACS, have been used to purify lymphoid cell subpopulations (*34,35*). One of the simplest techniques for negative selection involves complement-mediated lysis using a complement-fixing antibody against a surface determinant of the cell type to be depleted. Alternatively, an affinity column technique can employ noncomplement-fixing antibodies. Both of these techniques are very effective if carefully performed, and allow the separation of large numbers of cells in a relatively short time. The affinity column technique described here involves the separation of murine T-cells and CD4$^+$ or CD8$^+$ subpopulations from murine spleen tissue using columns manufactured by Pierce Laboratories. Other manufacturers (e.g., Biotex Laboratories) use slight variations that will be described in the manufacturer's instructions. The complete procedure for the separation of T-cell subpopulations involves several steps, namely the preparation of spleen cells, the purification of T-cells by depletion of B-cells, and the purification of CD4$^+$ T-cells by negative selection with the reciprocal anti-CD8 antibody. Alternatively, if the anti-mouse Ig used to deplete the B-cells crossreacts with rat Ig, CD4$^+$ T-cells can be separated from spleen cells in a single step by incubating the spleen cells with rat anti-CD8 prior to loading on the anti-Ig column.

### 3.3.1. Purification of Murine T-Cells on Anti-Ig Affinity Columns

This is a negative selection technique in which B-cells are removed by their binding, through surface Ig, to anti-Ig attached to plastic or glass beads in a column. Monocytes also adhere to the glass or plastic beads, and are retained on the column. However, the enriched T-cells are contaminated with natural killer (NK) cells, which can be removed by an additional step involving antibodies that are specific for NK cells.

1. Clamp the column (containing glass or plastic beads) and wash with 15 mL PBS. Drain the PBS to the top of the column bed, but not below, and close the column tap or clamp.
2. Add 10 mg polyclonal anti-mouse Ig in 1 mL of PBS, and allow it to enter the column.
3. Incubate for 1 h at room temperature.
4. Wash the column with 20 mL of PBS supplemented with 10% (v/v) FCS.
5. Adjust the flow rate for the particular column size (e.g., 6–8 drops/min for a standard Pierce column).
6. Resuspend viable mononuclear cells from murine spleen at approx $1 \times 10^8$/mL in PBS or RPMI medium supplemented with 10% (v/v) FCS and load onto reservoir of anti-Ig column.
7. Allow the cells to enter the column, and collect eluant into a fresh tube on ice.
8. Continue to top up reservoir with medium until a total of 20 mL has passed through the column.
9. Retain the eluant and centrifuge (200$g$ for 5–10 min) to recover the nonadherent cells (T-

cells plus null or NK cells).
10. Determine purity by FACSscan analysis with fluorescein isothiocyanate (FITC)-conjugated antibodies against mouse CD3 and Ig.

### 3.3.2. Purification of CD4⁺ T-Cells

1. Add the anti-CD8 rat MAb (preferably purified antibody, but diluted ascites or high-titer hybridoma supernatant can also be used) to the purified T-cell preparation.
2. After 30 min of incubation on ice, wash 3× and resuspend in RPMI medium.
3. Count cells and adjust concentration to $1 \times 10^8$/mL.
4. Load onto pre-prepared anti-rat Ig column.
5. Continue as in **steps 7–9** (**Subheading 3.3.1.**).
6. Check purity by FACScan analysis following labeling of cells with anti-CD4 and anti-CD8 antibodies.

### 3.3.3. Purification of B-Cells by Complement-Mediated Lysis of T-Cells and Adherence of Monocytes onto Plastic

1. Resuspend the mononuclear cells at $1 \times 10^7$/mL in medium containing the appropriate dilution of anti-CD3 or anti-Thy-1 (mouse only) antibody.
2. Incubate for 30 min at 4°C, shaking the cells periodically.
3. Centrifuge the cell mixture ($200g$ for 5 min) and resuspend at $1 \times 10^7$/mL in complement at the appropriate dilution in serum-free medium (*see* **Note 5**).
4. Incubate for 30–45 min at 37°C, shaking the cells periodically. (Cells can be checked for lysis after 30 min by removing a small aliquot and performing a viable count with EB/AO.)
5. Centrifuge the cells ($200g$, 5 min) and wash twice with RPMI-2 medium.
6. Resuspend in complete medium at $5 \times 10^6$, add 5 mL/dish to plastic Petri dishes (tissue-culture-grade, 9-cm diameter), and incubate at 37°C for 90–120 min.
7. Remove nonadherent cells with a Pasteur pipet after gently swirling the cell suspension in the dish.
8. Add 5 mL of fresh, complete medium prewarmed to 37°C to the Petri dish, swirl, and transfer to the nonadherent fraction.
9. Centrifuge ($200g$, 5 min) and resuspend in complete medium, perform a viable cell count, and check for purity by FACScan analysis with anti-CD3 and anti-Ig antibodies.

### 3.4. Preparation of APC

A variety of cell types can be used as APC. Normally, B-cells, macrophages, or DCs are present in spleen or PBMC samples in sufficient proportions to act as APC for the T-cells in these cell preparations. However, when using purified T-cells, T-cell subpopulations, or cultured T-cell lines or clones, it is necessary to add APC. Murine spleen cells or human PBMC, irradiated to prevent cell proliferation, are the most convenient source of APC. However, for specialized experiments, purified macrophages, B-cells, DCs, or Epstein-Barr virus (EBV)-transformed B-cells, L-cells, B-cell lymphoma, or fibroblast cell lines can also be used.

### 3.4.1. Irradiated Murine Spleen Cells

1. Prepare spleen cells (**Subheading 3.2.1.**) and suspend in PBS with 10% (v/v) FCS in a 10-mL plastic tube.
2. Place the tube within the chamber of a Cobalt-60, Cesium-137, or X-ray source, and expose to 15–30 Gy irradiation. (The dose required to prevent cell proliferation should be established for individual sources.)
3. Wash cells and resuspend in complete medium at a concentration of $4 \times 10^6$/mL (to be used at a final concentration of $2 \times 10^6$/mL in culture).

### 3.4.2. Preparation of EBV-Transformed Human B-Lymphoblastoid Cell Lines (BLCL) (see **Note 6**)

Human B-cells can be transformed by EBV, enabling them to grow continually in culture. **Caution:** EBV is a category 2 pathogen, and should be handled according to ACDP guidelines.

1. Grow the EBV-infected marmoset lymphoblastoid line B95-8 in RPMI supplemented with 15% (v/v) FCS in 250-cm$^2$ flasks kept flat in a $CO_2$ incubator at 37°C. Once the culture has been expanded to 50–100 mL at a cell density of $5 \times 10^5$/mL, leave for approx 10 d without replacing the medium. Harvest the supernatant containing the cell-free EBV by centrifugation at 300$g$ for 10 min. (This virus stock can be stored at –70°C until needed).
2. Prepare PBMC as described in **Subheading 3.2.3.**, centrifuge at 300$g$ for 5 min, and resuspend the pellet at $10^7$ cells/mL in complete medium.
3. Add an equal volume of undiluted B95-8 cell supernatant and incubate for 1–2 h at 37°C.
4. Wash the cells once with RPMI-2 and resuspend at $10^6$/mL in complete medium (15% [v/v] FCS). Plate out 200-µL vol in 96-well flat-bottomed microtiter plates.
5. Feed the cells sparingly (usually less frequently than once a week while the cell lines are becoming established) by removing 50–100 µL of medium and replacing with fresh medium. (The yellow color of an actively growing culture is a good guide to its need for feeding.)
6. Check for colony growth using an inverted microscope and expand confluent wells into wells of 24-well plates. Eventually expand cultures into 25-cm$^2$-tissue-culture flasks, which should be cultured upright.
7. Maintain the cultures by splitting 1:2-1:4 every 3–7 d, depending on the rate of growth.
8. Stocks of cells should be aliquoted and frozen in 10% (v/v) dimethyl sulfoxide (DMSO) in a liquid nitrogen freezing device.
9. For use as APC in proliferation assays, EBV-BLCL should be irradiated with 75 Gy as described for murine spleen cells (*see* **Subheading 3.4.1.**) and used at a final concentration of $1–2 \times 10^5$/mL in culture.

## 3.5. T-Cell Proliferation Assay

### 3.5.1. Coupling of Antigens to Latex Microspheres

In situations involving antigen preparations that are limiting or contaminated with agents that are toxic to cells (e.g., urea or detergents), coupling of the antigen to latex microspheres is a convenient method of purifying the antigen and of amplifying the proliferative response *(40)*. This approach has also been shown to be an effective means of enhancing T-cell responses to bacterial or viral antigens separated by sodium dodecyl sulfate-polyacrylamide gel electrophoresis (SDS-PAGE) *(40)*.

1. Wash latex microspheres (0.8-μm diameter) twice with 0.1 *M* glycine-NaOH buffer, pH 8.6, by centrifugation in a bench microfuge for 5 min.
2. Mix 100 μL of a 10% (w/v) suspension of latex microspheres in glycine buffer with 50–100 μg of antigen (at concentrations in the range of 0.2–10 mg/mL; can be in a variety of buffers), and bring the volume to 1 mL with glycine buffer.
3. Incubate at 4°C for 14–18 h with constant agitation.
4. Wash twice with PBS supplemented with 10% (v/v) FCS.
5. Block unbound sites by incubation in PBS supplemented with 10% (v/v) FCS at 4°C for 2 h.
6. Sterilize by exposure to UV light in a Petri dish.
7. Transfer to an Eppendorf tube, centrifuge, and resuspend in 1.0 mL of complete medium.
8. Store at –20°C in aliquots.

## 3.5.2. Proliferation Assay with Murine or Human Mononuclear-Cell Preparations

1. Prepare mononuclear-cell preparations: murine spleen cells at $4 \times 10^6$/mL in complete medium supplemented with 2% (v/v) normal mouse serum, human PBMC at $2 \times 10^6$/mL in complete medium supplemented with 10% (v/v) FCS, or human AB serum (*see* **Note 7**).
2. Prepare a range of antigen dilutions in complete medium: 0.1–100 μg/mL for soluble antigens or 10–1000 ng/mL for latex microsphere-coupled antigen (nominal concentration assumes 100% binding to microspheres of antigen from original preparation). The optimum range should be defined for individual antigens.
3. Plate out 100 μL of diluted antigen preparations, mitogen (2 μg/mL concanavalin A [Con A] for mouse cells or 20 μg phytohemagglutinin [PHA]/mL for human cells: positive control), and irrelevant antigen or medium alone (background control), into triplicate wells of 96-well flat-bottomed tissue-culture-grade microtiter plates (*see* **Note 8**).
4. Add 100 μL of mononuclear-cell preparation to each well and culture for 4 d (murine) or 6 d (human) in a 37°C incubator with 95% humidity and 5% $CO_2$.
5. Four to six hours prior to completion of the culture period, add 0.5 μCi of $^3$H-thymidine in 25 μL of complete medium to each well.
6. Following the 4–6-h pulse, harvest the wells onto glass-fiber filter paper with an automatic cell harvester.
7. Dry filters in oven at 60–80°C or under an infrared lamp.
8. Place complete filter sheets in bags or place punched-out disks in vials and add nonaqueous scintillation fluid.
9. Place vials in a conventional β-scintillation counter or bags in Betaplate (Wallac), microbeta (Wallac), or topcount (Packhard) counter, and count cpm for each well.
10. Express results as arithmetic mean of triplicate cultures in cpm per culture or as stimulation indices—thus, the ratio of counts in cultures with antigen divided by the response with medium alone or irrelevant antigen.

## 3.5.3. Proliferation Assay with Purified T-Cells, T-Cell Lines, or T-Cell Clones

1. Prepare responding T-cells at $4 \times 10^5$/mL in complete medium.
2. Prepare APC: irradiated murine spleen cells at $8 \times 10^6$/mL, or irradiated human PBMC at $2 \times 10^6$/mL in complete medium.
3. Prepare antigens as described in **Subheading 3.5.2.** and plate out 100 μL/well in 96-well microtiter plates.
4. Add 50 μL of T-cells and 50 μL APC/well.

5. Culture for 3 d (previously cultured T-cells) or 4–6 d (purified fresh T-cells).
6. Pulse, harvest, and count radioactivity as described in **Subheading 3.5.2.**

## 3.6. Detection of Thl/Th2/Th0/Tr1 Responses by Cytokine Production

The production of cytokines that are exclusive, or almost exclusive, to a particular T-cell population is a reliable method of demonstrating the induction of that T-cell population in vivo. Cytokines can be detected by a number of techniques, including the use of RT-PCR with specific primers to amplify cytokine mRNA *(41)*, intracellular staining of the cytokine *(42)*, or by the use of specific bioassays or immunoassays to detect the cytokine after specific antigen stimulation of T-cells in vitro *(43)*. Alternatively, the number of T cells secreting a particular cytokine can be enumerated using the enzyme-linked immunospot (ELIspot) assay. The range of cytokine assays that have been used for the detection of Thl/Th2/Th0/Tr cells are IFN-γ, TNF-β, TGF-β, IL-2, IL-4, IL-5, IL-6, and IL-10. Although IFN-γ is also produced by NK cells and CD8$^+$ T-cells, the production of IFN-γ without IL-4 or IL-5 is considered to be the most reliable indicator of a Thl response. Conversely, IL-4 and IL-5 production without IFN-γ was considered to be indicative of a Th2 response. However, it has recently been demonstrated that Tr1 cells secrete IL-5 as well as IL-10, but unlike Th2 cells, do not secrete IL-4 *(7,9)*. Therefore, IL-4 is probably the most important cytokine in the demonstration of a Th2 response. However, when compared with IL-5, IL-4 is often difficult to detect using ex vivo T-cells, but is readily detected from cultured T-cell lines or clones *(6,9)*.

### 3.6.1. Preparation of Cytokine-Conditioned Medium From In Vitro Antigen-Stimulated T-Cells

1. Prepare antigens, responding mononuclear cells; or T-cells and APC, and plate out in 96-well plates as described for the proliferation assay (*see* **Subheading 3.5.** and **Note 9**). Con-A is not a very potent stimulus for Th2 cytokines, and can be substituted by phorbal myristate acetate (PMA; 25 ng/mL) and soluble anti-CD3 antibody (2.0 µg/mL) as the positive control.
2. Remove supernatants after 24 h for IL-2 and 72 h for IL-4, IL-5, IL-6, IL-10, IFN-γ, TGF-β or TNF-β using a multichannel pipet, add to fresh microtiter plates, and store at –20°C. A minimum of 50 µL will be required for each cytokine assay (*see* **Note 10**).

### 3.6.2. Assessment of Cytokine Levels by Immunoassay

Two affinity-purified MAb, which are specific for different epitopes on the cytokine to be detected, are required to act as capture and detecting antibodies in the cytokine immunoassay. The detecting antibody is labeled with biotin.

1. Add 100 µL of anticytokine antibody (1–2 µg/mL in PBS) to the wells of 96-well maxisorb ELISA plates and incubate at 4°C overnight.
2. Discard excess antibody and wash the wells 3× with ELISA washing buffer.
3. Add 200 µL ELISA blocking buffer and leave at room temperature for 2 h.
4. Wash three times with ELISA washing buffer.
5. Prepare serial dilutions of standard cytokine (typical range 15–5000 pg/mL) in complete medium. The concentration of any in-house standard cytokine should be checked against

the international standard or international reference reagent (*see* **ref. 43**).

6. Add 50 µL of standards and test samples (supernatants) or medium alone to wells in triplicate, and incubate at 4°C overnight or at room temperature for 2 h.
7. Wash 6× with ELISA washing buffer.
8. Add biotin-conjugated anti-cytokine antibody (1–2 µg/mL in PBS supplemented with 0.1% [w/v)] BSA) and incubate at room temperature for 2 h.
9. Wash 6× with ELISA washing buffer.
10. Add alkaline phosphatase-conjugated streptavidin appropriately diluted (1/1000–1/5000 or as suggested by the suppliers), and incubate at room temperature for 1 h.
11. Wash 6× with ELISA washing buffer.
12. Add 100 µL phosphatase substrate solution and leave for 20–60 min until the color has developed.
13. Read absorbency at 405 nm on an ELISA plate reader.
14. Construct a standard curve of absorbance vs standard cytokine concentration, and read off cytokine concentrations of the samples from their absorbancy values.

### 3.6.3. IL-2 Bioassay Using the CTLL Cells

This bioassay exploits the IL-2 dependence of the CTL lines (CTLL) cells. Since the cell line also proliferates (weakly) in the presence of murine (but not human) IL-4, it is necessary to include a neutralizing anti-IL-4 antibody when assaying murine IL-2.

#### 3.6.3.1. MAINTENANCE OF CTLL CELLS

1. Obtain frozen or growing CTLL cells (from ATCC or another research laboratory), and culture in 10-mL vol of complete medium supplemented with IL-2 (5–10 U/mL recombinant IL-2 or 3% (v/v) rat Con A-activated spleen-cell supernatant *(33)* in 50-mL tissue flasks placed upright in a $CO_2$ incubator at 37°C.
2. Passage the cells after 2–3 d, when the cell density should have reached $1-2 \times 10^5$/mL; add 1 mL of the cell culture to a fresh flask containing 9 mL of fresh complete medium supplemented with IL-2 as described in **step 1**. (Passage on Monday, Wednesday, and Friday was found to be convenient.)

#### 3.6.3.2. IL-2 ASSAY

1. Wash the CTLL cells twice in complete medium, return to incubator for approx 1 h, and wash twice again.
2. Count CTLL cells and adjust concentration to $2 \times 10^4$/mL.
3. Prepare serial dilution of standard IL-2 in the range of 0.1–100 U/mL.
4. Thaw test samples and add 50 µL in triplicate to the wells of 96-well microtiter plates. Add, in triplicate, 50 µL of diluted standards or medium only (negative control) to remaining wells.
5. Add 25 µL of anti-murine IL-4 antibody (1.0 µg/mL of 11-B-11 or other anti-IL-4 neutralizing antibody) and incubate at 37°C for 30 min. (This step can be omitted when assaying human IL-2.)
6. Add 50 µL of CTLL cells to each of the wells.
7. Incubate for 24 h in a $CO_2$ incubator at 37°C.
8. Pulse with 0.5 µCi ³H-thymidine in 25 µL of complete medium/well and harvest 4–6 h later (as described in **Subheading 3.5.**).

9. Count incorporated $^3$H-thymidine (as described in **Subheading 3.5.3.**), prepare a standard curve of CPM vs IL-2 concentration, and read off concentration of unknown samples from the standard curve.

## 3.7. Quantification of Cytokine-Secreting Cells by ELISpot Assay (see Note 11)

Antigen-specific activation of ex vivo T cells from a primed host is usually accompanied by cytokine secretion, and this can be used as a measure of T-cell subtype induction in vivo. Detection of cyokines in supernatants (**Subheading 3.6.2.**) is one method that can be employed to quantify T cell responses and to discriminate Th1, Th2, and Tr1-type subtypes. However, it does not allow quantification of the number of responding T-cells. The ELISpot assay, originally used to determine the frequency of individual antibody-forming cells, has been adapted for the quantification of individual cytokine secreting T-cells. Cytokines secreted by T-cells stimulated by antigen in the presence of APC are captured by specific antibodies against cytokines (e.g., IFN-γ, IL-4, or IL-5) immobilized onto the wells of 96-well tissue-culture plates. The cytokine is detected by a second biotin-conjugated anti-cytokine antibody, followed by the addition of streptavidin-conjugated alkaline phosphatase or horseradish peroxidase (HRP). Following addition of a chromogenic substrate, the release of cytokine from individual cells can be detected as spots using a dissection microscope.

The ELISpot assay can be performed on unseparated murine spleen or lymph-node cells or human PBMC. Alternatively, T-cells can be purified from these cell preparations and stimulated with antigen in the presence of irradiated APC. Depending on the cell type and the frequency of responding cells, the cell concentration in culture must be varied in order to generate spots in the appropriate range for easy counting under the microscope. Ideally, cells should be cultured at a range of concentrations ($10^3$ to $10^6$/well). The number of antigen-specific cytokine-secreting cells is quantified by subtracting the number of spots obtained by cells incubated in the absence of antigen. Cells cultured with mitogen can act as positive controls. Here, the number of cells may need to be reduced, as the spots are usually difficult to count. The incubation time may also need to be varied for different cytokines; for example 16-18 h for IFN-γ and 30–40 h for IL-4 and IL-5. Some operators prestimulate the cells in conventional round-bottomed tissue-culture plates for 24–48 h prior to transfer to the nitrocellulose plates, and culture for a further 6–24 h.

1. Add 100 μL of anti-cytokine antibody (5–15 μg/mL in PBS or as recommended by suppliers) to the wells of 96-well nitrocellulose plates and incubate at 4°C overnight or for 2 h at 37°C.
2. Discard excess antibody and wash the wells 3× with sterile PBS.
3. Add 200 μL RPMI medium with 10% FCS and leave at room temperature for 2 h. Wash 3× with sterile PBS or RPMI medium.
4. Prepare antigens, responding mononuclear cells (or T-cells and APC), and add to antibody-coated 96-well plates as described for the proliferation assay (*see* **Subheading 3.5.** and **Note 9**). Use a single concentration of antigen (established from preliminary experiments with that antigen) and one or more concentrations of cells, determined from preliminary experiments; suggested concentrations: $2.5 \times 10^5$/mL ($5 \times 10^4$/well in 200-μL

wells of 96-well plate) for IFN-$\gamma$ and $1 \times 10^6$/mL ($2 \times 10^5$/well) for IL-4 or IL-5.

5. Culture at 37°C in a $CO_2$ incubator for 18 h (IFN-$\gamma$) or 30–40 h (IL-4 or IL-5). Do not disturb the plate during this incubation period.

6. Discard the cells and medium from the wells and wash 6× with ELISA washing buffer (nonsterile from this point on).

7. Add biotin-conjugated anti-cytokine antibody (1–5 µg/mL or as recommended by suppliers in PBS supplemented with 0.1% [w/v] BSA) and incubate at room temperature for 2 h.

8. Wash 6× with ELISA washing buffer.

9. Add streptavidin-alkaline phosphatase appropriately diluted (1/1000–1/5000 or as recommended by the suppliers), and incubate at room temperature for 1 h.

10. Wash 6× with ELISA washing buffer and drain well.

11. Add phosphate substrate solution (BCIP/TNB) and leave for 20–60 min until a blue color has developed.

12. Wash the plate under running water and allow to air-dry.

13. Count the spots by eye under a dissection microscope or using an automated counter.

14. Calculate frequency of antigen-specific cytokine-secreting cells by subtracting the number of detected spots in the absence of antigen from the frequency of spots obtained in the presence of relevant antigen.

### 3.8. Cytotoxic T-Cell Assay

The MHC-restricted cytotoxic activity of antigen-specific T-cells is usually measured using peptide-pulsed or virus-infected target cell lines, which are MHC-compatible with the responding T-cell. Tumor-cell lines expressing a range of murine MHC class I or class II molecules are available from the ATCC (e.g., P815 [*H-2^d*], EL4 [*H-2^b*], or A-20 [*H-2^k*]). CTL assays with human cells usually employ autologous or MHC-matched EBV-transformed B-cells or mouse L-cells transfected with the appropriate human MHC gene. In general, CTL assays are performed with antigen-restimulated bulk cultures established 5–10 d prior to assay. However, assays can also be performed using fresh spleen cells or PBMC or established T-cell lines. Because of the low frequency of responding T-cells, lysis may not be detectable when using fresh cells even at a high killer:target ratio (100:1 or 50:1). In contrast, established T-cell lines or clones should kill at effector:target ratios as low as 1:1.

### 3.8.1. Preparation of Murine CTL Effector Cells Using Bulk Cultures

1. Prepare spleen cells from virus-infected or immunized mice, and suspend at $2 \times 10^6$/mL in complete medium.

2. Culture cells with live virus (concentration to be established for each virus), vaccinia virus recombinant (1–5 PFU/cell), or specific peptide (1 µg/mL; previously shown to be recognized by mice of the corresponding haplotype) in 10–20 mL vol in 50-mL flasks (upright) at 37°C in a $CO_2$ incubator.

3. Add 5 U/mL of IL-2 after 3–4 d, and culture for a further 4–5 d or longer if fresh medium and IL-2 are added.

4. At the end of the culture period, centrifuge cells ($200g$, 5 min), and count the number of viable cells.

5. Resuspend at $2–4 \times 10^6$/mL in complete medium.

### 3.8.2. Preparation of $^{51}$Cr-Labeled Target Cells

1. Centrifuge $5 \times 10^6$ target cells and resuspend in 0.2–0.3 mL of serum-free medium.

2. Add 100 μCi $^{51}$Cr/5 × 10$^6$ cells and incubate for 60 min at 37°C.
3. Add 10 mL of RPMI-2, centrifuge (200$g$, 5 min), and discard supernatant into radioactive waste container. Repeat twice.
4. Resuspend in complete medium and count the number of viable cells.
5. Resuspend at 2 × 10$^5$/mL.

### 3.8.3. Killing Assay

1. Add antigen (peptide, live virus, or vaccinia virus recombinant, the optimum concentrations to be determined for individual antigens, or use a range of doses) to aliquots of the target cells. (The number and volume of aliquots will be determined by the number of test and control antigen preparations and the number of effector-cell samples to be tested) (*see* **Note 12**).
2. Prepare twofold dilutions of the effector cells in complete medium in triplicate wells of 96-well plates using a multichannel pipet.
3. Add 100 μL of target cells to each of the wells with effector cells and into 12 additional wells without effector cells. Add 100 μL of complete medium to six of these wells to measure spontaneous $^{51}$Cr release from target cells, and 100 μL of 1% (v/v) Triton X-100 to the other six wells to measure maximum $^{51}$Cr release from target cells.
4. Using plate carriers, centrifuge the plate(s) (150$g$, 1 min) to pellet the cells gently and allow interaction of CTL effector and target cells.
5. Incubate at 37°C for 4–6 h.
6. Centrifuge the plate(s) for 5 min at 250$g$.
7. Harvest 100 μL of supernatant/well, using a multichannel pipet, and transfer to a fresh plate or LP2 tubes for counting.
8. Count radioactivity of each sample in a γ-scintillation counter (tubes) or in a microbeta or topcount Beta scintillation counter (plates) after the addition of scintillation fluid.
9. Calculate the percentage cytotoxicity as follows:
   [($^{51}$Cr release in the presence of effector cells-spontaneous $^{51}$Cr release)/ (maximum $^{51}$Cr release-spontaneous $^{51}$Cr release)] × 100
10. If spontaneous release is >20%, the results may not be reliable.

## 3.9. Helper T-Cell Assay

This assay tests the capacity of antigen-stimulated T-cells to help B-cells to produce specific antibody, and is dependent on a source of antigen-primed T- and B-cells. For murine systems, an alternative in vivo helper assay can be used. This involves adoptive transfer of primed T- and B-cells into sublethally irradiated recipients, and evaluation of specific antibody levels in the serum 10–14 d later (**6**).

### 3.9.1. T- and B-Cell Culture

1. Prepare purified T-cells (as described in **Subheading 3.3.1.**) from mice immunized with the relevant antigen 10–14 d earlier, or use antigen-specific CD4$^+$ T-cell clones and resuspend at 4 × 10$^6$/mL in complete medium.
2. Prepare primed B-cells from immunized mice by depletion of T-cells with anti-Thy-l or anti-CD3 antibodies and complement (*see* **Subheading 3.3.3.**). Count and resuspend the B-cells at 4 × 10$^6$/mL.
3. Prepare irradiated spleen cells as APC (*see* **Subheading 3.4.1.**), and resuspend at 8 × 10$^6$/ mL in complete medium.
4. Add T-cells, B-cells, APC, and antigen in duplicate or triplicate to 2-mL wells of 24-well

tissue-culture plates, so that the APC and B-cell concentrations are constant at $2 \times 10^6/$ mL and $1 \times 10^6/$mL, respectively, and the concentration of T-cells is varied from $1 \times 10^5/$ mL to $1 \times 10^6/$mL, giving ratios of B-cells to T-cells from 1:1 up to 10:1. The antigen concentrations (range 0.1–10 µg/mL) should be determined for each antigen. Control wells should have B-cells or T-cells alone with antigen or T- and B-cells without antigen (*see* **Note 13**).

5. Culture in a humidified $CO_2$ incubator at 37°C.
6. After 7–10 d, remove supernatants and store at –20°C until ready to assay for antibody (*see* **Note 14**).

### 3.9.2. ELISA Antibody Assay

1. Coat the wells of 96-well maxisorb ELISA plates with antigen by adding 100 µL antigen (concentration in the range 1–5 µg/mL) in PBS or carbonate-bicarbonate coating buffer, and incubate at 4°C overnight (*see* **Note 15**).
2. Wash 3× with ELISA washing buffer.
3. Add ELISA blocking buffer and leave at room temperature for 1 h.
4. Wash 3× with ELISA washing buffer.
5. Add 100 µL of complete medium to the wells in rows 2–8 of the plate, and add 200 µL vol of test samples (neat culture supernatant or serum diluted 1/100) in triplicate to the first row of wells. This row should also have triplicate samples of a standard supernatant, or appropriately diluted serum or purified preparation known to contain antibodies against the antigen on the plate (positive control). Negative-control wells will have medium alone.
6. Using a multichannel pipet, make serial dilutions of the test and control samples by transferring 100 µL from row 1 to row 2, and so on down the plate, discarding 100 µL from row 8. (Alternatively, a wider range of dilutions can be performed by diluting across the plate.)
7. Incubate at room temperature for 2 h.
8. Wash 6× with ELISA washing buffer.
9. Add 100 µL of alkaline phosphatase-conjugated sheep/goat/rabbit anti-mouse IgG (or specific antibodies against Ig isotypes or IgG subclasses).
10. Incubate for 2 h at room temperature.
11. Wash 6× with ELISA washing buffer.
12. Add 100 µL phosphatase substrate solution.
13. Incubate for 20–40 min at room temperature and read absorbance at 405 nm on an ELISA plate reader.
14. Express results as endpoint antibody titers by linear regression from the straight part of the curve to 2 SD above the background control values.

## 4. Notes

1. All manipulations with cells in tissue-culture require rigid adherence to aseptic techniques. Almost all stages of the techniques should be performed in a class II laminar-flow cabinet, and the use of sterile disposable tissue-culture-grade plastics is almost mandatory. All glassware and instruments should be autoclaved at 121°C for 20 min. Long-term cell lines of T-cells derived from humans or mice, or cell lines used as APC or in cytokine assays, should be routinely screened for mycoplasma contamination.
2. Spleen-cell preparations can also be made by teasing the organ with scissors and forceps or using a glass homogenizer. However, in our experience, the highest yield of viable cells can be obtained using the wire or nylon gauze and plunger of a 5-mL syringe. The size of the pores in the gauze does not appear to be critical.
3. If a UV microscope is not available, viable cell counts can be performed using trypan

blue, which is taken up by dead cells and is visible under white light. However, it is more difficult for an inexperienced operator to perform accurate counts using this method, especially when the lymphoid cells are contaminated with red blood cells.

4. Purification of lymphocytes for functional studies should ideally be performed by negative enrichment through depletion procedures. Although positive enrichment usually yields the best purity and may be the only approach that is applicable, it should be noted that the binding of MAb to cells may influence their subsequent behavior in functional assays.

5. Fresh or lyophilized normal rabbit or guinea-pig serum can be used as a source of complement. Serum should be stored at –70°C and kept at 4°C following thawing prior to incubation with the cells. Each batch should be screened for toxicity against the cell type being used. Toxicity can be reduced by absorption with agarose.

6. Some workers have suggested that EBV-specific CTL, which are present in approx 90% of the adult population, may kill EBV-infected B-cells, and slow down or prevent the establishment of EBV-BLCL. This can be overcome by either removal of the T-cells by E-rosetting, or through the addition of cyclosporin A (0.5 μg/mL). One of the most common reasons for failure to establish BLCL is overzealous feeding of the cultures.

7. Fetal calf serum (FCS), usually at 10% (v/v), is the most widely used serum supplement used in T-cell assays. However, different batches of FCS need to be screened for optimum growth of T-cells without nonspecific stimulatory activity (because of the presence of endotoxin, cytokines, or xenoantigens). High-background spontaneous proliferation is often a problem with many sources of FCS. If a suitable batch cannot be obtained, pooled human AB serum or mouse serum can be substituted. The latter must be used at 2% (v/v) or less. Autologous serum has also been used in T-cell assays. However, when obtained from immunized or infected humans or mice, it is likely to contain antibodies against the antigen that will be used in the T-cell assay, and may therefore, affect the T-cell response to that antigen in a positive or negative fashion.

8. Although 200-μL vol in 96-well plates are the most commonly used cultures for proliferation and cytokine assays, cultures can be performed in 1–2-mL vol in 24-well plates, 20 μL vol in 384-well plates, or in 20-μL hanging drops in Teresaki plates *(44)*. The larger cultures are useful when the proliferation-type assay is established to generate supernatants for cytokine assays. Most automated equipment (harvesters, counters, and ELISA plate readers) are designed for compatibility with 96-well plates. However, many ELISA plate readers are now compatible with the 384-plate format.

9. Although coupling of antigens to latex microspheres enhances T-cell proliferative response to the antigen, and in many cases cytokine production, recent evidence from our laboratory suggests that the use of particulate latex-microsphere-coupled antigen or soluble antigens in vitro may preferentially stimulate Th1 or Th2 subpopulations, respectively *(45)*.

10. The stimulation of T-cells for the generation of supernatants for cytokine analysis can be performed in 200-μL vol in 96-well plates or using the same concentrations of T-cells, APC, and antigen in 1–2-mL vol in 24-well plates. When 24-well plates are used, the supernatants are transferred to sterile 1–2 mL tubes on the appropriate day and stored at –20°C until required for testing. Positive- and negative-control cultures should be included, when medium, mitogens, PMA and anti-CD3 are substituted for antigen.

11. All procedures up to discarding the cells from the plate (**step 8**) should to be carried out aseptically in a laminar flow hood using sterile reagents.

12. In certain situations, it may be necessary to pulse the target cells with antigen, in which

case the target cells are incubated with the antigen for 1–2 h, then washed twice, and resuspended to their original concentration ($2 \times 10^5$/mL). If vaccinia virus recombinants expressing the foreign antigen of interest are used for restimulating the effector cells in the bulk cultures, they should not be used in the read-out CTL assay, since the background vaccinia virus-specific responses will be very high.

13. When antigen-specific T-cell lines or clones are used, the numbers of T-cells in the helper assay should be reduced by 10- to 100-fold. The helper function of cultured Th1-cells may be undetectable because of their CTL activity against antigen-primed B-cells, especially at higher T:B-cell ratios.

14. Because of interference by residual antigen in the assaying of secreted antibody in some cases, it may be necessary to change the medium during the culture period. Some workers have recommended removal of most of the medium after 1–5 d, and adding fresh medium and culturing for an additional 5–7 d before removing the supernatants for antibody analysis. Care should be taken to avoid disturbing the cells during this procedure.

15. The binding of antigens to ELISA plates varies greatly between different antigen preparations. Many operators recommend carbonate-bicarbonate buffer at alkaline pH, but PBS (pH 7.2) appears to be adequate for most antigens. Synthetic peptides or short polypeptides often bind poorly, and in these cases, drying the antigen preparation onto the plate by placing in a nonhumidified 37°C incubator or on the bench overnight without the lid has worked well. However, this procedure may denature native proteins and thereby destroy certain conformational epitopes. Binding of certain viruses (e.g., poliovirus) has also been a problem, and an indirect binding procedure may be required; purified polyclonal antibody (or MAb) against the virus is first bound to the plate and used to capture the virus (*6*). This approach is also useful for specific binding of antigen from relative crude preparations.

## References

1. Mills, K. H. G. (1989) Recognition of foreign antigen by T cells and their role in immune protection. *Curr. Opin. Infect. Dis.* **2,** 804–814.
2. Jankovic, D., Liu, Z., and Gause, W.C. (2001) Th1- and Th2-cell commitment during infectious diseases: asymmetry in divergent pathways. *Trends Immunol.* **22,** 450–457.
3. Janeway, C.A. (2001) How the immune system works to protect the host from infection: a personal view. *Proc. Natl. Acad. Sci. USA* **98,** 6461–7268.
4. Mosmann, T. R. and Coffman, R. L. (1989) Th1 and Th2 cells: different patterns of lymphokine secretion lead to different functional properties. *Annu. Rev. Immunol.* **7,** 145–173.
5. Abbas, A. K., Murphy, K. M., and Sher, A. (1996) Functional diversity of helper T lymphocytes. *Nature* **383,** 787–793.
6. Mahon, B. P., Katrak, K., Nomoto, A., Macadam, A., Minor, P. D., and Mills, K. H. G. (1995) Poliovirus-specific Th1 clones with cytotoxic and helper activity mediate protective humoral immunity against a lethal poliovirus infection in a transgenic mouse model. *J. Exp. Med.* **181,** 1285–1292.
7. Groux, H., O'Garra, A., Bigler, M., Rouleau, M., Antonenko, S., De Vries, J. E., and Roncarolo, M. G. (1997) A CD4$^+$ T-cell subset inhibits antigen-specific T-cell responses and prevents colitis. *Nature* **389,** 737–742.
8. Chen, Y., Kuchroo, V. K., Inobe, I., Hafler, D. A., and Weiner, H. L. (1994). Regulatory T cell clones induced by oral tolerance: suppression of autoimmune encephalomyelitis. *Science* **265,** 1237–1240.
9. McGuirk, P., McCann, C., and Mills, K. H. G. (2002) Pathogen-specific T regulatory 1 (Tr1) cells induced in the respiratory tract by a bacterial molecule that stimulates IL-10

production by dendritic cells: a novel strategy for evasion of protective Th1 responses against *Bordetella pertussis. J. Exp. Med.* **195,** 221–231.

10. Schwartz, R. H. (1985) T-lymphocyte recognition of antigen in association with gene products of the major histocompatibility complex. *Annu. Rev. Immunol.* **3,** 237–261.

11. Zinkernagel, R. M. and Doherty, P. C. (1979) MHC restricted cytotoxic T cells: studies on the biological role of polymorphic major transplantation antigens determining T cell restriction specificity, function and responsiveness. *Adv. Immunol.* **27,** 51–77.

12. Mills, K. H. G. (1986) Processing of viral antigens and presentation to class II-restricted T cells. *Immunol. Today* **7,** 260–263.

13. Townsend, A. R. M., Gotch, F. M., and Davey, J. (1985) Cytotoxic T-cells recognise fragments of the influenza nucleoprotein. *Cell* **42,** 457–467.

14. Watts, C. and Powis, S. (1999) Pathways of antigen processing and presentation. *Rev. Immunogenet.* **1,** 60–74.

15. Morrison, L. A., Lukacher, A. E., Braciale, V. L., Fan, D. P., and Braciale, T. J. (1986) Differences in antigen presentation to MHC class I- and class II-restricted influenza virus-specific cytotoxic T lymphocyte clones. *J. Exp. Med.* **163,** 903–921.

16. Raychaudhuri, S. and Morrow, W. J. W. (1993) Can soluble antigen induce CD8$^+$ cytotoxic T cell responses? A paradox revisited. *Immunol. Today* **14,** 344–348.

17. Mills, K. H. G., Skehel, J. J., and Thomas, D. B. (1986) Conformational dependent recognition of influenza virus haemagglutinin by murine T-helper clones. *Eur. J. Immunol.* **16,** 276–280.

18. Mills, K. H. G., Burt, D. S., Skehel, J. J., and Thomas, D. B. (1988) Fine specificity of murine class-II-restricted T-cell clones for synthetic peptides of influenza virus haemaglutinin: heterogeneity of antigen interaction with the T-cell and the Ia molecule. *J. Immunol.* **140,** 4083–4090.

19. Czerkinsky, C. Anjuere, F., McGhee, J. R., George-Chandy, A., Holmgren, J., Kieny, M. P., et al. (1999) Mucosal immunity and tolerance: relevance to vaccine development. *Immunol. Rev.* **170,** 197–222.

20. Ryan, E. R., Daly, L., and Mills K. H. G. (2001) Immunomodulators and delivery systems for vaccination by mucosal routes. *Trends Biotechnol.* **19,** 293–304.

21. Moser, M. and Murphy, K. M. (2000) Dendritic cell regulation of TH1-TH2 development. *Nat. Immunol.* **1,** 199–205.

22. Whelan, M., Harnett, M. M., Houston, K. M., Patel, V., Harnett, M., and Rigley, K. P. (2000) A filarial nematode-secreted product signals dendritic cells to acquire a phenotype that drives development of Th2 cells. *J. Immunol.* **164,** 6453–6460.

23. Aguado, T., Engers, H., Pang, T., and Pink, R. (1999) Novel adjuvants in clinical testing November 2-4, 1998, Fondation Merieux, Annecy, France: a meeting sponsored by the World Health Organization. *Vaccine* **17,** 2321–2328.

24. Allison, A. C. and Byars, N. E. (1986) An adjuvant formulation that selectively elicits the formation of antibodies of protective isotypes and of cell-mediated immunity. *J. Immunol. Methods* **95,** 157–168.

25. Smith R. E., Donachie, A. M., and Mowat, A. M. (1998) Immune stimulating complexes as mucosal vaccines. *Immunol. Cell Biol.* **76,** 263–269.

26. Conway, M., Madrigal, L., McClean, S., Brayden, D. J., and Mills, K. H. G. (2001) Protection against *Bordetella pertussis* infection following parenteral or oral immunization with antigens entrapped in biodegradable polymers: effect of formulation and route of immunization on induction of Th1 and Th2 cells. *Vaccine* **19,** 1940–1950.

27. Mills, K. H. G., Kitchin, P. A., Mahon, B. P., Barnard, A. L., Adams, S. E., Kingsman, S.

M., et al. (1990) HIV p24-specific T cell clones from immunized primates recognize highly conserved regions of HIV-1. *J. Immunol.* **144,** 1677–1683.

28. Ribi, E. and Cantrell, J. (1985) A new immunomodulator with potential clinical applications: monophosphoryl lipid A, a detoxified endotoxin. *Clinical Immunol. News* **6,** 33–36.

29. Marinaro, M., Staats, H. F., Hiroi, T., Jackson, R. J., Coste, M., Boyaka, P. N., et al. (1995) Mucosal adjuvant effect of cholera toxin in mice results from induction of T helper 2 (Th2) cells and IL-4. *J. Immunol.* **155,** 4621–4629.

30. Ryan, E. J., McNeela, E., Murphy, G., Stewart, H., O'Hagan, D., Pizza, M., et al. (1999) Mutants of *Escherichia coli* heat labile toxin act as effective mucosal adjuvants for nasal delivery of an acellular pertussis vaccine: differential effects of the nontoxic AB complex and enzyme activity on Th1 and Th2 cells. *Infect. Immun.* **67,** 6270–6280.

31. Ogra, P. L. and Garofalo, R. (1990) Secretory antibody response to viral vaccines. *Prog. Med. Virol.* **37,** 156–189.

32. Mills, K. H. G., Cosgrove, C., McNeela, E. A., Sexton, A., Giemza, R., Jabbal-Gill, I., et al. (2003) Protective diptheria immunity induced in healthy volunteers by unilateral prime-boost intranasal immunization associated with restricted ispilateral mucosal secretory IgA. *Infect. Immun.* **71,** 726–732.

33. Mills, K. H. G. (2000) Murine T cell culture, in *Lymphocytes—A Practical Approach.* (Rowland Jones, S. and McMichael A., eds.) IRL Press, Oxford, pp. 95–134.

34. Mills, K. H. G. (1986) An indirect rosette technique for the identification and separation of lymphocyte subpopulations by monoclonal antibodies, in *Immunological Techniques, Methods in Enzymology, vol. 121. Immunochemical Techniques* (Langone, J. J. and van Vunakis, H., eds.), Academic Press, Boca Raton, FL, pp. 726–737.

35. Plebanski, M. (2000) Preparation of lymphocyte and identification of lymphocyte subpopulations, in *Lymphocytes—A Practical Approach* (Rowland Jones, S. and McMichael A., eds.) IRL Press, Oxford, pp 1–26.

36. Carmichael, A. (2000) Limiting dilution-analysis for the quantitation of antigen-specific T cells, in *Lymphocytes—A Practical Approach* (Rowland Jones, S. and McMichael A., eds.) IRL Press, Oxford. Pp. 179-196.

37. Ogg, G. S. (2000) HLA-peptide tetrameric complexes, in *Lymphocytes—A Practical Approach* (Rowland Jones, S. and McMichael A., eds.) IRL Press, Oxford. Pp. 197–208.

38. Mills, K. H. G., Skehel, J. J., and Thomas, D. B. (1986) Extensive diversity in the recognition of influenza virus hemagglutinin by murine T helper clones. *J. Exp. Med.* **163,** 1477–1490.

39. Dresser, D. (1986) Immunization of experimental animals, in *Handbook of Experimental Immunology,* 4th ed. (Weir, M., ed.), Blackwell Scientific, Oxford, pp. 8.1–8.21.

40. Katrak, K., Mahon, B. P., Jones, W., Brautigam, S., and Mills, K. H. G. (1992) Preparative separation of foreign antigens for highly efficient presentation to T cells in vitro. *J. Immunol. Methods* **156,** 247–254.

41. Melby, P. C., Damsel, B. J., and Tryon, V. V. (1993) Quantative measurement of human cytokine gene expression by polymerase chain reaction. *J. Immunol. Methods* **159,** 235–243.

42. Jung, T., Schauer, U., Heusser, C., Neumann, C., and Rieger, C. (1993) Detection of intracellular cytokines by flow cytometry. *J. Immunol. Methods* **159,** 197–207.

43. Thorpe, R., Wadhwa, M., Bird, C. R., and Mire-Sluis, A. R. (1992) Detection and measurement of cytokines. *Blood Rev.* **6,** 133–148.

44. Knight, S. (1987) Lymphocyte proliferation assays, in *Lymphocytes—A Practical Approach* (Klaus, G. G. B., ed.), IRL, Oxford, pp. 189–208.

45. Moore, A., McCarthy, L., and Mills, K. H. G. (1999) The adjuvant combination monophosphoryl lipid A and QS21 switches T cell responses induced with a recombinant HIV protein from Th2 to Th1. *Vaccine* **17,** 2517–2527.

# 17

## Construction of MHC Class I-Peptide Tetrameric Complexes for Analysis of T-Cell-Mediated Immune Responses

**Rachel V. Samuel and Tomáš Hanke**

## 1. Introduction

Tetrameric major histocompatibility complex (MHC) class I-peptide complexes (tetramers) are a powerful tool in the study of antigen-specific CD8[+] T cell responses *(1,2)*. Although the interaction of a monomeric MHC-peptide complex with the T-cell receptor is of a low affinity and fast off-rate, the avidity of multimeric complexes provides a relatively stable T-cell binding, which allows T-cell enumeration and phenotypic analysis. The tetramer approach is highly sensitive, with a detection limit of approx 0.02% of CD8[+] T cells, and the frequencies obtained correlate well with other T-cell assays. Tetramer analysis gives up to five- and 10-fold higher frequencies than the respective interferon-γ-based enzyme-linked immunospot (ELISpot) and limiting dilution assays, although these ratios may depend on the antigenic load. The use of tetrameric MHC-peptide complexes revealed, for the first time, massive clonal expansions of T-cells, which in the case of primary Epstein-Bar virus (EBV) infection reached 45% of circulating CD8[+] peripheral blood mononuclear cells (PBMC) (*see* **ref. 3**). The ease with which tetramer complexes are constructed depends on the particular MHC (called HLA for humans) molecule and the peptide ligand. For example, the HLA-A*0201 molecule folds relatively easily into a conformationally correct complex compared to the HLA-B57 molecule. A growing list of these reagents is available commercially and also from the National Institutes of Health, which provide tetramers free of charge, but for research purpose only (**Table 1**). The construction of MHC class II-peptide tetrameric complexes has proven to be more problematic than class I, with a fewer publications mainly involving mouse tetramers and no standard protocol.

From: *Methods in Molecular Medicine, Vol. 87: Vaccine Protocols, 2nd ed.*
Edited by: A. Robinson, M. J. Hudson, and M. P. Cranage © Humana Press Inc., Totowa, NJ

**Table 1**
**MHC Class I Alleles Available at the NIH Tetramer Facility (2001)**

| Human alleles | Murine alleles | Rhesus macaque alleles | Chimpanzee alleles |
|---|---|---|---|
| HLA-A*0101 | H-2D(b) | Mamu-A*01 | Patr-A*04 |
| HLA-A*0201 | H-2D(d) | Mamu-A*02 | Patr-B*13 |
| HLA-A*0205 | H-2D(k) | Mamu-A*11 | |
| HLA-A*0301 | H-2K(b) | Mamu-B*01 | |
| HLA-A*1101 | H-2K(d) | Mamu-B*03 | |
| HLA-A*2301 | H-2K(k) | Mamu-B*04 | |
| HLA-A*2402 | Qa1b | | |
| HLA-A*68012 | | | |
| HLA-A*7401 | | | |
| HLA-B*0702 | | | |
| HLA-B*0801 | | | |
| HLA-B*1501 | | | |
| HLA-B*2705 | | | |
| HLA-B*3502 | | | |
| HLA-B*3503 | | | |
| HLA-B*5101 | | | |

Here, a generalized recipe for preparation of MHC class I tetramers with suggested approaches to optimization for more troublesome heavy chains is described.

## 2. Materials

### 2.1. Cloning of the MHC Genes

1. PCR reagents as described in Sambrook et al. *(4)*.
2. IPTG-inducible expression vectors (e.g., pET vector [Novagen]).
3. DNA-sequencing equipment.

### 2.2. Expression of the Heavy Chain and $\beta_2$-Microglobulin ($\beta_2$-m)

1. Spectrophotometer.
2. Agar plates containing 100 µg/mL ampicillin.
3. Low Salt LB (LLB) medium: 10 g bacto-tryptone, 5 g bacto-yeast extract, and 5 g NaCl to 980 mL of distilled water. Sterilize by autoclaving.
4. 1 *M* isopropylthio-β-D-galactosidase (IPTG).
5. Ampicillin 0.1 g/mL (1000×).
6. *Escherichia coli* strains BL21 or HMS 174 (Novagen).

### 2.3. Purification of the Inclusion Bodies

1. Sonicator.
2. Homogenizer.
3. Centrifuge.

4. Triton wash buffer: 0.5% Triton X-100, 50 m*M* Tris-HCl pH 8.0, 100 m*M* NaCl, 0.1% sodium azide, 1 m*M* EDTA, 1 m*M* dithiothreitol (DTT).
5. Resuspension buffer: 50 m*M* Tris-HCl, pH 8.0, 100 m*M* NaCl, 1 m*M* ethylenediamine-tetraaceticacid (EDTA), 1 m*M* DTT.
6. Urea denaturant buffer: 8 *M* Urea, 0.1 m*M* DTT, MES, pH 6.5.
7. Commercial protein assay: e.g., Biorad Reagent.

## 2.4. In Vitro Refolding into MHC-Class I-Peptide Complex Monomers

1. Cold room.
2. Magnetic stirrer.
3. Refolding buffer: 100 m*M* Tris-HCl, pH 8, 400 m*M* L-arginine HCl, 5 m*M* reduced glutathione, 0.5 m*M* oxidized glutathione, 2 m*M* EDTA.

## 2.5. Concentration and Biotinylation of the Refolded Monomers

1. Nitrogen tank.
2. Stir cell (380 mL and 2,000 mL) and ultra-centrifugation membranes with 10-kDa membrane cut-off (Amicon).
3. Buffer exchange disposable columns PD-10 (Pharmacia).
4. BirA buffer (20 m*M* Tris-HCl, pH 8) filtered through 0.2-μm membrane before use.
5. Bir A enzyme 1 mg/mL (Avidity).
6. Biomixes A and B (Avidity).
7. Protease inhibitors: leupeptin 1 mg/mL (1000×) and pepstatin 1 mg/mL (1000×).

## 2.6. Two-Step Purification of MHC Class I-Peptide Complex Monomers

1. Gel filtration Superdex 75 Column (Pharmacia).
2. Anion-exchange column (Biocad, Pharmacia).
3. FPLC Buffer: 20 m*M* Tris-HCl, pH 8.0, 100 m*M* NaCl. Filter before use.

## 2.7. Estimation of MHC Class I-Peptide Complex Monomer Concentration by ELISA

1. ELISA reagents and special equipment, as described in *Current Protocols in Immunology (5)*.
2. W6/32 antibody *(6)* 5 μg/mL in phosphate-buffered saline (PBS).
3. 1% bovine serum albumin (BSA) in PBS.
4. Avidin-horseradish peroxidase (HRP; Sigma).
5. Colorimetric reagent for peroxidase: 3,3',5,5'-tetramethyl benzidine (Sigma).

## 2.8. Tetramerisation of MHC Class I-Peptide Complex

1. Streptavidin conjugated to e.g., phycoerythrin (PE).

## 2.9. Flow Cytometry

1. Fluorescence-activated cell sorter (FACS) machine.
2. Anti-CD8 antibody conjugated to e.g., Tricolor (Caltag) or fluorescein isothiocyanate (FITC) (Pharmingen).
3. FACS Wash Buffer (PBA): 0.05% BSA, 0.01% sodium azide in PBS.
4. FACS Fix: 2–3% formaldehyde, 0.05% BSA in PBS.

## 3. Methods

### 3.1. Cloning of the MHC Heavy- and Light-Chain Genes into an Expression Vector

#### 3.1.1. Modification of MHC Heavy Chain and $\beta_2$-m Genes

The gene for the extracellular domain of the MHC heavy chain is amplified from cDNA. The open reading frame is modified by a deletion of the sequence coding for the signal sequence at the 5'-end and an addition of a region coding for the biotinylation signal substrate peptide (BSP) to the 3'-end (*see* **Note 1**). PCR primers for amplification of the rhesus macaque heavy-chain molecule Mamu-A*01 are shown as examples:

1. The MHC gene is PCR amplified from cDNA (*7*) using an upstream primer: 5'-CCT GAC TCA GAC CAT ATG GGC TCT CAC TCC ATG and a downstream primer: 5'-G TGA TAA GCT TAA CGA TGA TTC CA CAC CAT TTT CTG TGC ATC CAG AAT ATG ATG CAG GGA TCC CTC CCA TCT CAG GGT GAG GGG C containing sites for restriction endonucleases NdeI and HindIII, respectively. The downstream primer codes for the BSP sequence.
2. Rhesus $\beta_2$-m is also amplified by PCR from cDNA (*see* **Note 2**).

#### 3.1.2. Cloning of Modified MHC Heavy Chain and $\beta_2$-m into Expression Vectors

The PCR products from both heavy chain and $\beta_2$-m are digested using their respective restriction endonucleases and cloned individually into the polylinker site of an expression vector such as pET.

### 3.2. Expression and Purification of the Heavy Chain and $\beta_2$-m Proteins

The following steps are performed for both the heavy chain and the $\beta_2$-m molecules.

#### 3.2.1. Transformation of BL21pLys with the Recombinant Expression Vectors

1. Add approx 1 µg of plasmid to 20 µL of competent BL21 stock and process according to the protocol for preparation of competent cells (*4*).
2. To obtain colonies, shake the transformed bacteria without ampicillin at 37°C for 1 h, plate them on agar supplemented with 100 µg/mL of ampicillin and leave overnight at 37°C.

#### 3.2.2. Induction of Protein Expression

The heavy chain and $\beta_2$-m will be expressed from pET expression vectors upon addition of IPTG.

1. Inoculate 30 mL of LLB, supplemented with ampicillin, with a single colony and leave agitating at 250 rpm overnight at 37°C.
2. Inoculate 30 mL of culture per 1-L flask of LLB medium and ampicillin (*see* **Note 3**).
3. Allow growth of bacterial culture till the OD 600 nm reaches 0.5. Add 0.5 mL of 1 *M* IPTG and leave shaking at 37°C for 4–6 h.
4. Flasks can be left overnight at 4°C or spun down at 3485*g* for 30 min and resuspended in 50–100 mL of ice-cold PBS.

### 3.2.3. Purification of Inclusion Bodies

Protein in the bacteria is expressed in insoluble inclusion bodies, which are isolated by several cycles of sonication followed by repeated homogenization and washes with detergent (Triton). Purified protein is solubilised in urea (*see* **Note 4**).

1. Sonicate in 30- to 60-s bursts while constantly cooling on ice. Since sonication generates heat, cooling the samples will reduce the degradation of inclusion body protein. Sonicate until the sample has a similar viscosity to water.
2. Spin at 7741$g$ (Beckman J-20) in polycarbon centrifuge tubes for 20 min. The resulting precipitate will be layered. The bottom-most layer is the inclusion body protein and has a chalky, tight consistency. The top layers contain unsonicated bacteria, and can be either removed by repeat sonications or discarded.
3. At least three Triton washes of the inclusion bodies should be performed. Transfer the inclusion body pellet into a homogenizer and resuspend in Triton buffer by ten strokes of the piston. Transfer the content back into the centrifuge tube and spin for 10 min at 27,000$g$. Three washes should be sufficient to obtain a tight, chalky, white pellet; however, more washes can be performed.
4. The detergent is removed by resuspending the pellet in Resuspension buffer. Spin again for 10 min at 27,000$g$.
5. The pellet is solubilised in Urea Buffer (*see* **Note 5**). If there is difficulty getting the pellet to solubilize, leave rotating overnight at 4°C before spinning at 27,000$g$ for 10 min to remove any undissolved material.
6. Small aliquots of the heavy and light chains can be run on sodium dodecyl sulfate-polyacrylamide gel electrophoresis (SDS-PAGE) to determine the purity of the preparation (**Fig. 1**).
7. Estimate protein concentration at Absorbancy (A) 695 nm using the BIORAD reagent or any commercial protein-estimation kit.
8. Make 10-mg aliquots and store at –70°C (*see* **Note 6**).

## 3.3. In Vitro Refolding into MHC Class I-Peptide Complex Monomers

The heavy chain, $\beta_2$-m and relevant peptide are refolded into conformationally correct MHC class I-peptide complexes by diluting urea into a large volume (0.5–1 L) of the refold buffer.

1. The refold is carried out at 4°C. Cool the refold buffer before slowly adding 15 mg of heavy chain (*see* **Note 7**).
2. Add 30 mg of $\beta_2$-m. This should go quite easily into solution.
3. Finally, add 8–10 mg of peptide, which can be first solubilised in around 50 µL of dimethyl sulfoxide (DMSO).
4. Leave stirring slowly (not to generate bubbles) overnight at 4°C.
5. Over the next 36–48 h, two additional 15-mg aliquots of heavy chain are added (*see* **Note 8**).

## 3.4. Biotinylation of the MHC Class I-Peptide Complex Monomers

The biotinylation reaction is a BirA enzyme-catalyzed addition of biotin to the C-terminus of the modified heavy-chain molecule.

1. Concentrate refold to 5 mL using stir cells (Amicon), which removes excess of solvent across a membrane (10 kDa cut-off) upon application of pressurized nitrogen.
2. Using two PD-10 columns, which bind the concentrated refolded monomer, the refold buffer is exchanged for a BirA buffer. The protein is eluted with 3.5 mL of buffer per column, e.g. a total of 7 mL.

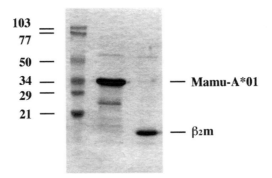

Fig. 1. SDS-PAGE gel stained with Coomassie blue G-250 showing the purified MHC heavy and light chains. Molecular mass markers are indicated in kDa.

3. For biotinylation, add to the eluent 800 µL (1/8th the eluent volume) of each of Biomixes A and B and 4 µL of the BirA enzyme. The protease-inhibitors pepstatin and leupeptin are also added to slow protein degradation (*see* **Note 9**).
4. The reaction is incubated overnight at room temperature.

## 3.5. Two-Step Purification of Biotinylated MHC Class I-Peptide Complex Monomers

The biotinylated monomeric complexes are purified sequentially by gel filtration and ion-exchange columns.

1. The samples are spun at 960*g* for 5 min to remove any precipitate from the biotinylation reaction. It is filtered before being loaded onto the equilibrated FPLC column.
2. The MHC class I-peptide complex is approximately 45 kDa, and should come off between 120 and 180 mL, depending on the calibration of the column using standard markers (**Fig. 2**).
3. The sample is diluted in 20 m*M* Tris-HCl, pH 8.0 to remove the FPLC buffer salt, and concentrated to 5–10 mL using a stir cell.
4. The sample is loaded onto an ion-exchange column, which will separate the biotinylated complex from the unbiotinylated (**Fig. 3**); (*see* **Note 10**).
5. The sample is further concentrated to 0.5–1 mL. Centriprep units with a 10-kDa cut-off membrane can be used.
6. Add protease inhibitors leupeptin and pepstatin, and EDTA, pH 8.0 to a final concentration of 4 m*M*. Store in glass vials in the dark at 4°C.

## 3.6. Estimation of Biotinylated MHC Class I-Peptide Complex Monomer Concentration by ELISA

Simple estimation of protein concentration might overestimate the actual concentration of biotinylated monomer leading to suboptimal tetramerization. Therefore, an enzyme-linked immunosorbent assay (ELISA) employing monoclonal antibody (MAb) W6/32, which is specific for the conformationally correct heavy chain, is used.

1. Coat an ELISA plate for 2-4 h at 37°C with 100 µL of 5 µg/mL of W6/32 antibody.
2. Block with 200 µL of 10% BSA including control wells without W6/32 overnight.

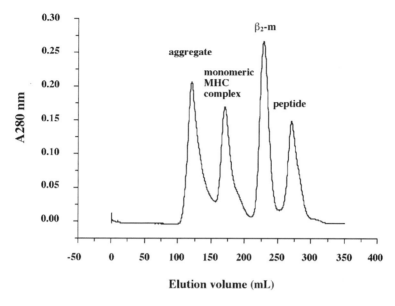

Fig. 2. Size purification and isolation of refolded monomeric complex on an FPLC column.

3. Add 3–4 μL of concentrated monomer to 100 μL of PBS and serially dilute three- or fourfold across the row. If available, include a biotinylated monomeric MHC class I-peptide complex added into wells with and without W6/32 as controls.
4. Wash 6× with PBS. Add 100 μL of avidin-HRP (1:2000 dilution) and incubate for 20 min at room temperature.
5. Wash 6× with PBS and develop with the appropriate HRP colorimetric reagent.
6. Estimate concentration by measuring the A at the relevant wavelength.

### 3.7. Tetramerization of MHC Class I-Peptide Monomers

1. From the estimated protein concentration of monomeric complexes, calculate the amount of streptavidin conjugate to give a 4:1 molar ratio of biotinylated monomer to streptavidin (*see* **Note 11**).
2. Add tenths of the calculated streptavidin volume at a time in 20-min intervals while rotating at 4°C.
3. Store at 4°C in the dark.

### 3.8. Cell Staining and Flow Cytometry

Fluorochrome-conjugated tetramers (*see* **Note 12**) are incubated with cell populations, and the tetramer-reactive cells can be visualized on a FACS machine.

1. One half to a million of PBMC are washed once in FACS wash buffer PBA and spun at 176*g* for 5 min.
2. Resuspend the cell pellet in 50 μL of PBA, add approx 1 μg of tetramer and incubate at 37°C for 20 min.
3. Add appropriate amount of conjugated anti-CD8 antibody and incubate on ice for a further 20 min (*see* **Note 13**).
4. Wash 3× with PBA buffer.

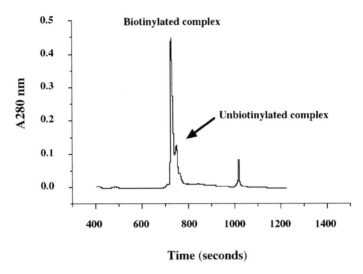

Fig. 3. Separation of biotinylated and unbiotinylated forms of refolded monomeric MHC class I complexes on an anion-exchange column.

5. Resuspend in 300–500 µL of FACS FIX.
6. Analyze on a FACS machine.

## 4. Notes

1. For more precise information regarding the cloning of individual HLA molecules, e.g. primer sequences, refer to the methods section of papers.
2. Human $\beta_2$-m can be used instead of rhesus macaque $\beta_2$-m to make macaque tetramers. Human $\beta_2$-m is generally used instead of mouse $\beta_2$-m in the construction of mouse tetramers, as it binds more strongly to the mouse heavy chain.
3. 15% glycerol stocks of the transformed bacteria can be made by inoculating a small (5 mL) vol of LB medium with a bacterial colony and culturing overnight at 37°C. Glycerol stocks should be stored at –70°C.
4. As protein expression might vary between MHC molecules, inoculate as many 1L flasks as required. Expression might range from 10–60 mg per L after purification.
5. In the protocol described, urea buffer at pH 6.5 is used. Alternatively, urea buffer at pH 8 (8 $M$ urea, 0.1 $M$ NaH$_2$PO$_4$, 0.01 $M$ Tris-HCl, pH 8, 0.1 m$M$ EDTA, 0.1 m$M$ DTT) can be used. The optimal pH is empirically determined. For example, check whether the protein precipitates less in the refold buffer with one pH compared to the other.
6. One-mL aliquots of purified protein are made because repeated freeze-thawing of a large volume-stock will result in increased degradation/precipitation of the protein stock upon each freeze-thaw cycle.
7. Direct addition of protein to the refold buffer may result in large amounts of the protein precipitating out. If this occurs, add approx 2–3 mL of refold buffer dropwise into the aliquot of heavy chain before adding the diluted sample to the large refold flask.
8. Adding smaller aliquots of heavy chain reduces the formation of aggregates of heavy chain thus allowing optimal accessibility to $\beta_2$-m and peptide.

9. EDTA should not be added to the biotinylation mix as this will inhibit the BirA enzymatic reaction.
10. The relative positions of the peaks containing the biotinylated and non-biotinylated monomers depend on the particular MHC-class I complex. Therefore, collect both peaks and check for biotinylation using the ELISA method described in **Subheading 3.6.**
11. Calculation of amount of streptavidin required for tetramerization: for every 1 mg of monomer, add 0.812 mg of streptavidin-PE.
12. Other fluorochromes, such as fluoroscein or anthophycocyanin, have also been used, but PE remains the fluorochrome of choice as it stains more brightly.
13. Other surface markers can also be used in conjunction for further characterization of the antigen-specific cells.

## Acknowledgments

The authors would like to thank Dr. Graham Ogg for his initial guidance. Both RVS and TH are supported by Medical Research Council of the United Kingdom.

## References

1. Altman, J. D., Moss, P. A. H., Goulder, P. J. R., Barouch, D. H., McHeyzer-Williams, M. G., Bell, J. I., et al. (1996) Phenotypic Analysis of Antigen-Specific T Lymphocytes. *Science* **274,** 94–96.
2. McMichael, A. J. and O'Callaghan, C. A. (1998) A new look at T cells *J. Exp. Med.* **187,** 1367–1371.
3. Tan, L. C., Gudgeon, N., Annels, N. E., Hansasuta, P., O'Callaghan, C. A., Rowland-Jones, S., et al. (1999) A re-evaluation of the frequency of CD8+ T cells specific for EBV in healthy virus carriers. *J. Immunol.* **162,** 1817–1835.
4. Sambrook, J., Fritsch, E. F., and Maniatis, T. (1989) *Molecular Cloning: A Laboratory Manual.* Cold Spring Harbor Laboratory, Cold Spring Harbor, NY.
5. Coligan, J. E., Kruisbeek, A. M., Marguiles, D. M., Shevach, E. M., and Strober, W. (1994) *Current Protocols in Immunology*, John Wiley & Sons, USA.
6. Brodsky, F. M. and Parham, P. (1982) Monomorphic anti-HLA-A,B,C monoclonal antibodies detecting molecular subunits and combinatorial determinants. *J. Immunol.* **128,** 129–135.
7. Hanke, T., Samuel, R. V., Blanchard, T. J., Neumann, V. C., Allen, T. M., Boyson, J. E., et al. (2000) Effective induction of SIV-specific CTL in Macaques using a multi-epitope gene and DNA-prime MVA-boost vaccination regimen. *J. Virol.* **73,** 7524–7532.

# 18

## Assessment of Functional Antibody Responses

### Ray Borrow and Paul Balmer

## 1. Introduction

For more than a century, humoral immunity has been recognized as the principal mechanism of defense against most bacterial infections. To evaluate the immunogenicity of vaccines, a variety of assays may be employed, although it is essential that the assay of choice should be a good surrogate for clinical protection. Both radioimmunoassay (RIA) and enzyme-linked immunosorbent assay (ELISA) accurately measure antibody levels to capsular polysaccharide and other antigens, for example, but these assays do not measure functional antibodies, and although useful, care is needed to ascertain that there are strong correlations with an appropriate functional assay. Problems may be encountered with antigen purity (1), which may be overcome with the use of highly purified antigens or adsorbing out crossreactive determinants, or low-avidity antibodies overcome by the use of chaotrophs (2).

Ultimately, a functional assay is required in order to validate these other laboratory surrogates, and this will allow parallels to be drawn with clinical protection. If good correlates are proven, then immunogenicity, backed with safety data, may be used instead of efficacy trials for the licensure of new vaccines. Recently, this was the case in the United Kingdom, where meningococcal serogroup C conjugate (MCC) vaccines were introduced, a decision underpinnned by immunogenicity data derived from serum bactericidal antibody titers (3).

Functional assays are utilized widely for measurement of immune responses to vaccines. For viral antibodies—for example, measles—these have been measured by testing end point serial dilutions of serum for hemagglutination-inhibition or virus neutralization using cytopathic effect induced by highly adapted measles virus (4) or by plaque reduction neutralization assays (5).

From: *Methods in Molecular Medicine, Vol. 87: Vaccine Protocols, 2nd ed.*
Edited by: A. Robinson, M. J. Hudson, and M. P. Cranage © Humana Press Inc., Totowa, NJ

This chapter focuses on two topical bioassays, a serum bactericidal assay for *Neisseria meningitidis* serogroup C and an opsonophagocytic assay for *Streptococcus pneumoniae*. Polysaccharide-protein conjugate vaccines have or are presently being introduced into the immunization schedules of various countries to prevent disease caused by these two bacteria.

## 1.1. Serum Bactericidal Assay for Serogroup C Meningococcal Vaccines

For meningococci, the role of circulating antibody and complement in protection from meningococcal disease was demonstrated in the 1960s *(6)*, and serum bactericidal antibody activity has been shown to highly correlate with immunity to meningococcal disease *(6,7)*. An inverse correlation was observed between the age-related incidence of disease and the age-specific prevalence of complement-dependent serum bactericidal activity *(6)*. Therefore, the induction of bactericidal antibodies after vaccination with meningococcal serogroup C polysaccharide or protein-polysaccharide conjugate vaccines is regarded as acceptable evidence of the potential efficacy of these vaccines *(8)*. In 1976, the World Health Organization (WHO) Expert Committee on Biological Standardization recommended a serum bactericidal assay (SBA) to meet the requirements for production and release of meningococcal polysaccharide vaccine *(9)*. A recent multi-laboratory study standardized the meningococcal serogroup C SBA and compared it to the recommended WHO procedure *(10)*. The standardized assay and the WHO-recommended assay differed only by selection of the target strains, growth of the target strains, and the final well volume of serum employed in the assay method. This assay was recently readdressed, with some further modifications suggested *(11)*. This modified assay will facilitate inter-laboratory comparisons of the functional antibody produced in response to current or developing MCC vaccines.

The original serological correlate of protection in military recruits was obtained using an SBA in which human sera was the exogenous source of complement (hSBA). However, because of difficulties with availability of suitable human sera, 3–4-wk-old baby rabbit serum is now recommended as an alternative complement source for the SBA (rSBA) *(10)*. It is generally accepted, however, that serogroup C meningococci are more susceptible to serogroup C-specific antibodies when using baby rabbit complement as opposed to human complement, resulting in higher SBA titers *(10)*. In the United Kingdom, correlates of protection for MCC vaccines have been re-evaluated with SBA titers as measured with baby rabbit complement (rSBA), being compared with titers using human complement (hSBA) as the "gold standard" *(3)*. This showed that rSBA titers of <8 predicted susceptibility and rSBA titers ≥128 predicted protection as measured by hSBA. The main uncertainty was therefore interpretation of rSBA titers between 8 and 64. In these cases, it was proposed that additional serological criteria would be required for presumption of protection, namely a fourfold rise in rSBA titer and/or demonstration of immunologic memory as evidenced by a typical booster response to a polysaccharide challenge and IgG-affinity maturation *(3)*. The main group of vaccinated individuals in whom substantial proportions had rSBA titers in the 8–64 range were toddlers age 12–14 mo and, to a lesser extent, preschool children age 3–4 yr. Both groups had received a single dose of MCC vaccine as part of the national catch-up program *(12)*. However, almost all toddlers with post-vaccination titers in the rSBA 8–64 equivocal range met the additional serological criteria required for presumption of protection *(3)*. The United Kingdom enhanced MCC surveillance program has subsequently allowed these proposed rSBA correlates of protection to be validated against the efficacy estimates obtained for MCC vaccines from post-licensure surveillance. Using age-specific vaccine efficacy estimates, and the percentage of vaccinated and unvaccinated individuals in different age groups with rSBA levels above various cut-offs, the most consistent predictor of protection for MCC vaccines is a cut-off of 1:4 or 1:8 as measured by rSBA *(13)*.

## 1.2. Opsonophagocytosis Assay for S. pneumoniae Vaccines

*S. pneumoniae* is an important bacterial pathogen of both children and adults worldwide. Host protection against invasive pneumococcal disease is primarily mediated by phagocytosis, requiring the presence of opsonic antibodies and an activated complement cascade *(14,15)*. Therefore, it is considered that an antibody titer determined by an in vitro opsonophagocytic assay (OPA) may be useful as a surrogate marker for protection against invasive pneumococcal disease.

The early OPAs were performed with fresh peripheral blood leukocytes (PBLs) as effector cells, and a variety of techniques—such as radioisotopic, flow cytometric, microscopic, and viability assays—were used to determine opsonophagocytic activity *(15–23)*. However, these assays are limited by the lack of standardization because of the variability in reagents preventing inter-laboratory comparison of opsonophagocytic titers. To overcome these problems, a standardized OPA for the measurement of functional antibody activity using differentiated HL-60 cells (human promyelocytic leukemia cells) and baby rabbit complement was established *(24)*. The use of cultured phagocytes eliminates the need for fresh PBLs and decreases the inter-assay variability that occurs with random PBL donors. The phagocytic activity of differentiated HL-60 cells is comparable to that of PBLs and the reproducibility of the OPA with HL-60 cells was found to be within one dilution of the median for most serotypes and serogroups of *S. pneumoniae* tested *(24)*. Complement-mediated opsonophagocytosis is dependent upon the level of expression of the appropriate cell-surface receptors. Differentiated HL-60 cells were found to have a similar pattern of expression of cell-surface receptors to that of PBL isolated from human donors *(24)*. The levels of expression of $Fc\gamma II$, CR1, and CD15 were comparable, but differentiated HL-60 cells express lower levels of $Fc\gamma I$, $Fc\gamma III$, and CR3. Although CR3 is considered to be one of the primary cell-surface receptors involved in opsonophagocytosis, the high effector cell:target-cell ratio used in the OPA appears to offset the low expression of CR3 by differentiated HL-60 cells. A multi-specific OPA has been developed using antibiotic-resistant pneumococci *(25)*. This reduces the volume of test sera required and increases the throughput of the assay, but there are obvious concerns about the use of antibiotic-resistant pneumococci and the simultaneous analysis of related serotypes (e.g., serotypes 6A and 6B or serotypes 9V and 9N).

The standardized OPA has been further developed to a rapid, semi-automated flow-cytometric OPA, which minimizes the handling of viable bacteria and is not influenced by the presence of penicillin in the test sera *(26)*. The flow-cytometric OPA utilizes nonviable *S. pneumoniae* labeled with 5,6-carboxyfluoroscein succinimidyl ester as bacterial targets and differentiated HL-60 cells as the effector-cells. For each sample, plus an effector cell control and baby rabbit complement control, the percent *S. pneumoniae* uptake for each dilution is plotted, and the opsonophagocytic titer is given as 50% of the maximal phagocytosis. The flow-cytometric OPA was found to be reproducible and serotype-specific with low crossreactivity, and had a good correlation with the manual, standardized OPA, which utilizes viable colony counts. The semi-automation of the OPA increases the daily throughput to approx 50 test sera per operator and decreased the assay time to approx 4 h. It is important to note that the level of capsular polysaccharide expression appears to influence the level of opsonophagocytosis; opaque pneumococci have 1.2–5.6-fold greater quantities of capsular polysaccharide than transparent pneumococci, and are more resistant to opsonophagocytosis *(26,27)*.

Determination of opsonophagocytic activity appears to be an appropriate serological correlate of protection because both natural and vaccine-induced immunity are mediated by the opsonic activity of anti-capsular polysaccharide antibodies. However, the flow-cytometric standardized OPA is still relatively labor-intensive and requires cell-culture facilities that make it unsuitable for large-scale immunogenicity studies of current and new pneumococcal vaccines. A standardized ELISA to detect anti-pneumococcal capsular polysaccharide IgG levels has been established *(28–31)*. Since the OPA detects functional antibody that has been reported to correlate well with serotype-specific vaccine efficacy *(32)*, there must be a sufficient correlation between the OPA and ELISA. The correlation between the OPA and the ELISA is serotype-specific *(33)*, but has been improved by adsorbing sera with pneumococcal C-polysaccharide and pneumococcal serotype 22F polysaccharide to remove nonfunctional antibodies *(34)*. This gives the antibody concentrations detected by ELISA a stronger correlation to the functional antibodies detected by OPA.

A seven-valent pneumococcal polysaccharide conjugate vaccine (Prev(e)nar®) has been recently licensed in the United States and United Kingdom. Immunogenicity studies of Prev(e)nar® in the United States demonstrated that an antibody level of 0.15 µg/mL correlated with the vaccine efficacy of 97.4% *(35,36)*. To date, a specific opsonophagocytic titer has not been defined as a predicted level of protection.

Recently, a multiplex OPA has been developed for *N. meningitidis* serogroups A, C, Y, and W-135 using capsular polysaccharide coated to beads with different fluorescent spectra *(37)*. Opsonophagocytosis of the beads by HL-60 cells is analyzed by flow cytometry, and has been shown to correlate well to the SBA. However, it must be noted that the multiplex OPA is capsular polysaccharide-specific, and does not measure the contribution of the response to other surface molecules such as outer membrane proteins (OMPs). This technique has the obvious advantage of not using viable bacteria, and can analyze multiple targets from one sample. A similar protocol is under development for *S. pneumoniae*, but the conjugation of the capsular polysaccharide to the beads is more complex than for meningococcal polysaccharides. The increased numbers of desired targets will also increase the complexity of the flow-cytometric analysis.

### 1.3. Principle of the Neisseria meningitidis SBA

This chapter describes in detail the SBA used for detection of functional antibody response to MCC vaccines.

Serogroup C target strains are lysed in the presence of meningococcal-specific antibody and complement (antibody-mediated, complement-dependent killing). Serial dilutions of human sera are incubated with appropriate target strains and complement. The serum bactericidal titer for each unknown serum is expressed as the reciprocal serum dilution, yielding ≥50% killing as compared to the total number of target.

## 2. Materials
### 2.1. Serum Samples

1. A positive serum sample of known SBA titer should be assayed on each run. Quality-control sera should be collected by the testing laboratories. The Centers for Disease Control and Prevention (CDC, Atlanta, GA, USA) can provide a limited amount of QC sera. A standard reference serum (CDC1992) collected from adults immunized with a quadrivalent polysaccharide vaccine is available from the National Institute for Biological Standards and Control (NIBSC, Blanche Lane, South Mimms, Potters Bar, Herts, UK) *(38)*.
2. The minimum volume of serum needed is 25 µL. This volume will allow one measurement of bactericidal activity for each serum.
3. Serum samples to be assayed should be stored frozen at –70°C and not be freeze/thawed more than 4×.

### 2.2. Bacteria

*See* **Note 1** for storage of strain aliquots.

The Serogroup C target strain, C11 (phenotype C:16:P1.7ᵃ,1) (also known as 60E) *(6)* may be obtained from the Food and Drug Administration (Rockville, MD, USA), the ATCC (10801 University Blvd., Manassas, VA, USA), CDC or Health Protection Agency (HPA) Meningococcal Reference Unit (Manchester, UK).

### 2.3. Rabbit Complement

Pooled baby rabbit serum (Pel Freeze Inc, Brown Deer, Wisconsin, USA; distributors in the UK are MAST Group Ltd., Mast House, Derby Road, Bootle, Merseyside, L20 1EA) may be used for serogroup C SBA. Keep at –70°C and transport on dry ice. Aliquot bottles, which must only be defrosted for a minimum of time, into small volumes (1–3 mL) that must also be kept frozen at –70°C and defrosted only immediately prior to use. If thawed, complement must be refrozen, quick freeze with ethanol and dry ice is recommended. New lots of rabbit complement must be assayed with low, medium, and high QC sera (*see* **Subheading 2.1.**), and titers must fall within one dilution either side of the established SBA titer. Previously tested sera (in addition to QCs) may also be assayed with titers being within one dilution of their previously established SBA titer. Assays should be performed in duplicate for this validation. All normal controls should still be checked.

### 2.4. Bactericidal Buffer

A variety of bactericidal buffers is available, and either of the following may be used. With all new batches of bactericidal buffer it should be determined that there is no decrease in viable cell count after 60 min.

1. Gey's balanced salts solution (Gibco BRL, Cat. no. 24260-028 or equivalent) with 0.5% bovine serum albumin (BSA, fraction V) (Sigma, Cat. no. A7906 or equivalent). Filter-sterilize (0.22 μm) and store at +4°C.
2. Dulbecco's PBS containing 0.5 m$M$ MgCl$_2$ and 0.9 m$M$ CaCl$_2$, pH 7.4 (Life Technologies, Cat. no. 14080 or equivalent) with 0.1% glucose (Sigma, Cat. no. G7528, or equivalent). Filter-sterilize (0.22 μm) and store at +4°C.
3. Hank's balanced salt solution (HBSS), pH 7.2, containing 4 m$M$ NaHCO$_3$ (Gibco-BRL, Cat. no. 14175-046 or equivalent) and 0.1% BSA (fraction V) (Sigma, Cat. no. A7906 or equivalent). Filter-sterilize (0.22 μm) and store at +4°C.

### 2.5. Agar Plates

1. Blood agar (Blood agar base no. 2 with defibrinated horse blood (5%), Oxoid, Cat. no. CM331 or equivalent.)
2. Brain heart infusion agar (Becton Dickenson, Cat. no. 4311065 or equivalent) with 1% horse serum (Life Technologies, Cat. no. 16050-098 or equivalent).

### 2.6. 96-Well Tissue-Culture Plates

1. U-bottomed plates are recommended, as small volumes collect at the center of each well, making plating out more facile.
2. 96-well U-bottomed tissue-culture plates (Sterilin, Cat. no. 611U96 or equivalent).

### 2.7. Specialized Equipment

1. Appropriate microbiological safety cabinet (Biosafety level 2 safety cabinet).
2. Colony counter (for "tilt" method) (Perceptive Instruments, Haverhill, Suffolk, UK or equivalent). (A modification of the Cardinal Automatic Colony Counting System).
3. Spectrophotometer. For adjusting meningococcal cell suspensions.
4. Incubators. Both +37°C incubators and 5% CO$_2$, +37°C incubators are required.

## 3. Methods

### 3.1. Safety

#### 3.1.1. Sera

All human sera may contain human immunodeficiency virus (HIV), Hepatitis B virus, and/or other human pathogens. Use universal precautions when handling any specimen from a human source. Immunization with Hepatitis B vaccine is highly recommended.

#### 3.1.2. N. meningitidis Isolates

Biosafety level 2 practices are generally recommended when working with *N. meningitidis*. However, the potential for generating aerosols using this bactericidal

**Table 1**
**Microtitration Plate Template**

| Assay | 1 | 2 | 3 | 4 | 5 | 6 | 7 | 8 | 9 | 10 | 11 | 12 |
|---|---|---|---|---|---|---|---|---|---|---|---|---|
| Bactericidal buffer | 20 | 20 | 20 | 20 | 20 | 20 | 20 | 20 | 20 | 20 | 20 | *See* below |
| Patient serum (µL) | Nine twofold serial serum dilutions Transfer 20 µL from columns 1–9, mix 6×, and discard 20 µL from column ≠9 | | | | | | | | | 0 | 0 | |
| Complement (µL) | 10 | 10 | 10 | 10 | 10 | 10 | 10 | 10 | 10 | 10 | 10* | |
| Cells (µL) | 10 | 10 | 10 | 10 | 10 | 10 | 10 | 10 | 10 | 10 | 10 | |
| Final volume (µL) | 40 | 40 | 40 | 40 | 40 | 40 | 40 | 40 | 40 | 40 | 40 | |
| Reciprocal final serum dilution | 4 | 8 | 16 | 32 | 64 | 128 | 256 | 512 | 1024 | | | |

Column ≠12: Add 10 µL of bactericidal buffer, 10 µL of heat-inactivated serum, 10 µL of heat-inactivated complement and 10 µL of working solution of organisms (*see* **Note 2**).
  Column ≠11: * heat-inactivated complement.

procedure increases the risk of exposure, so biosafety level 3 practices should be considered, and an appropriate microbiological safety cabinet is essential. Immunization with serogroup C protein-polysaccharide conjugate vaccine should be considered but should only be used with, and not in place of, the previous recommendations.

### 3.2. Day 1

1. Preparation of target strain
   An aliquot of the target strain should be defrosted and plated out overnight at 37°C with 5% $CO_2$ on blood agar or brain heart infusion (with 1% horse serum) agar.

### 3.3. Day 2

1. Approximately 10–20 meningococcal colonies are picked from the overnight culture and spread out over an agar plate and cultured for 3–4 h at 37°C with 5% $CO_2$.
2. After 4 h, working in the safety cabinet, cells are suspended in bactericidal buffer at an optical density (OD) of 0.1 at 650 nm, with a cuvet of path length 10 mm. The cell suspension is then diluted in 5 mL bactericidal buffer (*see* **Subheading 2.4.**) to yield approx 50–60 colony-stimulating unit (CFU)/10 μL. Fill wells of columns 1–11 of a sterile U-bottomed 96-well plate with 20 μL of bactericidal buffer (equilibrated to room temperature). Add 10 μL of buffer to column 12. *See* **Table 1** for microtitration plate template.
3. Following the template, add 20 μL of each heat inactivated (56°C for 30 min) serum to the rows in column 1. Using a multi-channel pipet, serially dilute the 8 test sera twofold in the microtiter wells by removing 20 μL from the wells of column 1, transferring to the wells of column 2, and mixing 6×. Continue diluting through to column 9. Withdraw 20 μL from column 9 and discard.
4. Add 10 μL of test serum (heat-inactivated) to the corresponding well of column 12.
5. Add 10 μL of the working solution of bacteria to every well.
6. Add 10 μL of heat-inactivated (56°C for 30 min) complement to all wells of columns 11 and 12.
7. Add 10 μL of complement (removed 10 min previously from the –70°C freezer) to columns 1 to 10 and gently tap plates to mix.
8. Using the "tilt" method, plate out 10 μL from all wells of column 11 to determine $T_0$. For the "tilt" method, the agar plate is tilted through 45°C to allow the drops to run down the plate.
9. Seal the plates with plate sealers before transferring to the 37°C incubator.
10. Incubate the plates for 1 h at 37°C (without $CO_2$).
11. 10 μL drops are plated out from every well, using the tilt method, and incubated overnight at 37°C with 5% $CO_2$ for $T_{60}$.

### 3.4. Day 3

1. Count the number of colonies for $T_0$ and $T_{60}$. The number of colonies in column 11 is the number of viable cells. Column 12 is a test for complement-independent killing (*see* **Note 2**). Column 10 is a complement control (*see* **Note 3**).
2. The serum bactericidal titer is reported as the reciprocal serum dilution yielding ≥50% killing at $T_{60}$ as compared with the number of viable cells.
3. In order to assign a titer, the following conditions must be met:
   a. Target cell growth in column 12 (the serum control well) is ≥80% of the CFU in column 11.

b. The test serum must have a clearly defined SBA titer. In order to assign a titer at 50% reduction in CFU, at least two consecutive serial dilutions of the test serum must have a cell count <20% of the CFU per well compared to the CFU in column 11.

Serum, which does not fulfill condition 3(a) should be retested. If growth in the serum control well is <20% of the CFU per well compared to the CFU in column 11 after repeat testing, then the titer must be reported as "Not determined due to reduction in the control well."

A serum that does not fulfill condition 3(b) should be retested. If there are not at least two consecutive serial dilutions of the test serum with cell counts <20%, then the titer should be reported as <8.

Sera that give >50% of CFU per well compared to the CFU in column 11 in the test serial dilution must be reported to have a SBA titer of <4.

## 4. Notes

1. Target Strain Stocks. Multiple aliquots (0.5 mL) of the target strain(s) must be stored to prevent subculturing. Recommended storage medium is Glycerol Broth (Nutrient Broth (Becton Dickenson, Cat. no. 4311479 or equivalent) with 15% in glycerol). The stock of glycerol broth was prepared by taking a swab of an overnight meningococcal culture from a blood agar plate or brain heart infusion (with 1% horse serum) plate and emulsifying in the glycerol broth to make a heavy suspension. This is then aliquoted into 0.5 mL volumes in sterile plastic vials and immediately stored frozen at –70°C.

2. Decrease in CFU in Column 12. Column 12 is a control column to measure noncomplement-mediated lysis of cells. Serum samples may contain antibiotics, and as a result, the number of CFUs in column 12 is decreased. The β lactam family (containing penicillin) can be overcome with the use of β lactamase (Merck Ltd., Cat. no. 39084 3G or equivalent). The dilution in this serum control well must always be 1:4, regardless of the initial dilution in the serial diluted serum wells. The serum used in this control well must be heat-inactivated.

3. Decrease in CFU in Column 10. Column 10 is a control column to measure the complement resistance of the target strain. If the number of CFUs decreases as compared with column 11, this is as a result of the target strain becoming complement-sensitive.

## References

1. Sikkema, D. J., Friedman, K. E., Corsaro, B., Kimura, A., Hildreth, S. W., Madore, D. V., et al. (2000) Relationship between serum bactericidal activity and serogroup-specific immunoglobulin G concentration for adults, toddlers, and infants immunized with *Neisseria meningitidis* serogroup C vaccines. *Clin. Diagn. Lab. Immunol.* **7,** 764–768.

2. Granoff, D. M., Maslanka, S. E., Carlone, G. M., Plikaytis, B. D., Santos, G. F., Mokatrin, A., et al. (1998) A modified enzyme-linked immunosorbent assay for measurement of antibody responses to meningococcal C polysaccharide that correlate with bactericidal responses. *Clin. Diagn. Lab. Immunol.* **5,** 479–485.

3. Borrow, R., Andrews, N., Goldblatt, D., and Miller, E. (2001) Serological basis for use of meningococcal serogroup C conjugate vaccines in the United Kingdom: a re-evaluation of correlates of protection. *Infect. Immun.* **69,** 1568–1573.

4. Enders-Ruckle, G. (1965) Methods of determining immunity, duration and character of immunity resulting from measles. *Arch. Virusforsch* **16,** 182–207.

5. Albrecht, P., Herrmann, K., and Burns, G. R. (1981) Role of virus strain in conventional and enhanced measles plaque neutralization test. *J. Virol. Methods* **3,** 251–260.

6. Gotschlich, E. C., Goldschneider, I., and Artenstein M. S. (1969) Human immunity to the meningococcus IV. Immunogenicity of serogroup A and serogroup C polysaccharides in human volunteers. *J. Exp. Med.* **129,** 1367–1384.

7. Goldschneider, I., Gotschlich, E. C., and Artenstein, M. S. (1969) Human immunity to the meningococcus II. Development of natural immunity. *J. Exp. Med.* **129,** 1327–1348.

8. Goldschneider, I., Gotschlich, E. C., and Artenstein, M. S. (1969) Human immunity to the meningococcus. I. The role of humoral antibodies. *J. Exp. Med.* **129,** 1307–1326.

9. World Health Organization (1976) Requirements for meningococcal polysaccharide vaccine. World Health Organization technical report series, no. 594. World Health Organization, Geneva.

10. Maslanka, S. E., Gheesling, L. L., LiButti, D. E., Donaldson, K. B. J., Harakeh, H. S., Dykes, J. K., et al. (1997) Standardization and a multilaboratory comparison of *Neisseria meningitidis* serogroup A and C serum bactericidal assays. *Clin. Diagn. Lab. Immunol.* **4,** 156–167.

11. Borrow, R. and Carlone, G. M. (2001) Serogroup B and C serum bactericidal assays. In: Meningococcal Vaccines. *Methods in Molecular Medicine,* (Pollard, A. J. and Maiden, M. C. J., eds.). 2001. Humana Press, Totowa, NJ, pp. 289–304.

12. Miller, E., Salisbury, D., and Ramsay, M. (2002) Planning, registration, and implementation of an immunisation campaign against meningococcal serogroup C disease in the UK: a success story. *Vaccine* **20,** S58–S67.

13. Andrews, N., Borrow, R., and Miller, E. Validation of serological correlate of protection for meningococcal C conjugate vaccine using efficacy estimates from post-licensure surveillance in England. Submitted to *Clin. Diag. Lab. Immunol.*

14. Musher, D., Chapman, A. J., Goree, A., Jonsson, S., Briles, D. E., and Baughn, R. E. (1986) Natural and vaccine-related immunity to *Streptococcus pneumoniae. J. Infect. Dis.* **154,** 245–256.

15. Vioarsson, G., Jonsdottir, I., Jonsson, S., and Validmarsson, H. (1994) Opsonisation and antibodies to capsular and cell wall polysaccharides of *Streptococcus pneumoniae. J. Infect. Dis.* **170,** 592–599.

16. De Velasco, A. E., Verheul, A. F. M., Van Steijn, A. M. P., Dekker, H. A. T., Feldman, R. G., Fernandez, I. M., et al. (1994) Epitope specificity of rabbit immunoglobulin G (IgG) elicited by pneumococcal type 23F synthetic oligosaccharide and native polysaccharide-protein conjugate vaccines: comparison with human anti-polysaccharide 23F IgG. *Infect. Immun.* **62,** 799–808.

17. Esposito, A. L., Clark, C. A., and Poirier, W. J. (1990) An assessment of the factors contributing to the killing of type 3 *Streptococcus pneumoniae* by human polymorphonuclear leukocytes in vitro. *APMIS* **98,** 111–121.

18. Guckian, J. C., Christensen, G. D., and Fine, D. P. (1980) Role of opsonins in recovery from experimental pneumococcal pneumonia. *J. Infect. Dis.* **142,** 175–190.

19. Kaniuk, A., Lortan, J. E., and Monteil, M. A. (1992) Specific IgG subclass antibody levels and phagocytosis of serotype 14 pneumococcus following immunization. *Scand. J. Immunol.* **36 (Suppl. 11),** 96–98.

20. Lortan, J. E., Kaniuk, A. S., and Monteil, M. A. (1993) Relationship of an in vitro phagocytosis of serotype 14 *Streptococcus pneumoniae* to specific class and IgG subclass antibody levels in healthy adults. *Clin. Diagn. Lab. Immunol.* **91,** 54–57.

21. Obaro, S. K., Henderson, D. C., and Monteil, M. A. (1996) Defective antibody-mediated opsonisation of S. pneumoniae in high risk patients detected by flow cytometry. *Immunol. Lett.* **49,** 83–89.

22. Sveum, R. J., Chused, T. M., Frank, M. M. and Brown, E. J. (1986) A quantitative fluorescent method for measurement of bacterial adherence and phagocytosis. *J. Immunol. Methods* **90,** 257–264.

23. Wilkelstein, J. A., Smith, M. R., and Shin, H. S. (1975) The role of C3 as an opsonin in the early stages of infection. *Proc. Soc. Exp. Biol. Med.* **149,** 397–401.

24. Romero-Steiner, S., Libutti, D., Pais, L. B., Dykes, J., Anderson, P., Whitin, J. C., et al. (1997) Standardization of an opsonophagocytic assay for the measurement of functional antibody activity against *Streptococcus pneumoniae* using differentiated HL-60 cells. *Clin. Diagn. Lab. Immunol.* **4,** 415–422.

25. Nahm, M. H., Briles, D. E., and Yu, X. (2000) Development of a multi-specificity opsonophagocytic killing assay. *Vaccine* **18,** 2768–2771.

26. Martinez, J. E., Romero-Steiner, S., Pilishvili, T., Barnard, S., Schinsky, J., Goldblatt, D., et al. (1999) A flow cytometric opsonophagocytic assay for measurement of functional antibodies elicited after vaccination with the 23-valent pneumococcal polysaccharide vaccine. *Clin. Diagn. Lab. Immunol.* **6,** 581–586.

27. Kim, J. O., Romero-Steiner, S., Sorensen, U. B. S., Blom, J., Carvalho, M., Barnard, S., et al. (1999) Relationship between cell surface carbohydrates and intrastrain variation on opsonophagocytosis of *Streptococcus pneumoniae*. *Infect. Immun.* **67,** 2327–2333.

28. Koskela, M. (1987) Serum antibodies to pneumococcal C polysaccharide in children: response to acute pneumococcal otitis media or to vaccination. *Pediatr. Infect. Dis J.* **6,** 519–526.

29. Quataert, S. A., Kirsch, C., Wiedl, L. J., Phipps, D. C., Strohmeyer, S., Cimino, C.O., et al. (1995) Assignment of weight based antibody units to human pneumococcal standard reference serum. *Clin. Diagn. Lab. Immunol.* **2,** 590–597.

30. Siber, G. R., Priehs, C., and Madore, D. (1989) Standardization of antibody assays for measuring the response to pneumococcal infection and immunization. *Pediatr. Res.* **8,** S84–S91.

31. Phipps, D. C., Strohmeyer, S., Quataert, S. A., Siber, G., and Madore, D. V. (1990) Standardization of ELISA for the quantitation of antibodies to S. pneumoniae capsular polysaccharides (PnPs). *Pediatr. Res.* **27,** 179A.

32. Wenger, J. D., Steiner, S. R., Pais, L. B., Butler, J. C., Perkins, B., Carlone, G. M., et al. (1996) Laboratory correlates for protective efficacy of pneumococcal vaccines: how can they be identified and validated? Abstr. G37, p150, in Program and abstracts of the 36th Interscience Conference on Antimicrobial Agents and Chemotherapy. American Society for Microbiology, Washington, DC.

33. Vernacchio, L., Romero-Steiner, S., Martinez, J. E., MacDonald, K., Barnard, S., Pilishvili, T., et al. (2000) Comparison of an opsonophagocytic assay and IgG ELISA to assess responses to pneumococcal polysaccharide and pneumococcal conjugate vaccines in children and young adults with sickle cell disease. *J. Infect. Dis.* **181,** 1162–1166.

34. Concepcion, N. F. and Frasch, C. E. (2001) Pneumococcal type 23F absorption improves the specificity of a pneumococcal-polysaccharide enzyme-linked immunosorbent assay. *Clin. Diagn. Lab. Immunol.* **8,** 266–272.

35. Shinefield, H.R., Black, S., Ray, P., Chang, I.H., Lewis, N., Fireman, B., et al. (1999) Safety and immunogenicity of heptavalent pneumococcal $CRM_{197}$ conjugate vaccine in infants and toddlers. *Pediatr. Infect. Dis. J.* **18,** 757–763.

36. Black, S. B., Shinefield, H. R., Hansen, J., Elvin, L., Lauffer, D., and Malinoski, F. (2001) Post licensure evaluation of the effectiveness of seven valent pneumococcal conjugate vaccine. *Pediatr. Infect. Dis. J.* **20,** 1105–1107.

37. Martinez, J., Pilishvili, T., Barnard, S., Caba, J., Spear, W., Romero-Steiner, S., et al. (2002) Opsonophagocytosis of fluorescent polystyrene beads coupled to *Neisseria*

*meningitidis* serogroup A, C, Y, or W135 polysaccharide correlates with serum bacteri-cidal activity. *Clin. Diagn. Lab. Immunol.* **9,** 485–488.

38. Holder, P. K., Maslanka, S. E., Pais, L. B., Dykes, J., Plikaytis, B. D., and Carlone, G. M. (1995) Assignment of *Neisseria meningitidis* serogroup A and C class-specific anticapsular antibody concentrations to the new standard reference serum CDC 1992. *Clin. Diagn. Lab. Immunol.* **2,** 132–137.

# 19

## The Use of Complete Genome Sequences in Vaccine Design

### Nigel J. Saunders and Sarah Butcher

## 1. Introduction

### 1.1. Academic and Commercial Approaches

The availability of complete genome sequences offers a new position from which to approach vaccine and drug design. Indeed, in some instances, genome-sequencing projects have been initiated with these motives. It is true that every drug target and vaccine candidate is either coded directly by genes present within the genome or produced by the gene products. It follows that there is extensive information with respect to both protein targets with vaccine potential and the synthesis of other surface components. This is a new field, and the selection of vaccine candidates from genome sequences has not yet generated a new vaccine for use in clinical practice. The way in which this is likely to be approached by commercial and academic groups with different resources and areas of expertise is likely to differ, and to bring various perspectives and strengths to this area of research.

It is not yet clear which approach is likely to be most successful. Certainly, large-scale genome-led screening-orientated approaches, as exemplified by the strategies of commercial companies, are most likely to lead to new candidates in the shortest timeframe if they are successful. Such an approach can be likened to a reverse of the traditional mass-screening procedures that are familiar for antibiotic discovery and other drug-screening processes. In a vaccine-hunting study, many targets are pursued in a way that is similar to that in which a large number of chemicals might be screened against a particular candidate antimicrobial target. However, bacterial surfaces are the product of prolonged evolution in the presence of selective immune responses, and it is possible that organisms that do not typically cause a single infection or colonization

From: *Methods in Molecular Medicine, Vol. 87: Vaccine Protocols, 2nd ed.*
Edited by: A. Robinson, M. J. Hudson, and M. P. Cranage © Humana Press Inc., Totowa, NJ

followed by robust immunity may not yield to the screening-oriented approach. Likewise, the use of single or a small number of genome sequences in vaccine design may result in the identification of a majority of relatively strain-specific antigens that may either result in partial coverage or a vaccine with a short useful life that is compromised by "escape" strains. It may be that the more specific problem-oriented strategies that can be pursued within smaller research groups may yet make seminal progress in this regard. In each instance, the use of complete genome-sequence information can provide a foundation that influences the nature of the questions that can be addressed and the methods that can be used.

## 1.2. The Nature of Genome-Sequence Information

It is important to be clear about the nature of the information that is being used. A genome sequence is the chromosomal sequence of a subculture of an isolate of a strain of a species. It does contain the complete information for the coding potential of the sequenced organism, but this should be regarded as a singular example rather than as a representative set of information for the species. All vaccines must be directed against the entire pathogenic population, and as such, the origin of the sequenced strain and the nature of the population structure and composition must also ultimately be addressed. As more genome-sequenced strains become available from pathogenic species, their combined use will inevitably provide a far more comprehensive and robust framework for this type of investigation. However, they will remain a collection of examples, and many sequences from a single species may be required before we can approach the availability of representative information. This subject and the ways in which it can be addressed are examined later in this chapter, but it should be considered from the outset in any of vaccine design.

## 1.3. Working with Finished and Unfinished Sequences

Strategies vary depending upon whether the investigation will proceed during the sequencing project itself—and thus with sequence information in varying states of completeness—or with finished sequence data. It is important to remember that all sequences and annotations inevitably include errors, and that the reduction in their abundance as a project is completed is probably only one of degree. Clearly, if investigations are to be based on an extension of an existing research and vaccine-development approach, this will determine the way in which the sequence information is addressed. However, regardless of a laboratory's particular strategy, the first step is to address the genome sequence in a way that can identify the information that is potentially useful, and to focus upon this. The potential pitfalls of this process are frequently only evident after the fact, but there are ways in which they can be minimized. However, in the end a process of triage is necessary, in which the bulk of information that will not be pursued is separated from the genes that will be considered in greater detail.

## 1.4. Sources of Error in Sequence Data and Annotations

Most investigators will begin from a position in which one or more fully annotated sequences are available. This provides an important starting framework. However, the approach from a starting point of an annotated and an unannotated sequence should not be very different. All genome annotations are subject to errors derived from a variety of sources. The limits of most coding regions have not been demonstrated experimentally. Point mutations in the sequenced strain (in addition to occasional unresolved sequencing errors) may lead to disruption of the actual open reading frames. Most annotations are based upon similarities to genes that have been already described. As such, they are influenced by what has already been studied and submitted to the databases, and also upon the potentially erroneous interpretation of other researchers. As genomes are increasingly annotated on the basis of similarities to other annotated genome sequences, the possibility for repetition of mistakes increases, and thus the consistent annotation of similar sequences in multiple genomes cannot necessarily be regarded as additional evidence of their veracity. There is also a real danger of "circular annotation catastrophe" in which similarity between a part of "gene A" is used to annotate "gene B," similarity between part of "gene B" and part of "gene C" is used to annotate "gene C"—but when genes A and C are compared, they do not share any significant homology because different parts of the genes were used at each stage of the process. A genome annotation should most healthily be considered to be the "best guess on the basis of the available evidence at the time" of the annotating team. A researcher with a specific interest in a specific pathogen, or pathogen behavior, is likely to have at least as good an insight with regard to their area of expertise as that of the annotation team. So, although it is reasonable to use an annotation as a guide for research, its potential flaws should be considered. Before actually pursuing a gene of interest experimentally, it is necessary to repeat a basic bioinformatic analysis of the sequence of interest, if only to bring such an annotation up to date with respect to new and continually revised public information.

## 2. Selection of Vaccine Candidates From the Genome

The purely genome-led selection of vaccine candidates can be divided into two broad categories. The first—and the one most similar to approaches used prior to the availability of genome sequences—is selection of candidates on the basis of their putative function, which is determined by their similarity to other proteins for which some information is already available. The second strategy is based upon some particular characteristic of a gene that suggests candidature as a vaccine antigen—such as surface location—which can be predicted in the absence of previous knowledge of the function of the encoded protein or its similarity to others. A combination of these two approaches is common, and this is described in the following two sections.

## 3. Evaluation of Potential Gene Function

For a potential coding region of interest, the first step is to evaluate it by a homology method, typically a database similarity search of some type. When the work involves sequence data that are not in the public domain, these searches should not be performed over the Internet, since sending a query sequence to a non-secure public server may be considered a form of public data release that may compromise subsequent patent applications. The particular analyses performed are a matter of personal choice, and the most frequently used are either the BLAST suite of programs (available from:ftp://ncbi.nlm.nih.gov) *(1,2)* or FASTA (available from:ftp://ftp.virginia.edu/pub/fasta/) *(3)*.

## 3.1. BLAST and FASTA

Although programs in both BLAST and FASTA allow the comparison of a query sequence (or sequences) against sequences in a database (or databases), their underlying algorithms and statistical scoring methods differ, and so using both is a reasonable strategy. Equivalent BLAST searches are usually quicker, but FASTA searches can be more sensitive. The first homology analysis should usually be a nucleotide similarity search, such as a BLASTN analysis *(1)*. It should be noted that individual programs within both suites allow the comparison of nucleotide query sequences with nucleotide databases, protein queries with protein databases, or a variety of protein vs protein searches utilizing translation of nucleotide sequences in either query or database (or both) as required. One advantage of performing such a search is that it will reveal whether or not there are matches to sequences on the reverse-complement of the selected strand. This can be important, especially since open reading frames on the reverse-complement of the coding strand can be shown by some prediction methods to contain features of surface proteins based upon characteristics of membrane-spanning regions. A nucleotide search using a high threshold (e.g., >90% identity) is also a useful tool for high specificity, although nucleotide searches are less effective in identifying remote homologs than protein-based searches. It should be remembered that full consideration should be given to the statistical scores provided by the searching programs of choice (e values or Z scores, for instance) and suitable cut-off points selected for determining which matches may have no biological significance. The absolute values selected at this point will depend upon what the search is attempting to accomplish.

The major differences between different protein-based BLAST and FASTA programs are in the ways that frameshifts are handled—either in query or database sequences. As already mentioned, the nucleotide sequence of interest may not be perfect, and missing or additional nucleotides may introduce frameshifts or change the position of stop codons. Similarly, sequences in public databases may also contain sequencing error-induced frameshifts or incorrectly positioned stop codons. A combination of searches against a well-annotated but incomplete database, such as Swissprot *(4)*, and a larger database that may include fully automated annotation (e.g., TrEMBL or Genpept) using amino-acid based searches such as BLASTP, BLASTX (translation of query may reveal frameshift errors in query but not database) and TBLASTN (translation of nucleotide database entries) or equivalents FASTX/Y and TFASTX/Y, can then be used with lower thresholds to perform searches with greater sensitivity. Protein databases in which some level of filtration has been employed to remove redundancy are also useful resources, as these may decrease the likelihood of remote matches being hidden by multiple matches to more closely related proteins. Examples of these include databases built using the NRDB (non-redundant database) utility distributed with the University of Washington's BLAST (http://blast.wustl.edu/pub/nrdb) or NRDB90 (http://www.ebi.ac.uk/~holm/nrdb90/) *(5)*. It is vitally important in all of these searches that query sequences are checked for repeat or low complexity content, and filtered or masked appropriately, to prevent irrelevant matches to these over-represented regions. Suitable programs are an integral part of BLAST and include the DUST program of Tatusov and Lipman used for BLASTN (unpublished), and the SEG program of Wootton and Federhen *(6)*.

### 3.2. Presentation of Homology Data

In all cases, consideration must be given to the optimal presentation of results for easy assimilation and interpretation. It quickly becomes apparent that the interpretation of biological relevance of matches is vastly improved by some method of sorting matches, either by score or percentage identity, a graphical representation of where matches correspond to the query sequence, and a direct viewing of alignments. This is often integrated into proprietary software and some websites, and is typified by freely available programs such as MSPcrunch and Blixem *(7)*.

### 3.3. Increasing Homology Search Sensitivity and Its Risks

The actual parameters used as cutoffs vary depending upon the context of the search. For a general amino acid-based search with a reasonable balance of sensitivity and specificity, a threshold in the region of 40% identity may be appropriate for BLAST. However, if in a search for a protein that on biological grounds has been determined to be definitely present, then the search parameters may reasonably be relaxed until a homolog is identified. It is also reasonable to use other, more sophisticated homology searching methods in an attempt to identify more remote protein homologs. One such program in common use is PSI-BLAST (Position-Specific Iterated BLAST) *(2)*. PSI-BLAST performs an initial search against the database of choice and then retrieves and aligns significant matches. These matches are used to build a score model for the next round. A profile generated from the alignment is then used as a "query" to perform iterative searches of the same database, and the results of each are used to refine the next. Although the interpretation of the results should be increasingly circumspect when several iterations have been performed, this can be a most useful tool when remote members of a particular protein family are being sought. It is particularly important to remember the modular architecture of proteins when interpreting such search results, since the presence of a well-conserved but relatively common domain in an initial round may act as a bridge to produce hits against other proteins with completely unrelated function, which simply happen to share the presence of that one domain. In terms of sensitivity, it can be considered as sitting midway between traditional sequence-based BLAST and FASTA methods and full profile-based homology searching methods, where the initial query consists of a profile built from a carefully constructed multiple sequence alignment of related nucleotide or protein sequences. It is equally important to remember that a single amino-acid change near an active site may potentially alter the substrate specificity or enzymatic activity of an enzyme, although two such sequences could share >99% identity. The identification of gene function using sequence similarity is actually only based upon a prediction of similarity of protein structure, and reflects common ancestry. Conservation of sequence is not, in itself, evidence of conservation of function—although it is frequently a reasonable basis for this type of inference.

### *3.4. Tracking the "Annotation Trail"*

It follows that the identification of sequence similarities should be only the first step in determining the potential function of a protein, even before the stage of experimental investigation. An attempt should be made to track the "annotation trail" of the similarities that are identified. If genome annotations have made a chain of consistent functional attributions, this should be considered only as a single piece of evidence (as opposed to the sum of each of the individual hits). If a gene with references to experimental work is identified, this should be pursued directly. If an initial gene is found from which the other annotations follow, this should be compared directly with the sequence of interest, and a similarity search with this sequence should be performed to find the basis of this original annotation. Once a link to an experimental source can be established, the specific region of the similarity should be considered, and the existing evidence evaluated. This is important, as alluded to earlier, because it should be recognized that similarity based upon a single protein component, such as an ATP-binding domain, is not evidence that the function of other, possibly quite dissimilar, regions are related. Also, many database submissions include a function-associated annotation determined for one coding region, but which has been applied to several that were simultaneously submitted in a larger sequence for which there is actually no experimental evidence of a function. A superficially annotated gene may actually be of unknown function.

## 4. Surface Protein Identification

A vaccine candidate should be a target that is accessible to the immune response. Therefore, a normal starting point will be the consideration of surface proteins as vaccine candidates. This does not exclude the potential importance of other surface structures, but the information in genome sequences provides information on the protein components most directly. The methods that are used at this point can vary, and may or may not be purely informatics-based. There are several surface protein prediction methods, and at this stage, if inclusivity is important, it may be advisable to use more than one method and to compare and combine the results. This is particularly important when one is considering that most feature prediction methods are not infallible and that each program may have its own inherent strengths and weaknesses. Furthermore, some methods are more specific in nature than others, and can only be identified by combining evidence gleaned from more than one method.

### *4.1. Identification on the Basis of Transmembrane Regions*

The presence of putative transmembrane (TM) helices within a protein may suggest that the protein is membrane-associated, but alone it does not allow for discrimination between proteins that associate with intracellular and cell-surface membranes. If that same protein also shows a putative secretory signal peptide, then this can help to suggest that this protein is indeed surface-expressed. A number of programs are available specifically for the prediction of TM helices, and have recently been reviewed elsewhere *(8)*. These rely on hidden Markov Models (e.g., TMHMM v.2, http://www.cbs.dtu.dk/services/TMHMM-2.0/) *(9)*, neural networks (e.g., the PHDhtm subset of the PredictProtein server (at http://www.embl-heidelberg.de/predictprotein/predictprotein.html) *(10,11)*, or other methods such as Dense Alignment Surface (DAS) utilized in a program called DAS written specifically for predicting TM helices in prokaryotic membrane proteins (available as a server at http://www.sbc.su.se/~miklos/DAS/maindas.html) *(12)*. It should be noted that these methods are not infallible. The position and length of predicted TM helices may be inaccurate, and the N-terminal hydrophobic region of a signal sequence may itself be incorrectly interpreted as a TM helix.

The ability to plot amino acid properties of putative proteins as a sliding-window analysis may be helpful in identifying candidates of interest. A sliding-window analysis calculates a moving average score along the protein for the property being considered, and the window size may be varied to allow the adjustment of relative sensitivity vs signal noise. Trends of particular interest include charge and hydrophobicity. One commonly used calculation of hydrophobicity is that of Kyte & Doolittle *(13)*. The method relies on the assignment of amino acids onto a relative hydrophobicity scale, based on a number of physical characteristics, with higher positive scores indicating more hydrophobic properties. Programs that calculate and plot a moving average of hydropathic index along a protein include TGREASE from the Fasta 2 package (ftp.virginia.edu) and octanol from the EMBOSS package (available from ftp://ftp.uk.embnet.org/pub/EMBOSS/) *(14)*. Another program typifying the type of simple metrics that may be plotted by these types of programs is pepinfo, again from the EMBOSS package. This program plots a histogram of the presence of residues with the physico-chemical properties: Tiny, Small, Aliphatic, Aromatic, Non-polar, Polar, Charged, Positive, and Negative, as well as producing hydrophobicity plots using three alternative methods. Another program within the EMBOSS package which may be of interest in this context is Charge, which calculates a sliding window plot of charge along a protein.

## 4.2. Identification on the Basis of Protein-Transport Motifs

Another strategy for the identification of surface proteins is based upon the presence of motifs associated with transport, such as signal peptidase sequences or cell wall anchoring characteristics. In addition, if species-specific information on common characteristics of surface proteins is known, such as attachment to phosphorylcholine in cell wall teichoic acid, these can also be used. These characteristics were used by Wizemann et al. *(15)* in the primary vaccine candidate selection for *Streptococcus pneumoniae*, leading to an initial list of approx 100 genes for further study. A similar approach was used by Adamou et al., *(16)* in which a family of proteins was identified as potential vaccine candidates on the basis of their hydrophobic leader sequence that is believed to target them to the cell surface. Specific features of a "typical" signal peptide may be identified by their secondary structure, and include a positively charged amino-terminal region followed by a stretch of 11–15 hydrophobic residues and a specific leader peptidase (Lpp or LppII for lipoproteins) *(17)*.

A commonly used program for identifying putative signal peptide sequences is SignalP (http://www.cbs.dtu.dk/services/SignalP) *(18)*. SignalP uses a neural network-based approach, and users are required to choose between network assemblies trained on Gram-positives, Gram-negatives, or eukaryotes as appropriate for the sequence under study. SignalP is capable of distinguishing between secretory signal peptides and those associated with intracellular signal transduction, and thus is a most useful tool. Coiled coil regions, a feature commonly found in Gram-positive surface proteins, may be identified using the Coils program *(19)*. Furthermore, a number of different programs will readily identify short primary amino acid-sequence motifs of interest, either as perfect matches or with different levels of degeneracy. Typically, programs use a defined regular expression syntax for pattern description, often based on that used by the PROSITE database *(20)*. For example, standard IUPAC one-letter codes for amino acids are used, "x" being used for a position in which any amino acid is accepted. Ambiguities are indicated either by listing the acceptable amino acids for a given position between square parentheses, or by listing unacceptable amino acids within curly braces. Elements are separated by a hyphen, and repetitions of an element may be indicated by following the element with a number or range of numbers within brackets, showing the number of repetitions. Patterns restricted to either the N- or C-terminus of a sequence are indicated with a "<" symbol or "\", respectively. Program examples include Fuzznuc (patterns in nucleotides), Fuzzpro and Dreg (uses more standard regular expressions) from the EMBOSS package (available from: ftp:// ftp.uk.embnet.org/pub/EMBOSS/) *(14)*. Query motifs may either be constructed by the user or may be derived from a database of previously described functional motifs and patterns—such as the PROSITE database *(20)*.

## 5. The Early Inclusion of Experimental Data

The genome-based analysis should not be confined to the initial stages of a project. For example, common features of genes that are selected after experimental stages can be sought, and these can be used as the basis for further candidate hunting. In addition to *in silico* predictions, the information from experiments can be incorporated at any stage. The importance of early pursuit of supportive experimental data cannot be over-emphasized. Each stage of the genome sequence-analysis process is one of potentially error-prone hypothesis generation. Each subsequent step that is based upon previous informatics analyses becomes increasingly vulnerable to the influence of mistakes that have occurred in previous stages. For this reason, wherever possible, analyses should be performed on the original sequence data, rather than on results derived from them, and complementary independent analyses should be combined to provide a degree of corroboration between results. The nature of suitable experiments is so dependent upon the specific direction of a particular research strategy that it is not possible to expand upon this in this chapter. However, it is usually advisable to experiment early.

Once the first list of potential vaccine candidates has been defined, it is then necessary to evaluate them in more detail. In the context of a screening-based strategy, this includes a series of steps, which serve to identify the more promising candidates, and to progressively focus upon a smaller and more tractable number of proteins. This process is illustrated by the first publication to describe this genomic approach using *Neisseria meningitidis (21)*, and this is similar to the strategies that have been adopted by other companies seeking similar results in other species. The main preliminary steps are:

1. Identification of an inclusive list of candidates.
2. Cloning and expression of the candidate genes.
3. Assessment of their antigenicity.
4. Evaluation of the ability of raised antibodies to bind to bacterial surface structures and mediate opsonization and/or bactericidal activity.
5. Assessment of antibody effectiveness in passive protection studies.

## 6. Particular Issues Related to a High-Throughput Strategy

An investigator must be concerned about mistakenly excluding a potentially successful vaccine candidate, but, in the absence of limitless resources, decisions on inclusion and exclusion must be made continuously. Clearly, the basis of these decisions is of paramount importance, although it is also true that, if the strategy is successful, then only a small number of final vaccine components are probably needed. In addition, the interpretation of data that support a candidate must be particularly cautious. This is because one's theoretical framework and the nature of the data collected are different from that typical of most smaller problem-oriented studies. Most obviously, one is frequently investigating genes for which there is little or no existing experimental information about function, and as such there is no framework for interpreting the results obtained. This is in the context of a project motivated by a desire to obtain "positive" results. In an environment in which results are pursued rather than hypotheses tested, there is an inherent vulnerability to false-positive results or optimistic interpretation of experiments. This is in the context of studies in which potentially hundreds of candidates will be pursued, but data and—where possible—statistical analysis will be pursued on a case-by-case basis. When dealing with an interaction as complex as that between bacterium, host, and the immune response, especially since model systems with their inherent flaws are inevitably involved, great care is needed in this regard. There is no intention to suggest that such a genome-based approach is not extremely valuable and robust—it is simply necessary to highlight some of its complexities.

## 7. An Example of the Use of a Genome-Based Strategy and Its Novel Complications

The *N. meningitidis* strain MC58 project conducted by Chiron serves to illustrate both the general strategy and a potential problem of the type described here. Unfortunately, most other researchers in this area have not published their results, but based upon their presentations at meetings, their experimental approaches are similar, and they are likely to have encountered similar problems. The meningococcal genome was sequenced *(22)*, and was used to directly feed a vaccine-candidate identification research project *(21)*. Using a combination of prediction methods including PSORT (http://psort.nibb.ac.jp) and PEPPLOT (Wisconsin Package Version 10.0, Genetics Computer Group (GCG), Madison, WI), 350 genes identified as potentially encoding surface-located or secreted proteins were systematically cloned into expression vectors, and the purified recombinant proteins were used to immunize mice. The expression, surface localization, and immunogenicity of each were then determined using a combination of enzyme-linked immunosorbent assay (ELISA), Flow cytometry, and bactericidal assays. Twenty-five proteins that had positive results in these assays were selected for further evaluation, and some were shown to be highly conserved in sequence-based analysis of these genes in other unrelated meningococcal strains. Using a similar strategy with *Chlamydia pneumoniae*, 147 surface proteins were identified, of which 98% were cloned and expressed and 58 generated antibodies that bind the *C. pneumoniae* elemental bodies *(23)*.

GNA33 was an interesting vaccine candidate from *N. meningitidis* strain MC58 and serves to illustrate problems related to high-throughput experiments that might be less likely to complicate more directed approaches. GNA33 is a conserved protein that elicited serum bactericidal antibody responses in mice and showed homology with membrane-bound lytic murein transglycosylase from *E. coli* and *Synechocystis* sp. Mice immunized with recombinant protein generated high serum bactericidal antibody titers, and binding to the cell surface could be readily demonstrated. Therefore, this was one of the most promising initial candidates. Although it seemed surprising for a protein expected to be predominantly located in the periplasm, ways in which it might be exposed to the surface were envisaged. However, in reality, the candidature of GNA33 was artefactual. GNA33 acts as a mimetic for a surface-exposed epitope of loop 4 of porin A (PorA) of strains with the P1.2 subserotype *(24)*, a previously investigated vaccine candidate with a tendency to produce strain-specific protection. It is fortunate for the field of vaccine development that this mimicry has been studied and reported, and can thus serve to illustrate this type of issue.

## 8. Evaluation of Vaccine Candidate Conservation in the Population

As emphasized at the beginning of this chapter, a genome sequence is a singular example from a species being investigated. The meningococcal vaccine development paper addressed this quite robustly, and should serve as an example of the level of assessment that should be generally presented *(21)*. The investigation of the presence, conservation, and possibly also the essentiality of the most promising candidates is needed before their true value in a vaccine can be appraised. It is pointless to have a potent immunogenic vaccine that does not cover a significant portion of the disease-associated population. It is necessary to base this stage of the investigation on a robust understanding of the population biology of the particular organisms under investigation. For example, if one is dealing with a relatively panmictic, naturally transformable population, there is a greater need for awareness of variant sequences, in addition to gene presence and absence information, since horizontal transfer and the formation of gene mosaics may potentially compromise a vaccine more quickly than in a more clonal species. Strictly speaking, this is an aspect that extends beyond the remit of a sequence-based vaccine-design strategy, and is not discussed in further detail here. It is mentioned here to emphasize the importance of recognizing the true nature of the information that is the framework of a genome-based approach.

## 9. The Use of Genome-Based Secondary Screening in Model Systems for Candidate Selection

Other approaches that incorporate methods that address the whole organism in different ways also depend upon genome sequences. Like the methods applied for the identification of surface proteins, these can be used to select candidates that have not previously been studied, and for which a potential function is not required to be known at the outset. Although signature-tagged mutagenesis (STM) and in vitro expression technology (IVET) make passing use of genomes for the identification of the coding sequences associated with the insertion sites, they can equally be performed in species and strains for which there are no complete genome sequences; thus, they are not addressed here. The two main methods that require and make use of the genome-sequence information that can be used to select candidates for investigation as vaccine candidates are DNA microarrays and protein-expression profiling that depends upon mass-spectrometric protein sequencing. Using both methods, experiments can be done that determine the alterations in gene expression associated with potentially critical stages of the bacterium-host interaction, and candidates identified in this way can be pursued with similar strategies to those used to investigate genes from *in silicio* analyses.

## Acknowledgment

NJS is supported by a Wellcome Trust Advanced Research Fellowship.

## References

1. Altschul, S. F., Gish, W., Miller, W., Myers, E. W., and Lipman, D. J. (1990) Basic local alignment search tool. *J. Mol. Biol.* **215,** 403–410.
2. Altschul, S. F., Madden, T. L., Schäffer, A. A., Zhang, J., Zhang, Z., Miller, W., et al. (1997) Gapped BLAST and PSI-BLAST: a new generation of protein database search programs. *Nucleic Acids Res.* **25,** 3389–3402.
3. Pearson, W. R. and Lipman, D. J. (1988) Improved tools for biological sequence comparison. *Proc. Natl. Acad. Sci. USA* **85,** 2444–2448.
4. Bairoch, A. and Apweiler, R. (2000) The SWISS-PROT protein sequence database and its supplement TrEMBL in 2000. *Nucleic Acids Res.* **28,** 45–48.
5. Holm, L. and Sander, C. (1998) Removing near-neighbour redundancy from large protein sequence collections. *Bioinformatics* **14,** 423–429.
6. Wootton, J. C. and Federhen, S. (1996) Analysis of compositionally biased regions in sequence databases. *Methods Enzymol.* **266,** 554–571.
7. Sonnhammer, E. L. L. and Durbin, R. (1994). A workbench for Large Scale Sequence Homology Analysis. *Comput. Appl. Biosci.* **10,** 301–307.
8. Moller, S., Croning, M. D. R., and Apweiler, R. (2001) Evaluation of methods for the prediction of membrane spanning regions. *Bioinformatics* **177,** 646–653.
9. Krogh, A., Larsson, B., von Heijne, G., and Sonnhammer, E. L. L. (2001) Predicting transmembrane protein topology with a hidden Markov model: Application to complete genomes. *J. Mol. Biol.* **305,** 567–580.

10. Rost, B. (1996) PHD: predicting one-dimensional protein structure by profile based neural networks. *Methods Enzymol.* **266,** 525–539.

11. Rost, B., Fariselli, P., and Casadio, R. (1996) Topology prediction for helical transmembrane proteins at 86% accuracy. *Protein Sci.* **7,** 1704–1718.

12. Cserzo, M., Wallin, E., Simon, I., von Heijne G., and Elofsson A. (1997) Prediction of transmembrane alpha-helices in prokaryotic membrane proteins: the Dense Alignment Surface method. *Protein Eng.* **10,** 673–676.

13. Kyte, J. and Doolittle, R. F. (1982) A simple method for displaying the hydrophobic character of a protein. *J. Mol. Biol.* **157,** 105–132.

14. Rice, P., Longden, I., and Bleasby, A. (2000) EMBOSS: The European Molecular Biology Open Software Suite. *Trends Genet.* **16,** 276–277.

15. Wizemann, T. M., Heinrichs, J. H., Adamou, J. E., Erwin, A. L., Kunsch, C., Choi, G. H., et al. (2001) Use of a whole genome approach to identify vaccine molecules affording protection against *Streptococcus pneimoniae* infection. *Infect. Immun.* **69,** 1593–1598.

16. Adamou, J. E., Heinrichs, J. H., Erwin, A. L., Walsh, W., Gayle, T., Dormitzer, M., et al. (2001) Identification and characterization of a novel family of pneumococcal proteins that are protective against sepsis. *Infect. Immun.* **69,** 949–958.

17. Von Heijne, G. (1986) A new method for predicting signal sequence cleavage sites. *Nucleic Acids Res.* **14,** 4683–4690.

18. Nielsen, H., Engelbrecht, J., Brunak, S., and von Heije, G. (1997) Identification of prokaryotic and eukaryotic signal peptides and prediction of their cleavage site. *Protein Eng.* **10,** 1–6.

19. Lupas, A., Van Dyke, M., and Stock, J. (1991) Predicting coiled coils from protein sequences. *Science* **252,** 1162–1164.

20. Bairoch A., Bucher, P., and Hoffman, K. (1997) The PROSITE database: its status in 1997. *Nucleic Acids Res.* **25,** 217–221.

21. Pizza, M., Scarlato, V., Masignani, V., Giuliani, M.M., Arico, B., Comanducci, M., et al. (2000) Identification of vaccine candidates against serogroup B meningococcus by whole-genome sequencing. *Science* **287,** 1816–1820.

22. Tettelin, H., Saunders, N. J., Heidelberg, J., Jeffries, A. C., Nelson, K. E., Eisen, J. A., et al. (2000) Complete genome sequence of *Neisseria meningitidis* serogroup B strain MC58. *Science* **287,** 1809–1815.

23. Grandi, G. (2001) Antibacterial vaccine design using genomics and proteomics. *Trends Biotechnol.* **19,** 181–188.

24. Granoff, D. M., Moe, G. R, Guiliani, M. M., AduBobie, J., Santini, L., Brunella, B., et al. (2001) A novel mimetic antigen eliciting protective antibody to *Neisseria meningitidis*. *J. Immunol.* **167,** 6487–6496.

# 20

## Severe Combined Immunodeficient (SCID) Mice in Vaccine Assessment

### Michael J. Dennis

## 1. Introduction

### 1.1. Advantages of Immunodeficient Mice for Vaccine Assessment

New or improved vaccines require testing before they are licensed for use in the general population. Although toxicity and immunological data can be obtained from Phase I human trials, in the vast majority of cases it is not possible to demonstrate efficacy by challenging vaccine recipients with the specific infectious agent. Therefore, prior to large-scale production of vaccines and their assessment in Phase II and III clinical trials, there is a requirement for in vivo studies that can predict the level of protection that may be expected from a vaccine. Although many animal models are available for infectious disease studies, they all rely on the animal's own immune system for the generation of the protective responses, and these may not reflect the immunological responses generated in humans. The route of challenge that must be used in order to achieve infection is often not the same as the one that occurs in human disease, and this further confounds the relevance of the animal model. In addition, some infections are specific to humans, and it is sometimes impossible to find a suitable animal species that human pathogens will infect. This may be because of the lack of appropriate receptors, the presence of a functional immune system able to eliminate the pathogen, or the fact that models cannot always be relied on to re-create the normal pathophysiology. In some cases, this resistance to infection can be overcome by the development of a transgenic animal in which the appropriate receptors are expressed. The development of transgenic models has been directed toward genetic disorders or dissection of the immune system by gene-knockout technology.

Since the first reports of the discovery of a mutant mouse lacking a functional immune system *(1,2)*, the Severe Combined Immunodeficient (SCID) mouse has played

From: *Methods in Molecular Medicine, Vol. 87: Vaccine Protocols, 2nd ed.*
Edited by: A. Robinson, M. J. Hudson, and M. P. Cranage © Humana Press Inc., Totowa, NJ

an important role in the study of human infection and immunity. In many cases, the lack of immunity has allowed the establishment of a range of viral, bacterial, and protozoal infections to which normal mice are resistant. Most importantly, however, the capacity of these mice to accept xenografts from a range of other species, including man, has resulted in the development of a number of mouse models using agents that are restricted to replication in human cells or in which the typical pathology can be reproduced in these human/mouse chimeras. Soon after their discovery, the ability of these animals to allow reconstitution with human immune cells was exploited (3–6). These models could be used for the study of the pathology of infection, and they also found application in the evaluation of prophylactic and therapeutic treatment of human disease (7,8).

Classically, the SCID mouse has been reconstituted by one of two methods. In the first, small pieces of human fetal thymus, liver, spleen, bone marrow, or lymph node have been implanted under the kidney capsule or in the mammary fat pad (1). In the second, human adult peripheral blood cells (PBL) have been inoculated into the peritoneal cavity (2). When grafted with human fetal cells, the mice are termed SCID-hu, whereas mice reconstituted with adult PBL are termed Hu-PBL-SCID. In both cases, long-term reconstitution of these mice with functional human lymphoid cells has been reported (9,10). Both models have limitations, as discussed later in this chapter. Because adult PBLs are more readily available than fetal tissue and to the wide range of possibilities for pre-priming or for selecting subpopulations of blood cells prior to engraftment, the majority of work has been conducted using the Hu-PBL-SCID model.

Other fetal tissues have also been successfully engrafted into SCID mice to provide models for diseases that are highly tissue-specific. Engrafted human gut tissue has been successfully infected with *Shigella*, and typical lesions have been demonstrated (11). Similarly, we have demonstrated that sections of fetal primate gut can be engrafted beneath the skin of SCID mice, which retain its villous structure for a minimum of 12 wk (12) (**Fig. 1**). The engrafted gut segments were subsequently infected with *Campylobacter jejuni* by injection into the lumen. Other workers have engrafted SCID mice with human skin, with retinal, liver, or vaginal tissue, and have observed infection and pathology that parallels that seen in man (13–16).

The adoptive transfer of primed human lymphocytes to mice can result in the expression of specific human immunoglobulins in mouse serum and to the establishment of a corresponding protective immunity in these mice. There are now several reports of both primary and secondary immune responses elicited in reconstituted mice (17–25).

The reconstitution of mice with human immune cells from convalescent patients has led to the detection of pathological processes, directed against the microorganism, which are not seen in non-reconstituted animals (2,26). Not only does this model have a vast potential for the study of the pathology of infections, but it has also found application in the evaluation of prophylactic and therapeutic treatments of human infectious diseases. One well-explored area of research is the study of human immunity in SCID mice that have been engrafted with a functional human immune system from vaccine recipients. Disease models using immunodeficient mice are summarzied in **Table 1**.

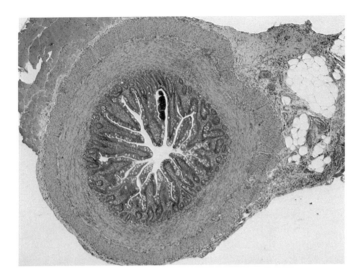

Fig. 1. Cross-section of primate ileum grafted into C.B-17 SCID-beige mouse 12 wk after insertion.

This chapter focuses on the Hu-PBL-SCID model, since this system can be used with blood samples from vaccine recipients. The adoptive transfer of primed human lymphocytes to mice can result in the expression of specific human immunoglobulins in mouse serum and the establishment of a corresponding protective immunity in these mice *(27)*. There is evidence that both primary *(18,19)* and secondary *(23)* immune responses can be elicited in SCID mice that have been reconstituted with human lymphocytes or tissues *(20)*, and the induction of protection against specific human pathogens has been demonstrated after the immunization of animals with appropriate vaccine preparations *(28)*. The Hu-PBL-SCID model has also been used to demonstrate the ability of cytokine therapies to induce specific cellular immunity *(29)*. SCID mice can also be used for the passive transfer of human immunoglobulins for the evaluation of protective antibodies *(30–32)*.

### 1.2. Mouse Strains and the Nature of Immunological Defects

The murine *scid* mutation was first recognized in C.B-17 mice *(33)*, and is defined as an autosomal recessive mutation that results in a general absence of mature B- and T-lymphocytes. The mutation manifests as an impairment in the Variable, Diversity and Joining (V(D)J) recombination process that normally leads to functional immunoglobulin and T-cell receptor (TCR) variable-region gene products. Recent studies suggest that the SCID defect lies in the gene encoding the catalytic subunit of the DNA-dependent protein kinase. This is a nuclear protein made up of two subunits (Ku70 and Ku86) as well as the large catalytic subunit DNA PKcs *(34)*. This leads to an inability to repair double-stranded DNA breaks, which is also inferred from an observed increased sensitivity to ionizing radiation. Experimental inactivation of Prkdc

**Table 1**
**Disease Models in Immunodeficient Mice**

| Disease/organism | Reconstitution | Model | References |
|---|---|---|---|
| HIV-1 | Human PBL | Blocking of HIV entry into CD4+ T-cells | 60 |
| | Human PBL | Vaginal infection | 61 |
| | Human PBL | Reduction of viral loads with immunomodulators | 62 |
| | Human PBL | Uninfected CD4+ T-cells undergo apoptosis in infected lymphoid organs | 63 |
| | Human thymus/liver | HIV latency model (resting T-cells) | 64 |
| Hepatitis C | Human hepatocytes | Prolonged HCV infection | 65 |
| | Human liver tissue | HCV viremia-reduction in viral loads | 15 |
| CMV | Human retinal tissue | Human ocular infection, pathogenesis, infection kinetics | 14 |
| Varicella-zoster | Human skin | Virulence of mutant virus | 66 |
| Langat flavivirus | None | Comparison of neuroinvasion in deletion mutants | 67 |
| Rotavirus | None | 100-fold increase in chronic virus shedding compared with other models | 68 |
| Vaccinia | None | Lethal infection model | 69 |
| E. coli-induced inflammatory bowel disease | Mouse CD4+ cells | Subacute colitis | 70 |
| Crohn's disease | Mouse CD62L+CD4+ T-cells | LI-18 upregulated in inflamed colon | 71 |
| Muscular dystrophy | Human myoblasts | Detection of dysferlin proteins | 72 |
| Streptococcal impetigo | Human foreskin | Pathology of infection parallels human disease | 13 |
| Shigella | Human intestine | Inflammation and mucosal damage. Importance of neutrophils | 11 |
| Campylobacter jejuni | None | Colonization and disease | 73 |
| Legionella pneumophila | Human PBL | Lung infection | 59 |
| Mycobacterium tuberculosis | None | Virulence of vaccine candidate auxotrophic mutants | 74 75 |
| Ehrlichia chaffeensis | None | Persistent infection and disease | 76 |
| Brugia malangi /pahangi | None | B-cells required for protection | 77 |

has reproduced the SCID phenotype *(34)*, showing that *Prkdc* and *scid* are allelic, and the SCID mouse is often be referred to as *Prkdc^{scid}* in the literature.

### 1.2.1. Limitations and Refinements

Some SCID mice can develop populations of peripheral mature lymphocytes in a time- and strain-dependent manner. This "leakiness" may be the result of somatic reversion events or rescue of the liberated coding regions in *scid* pre-lymphocytes by an alternative recombination mechanism. The impact of increasing age upon immuno-globulin production and B-lymphocyte generation in "leaky" SCID mice has recently been investigated *(35)*.

Long-term studies using Hu-PBL-SCID mice have shown that human T-cells from these mice become anergic and unresponsive to stimulation. This anergy may result from either a graft-versus-host disease (GvHD) or reflect the lack of an appropriate microenvironment that might support normal lymphocyte trafficking and differentia-tion *(19)*. The macrophages, polymorphonuclear cells, and natural killer (NK) cells in the SCID mouse have a normal or enhanced activity, leading to destruction of the graft. The published reports on hu-PBL reconstitution are not consensual. The numbers and characteristics of human cells re-populating SCID mice are often different, depending on the organs screened and the time of engraftment. The kinetics of intraperitoneal (ip) engraftment are believed to consist of two phases: during the first phase, most of the injected cells remain in the peritoneal cavity and then dramatically disappear. During the second phase, selected clones of human T-cells proliferate and repopulate several peripheral organs. The Vβ profiles show that the T-cell repertoire is severely restricted compared to the number of subsets in the original donor *(36)*. This skewed repertoire is probably the result of an antigenic activation in the SCID environment.

During the past few years, new strains of mice with additional defects of the innate immune system have been developed to further optimize the Hu-PBL-SCID model.

The *scid* mutation has been introduced into the C3H strain of mice, which has been reported to produce very low levels of spontaneously leaky individuals *(37,38)*.

The spontaneous beige mutation is an analog of the human Chediak-Higashi syn-drome, and is associated with neutropenia and a lack of NK cytotoxic activity. Thus, the production of the double-mutant SCID-beige mouse has resulted in experimental animals that lack mature B- and T-cells, and also have defective NK cells *(39)*. The *beige* defect, which causes a defect in lysosomal membranes and granule formation, facilitates the acceptance of xenografts and may also render animals more susceptible to viral infections. In addition, these mice have been shown to be much less prone to develop "leaky" individuals compared to *scid/scid* mice *(40)*. The *beige* mutation has been introduced into several parent mouse strains, including Balb/c, SCID-beige *(41)*, and C.B.-17 SCID-beige *(42)*.

Back-crossing the SCID mutation into the Non-Obese Diabetic (NOD/Lt) strain of mice has resulted in the NOD-SCID mouse, which has reduced NK activity, macroph-age function, and serum hemolytic complement activity, in addition to the lack of B- and T-cells *(43)*. These mice have been shown to support PBL engraftments fivefold higher than CB-17 SCID mice, and show no age-related leakiness. Many publications describe the use of this mouse model, and it is now used as a standard assay for primitive human hematopoietic cells (SCID re-population cells are known as SRCs) *(44–46)*. Reported lack of T-cell development in this model has been addressed by treatment of the NOD-SCID mice with a monoclonal antibody (MAb) against the murine interleukin-2R beta, known to decrease killer-cell activity. This increased phenotypically normal T-cell development. Furthermore, analysis showed the emergence from the thymus of the naïve phenotype CD45RA+ *(47)*. The importance of this population is discussed in **Subheading 1.3.** Recent studies *(48,49)* have compared the engraftment of human cord blood subpopulations into NOD-SCID mice, and showed that CD34+/CD38+ cells repopulate rapidly but survive for only 12 wk, whereas CD34+/CD38– cells repopulate more gradually but maintain significant numbers for more than 20 wk. This subpopulation contains more T-cell precursors.

A third type of immunodeficient mice carries a germline mutation in which a large portion of the Recombination Activating Genes 1 or 2 (RAG-1,2) coding region is deleted *(50)*. This leads to a novel SCID phenotype from which no "leaky" mice are produced. However, recent reports suggest that RAG-2 mice may not reconstitute with human PBLs as well as SCID mice. A comparative study evaluating successful human lymphocyte engraftment by measuring CD3+ cells and human Ig showed reconstitution to be excellent in SCID-beige and NOD-SCID mice, but poor in RAG⁻ mice *(51)*. However, in this study, GVHD was reported in many of the successfully reconstituted animals. The NOD/LtSz-*Rag-1^null* has been reported to have a longer life-span than the NOD/LtSz-*scid* mouse, to have low NK activity, and to support high levels of engraftment with human lymphoid cells and hemopoietic stem cells.

## 1.3. The Potential of SCID Mice for Vaccine Studies

### 1.3.1. Primary Immunization

The Hu-PBL-SCID mouse system has long been shown to be capable of supporting antigen-specific antibody production. A secondary immune response can be readily induced in mice reconstituted with cells from human donors with pre-existing antibodies to diphtheria-tetanus and tetanus toxoids *(20,23)*, Hepatitis B surface antigen (HBsAg) *(25)*, HIV-1 gp160 *(3)*, influenza hemagglutinin *(21)*, or pneumococcal polysaccharide *(52)* by immunization with the relevant antigen. A more useful model, would be the ability to generate a primary immune response to an antigenic stimulus followed by an amnestic response to booster immunizations. With few exceptions *(24)*, this has proven to be difficult to achieve. For summary, *see* **Table 2.**

One possible reason for the difficulty in generating a primary immune response in reconstituted SCID mice is the loss of naive CD45RA+ cells following introduction into the mouse, with the subsequent loss of the T-cell repertoire. The majority of cells examined from all sites 2 wk after reconstitution are of the CD45RO+ type—e.g. memory, or helper/inducer-type, which are already pre-primed and cannot recognize novel antigens. This has led to the suggestion that secondary immune responses can only be generated in this system using cells taken from individuals who have been previously exposed to antigen. However, recent publications have indicated that RO+ to RA+ reversion can occur in vivo *(53–55)*, or can be induced in reconstituted mice

**Table 2**
**Primary/Secondary Response Models in Immunodeficient Mice**

| Disease/organism | Reconstitution | Model | Reference |
|---|---|---|---|
| HIV-1 | Human PBL | Chimeric plant virus produces anti-gp41 primary response | *18* |
| | Human PBL/Skin | APC aided primary Th1 response to gp160 | *19* |
| | Human PBL | Primary anti-nef CTL | *17* |
| Hepatitis B | Human PBL | Secondary response to HB surface antigen | *25* |
| Influenza | Human PBL | Protective secondary CTL response | *21* |
| RSV | Human PBL | RSV-F specific responses | *28* |
| EBV | Human PBL | Cytokines induce specific cellular immunity, prevent EBV-LPD | *29* |
| Tetanus toxin | Human PBL | Protective response to lethal dose | *83* |
| Tetanus toxoid | Human tonsil | Long-lasting secondary response | *20* |
| Diphtheria-tetanus toxoid | Human PBL | CD40 promotes secondary response | *23* |

by treatment with appropriate anti-interleukin monoclonals *(47)*. SCID mice transplanted with human fetal thymus and liver under the kidney capsule sustain human T-cell lymphopoiesis for over 1 yr, but do not generate mature B-cells. In contrast, mice engrafted with human fetal bones generate B-cells but not T-cells *(56)*. Simultaneous engraftment with thymus and bone results in mice that generate all classes of IgG, but are still unable to mount an antigen-specific antibody response. The additional implantation of human skin and lymph-node tissues results in mice capable of mounting specific responses IgG and IgM against tetanus toxoid *(10)*.

## 1.3.2. Adoptive Transfer of Immunity

Several studies have used PBLs taken from human vaccinees for the evaluation of vaccine efficacy in SCID mice. As part of a clinical trial of candidate HIV vaccines, sero-negative volunteers were immunized with a recombinant vaccinia expressing HIV-$1_{LAV/Bru}$ 160-kDa-envelope glycoprotein and subsequently boosted with recombinant gp160 protein *(57)*. For evaluation purposes, PBLS taken at intervals of between 4 wk and 72 wk after the booster injections were obtained and used to construct Hu-PBL-SCID mice. The reconstituted animals were challenged with $10^2$–$10^3$ minimal animal-infectious doses of HIV-$1_{IIIB}$. The PBLs from three of four immunized donors protected reconstituted SCID mice from challenge, as determined by the failure to isolate or detect HIV in mouse tissues by in vitro culture or polymerase chain reaction (PCR) amplification, respectively. This resistance to HIV-l challenge diminished over time, but PBL

**Table 3**
**Passive Protection/Adoptive Transfer Models in Immunodeficient Mice**

| Disease/organism | Reconstitution | Model | References |
|---|---|---|---|
| Ebola | None | Immune serum gave 100% protection | *30* |
| HIV-1 | Human PBL | CD4 immunoglobulin protects against infection | *31* |
| HSV-2 | None | Immune sera reduce incidence and severity of disease | *78* |
| Vaccinia | Murine CTL | High-avidity CTL reduced viral loads | *79* |
| Hepatitis B | HuPBL into spleen | HB core antigen binding inhibited | *80* |
| *Trypanosoma cruzi* | None | Th1 immunity protects against systemic infection | *81* |
| *Bacillus anthracis* | None | AntiPA-specific antibodies give protection | *32* |
| *Borrelia burgdorferi* | None | Passive protection with outer-surface protein anti-sera | *82* |
| *Ehrlichia chaffeensis* | None | B-cell-derived antibody | |

from one patient gave partial protection (50% of mice protected) at 41 wk post-boost. More recently, HIV-1 seronegative subjects were vaccinated with an HIV-1 p17 synthetic peptide vaccine. PBMC from subjects showing significant increase in antibody titers were injected into SCID mice, which were subsequently challenged with $10^3$ $TCID_{50}$ of HIV-1. Of these mice, 78% were protected from infection *(27)*. For a summary, *see* **Table 3**.

This chapter describes the basic steps required for the use of SCID mice, including requirements for handling mice, screening for the immunodeficient state, reconstitution with human PBL, and checks for successful reconstitution.

## 2. Materials

### 2.1. Maintenance of SCID Mice

Because of the severe immunodeficiency of SCID and related mice, these animals require special housing and handling. The mice must be kept in conditions that ensure that they are protected from possible opportunistic pathogens in the environment. The necessary equipment includes independently ventilated cages (IVCs) or plastic film isolators fitted with High-Efficiency Particulate Air (HEPA) filters (specially designed housing and manipulation equipment are available from a number of suppliers). For breeding or for non-infectious studies, the equipment should be maintained at positive pressure, whereas for experiments involving the use of infectious agents, negative pressure systems are more appropriate. SCID mice should be kept far away from conventional rodents, and should not share room space or ancillary equipment with such animals. Well-conceived protocols should be produced for maintenance and handling, and these should be rigorously adhered to by trained staff. All supplies of bedding, diet, drinking water, and ancillary equipment should be pre-sterilized by γ-irradiation, autoclaving, or filtration as appropriate, and class II (or class III if appropriate) cabinets should be used for carrying out all procedures, such as changing bedding, feeding, and experimental manipulation. It should also be noted that in some countries the breeding of mice with potentially harmful genetic defects may be governed by welfare legislation—for example, in the United Kingdom, a specific project license is required.

## 2.2. Assay of Mouse Immunoglobulin in the Sera of SCID Mice

1. Phosphate-buffered saline (PBS) + 0.05% (v/v) Tween 20 (PBST).
2. Blocking solution: PBST, 1% (w/v) bovine serum albumin (BSA) (Sigma, St. Louis, MO), 0.5% (v/v) fish gelatin (Sigma).
3. Rabbit anti-mouse IgG + IgM (heavy [H] + light [L] chain-specific), minimum crossreactivity to human serum proteins (Jackson ImmunoResearch Labs., Inc., West Grove, PA), diluted 1:5000 in PBS. For storage, dilute neat reagent 1:1 with glycerol and store at –20°C.
4. Rabbit anti-mouse IgG + IgM (H+L)-peroxidase conjugate, minimum crossreactivity to human serum proteins (Jackson ImmunoResearch Labs., Inc.); dilute 1:5000 in blocking solution. For storage, dilute neat reagent 1:1 with glycerol, and store at –20°C.
5. Chromopure mouse Ig (Jackson ImmunoResearch Labs., Inc.)-mouse Ig standard. For storage, dilute neat reagent 1:1 with glycerol and store at –20°C.
6. Substrate: AP-Yellow pNPP alkaline phosphatase (Microwell phosphatase substrate, BioFX Laboratories Inc., Randallstown, MD, USA) supplied as a one-component ready-to-use solution. Store at 2°–8°C, and allow to reach room temperature before use.
7. Stop solution: 3 $N$ sodium hydroxide.

## 2.3. Staining for the Beige Marker

1. 16% (w/v) Paraformaldehyde (prepare in fume hood).
2. Sudan black B (SBB): Dissolve 0.45 g SBB in 150 mL 100% ethanol. While stirring, add 12.3 g crystalline phenol dissolved in 23 mL 100% ethanol and 0.107 g of $Na_2PO_4 \cdot 7H_2O$ dissolved in 77 mL of double-distilled water. Filter through #4 Whatman filter paper.
3. Gill's hematoxylin (Sigma).
4. 50% (v/v) ethanol.

## 2.4. Isolation of Human Peripheral Blood Lymphocytes

1. RPMI-1640.
2. Lymphoprep (Nycomed, Birmingham, UK).
3. Complete medium: RPMI-1640, 10% (v/v) fetal calf serum (FCS), 1 m$M$ glutamine, 10 m$M$ HEPES, 50 µg/mL gentamicin.
4. 0.25% (w/v) Trypan blue in PBS (trypan blue is carcinogenic, and gloves must be worn). Trypan blue is stable at room temperature for several years if kept sterile.

## 2.5. Measurement of Human Immunoglobulins in Reconstituted SCID Mice

1. Reagents listed in **Subheading 2.2.**, **items 1**, **2**, **6**, and **7**.
2. Rabbit anti-human IgG + IgM (H+L), minimum crossreactivity with mouse serum proteins, diluted 1: 5000 (Jackson ImmunoResearch Labs., Inc.).
3. Chromopure human Ig (Jackson ImmunoResearch Labs., Inc.).

4. Rabbit antihuman IgG + IgM (H+L)-peroxidase conjugate, minimum crossreactivity with mouse serum proteins, diluted 1:5000 (Jackson ImmunoResearch Labs., Inc.).

## 2.6. Immunohistological Staining of Paraffin-Embedded Mouse Tissues

1. Xylene.
2. Ethanol 100%, 95% (v/v), 80% (v/v).
3. PBS.
4. Trypsin (Sigma): 0.1% (w/v) in 20 mM Tris-HC1, pH 7,6, containing 0.1% (w/v) $CaCl_2$. Make fresh each time.
5. $H_2O_2$ 3% (v/v) in methanol. Make fresh each time.
6. Normal animal serum (same species as biotin conjugate).
7. Monoclonal antibodies (MAb) diluted to predetermined titer, e.g.:
   a. DAKO (Carpenteria, CA) antihuman leukocyte common antigen (LCA, clones PD7/26 and 2BII) 1:50.
   b. DAKO CD 43 (T-cell clone DF-T1) 1:100 (or can be purchased prediluted from DAKO).
   c. DAKO CD 20 (B-cell clone L26) neat (purchased prediluted from DAKO).
   d. DAKO CD 68 (Mφ clone PG-M1) 1:100 (tissue must be trypsinized).
8. Rabbit anti-mouse IgG-biotin (DAKO).
9. Histostain-SP kit (Zymed [South San Francisco, CA]: the kit contains substrate buffer, amino-ethyl-carbazole [AEC], hydrogen peroxide, hematoxylin, cover slip mountant).
10. Streptavidin-peroxidase (Jackson ImmunoResearch, Inc.).

## 2.7. FACS Analysis of Reconstituted Mice

All antibodies and conjugates should be titrated against positive control samples before use.

1. PBS containing 0.1% (w/v) sodium azide (PBSA).
2. Fluorescein-conjugated MAb to human CD45 (DAKO clone no. T29/33).
3. Mouse anti-mouse $H-2K^d$-biotin (Pharmingen [San Diego, CA] clone SF1-1.1; alternatively, phycoerythrin (PE)-coupled rat anti-mouse $H-2K^d$ is available from the same supplier for single-step staining) (see **Note 1**).
4. Streptavidin-PE: (Becton Dickinson, San Jose, CA).
5. Paraformaldehyde stock solution 2% (w/v): Add 2 g paraformaldehyde to 100 mL PBS. Heat to 56°C in a water bath in a fume hood until the paraformaldehyde dissolves (approx 1 h). Allow the solution to cool to room temperature, and adjust pH to 7.4 using 0.1 *M* NaOH or 0.1 *M* HCl. Store at 4°C.
6. Paraformaldehyde working solution 0.5% (w/v): Add 10 mL 2% (w/v) solution to 30 mL PBS. Store at 4°C. Stable for 1 wk.

## 3. Methods

### 3.1. Handling of Immunodeficient Mice

All personnel involved in the handling of these mice should be trained in the required precautions and should use "barrier" methods, such as the use of disposable protective clothing, face-masks, and hair caps. It is also important that a health-monitoring program for the mice is implemented so that early recognition of problems is possible. Since SCID mice do not produce immunoglobulins, it is not possible to screen for the presence of virus- or bacteria-specific antibodies directly. Tissues can be taken from SCID mice and injected into pathogen-free mice, which are subsequently screened for the development of pathogen-specific antibodies. Similarly, sentinel mice can be housed with selected SCID mice prior to screening for pathogens. Diagnostic services are available from a range of laboratories, and some animal breeders can also supply enzyme-linked immunosorbent assay (ELISA) plates coated with antigens for "in-house" screening of specific antibodies. In order to maintain good-quality breeding stock, it is also advisable to rederive the colony from Caesarean-produced fetuses once a year. Most commercial animal breeders also now offer an embryo cryopreservation and storage service. This will provide insurance against the breakdown of an in-house breeding colony, and is particularly useful if the colony is unique in some way. This facility also offers a way to avoid the expense and waste of maintaining a breeding colony if there is a temporary lull in demand.

## 3.2. Screening of the Immunodeficient State of Mice

### 3.2.1. Assay of Mouse Immunoglobulin in Sera of SCID-Beige Mice

As stated in **Subheading 1.2.**, a certain proportion of SCID and SCID-beige mice become "leaky," and therefore, various checks must be carried out before the mice are introduced into experimental protocols (*see* **Note 2**). Since both the T- and B-cell defects are caused by the same mechanism, the simplest check for the loss of the *scid* phenotype is to look for the presence of mouse immunoglobulin in the serum of SCID or SCID-beige mice by ELISA (*see* **Note 3**).

1. Coat 96-well ELISA plates (NUNC Maxisorb) with rabbit anti-mouse IgG + IgM diluted 1:5000 in PBS for 16 h at 4°C (50 µL/well).
2. Wash plate 3× (5 min each wash) with PBST.
3. Block plate with PBST + 1% (w/v) BSA + 0.5% (v/v) (100 µL/well) fish gelatin for 1 h at 37°C.
4. Wash as in **step 2**.
5. Dilute mouse sera samples 1:50 in blocking solution, and add 100 µL to the first well of a row. Add 50 µL of blocking solution to all other wells of the row, and double-dilute samples across plate (*see* **Note 4**). Include a row of double-diluted mouse Ig standard (starting at 1 µg/mL). Incubate plate at 37°C for 90 min.
6. Wash plate as in **step 2**.
7. Dilute rabbit anti-mouse Ig-peroxidase (Px) conjugate 1:5000 in blocking solution and add 50 µL to each well. Incubate for 30 min at 37°C.
8. Wash plate as in **step 2**.
9. Add 50 µL. AP-Yellow substrate to each well and incubate for 60 min at room temperature.
10. Stop reaction with 3 *M* NaOH (50 µL/well) and read plate at 405–410 nm.
11. Use standard graph constructed using Hill kinetics (available on computer programs, such as Fig P; Biosoft) to calculate level of mouse Ig present in serum samples. Mice with levels Ig >10 µg/mL are considered leaky, and should not be used for experiments.

### 3.2.2. Sudan Black Staining for the Beige Marker (NK-Cell Marker)

The *beige* defect is confirmed by the staining of blood smears with Sudan black, which stains lysogenic granules. In blood smears from normal mice, the granules within neutrophils are small and numerous, whereas in Beige mice they are extremely large and few in number. The following method was kindly supplied by Anne Croy and Janice Greenwood (University of Guelph, Ontario, Canada).

1. Obtain fresh blood smears on glass slides from mouse tail vein (do not let smear become too thick) (*see* **Note 5**).
2. Fix smears in paraformaldehyde vapors by pouring a *small* amount of 16% (w/v) paraformaldehyde into the bottom of a glass slide bucket and placing slides in bucket for 10 min with the bucket closed. Carry out in fume hood.
3. Wash in running water for 10 min.
4. Stain with SBB for 1 h (keep bucket covered).
5. Dip in 50% (w/v) ethanol 5 × 5 s.
6. Wash in running tap water for 5 min.
7. Air-dry.
8. Counterstain in Gill's hematoxylin for 3 min.
9. Wash in running tap water 2–3 min.
10. Air-dry.
11. Read slides under oil immersion when dry. Beige granules seen in neutrophils are large and dark brown/black (**Fig. 2**). Count between 5 and 10 granulocytes, and every cell must have large granules to count as a *beige* mouse.

### 3.3. Human Leukocyte Preparation and Reconstitution of Immunodeficient Mice

Approximately $2 \times 10^7$ human PBLs are required for the reconstitution of each immunodeficient mouse (*see* **Note 6**). Higher numbers of cells can lead to the early production of EBV-induced tumors (unless Epstein-Barr virus (EBV)-negative blood is used). It has been demonstrated that tumor development in Hu-PBL-SCID mice can be prevented by administration of daily low doses of IL-2, but protection is lost if murine NK cells are depleted *(8)*. More recently, combined treatment with human granulocyte macrophage-colony-stimulating factor (GM-CSF) and low-dose IL-2 has been shown to be effective, even in mice depleted of murine NK cells *(29)*. The use of fewer cells reduces the number of mice that are successfully reconstituted. The most convenient source of normal PBLs—e.g. from nonimmunized volunteers—is in the form of buffy-coat concentrates that are sometimes available from blood transfusion centers. All human bloods should be handled with extreme care, and all personnel involved in the processing of human bloods should be offered vaccination against Hepatitis B. All of the following procedures must be carried out aseptically.

1. If possible, remove some plasma, and store at –20°C for future use.
2. Mix blood sample 1:1 (v/v) with RPMI-1640 at room temperature.
3. Add 15 mL of Lymphoprep to a 50-mL centrifuge tube.
4. Carefully layer 35 mL of the blood/RPMI mixture onto the Lymphoprep.
5. Centrifuge at 800*g* for 25 min at 20°C with the brake off.
6. Remove the buffy coat (white layer at the RPMI/plasma interface) to another centrifuge tube using a sterile pipet.
7. Top up the centrifuge tube with RPMI-1640 and wash the leukocytes twice by centrifugation at 250*g* for 5 min at 20°C with the brake on.

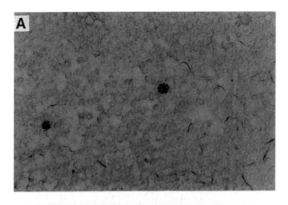

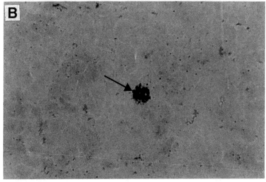

Fig. 2. Example of granules within neutrophils stained with Sudan black (**Subheading 3.2.2.**) taken from a Balb/c mouse (**A**) or a SCID-beige mouse (**B**). Arrow indicates giant granules.

8. Pour off supernatant, and resuspend leukocyte pellet in complete RPMI. Check the viability and numbers of leukocytes by mixing a small sample with an equal volume of 0.25% (w/v) trypan blue, and count using a hemacytometer.
9. Resuspend human leukocytes to $2 \times 10^7$ cells/0.25 mL in complete RPMI medium and inject 0.25 mL into the peritoneal cavity of each 4–6-wk-old immunodeficient mouse to generate Hu-PBL-SCID mice.

## 3.4. Checks for Successful Reconstitution

### 3.4.1. Measurement of Human Antibody Levels

Human antibodies are detectable in the sera of reconstituted mice from about 7d post-reconstitution, and continue to rise over the next few months (**Fig. 3**). In SCID-beige mice, we have seen maximum levels of about 3 mg/mL at 5 wk post-reconstitution (*see* **Note 7**). Mice with human Ig levels >10 μg/mL at 2 wk post-reconstitution are considered to be reconstituted (*see* **Note 8**).

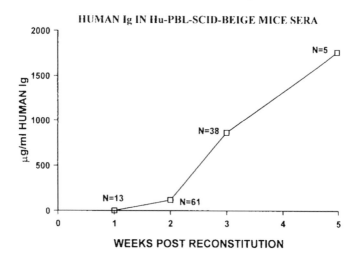

Fig. 3. Human immunoglobulin levels in SCID-beige mice following reconstitution with 2 × $10^7$ human PBLs. Antibody levels were measured as described in **Subheading 3.4.1.** N = number of mice examined at each time-point.

The method for detection of human Ig in mouse sera is the same as described in **Subheading 3.2.1.**, except that in stages 1, 5, and 7, the immunological reagents are replaced with rabbit anti-human IgG + IgM (H + L, minimum crossreactivity with mouse serum proteins) diluted 1:5000, Chromopure human Ig, and rabbit anti-human IgG + IgM (H+L)-peroxidase conjugate (minimum crossreactivity with mouse serum proteins), diluted 1:5000.

### 3.4.2. Immunohistological Staining of Paraffin-Embedded Mouse Tissues

The level of reconstitution can be evaluated from immunohistological examination of mouse tissues (**Fig. 4**). Careful control of nonspecific staining is required, and controls should include similar tissues from nonreconstituted immunodeficient mice, use of normal mouse serum instead of MAb to human CD markers, and normal human tonsil tissue as a positive control.

1. Deparaffinize sections with the following sequence:
   a. Xylene, 5 min.
   b. 100% ethanol, 5 min.
   c. 95% (v/v) ethanol, 1 min.
   d. 80% (v/v) ethanol, 1 min.
   e. PBS, 1 min.
   To enable easier staining, draw a circle around the section with a water-repellent stick or nail varnish. In all stages, 100 µL of reagent are added to each section. NB: At no time should the sections be allowed to dry out.
2. Incubate sections requiring trypsinization with the trypsin solution (**Subheading 2.6.**, **item 4**) for 30 min at room temperature.
3. Wash trypsinized sections with PBS for 5 min.

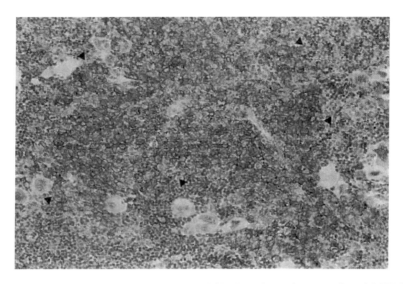

Fig. 4. Demonstration of human leukocytes within the spleen of a reconstituted SCID-beige mouse immunostained with a MAb to CD45 as described in **Subheading 3.4.2.** Arrows indicate human cells around an arteriole.

4. Incubate all sections with 3% (v/v) $H_2O_2$ in methanol for 5 min at room temperature and then wash with PBS.
5. Incubate sections with a 1:10 dilution of normal animal serum in PBS for 20 min at room temperature.
6. Drain sections (do not wash) and incubate with the appropriately diluted MAb for 45 min at 37°C or for 16 h at 4°C.
7. Wash sections in PBS, and incubate with a 1:300 dilution (in PBS) of rabbit anti-mouse IgG-biotin for 45 min at room temperature.
8. Wash sections in PBS for 5 min and incubate with a 1:500 dilution (in PBS) of streptavidin-peroxidase for 45 min at room temperature.
9. Wash sections in PBS for 5 min and incubate with AEC (made up from Zymed kit) for 10–15 min.
10. Wash sections in PBS for 5 min, rinse in distilled water, and counterstain with hematoxylin for 2 min at room temperature. Wash sections with tap water until clear and then with PBS until blue (approx 30 s). Finally, wash sections in distilled water for 5 min and apply cover slips with mountant from Zymed kit.

### 3.4.3. Flow Cytometric Analysis

Analysis of human cells within mouse tissues, such as spleen, by flow cytometry can be problematic because murine cells may stain nonspecifically for human markers (*see* **Note 1**) *(4)*. To exclude this possibility, two-color analysis must be carried out using a marker for human leukocytes (CD45) and a marker for the appropriate mouse histocompatibility antigen (e.g., anti-$H$-$2K^d$). Controls should include cells from the same tissues taken from non-reconstituted immunodeficient animals, isotype control

MAb (negative controls), human leukocytes (human positive control), and mouse leukocytes—e.g., Balb/c (mouse positive control).

1. Prepare single-cell suspension of mouse tissue—e.g., spleen or heparinized peripheral
   blood in PBS. (Do not use biotin-containing medium, such as RPMI.)
2. Adjust cell suspension to $1 \times 10^7$ cells/mL in PBSA containing 2% (v/v) normal mouse
   serum, and add 100 µL ($1 \times 10^6$ cells) to plastic round-bottomed tubes.
3. Add 10 µL of mouse antihuman CD45-fluorescein isothiocyanate (FITC) and 10 µL of
   mouse anti-mouse $H2\text{-}K^d$ biotin, mix, and incubate on ice for 45 min in the dark.
4. Add 2 mL of ice-cold PBSA + 2% BSA (w/v) and spin tubes at 300$g$ for 5 min at 4°C.
   Carefully aspirate supernatant from cell pellet. Repeat wash.
5. Add 50 µL of streptavidin-PE diluted 1:5 in PBSA and incubate for 45 min on ice in
   the dark.
6. Wash as in **step 4**.
7. Fix cells with 0.3–1.0 mL ice-cold 0.5% (w/v) paraformaldehyde, and analyze within
   1 wk.

## 4. Notes

1. The blocking of nonspecific binding when using tissue samples from reconstituted mice
   can be problematic. An alternative blocking system, described by Van Kuyk et al. *(58)*
   when using mouse anti-human CD45 and rat anti-mouse $H\text{-}2K^d$ consists of 17% rat anti-
   mouse Fcλ receptor, 15% purified rat IgG1, and 17% (v/v) normal mouse serum in HBSS
   containing 3% FBS, 0.1% sodium azide, and 10 m$M$ HEPES.
2. Although the "leakiness" of SCID and SCID-beige mice cannot be bred out, we have found
   that "leakiness" appears to be increased by the pairing of leaky parents. Thus, it is important that only nonleaky pairs (mouse immunoglobulin levels <10 µg/mL) be used for the
   breeding colony, and that their immunological status be monitored regularly. New breeding pairs should be established regularly so that breeders are only used at a young age.
   The number of SCID mice that become leaky varies with the mouse strain and the conditions under which the mice are kept (high-quality containment appears to produce fewer
   leaky mice). C.B.-17 SCID-beige mice produce approx 5–10% leaky individuals (which
   does not appear to change with age). Approximately 30% of Hu-PBL-SCID mice appear
   to become leaky—e.g. produce mouse Ig, after reconstitution with human PBLs. It has
   been reported that these mice are less likely to develop EBV-induced tumors than mice
   that are nonleaky.
3. It is also possible to look for mature mouse B- and T-cells in blood samples using flow-
   cytometry analysis in combination with specific antibody markers. Alternatively, the presence of mature mouse T- and B-lymphocytes can be determined by measuring the specific
   increased uptake of tritiated thymidine after stimulation of PBL in culture with PHA and
   LPS, respectively.
4. In order to prevent antibodies from binding to the coating in the first well before being
   diluted across, the dilutions can be made on a separate nonbinding plate. Make a 1/50
   dilution in the first well, and then double dilute across the plate. Then transfer 100 µL
   from dilution plate to coated plate, starting with the highest dilution.
5. It is important that slides of blood films be taken from fresh cuts. Heparinized blood in
   microhematocrit tubes is altered, and is unreliable for Sudan black staining. All staining
   procedures should be carried out in a chemical fume hood, and gloves must be worn.
6. In order to improve the production of human antibodies, various treatments of both the
   host and donor cells have been attempted. NK cells and CTLs can be removed from human

PBLs by pre-treatment with 250 $\mu M$ leucyl-leucine-methyl ester in serum-free RPMI for 20 min at room temperature (do not carry out at 37°C). The removal of CD8+ cells may increase the production of EBV tumors. NK-cell activity in SCID mice can be depleted by ip injection of anti-ASGM1 antibodies (Wako Chemicals, Dallas, TX) 1 d prior to human PBL injection. Engraftment with human PBL has been reported to be greatly improved by irradiating the mice with 3 Gy γ-irradiation, by injection of a MAb TMβ-1, or a combination of both treatments immediately prior to injection of the PBLs.

7. The level of human immunoglobulin in the sera of reconstituted SCID mice varies between mice, even if given the same batch of PBLs. Levels as high as 20 mg/mL have been reported. Although reports vary, in general, GVHD is not a frequent occurrence in reconstituted mice.

8. Although mice with human Ig levels >10 µg/mL are considered to be reconstituted successfully, mice with levels less than this may still be used in some cases. One of the SCID-beige strains of mice we use apparently reconstitutes poorly, producing human Ig levels of approx 1 µg/mL. However, the reconstituted mice, unlike unreconstituted mice, were susceptible to *L. pneumophila* infection.

Some mice do not become reconstituted, even when using the same donor. In our experience, approx 90% of mice reconstitute successfully (human Ig >10 µg/mL) when using 2 × 10⁷ human PBL/mouse (C.B.-17 SCID-beige).

## References

1. McCune, J. M., Namikawa, R., Kaneshima, H., Shultz, L. D., Lumberman, M., and Welshman, I. L. (1988) The SCID-Hu mouse: murine model for the analysis of human hematolymphoid differentiation and function. *Science* **241,** 1632–1639.
2. Mosier, D. E. (1990) Immunodeficient mice xenografted with human lymphoid cells: new models for in vivo studies of human immunobiology and infectious diseases. *J. Clin. Immunol.* **10,** 185–191.
3. Mosier, D. E., Gulizia, R. J., MacIsaac, P., Mathieson, B. J., Smith, G., Hu, S. L., et al. (1992) Evaluation of gp160 vaccinees in the hu-PBL-SCID mouse model. *AIDS Res. Hum. Retrovir.* **8,** 1387.
4. Mosier, D. E., Gulizia, R. J., Baird, S. M., Wilson, D. B., Spector, D. H., and Spector, S. A. (1991) Human immunodeficiency virus infection of human-PBL-SCID mice. *Science* **251,** 791–794.
5. Torbett, B. E., Picchio, G., and Mosier, D. E. (1991) Hu-PBL-SCID mice-a model for human immune function, AIDS, and lymphomagenesis. *Immunol. Rev.* **124,** 139–164.
6. Mosier, D. E., (1996) Viral pathogenesis in hu-PBL-SCID mice. *Semin. Immunol.* **8,** 255–262.
7. Levine, B., Hardwick, J. M., Trapp, B. D., Crawford, T. O., Bollinger, R. C., and Griffin, D. E. (1991) Antibody-mediated clearance of alphavirus infection from neurons. *Science* **254,** 856–860.
8. Baiocchi, R. A. and Caligiuri, M. A. (1994) Low dose interleukin 2 prevents the development of Epstein-Barr virus (EBV) associated lymphoproliferative disease in scid/scid mice reconstituted i.p. with EBV-seropositive human peripheral blood lymphocytes. *Proc. Natl. Acad. Sci. USA* **91,** 5577–5581.
9. Berney, T., Damarism Molano, R., Pileggi, A., Cattan, P., Li, H., Ricordi, C., and Inverardi, L. (2001) Patterns of engraftment in different strains of mice reconstituted with human peripheral blood lymphocytes. *Transplantation* **72,** 133–140.

10. Carballido, J. M., Namikawa, R., Carballido-Perrig, N., Antonenko, S., Roncarolo, M. G., and de Vries, J. E. (2000) generation of primary antigen-specific human T-and B-cell responses in immunocompetent SCID-hu mice. *Nat. Med.* **6,** 103–106.

11. Zhang, Z., Jin, L., Champion, G., Seydel, K. B., and Stanley S. L. (2001) *Shigella* infection in a SCID mouse-human intestinal xenograft model: a role for neutrophils in containing bacterial dissemination in human intestine. *Infect. Immun.* **69,** 3240–3247.

12. Hall, G. A, Hodgeson, A. E, Leach, S. A, Dennis, M. J., Cawthraw, S., and Newell, D. (1999) Experience with intestinal xenografts to model *Campylobacter* infection. *European Soc. Vet. Pathol.* 17th meeting, Nantes, p. 167.

13. Scaramuzzino, D. A., McNiff, J. M., and Bessen, D. E. (2000) Humanized in-vivo model for streptococcal impetigo. *Inf. Immun.* **68,** 2880–2887.

14. Bidanset, D. J., Ryback, R. J., Hartline, C. B., and Kern, E. R. (2001) Replication of human cytomegalovirus in severe combined immunodeficient mice implanted with human retinal tissue. *J. Infect. Dis.* **184,** 192–195.

15. Ilan, E., Arazi, J., Nussbaum, O., Zauberman, A., Erin, R., Lubin, I., et al. (2002) The Hepatitis C virus (HCV)-trimera mouse: A model for evaluation of agents against HCV. *I. Infect. Dis.* **185,** 153–161.

16. Kish, T. M., Budgeon, L. R., Welsh, P. A., and Howett, M. K. (2001) Immunological characterization of human vaginal xenografts in immunocompromised mice: development of a small animal model for the study of HIV-1 infection. *Am. J. Pathol.* **159,** 2331–2345.

17. Segall, H., Lubin, I., Marcus, H., Canaan, A., and Reisner, Y. (1996) Generation of primary antigen-specific human CTL in human/mouse radiation chimera. *Blood* **88,** 721–730.

18. Marusic, C., Rizza, Lattanzi, L., Mancini, C., Spada, M., Bellardelli, F., et al. (2001) Chimeric plant virus particles as immunogens for inducing murine and human immune responses against HIV-1. *J. Virol.* **75,** 8434–8439.

19. Delhem, N., Hadida, F., Gorochov, G., Carpentier, F., de Cavel, J. P., Andreani, J. F., et al. (1998) Primary Th1 cell immunization against HIVgp160 in SCID-hu mice co-engrafted with peripheral blood lymphocytes and skin. *J. Immunol.* **161,** 2060–2069.

20. Duchosal, M. A., Fuzzati-Armentero, M. T., Baccala, R., Layer, A., Gonzalez-Quintial, R., Leturq, M. R., et al. (2000) Human adult tonsil xenotransplantation into SCID mice for studying human immune responses and B-cell lymphomagenesis. *Exp. Hematol.* **28,** 177–192.

21. Albert, S. E., McKerlie, C., Pester, A., Edgell, B. J., Carlyle, J., Petric, M., et al. (1997) Time-dependent induction of protective anti-influenza immune responses. *J. Immunol.* **159,** 1393–1403.

22. Holscher, C., Hasch, G., Joswig, N., Stauffer, U., Muller, U., and Mossman, H. (1999) Long-term substitution and specific immune responses after transfer of bovine peripheral blood lymphocytes into severe combined immunodeficient mice. *Vet. Immunol. Immunopathol.* **70,** 67–83.

23. Murphey, W. J., Funarkoski, S., Fanslow, W. C., Rager, H. C., Taub, D. D., and Longo, D. L. (1999) CD40 stimulation promotes human secondary immunoglobulin reponses in HuPBL-SCID chimeras. *Clin. Immunol.* **90,** 22–27.

24. Sandhu, J., Shpitz, B., Gallinger, S., and Hozumi, N. (1994) Human primary immune response in SCID mice engrafted with human peripheral blood lymphocytes. *J. Immunol.* **152,** 3806–3813.

25. Tournoy, K. G., Depraetere, S., Pauwels, R. A., and Leroux-Roels, G. G. (2000) Mouse strain and conditioning regimen determine survival and function of human leucocytes in immunodeficient mice. *Clin. Exp. Immunol.* **119,** 231–239.

26. Mead, J. R., Arrowood, M. J., Healey, M. C., and Sidwell, R. W. (1991) Cryptosporidial infections in SCID mice reconstituted with human or murine lymphocytes. *J. Protozool.* **38**, 59S–61S.

27. Sarin, P. S., Talmadge, J. E., Heseltine, P., Murcar, N., Gendelman, H. E., Coleman, R., et al. (1999) Booster immunization of HIV-1 negative volunteers with HGP-30 vaccine induces protection against HIV-1 virus challenge in SCID mice. *Vaccine* **17**, 64–71.

28. Nguyen, H., Hay, J., Mazzuli, T., Gallinger, S., Sandhu, J., Teng, Y-T. A., and Hozumi, N. (2000) Efficient generation of respiratory syncitial virus (RSV)-neutralizing human MoAbs via human peripheral blood lymphocyte (huPBL)-SCID mice and scFv phage display libraries. *Clin. Exp. Immunol.* **122**, 85–93.

29. Baiocchi, R. A., Ward, J. S., Carrodeguas, L., Eisbeis, C. F., Peng, R., Roychowdhury, S., et al. (2001) GM-CSF and IL-2 induce specific cellular immunity and provide protection against Epstein-Barr virus lymphoproliferative disorder. *J. Clin. Investig.* **108**, 887–894.

30. Gupta, M., Mahanty, S., Bray, M., Ahmed, R., and Rollin, P. E. (2001) Passive transfer of antibodies protects immunocompetent and immunodeficient mice against lethal Ebola virus infection without complete inhibition of viral replication. *J. Virol.* **75**, 4649–4654.

31. Gaudin, M. C., Allaway, G. P., Olson, W. C., Weir, R., Maddon, P. J., and Koup, R. A. (1998) CD4-immunoglobulin G2 protects Hu-PBL-SCID mice against challenge by primary human immunodeficiency virus type 1 isolates. *J. Virol.* **72**, 3475–3478.

32. Fowler, K., McBride, B. W., Turnbull, P. C., and Baillie, L. W. (1999) Immune correlates of protection against anthrax. *J. Appl. Microbiol.* **87**, 305.

33. Bosma, M. J. and Carroll, A. M. (1991) The SCID mouse mutant: definition, characterization, and potential uses. *Annu. Rev. Immunol.* **9**, 323–350.

34. Jhappan, C., Morse, H. C., Fleischmann, R. D., Gottesman, M. M, and Merlino, G. (1997) DNA-PKcs: a T-cell tumour suppressor encoded at the mouse scid locus. *Nat. Genet.* **17**, 483–486

35. Hinkley, K. S., Chiasson, R. J., Prior, T. K., and Riggs, J. E. (2002) Age-dependent increase of peritoneal B-1b B-cells in SCID mice. *Immunology* **105**, 196–203.

36. Garcia, S., Dadaglio, G., and Gougeon, M. L. (1997) Limits of the Human-PBL-SCID mice model: severe restrictions of the Vβ T-cell repertoire of engrafted human T-cells. *Blood* **89**, 329–336.

37. Nonoyama, S., Smith, F. O., Bernstein, I. D., and Ochs, H. (1993) Strain-dependent leakiness of mice with severe combined immune deficiency. *J. Immunol.* **150**, 3817–3824.

38. Anderson, M. R. and Tary-Lehmann, M. (2001) Staphylococcal enterotoxin-B-induces lethal shock in mice is T-cell dependent but disease susceptibility is defined by the non T-cell compartment. *Clin. Immunol.* **98**, 85–94.

39. MacDougall, J. R., Croy, B. A., Chapeau, C., and Clark, D. A. (1990) Demonstration of a splenic cytotoxic effector cell in mice of genotype SCID/SCID.BG/BG. *Cell. Immunol.* **130**, 106–117.

40. Mosier, D. E., Stell, K. L., Gulizia, R. J., Torbett, B. E., and Gilmore, G. L. (1993) Homozygous scid/scid-beige/beige mice have low levels of spontaneous or neonatal T-cell-induced B-cell generation. *J. Exp. Med.* **177**, 191–194.

41. Froidevaux, S. and Loor, F. (1991) A quick procedure for identifying doubly homozygous immunodeficient scid beige mice. *J. Immunol. Methods* **137**, 275–279.

42. Shultz, L. D., Schweitzer, P. A., Christianson, S. W., Gott, B., Schweitzer, I. B., Tennent, B., Mckenna, S., Mobraaten, L., Rajan, T. V., and Geiner, D. L. (1995) Multiple defects in innate and adaptive immunologic function in NOD/LtSz-scid mice. *J. Immunol.* **154**, 180–191.

43. Greiner, D. L. and Shultz, L. D. (1998) The use of NOD/LtSz-scid/scid mice in biomedical research, in *NOD Mice and Related Strains: Research Applications in Diabetes, AIDS, Cancer and Other Diseases*. (Leiter, E. and Athinson, M., eds.) Landes Bioscience, Austin, TX pp. 173–203.

44. Dick, J. E., Guenechea, G., Gan, O. I., and Dorrell, C. (2001) In vivo dynamics of human stem cell repopulation in NOD/SCID mice. *Ann. NY Acad. Sci.* **938,** 184–190.

45. Lapidot, T. (2001) Mechanism of human stem-cell migration and repopulation of NOD/SCID and B2mnull mice: The role of SDF-1/CXCR4 interactions. *Ann. NY Acad. Sci.* **938,** 83–95.

46. Kollet, O., Peled, A., Byk, T., Ben-Hur, H., Greiner, D., Shultz, L., and Lapidot, T. (2000) β2 microglobin-deficient (B2m$^{null}$) NOD/SCID mice are excellent recipients for studying human stem cell function. *Blood* **95,** 3102–3105.

47. Kerre, T. C., De Smet, G., De Smet, M., Zippelius, A., Pittet, M. J., Langerak, A. W., de Bosscher, J., Offner, F., Vanderkerchove, B., and Plum, J. (2002) Adapted NOD/SCID model supports development of phenotypically and functionally mature T-cells from human umbilical cord blood CD34(+) cells. *Blood* **99,** 1620–1626.

48. Hogan, C. J., Shpall, E. J., McNulty, O., McNiece, I., Dick, J. E., Shultz, L. D., and Keller, G. (1997) Engraftment and development of human CD34(+)-enriched cells from umbilical cord blood in NOD/LtSz-scid/scid mice. *Blood* **90,** 85–96.

49. Hogan, C. J., Shpall, E. J., McNiece, I., and Keller, G. (1997) Multilineage engraftment in NOD/LtSz-scid/scid mice from mobilized human CD34(+) peripheral blood progenitor cells. *Biol. Blood Marrow Transplant* **3,** 236–246.

50. Shinkai, Y., Rathbun, G., Lam, K.-P., Oltz, E. M., Stewart, V., Mendelsohn, M., et al. (1992) RAG-2-Deficient mice lack mature lymphocytes owing to inability to initiate V(D)J rearrangement. *Cell* **68,** 855–867.

51. Shultz, L. D., Lang, P. A., Christianson, S. W., Gott, B., Lyons, B., Umeda, S., et al. (2000) NOD/LtSz-Rag/null mice: an immunodeficient and radio-resistant model for engraftment of human hematolymphoid cells, HIV infection and adoptive transfer of NOD mouse diabetogenic T-cells. *J. Immunol.* **164,** 2496–2507.

52. Aaberge, I. S., Michaelsen, T. E., Rolstad, A. K., Groeng, E. C., Solberg, P., and Lovik, M. (1992) SCID-Hu mice immunized with a pneumococcal vaccine produce specific human antibodies and show increased resistance to infection. *Infect. Immunol.* **60,** 4146–4153.

53. He, X., Weyand, C. M., Goronzy, J. J., Zhong, W., and Stuart, J. M. (2002) Bi-directional modulation of T-cell-dependent antibody production by prostaglandin E(2) *Int. Immunol.* **14,** 69–77.

54. Wedderburn, L. R., Jeffery, R., White, H., Patel, A., Vaarsini, H., Lind, D., et al. (2001) Autologous stem cell transplantation for paediatric-onset polyarthritis nodosa: changes in autoimmune phenotype in the context of reduced diversity of the T- and B-cell repertoires and evidence for reversion from CD45RO(+) to RA(+) phenotype. *Rheumatology* **40,** 1299–1307.

55. Giorgi, J. V., Hausner, M. A., and Hultin, L. E. (1999) Detailed immune phenotype of CD8+ memory cyotoxic T-lymphocytes (CTL) against HIV-1 with respect to expression of CD45RA/RO, CD62L and CD28 antigens. *Immunol. Lett.* **66,** 105–110.

56. Roncarolo, M. G., Carballido, J. M., Rouleau, M., Namikawa, R., and de Vries, J. E. (1996) Human T- and B-cell functions in SCID-hu mice. *Semin. Immunol.* **8,** 207–213.

57. Mosier, D. E., Gulizia, R. J., MacIsaac, P. D., Corey, L., and Greenberg, P. D. (1993) Resistance to human immunodeficiency virus 1 infection of SCID mice reconstituted with

peripheral blood leukocytes from donors vaccinated with vaccinia gpl60 and recombinant gpl60. *Proc. Natl. Acad. Sci. USA* **90**, 2443–2447.

58. Van Kuyk, R., Torbett, B. E., Gulizia, R. J., Leath, S., Mosier, D. E., and Koenig, S. (1994) Cloned human CD8+ T lymphocytes protect human peripheral blood leukocyte-severe combined immunodeficient mice from HIV-l infection by an HLA-unrestricted mechanism. *J. Immunol.* **153**, 4826–4833.

59. Williams, A., McBride, B. W., Hall, G., Fitzgeorge, R. B., and Farrar, G. H. (1995) Experimental legionnaires disease in SCID-Beige mice reconstituted with human leukocytes. *J. Med. Microbiol.* **42**, 433–441.

60. Ono, M., Wada, Y., Wu, Y., Nemori, R., Jinbo, Y., Wang, H., et al. (1997) FP-21399 blocks HIV envelope protein-mediated membrane fussion and concentrates in lymph nodes. *Nat. Biotechnol.* **15**, 343–348.

61. Di Fabio, S., Giannini, G., Lapenta, C., Spada, M., Binelli, A., Germinario, E., et al. (2001) Vaginal transmission of HIV in hu-SCID mice: a new model for the evaluation of vaginal microbicides. *AIDS* **15**, 2231–2238.

62. Bahr, G. M., Darcissac, E. C., Casteran, N., Amiel, C., Cocude, C., Truong, M. J., et al. (2001) Selective regulation of human immunodeficiency virus-infected CD4(+) lymphocytes by a synthetic immunomodulator leads to potent virus suppression in vitro and in hu-PGL-SCID mice. *J. Virol.* **75**, 6941–6952.

63. Miura, Y., Misawa, N., Maeda, N., Inagaki, Y., Tanaka, Y., Ito, M., et al. (2001) Critical contribution of tumour necrosis factor-related apoptosis-inducing ligand (TRAIL) to apoptosis of human CD4+ T-cells in HIV-1 infected hu-PGL-NOD-SCID mice. *J. Exp. Med.* **193**, 651–660.

64. Brooks, D. G. and Zack, J. A. (2002) Effect of latent human immunodeficiency virus infection on cell surface phenotype. *J. Virol.* **76**, 1673–1681.

65. Mercer, D. F., Schiller, D. E., Elliott, J. F., Douglas, D. N., Hao, C., Rinfret, A., et al. (2001) Hepatitis C virus replication in mice with chimeric human livers. *Nat. Med.* **7**, 890–891.

66. Santos, R. A., Hatfield, C. C., Cole, N. L., Padilla, J. A., Moffat, J. F., Arvin, A. M., et al. (2000) Varicella-zoster virus escape mutant VZV-MSP exhibits an accelerated cell-to cell spread phenotype in both infected cell cultures and SCID-hu mice. *Virology* **275**, 306–317.

67. Pletnev, A. G. (2001) Infectious cDNA clone of attenuated Langat tick-borne flavivirus (strain E5) and a 3' deletion mutant constructed from it exhibit decreased neuroinvasiveness in immunodeficient mice. *Virology* **282**, 288–300.

68. VanCott, J. L., McNeal, M. M., Flint, J., Bailey, S. A., Choi, A. H., and Ward R. L. (2001) *Eur. J. Immunol.* **31**, 3380–3387.

69. Neyts, J. and De Clerq, E. (2001) Efficacy of 2-amino-7-(1,3-dihydroxy-2-propoxymethyl) purine for treatment of Vaccinia virus (Orthopoxvirus) infections in mice. *Antimicrob. Agents. Chemother.* **45**, 84–87.

70. Yoshida, M., Watanabe, T., Usui, T., Matsunaga, Y., Shirai, Y., Yamori, M., et al. (2001) CD4 T-cells monospecific to ovalbumin produced by *Escherichia coli* can induce colitis upon transfer to Balb/c and SCID mice. *Int. Immunol.* **13**, 1561–1570.

71. Wirtz, S., Becker, C., Blumberg, R., Galle, P. R., and Neurath, F. (2002) Treatment of T-cell-dependent experimental colitis in SCID mice by local administration of an adenovirus expressing LI-18 antisense m RNA. *J. Immunol.* **168**, 411–420.

72. Leriche-Guerin, K., Anderson, L. V., Wrogemann, K., Roy, B., Goulet, M., Tremblay, J. P. (2002) Dysferlin expression after normal myoblast transplantation in SCID and in SJL mice. *Neuromuscul. Disord.* **12**, 167–173.

73. Hodgeson, A. E., McBride, B. W., Hudson, M. J., Hall, G., and Leach S. A. (1998) Experimental campylobacter infection and diarrhoea in immunodeficient mice. *J. Med. Microbiol.* **47**, 799–809.

74. Hondalus, M. K., Bardarov, S., Russell, R., Chan, J., Jacobs, W. R., and Bloom, B. (2000) Attenuation of and protection induced by a leucine auxotroph of *Mycobacterium tuberculosis*. *Infect. Immun.* **68**, 2888–2898.

75. Smith, D. A., Parish, T., Stoker, N. G., and Bancroft, G. J. (2001) Characterization of auxotrophic mutants of *Mycobacterium tuberculosis* and their potential as vaccine candidates. *Infect. Immun.* **69**, 1142–1150.

76. Winslow, G. M., Yager, E., Shilo, K., Volk, E., Reilly, A., and Chu, F. K. (2000) Antibody-mediated elimination of the obligate intracellular bacterial pathogen *Erlichia chaffeensis* during active infection. *Infect. Immun.* **68**, 2187–2195.

77. Paciorkowski, N., Porte, P., Shultz, L. D., and Rajan, T. V. (2000) B1 B lymphocytes play a critical role in host protection against lymphatic filarial parasites. *J. Exp. Med.* **191**, 731–735.

78. Morrison, L. A., Zhu, L., and Thebeau, L. G. (2001) Vaccine-induced serum immunoglobulin contributes to protection from herpes simplex virus type 2 genital infection in the presence of immune T-cells. *J. Virol.* **75**, 1195–1204.

79. Derby, M. A., Alexander-Miller, M. A., Tse, R., and Berkofsky, J. A. (2001) High-avidity CTL exploit two complementary mechanisms to provide better protection against viral infection than low-avidity CTL. *J. Immunol.* **166**, 1690–1697.

80. Cao, T., Meuleman, P., Deambere, I., Sallberg, M., and Leroux-Roels, G. (2001) In vivo inhibition of anti-hepatitis B virus core antigen (HbcAg) immunoglobulin G production by HbcAg-specific CD4(+) Th1-type T-cell clones in a hu-PBL-NOD/SCID mouse model. *J. Virol.* **75**, 11,449–11,456.

81. Hoft, D. F., Schnapp, A. R., Eickhoff, C. S., and Roodman, S. T. (2000) Involvement of CD4+ Th1 cells in systemic immunity protective against primary and secondary challenges with *Trypanosma cruzi*. *Infect. Immun.* **68**, 197–204.

82. Zhong, W., Gern, L., Stehle, T., Museteanu, C., Kramer, M., Wallich, R., and Simon, M. M. (1999) Resolution of experimental and tick-borne *Borrelia burgdorferi* infection in mice by passive but not active immunization using recombinant OspC. *Eur. J. Immunol.* **29**, 946–957.

83. Naito, S., Okada, Y., Takahashi, M., Kato, H., Taneichi, M., Ami, Y., et al. (2000) Anti-tetanus toxoid antibody production and protection against lethal doses of tetanus toxin in hu-PBL-SCID mice. *Int. Arch. Allergy Immunol.* **123**, 149–154.

# 21

# Clinical Trials

## Paddy Farrington and Elizabeth Miller

## 1. Introduction

The transition from laboratory testing to evaluation in humans marks an important stage in vaccine development. Concerns about safety and benefit to the patient and to the community may raise complex ethical issues, whereas the inherent variability of human responses must be taken into account to obtain valid estimates of vaccine effect. This latter requirement explains why a coherent statistical framework for the design, analysis, and interpretation of clinical trials is regarded as essential today. A vast body of experience and methodology has been developed since the 1940s, when the scientific method was first applied systematically to the evaluation of vaccines. One striking feature of clinical trial research is its broad collaborative nature, involving laboratory, epidemiological, clinical, and statistical skills. As a result, rather than attempt to describe in detail the planning and conduct of clinical trials, this chapter will review the broad principles and stages involved in evaluating vaccines in humans, using examples from the literature. Details of methodological and other issues of particular relevance to vaccine evaluation are provided in **Subheading 3**. In the UK and elsewhere, the Clinical Trials Directive 2001/20/EU will be implemented by May 2004 to provide legislation that will standardize clinical trials throuhgout the European community.

## 2. The Evaluation Process

Vaccines are evaluated in a sequence of clinical trials, which provide increasingly stringent tests of the vaccine's safety, immunogenicity, and protective efficacy. Successful completion of the first three experimental phases is normally required for licensure, after which further observational studies are undertaken to monitor the performance of the vaccine in the field. The main features of these various phases are compared in **Table 1**. However, these categorizations are not rigid. Vaccine evalua-

From: *Methods in Molecular Medicine, Vol. 87: Vaccine Protocols, 2nd ed.*
Edited by: A. Robinson, M. J. Hudson, and M. P. Cranage © Humana Press Inc., Totowa, NJ

**Table 1**
**The Evaluation Process**

| | | Main characteristics | | |
|---|---|---|---|---|
| Stage | Rationale | Primary outcome | Subjects | Design |
| Phase I | First trials in humans | Safety and immunogenicity | Adult volunteers Typical study size: 10–100 | Controlled or uncontrolled |
| Phase II | Initial evaluation in target population | Safety and immunogenicity | Target population Typical study size: 50–500 | Randomized, double-blind controlled trial |
| Phase III | Full evaluation in target population | Protective efficacy | Target population Typical study size: 1000–50,000 | Randomized, double-blind controlled trial |
| Phase IV | Post-licensure surveillance | Safety and effectiveness | Vaccinees Variable study size | Epidemiologic studies |

tion strategies will vary according to different circumstances, as in the context of the AIDS epidemic *(1)*.

Clinical trials are undertaken in accordance with a protocol that sets out the rationale for the study and the detailed plan of the investigation. **Fig. 1** shows typical headings for a vaccine trial protocol, which may be expanded in suitable appendices to include model letters and forms, laboratory protocols, and details of other procedures. The protocol forms the basis of the submission to ethical committees and thus must demonstrate that the study meets ethical requirements (*see* **Note 1**).

## 2.1. Phase I Trials

These are the first trials in which the experimental vaccine is used in humans, and are typically conducted in adult volunteers. Phase I trials are generally small, and increase in size as experience with the vaccine grows: One trial of a new live oral typhoid fever vaccine was conducted on a sample of only three *(2)*. The primary goal of such trials is to accrue initial data on the tolerability and immunogenicity of the vaccine prior to conducting larger Phase II studies. The safety data available from Phase I trials is necessarily limited to documenting the more common reactions and identifying serious or unusual adverse side effects. In some cases, prior exposure to the infectious agent may present special problems. In a trial of a diphtheria conjugate meningococcal A and C vaccine, 80 adult volunteers were recruited, but only 8 had sufficiently low antidiphtheria antibody titers to allow them to receive the vaccine, and an additional 8 were given a placebo *(3)*.

A further problem with some vaccines—particularly polysaccharide vaccines—is that the immune response is age-dependent *(4)*, thus limiting the value of antibody data collected on adults. For the common childhood infections, few if any adults are

```
┌─────────────────────────────────────────────┐
│                                             │
│          Protocol Headings                  │
│                                             │
│   1.  Introduction                          │
│       Background and rationale              │
│                                             │
│   2.  Aims and objectives                   │
│       Primary and secondary objectives      │
│                                             │
│   3.  Study design                          │
│       Outcome measures. hypotheses,         │
│       plan of study, trial size             │
│                                             │
│   4.  Study population                      │
│       Inclusion and exclusion criteria      │
│                                             │
│   5.  Methods and Procedures                │
│       Recruitment, vaccine handling.        │
│       vaccine delivery, follow-up, laboratory│
│       methods, statistical analysis         │
│                                             │
│   6.  Trial Monitoring                      │
│       Data monitoring, quality assurance    │
│       of data and laboratory methods        │
│                                             │
│   7.  Timetable                             │
│       Start and end of recruitment, end of  │
│       follow-up, date of report             │
│                                             │
│   8.  Ethical approval                      │
│                                             │
└─────────────────────────────────────────────┘
```

Fig. 1. Protocol headings.

likely to remain susceptible. In this case, immune responses may reflect secondary rather than primary responses, as was found in a Phase I trial of an acellular pertussis vaccine in which, prior to the trial, only 8 of 54 participants lacked detectable antibody to one of the three antigens in the vaccine *(5)*. In some cases, more detailed investigations on optimal dosage and delivery may be undertaken in Phase I trials. For example, a trial of a vaccine against tick-borne encephalitis demonstrated a clear dose-to-antibody response relationship in 56 healthy volunteers randomized to five different doses of antigen *(6)*. Occasionally, Phase I trials can help to elucidate the biological mechanisms involved in a vaccine's effect. A randomized placebo-controlled Phase I trial of vaccine therapy in 28 patients with acquired immunodeficiency syndrome (AIDS) or AIDS-related complex (ARC), for instance, suggested that the clinical improvements observed in immunized patients were attributable to a nonspecific effect of the vaccine on boosting natural resistance rather than to antiHIV immunity *(7)*.

Uncontrolled studies may be adequate, especially in earlier Phase I trials, particularly because comparisons of reaction rates between necessarily small and possibly atypical groups may be biased, and certainly lack power (*see* **Note 2**). For instance, in the trial of meningococcal A and C vaccine mentioned previously *(3)*, 6/8 vaccinees and 2/7 placebo recipients experienced local pain after the second dose. The difference of 46% in reaction rates is not significant ($p = 0.13$), but the power to detect such a difference, if genuine, is only 40% with this sample size. The use of a control group, preferably randomized, is nevertheless valuable in generating hypotheses to be tested in subsequent trials.

## 2.2. Phase II Trials

Following successful completion of Phase I studies, the vaccine may be evaluated in those individuals for whose benefit it was developed. The vaccine is now being administered for its potential prophylactic effect, and its use in the United Kingdom is regulated by the Medicines Act (1976) and a Clinical Trial Certificate (CTC) or Exemption (CTX) is required. Information on the method of manufacture, the results of toxicity and immunogenicity testing in animals, evidence of protection in an animal model, and data from Phase I studies are fully considered before approval is given. Similar regulatory control over prelicensing use of vaccines exists in other countries— for example, the Federal Food, Drug and Cosmetic Act in the United States.

The primary objective of Phase II trials is to evaluate the safety and reactogenicity of one or several vaccine preparations in their target population (*see* **Note 3**). This evaluation is usually comparative, and Phase II trials typically involve one or more vaccines and a control group. The sample sizes should be sufficient to identify clinically important differences in reaction rates and immune responses, a requirement that seldom necessitates more than a few hundred participants (*see* **Note 4**). Careful design and analysis, with due attention to statistical issues, are required to avoid biased comparisons and invalid inferences. In particular, a random allocation of participants to vaccine groups is recommended (*see* **Note 5**). Ideally, group membership should be unknown to both the participant and the clinician, and indeed the laboratory staff that undertake the serological testing. However, such "double blinding" is not always possible. For example, in a trial of diphtheria-tetanus-pertussis (DTP) and *Haemophilus influenzae b* (Hib) vaccines given separately or combined to infants in a single vaccine, it was clearly impossible to mask group membership *(8)*.When two vaccines were given separately, parents were not told which was administered to which arm, so that an element of single-blinding was maintained. A further comparison, again necessarily unblinded, was also made between injection sites—all injections in the first half of the study were administered into the thigh, and all in the second half into the arm. This study also illustrates the economy of so-called factorial designs (*see* **Note 6**); the two comparisons (between vaccine groups and injection sites) were achieved without the need to increase the sample size over that required for each one separately. In this example, any bias caused by the lack of double-blinding could have been eliminated by use of a placebo. However, this was considered unethical, since both vaccines have proven benefits.

Ethical issues of this nature are likely to become increasingly common as new vaccines (or combinations of vaccines) are developed to replace existing ones. In such situations, the appropriate control is the existing vaccine rather than a placebo, and the trial can only be justified on ethical grounds if the new preparation presents some additional benefit, at least in principle. For example, in a Phase II trial of acellular pertussis vaccines in the United Kingdom, the control was the existing whole-cell vaccine and the ethical justification of the trial rested on the positive benefit of reduced reactogenicity from the acellular preparation *(9)*. When ethically justified, use of a placebo control group is recommended, since it provides insurance against unexpected events. For instance, a placebo-controlled Phase II trial of rotavirus vaccine in the United States failed to demonstrate any difference in the serological response rates in vaccine and placebo recipients, which the investigators attributed to an unexpectedly high incidence of asymptomatic wild-type infection *(10)*. This would not have been picked up if the study had not included placebo controls.

When the purpose of the trial is to compare vaccine groups, or vaccine and placebo groups, it is important to select a sample size large enough to distinguish systematic differences between groups from fluctuations resulting from the random variability in individual responses (such as reactions) and measurements (such as rectal temperatures or antibody levels). In order to calculate the sample size, *a priori* estimates of the magnitude of the background variability of the quantities to be measured are required. For quantities expressed as proportions, an estimate of this proportion is needed. For quantitative measurements, an estimate of the standard deviation is required. These initial estimates may be obtained from earlier Phase I studies or from the literature. The statistical issues involved in calculating sample sizes are discussed in **Note 4**.

In view of their appreciable size, Phase II trials require careful attention to logistical issues. In particular, clear procedures are required for handling vaccines, including their labeling, storage, and transport. The condition of the vaccines should be monitored, for instance, using temperature-sensitive (ts) devices to identify any that may have been exposed to temperatures outside the recommended range during storage or distribution. More generally, strict quality-control procedures are required (*see* **Note 7**).

Most Phase II trials may be regarded as preliminary investigations, laying the groundwork for Phase III protective efficacy trials. Some trials are used to identify the most promising preparations, dosages, and schedules for evaluation in a Phase III trial. In some cases, however, Phase II type studies take on a different purpose because they are used to support major decisions about vaccination policy. For instance, this is the case when a vaccine has already undergone a successful evaluation in a Phase III trial, possibly in another country; additional data are required to support the introduction of the vaccine in a different population, and possibly under a different immunization schedule from that used in the Phase III trial. Such Phase II trials may be described as confirmatory rather than exploratory. Thus, confirmatory Phase II trials of acellular pertussis vaccine were planned in the United Kingdom to evaluate those preparations for which efficacy, relative to whole-cell vaccine, had been demonstrated in Phase III trials conducted in countries with a higher incidence of pertussis than the United Kingdom.

The recent introduction of meningococcal C conjugate vaccine into the UK primary immunization schedules provides an excellent example of how Phase II trials can be designed to support licensure of vaccines and underpin policy decisions. This was the rationale for the coordinated series of Phase II trials that preceded the implementation of the national meningococcal C conjugate vaccination program in the United Kingdom *(11)*. Because a correlate of protection based on the serum bactericidal assay already existed for C polysaccharide vaccines *(12)*, formal efficacy trials of the C conjugate vaccines were not considered necessary for licensure by the UK Medicines Control Agency. However, a number of key policy-related questions needed to be answered in Phase II trials before a national campaign with these vaccines could be planned in the target high-risk population (namely, all individuals under 18 yr of age). These were as follows: What is the minimum number of doses required for immunization of children 1 yr of age and above? Are there any interactions between the diphtheria and tetanus proteins used in the conjugate vaccines and other diphtheria and tetanus-containing vaccines given to the target population? What is the safety profile of the vaccine in a school-age population? What is the response in children who have already received the unconjugated meningococcal C vaccine? An integrated series of phase II trials, funded by the Department of Health, was therefore designed to answer these questions and to provide comparative immunogenicity and safety data on different manufacturers' vaccines *(11)*. The DH-funded trials were carried out in tandem with the manufacturer-sponsored trials designed to provide the immunogenicity and safety data needed to support a license application.

### 2.3. Phase III Trials

The primary purpose of a Phase III trial is to assess the protective efficacy of the vaccine in the target population. Vaccine efficacy (VE) is defined as the percentage reduction in the incidence rate of disease in vaccinated compared to unvaccinated individuals. Thus:

$$VE = 100 \times (IRU - IRV)/IRU \qquad (1)$$

where IRU denotes the incidence rate in unvaccinated and IRV the incidence rate in vaccinated individuals. Very rarely, other indices of vaccine efficacy may be used. For instance, in a therapeutic trial of herpes simplex virus vaccine in patients with chronic, recurrent genital herpes, efficacy was defined as the absolute reduction in the average number of recurrences per month *(13)*.

The incidence rates IRU and IRV are usually calculated as numbers of events per total person-time of follow-up, thus allowing for different observation times between individuals. For recurrent infections, the numerators may include either only the first or the total number of distinct episodes. These various definitions have been used in trials of the SPf66 malaria synthetic vaccine *(14,15)*. For the particular circumstances of measles vaccine trials in developing countries, it has been argued that it is more appropriate to use total mortality from any cause, rather than measles morbidity, as the primary outcome *(16)*, since the effect of vaccination may have nonspecific immunologic consequences. This raises the important issue of whether Phase III trials should be experimental (conducted under controlled conditions to measure a biological effect) or practical (undertaken in conditions similar to those in which the vaccine will be routinely administered to evaluate the impact on public health). The emphasis will vary according to circumstances, but the issue is all the more important because once a trial has been completed, for ethical reasons it may be impossible to repeat it.

Phase III trials may be large, especially when the disease concerned is rare. The 1954 field trial of the Salk polio vaccine involved 1.8 million children in the United States, of whom over 400,000 were randomly assigned to vaccine or placebo, and a much larger number enrolled in an open study *(17)*. Trials on such a gigantic scale are rare, but many nevertheless require sample sizes running into the thousands. Whatever their size, Phase III trials require careful design in order to avoid the potential biases that may arise from variations in disease incidence and case ascertainment. Phase III trials must therefore, as a general rule, involve a randomized control group with double-blind treatment allocation, and will require careful management and the application of quality-control procedures (*see* **Notes 5** and **7**). In addition, procedures for handling protocol violations and losses to follow-up should be clarified prior to starting the trial, since these can have a substantial impact on the results (*see* **Notes 8** and **9**).

The first stage in planning a Phase III trial is to define the outcome of primary interest. Many vaccines—e.g., those against pertussis *(18)* or rotavirus *(19)*—alter the clinical course of disease. Thus, a vaccine that is effective in preventing clinically typical disease may have a considerably lower efficacy against milder or asymptomatic infection. Clarity about the purpose of the trial and the intended use of the vaccine is, therefore essential from the start in order to avoid confusion resulting from contradictory interpretations of the trial results.

These considerations will guide the choice of primary case definition, which should be chosen with care and with due regard to possible biases. Clinical case definitions may lack specificity, unless corroborated by laboratory evidence. Nonspecific case definitions will bias vaccine-efficacy estimates toward zero, since the vaccine cannot be expected to protect against infections other than that for which it was developed. This problem arises particularly for relatively rare infections. Thus, although the original MRC trials of pertussis vaccine could make use of a purely clinical case definition in the 1940s and 1950s, when whooping cough was widespread *(20)*, such an approach would no longer be appropriate today, when vaccination has greatly reduced the proportion of pertussis-like episodes attributable to *Bordetella pertussis*. This illustrates the important point that the specificity and predictive value of case definitions are not absolutes, but depend on epidemiological factors, such as the disease incidence and the incidence of infections with similar clinical manifestations *(21)*. The specificity of a clinical case definition may be improved by laboratory confirmation. However, the use of laboratory methods for this purpose should be validated, since the sensitivity of the method may vary between vaccinated and unvaccinated cases. For example, there is some evidence that bacterial isolation rates of *B. pertussis* are lower in vaccinated than unvaccinated cases *(22,23)*, which would result in an artificially high estimate of vaccine efficacy. This was apparent in the first Swedish Phase III trial of two acellular pertussis vaccines against placebo, which used cough plus isolation of *B. pertussis* as the primary case definition and produced estimated efficacies of 54% and 69% *(24)*. Subsequent reanalysis, however, using serological markers as laboratory evidence of infection, suggested that these estimates could have been seriously biased upward by differential sensitivity of the culture method, but that high efficacy was nevertheless achieved against clinically typical pertussis *(23)*. Subsequent clinical trials in Sweden have used a revised case definition encompassing clinically typical, laboratory-confirmed pertussis. Clearly, restricting the focus to more severe disease may require larger sample sizes, since the number of cases will be reduced.

Phase III trials should be designed with a clear primary goal, to ensure the statistical validity of the results and avoid problems of interpretation arising from the use of multiple end points (*see* **Note 10**). This primary goal will vary according to different circumstances. Thus, for example, if the vaccine is the first available preparation against a serious disease, the trial should be designed to detect any evidence of protective efficacy. This would be the case with an AIDS vaccine trial. Difficult ethical issues surround the dilemma of whether such a trial should be interrupted and vaccine offered to all who are at risk once some protective efficacy has been demonstrated—or whether the study should be continued to obtain more precise estimates of vaccine efficacy and information on longer-term protection. This issue arose in a trial of Zidovudine in HIV-infected patients *(25)*. Provisions for interim analyses to be undertaken by an independent Data Monitoring Committee with the power to break the randomization code should therefore be made in the trial protocol, along with a statement regarding their statistical implications. For less serious diseases, such as rotavirus infection in developed countries, a vaccine may be required to demonstrate a substantial protective effect (for example, VE >70%) before it would be considered for widespread use.

Recent Phase III trials of a heptavalent pneumococcal conjugate vaccine in the United States had the primary outcome measurement of protective efficacy against invasive pneumococcal disease in infants caused by the serotypes included in the vaccine *(26)*. Secondary outcomes were protection against invasive pneumococcal disease regardless of serotype, effectiveness against clinical otitis media visits and episodes, and the impact on frequent and severe otitis media and ventilatory-tube replacement. High efficacy (97.4%) was demonstrated for the primary outcome, and lower but informative efficacies for the secondary outcomes were demonstrated. The conclusion was that the vaccine was highly effective in preventing invasive pneumococcal disease, and had a significant impact on otitis media.

Particular problems surround the evaluation of protective efficacy for second-generation or subsequent vaccines. Thus, acellular pertussis vaccines could only be introduced for primary immunization in the United Kingdom if they were shown to offer equivalent protection to the whole-cell vaccines in Phase III trials, their added benefit deriving from much reduced reactogenicity. The relevant comparison in this case is not between acellular vaccine and placebo—which in any case might raise ethical difficulties—but between acellular and whole-cell vaccine, with the goal of showing that the efficacies of the two vaccines do not differ by more than a specified amount. Occasionally, trials may be designed for both vaccine-placebo and vaccine-vaccine comparisons, as in the case of the randomized placebo-controlled trial of two formulations of typhoid vaccine (capsules and liquid) in Indonesia *(27)*. This trial was designed to show that a vaccine with VE = 50% was significantly better than placebo, and that a vaccine with VE = 75% was significantly better than one with VE = 50%. Two placebo groups (capsule and liquid) were used to maintain blindness, with over 5000 participants in each of the four groups.

The Data Monitoring Committee has the task of reviewing safety data as the trial progresses. Ideally, the background incidence of serious adverse events should have been documented prior to the trial, since in large trials, one or more deaths or serious events are likely to occur purely by chance. The Data Monitoring Committee may decide to stop the trial if the evidence supports a causal link with the vaccine. In the 1986 Swedish placebo-controlled trial of acellular pertussis vaccines, three deaths caused by invasive bacterial infection occurred in one of the two vaccine groups. The Data Monitoring Committee initiated further studies while the trial continued, but found no evidence of a causal link *(28)*. It is advisable to continue monitoring of the trial cohort after the trial has ended. Thus, in the Senegal randomized trial of high-titer measles vaccines given at 5 mo compared to standard vaccine given at 10 mo, a significantly higher late mortality was found in high-titer vaccine recipients than in the standard vaccine control group *(29)*.

Phase III trials also provide an opportunity to establish laboratory correlates of protection. These are required in order to verify the potency of future batches of a vaccine that has been shown to be effective in a Phase III trial, and to enable similar vaccines to be licensed without direct evidence of protective efficacy. Laboratory measures that might be correlated with protection in humans are antibody levels in vaccinees to one or more vaccine antigens, or antibody levels or protection in an appropriate challenge test in immunized animals. In the case of whole-cell pertussis vaccines, both the agglutinin response in children and protection in a mouse intracerebral challenge test have been found to predict protection under conditions of household exposure *(30)*. The latter test, standardized to appropriate international units, has provided a means of calibrating the potency of whole-cell pertussis vaccines throughout the world. In contrast, acellular pertussis vaccines do not pass this test; thus, there is an urgent need to establish new correlates of protection. It was disappointing that during the first controlled trial of acellular pertussis vaccines, no correlation between antibody levels to vaccine antigens in children and the subsequent development of pertussis was found *(24)*.

## 2.4. Phase IV Trials

Following licensure of the vaccine, further studies are conducted to monitor its performance under field conditions. Such observational studies differ fundamentally from randomized controlled trials because a randomized control group is no longer available. Therefore, these studies are subject to potential biases (**Note 9**) and may be difficult to interpret. Nevertheless, they constitute an essential part of the process of vaccine evaluation and development. Many of the methods used are variants of standard epidemiological tools, such as case-control and cohort studies *(31,32)*, and will not be described in detail here.

Phase IV post-licensure studies are undertaken to monitor vaccine effectiveness and document the less frequent adverse reactions. The term "effectiveness," rather than "efficacy," is used to emphasize the transition from controlled experimental to field evaluation, in which such factors as vaccine storage, variability of schedules, and delivery may intervene. In addition, if the vaccine is widely administered, herd immunity effects will enhance the vaccine's effectiveness. Such studies are essential for the identification of changes in the epidemiology of a disease, which may have implications for the vaccination program. For example, in the late 1960s, epidemiological studies revealed that the effectiveness of whole-cell pertussis vaccine had dropped considerably, and this was attributed to changes in the predominant pertussis genotypes *(33)*. The composition of the vaccine was thus revised to include all genotypes, and subsequent studies demonstrated a protective effectiveness of more than 80% *(22)*.

Studies of rare adverse reactions attributable to vaccines given as part of routine vaccination programs are of particular importance. Rare reactions cannot be investigated with any substantial power in Phase II or III clinical trials, even with sample sizes in the tens of thousands. For example, an association between intussusception and administration of an oral rotavirus vaccine, which indicated a causal relationship, was observed following adverse event reports after licensure of the vaccine *(34)*; the vaccine was subsequently withdrawn from use in 1999. On the other hand, passive reports of possible vaccine reactions (the "Yellow Card" system used in the United Kingdom) inevitably underestimate the true absolute risks. Moreover, for nonspecific events, such as febrile convulsions, passive reports of events potentially attributable to vaccine cannot be used to estimate relative risks, since some temporally associated events may occur by chance. More sophisticated methods of active surveillance are therefore required. In 1992, a laboratory-based study involving an active retrospective search for cases of aseptic meningitis identified an increased rate 15–35 d after vaccination with licensed measles,mumps,rubella vaccine (MMR) containing the Urabe strain of the mumps virus *(35)*. These vaccines were replaced by ones containing the Jeryl-Lynn strain of mumps. More recently, a new method that only uses data from cases has been developed, enabling the proportion of adverse events attributable to the vaccine to be determined for any specified time interval after vaccination. Using this method, it was shown that 67% of febrile convulsions occurring 6–11 d after MMR vaccination was attributable to the measles component of the vaccine *(36)*.

## 3. Notes

1. Ethical issues: Participation in the trial must be on the basis of informed consent. This is obtained from the participant or, in the case of a child, from his or her parent or guardian. Informed consent should preferably be obtained in writing, after the potential participant has had an opportunity to consider the issues involved. These may be presented in a leaflet, booklet, or video. The trial investigators should take all reasonable steps to minimize any risk to participants and to guarantee their anonymity. The ethical requirement to minimize risks to patients may have a profound influence on the design of the study. For instance, the existence of vaccines with proven efficacy may preclude the use of a placebo group; other examples are given in the main text.

Trial participants who receive unlicensed products should be provided with adequate guarantees of compensation. The current UK legislation, under which the right to compensation is dependent on proof of negligence, is recognized as providing inadequate coverage in the context of Phase I–III clinical trials *(37)*. For Phase I studies in healthy volunteers, a separate compensation contract with each volunteer is feasible, and a suitable draft contract has been recommended by the Association of the British Pharmaceutical Industry (ABPI). For Phase II and III trials, commercial manufacturers of unlicensed vaccines should accept "no fault" liability for their products in accordance with the guidelines issued by the ABPI *(38)*. With these agreements, the manufacturers accept liability under certain conditions without the requirement for negligence to be proven against the company.

Ethical issues are involved at every stage of a clinical trial. Failure to publish the results is considered unethical, since it negates the entire basis of the trial—namely, to further medical knowledge. A general discussion of medical ethics in the context of clinical trials may be found in Pocock (*see* Chapter 7, in **ref. *39***).

2. Hypotheses, estimation, and power: The purpose of a trial is usually twofold: first, to test a specific null hypothesis about the vaccine (for instance, "this vaccine gives no protection against infection"), and second, to estimate the effect of the vaccine. These goals are closely linked, but differ in emphasis. The first is achieved by a $p$-value, and the second by an estimate and its confidence interval. The two emphases should be regarded as complementary. The hypothesis-testing framework helps to clarify the primary goal of the trial, whereas the estimation approach provides a quantitative assessment of the vaccine. Because hypotheses can only be disproved, a so-called null hypothesis is formulated about the vaccine; for instance, VE = 0%, and this is rejected if the data are found to be incompatible with it in a precisely defined statistical sense. The power of the trial is the probability of rejecting the null hypothesis when it is false. Thus, power can be considered as a statistical version of sensitivity, and depends on the magnitude of the true effect and the sample size. Although the hypothesis-testing framework is invaluable for clarifying the key design issues in a trial, when it comes to the analysis, the raw statistical assessment of "significance" contained in a $p$-value may bear little relationship to clinical or epidemiological importance. This is best evaluated using an effect estimate (e.g., vaccine efficacy or difference in reaction rates) and its confidence interval. For example, a recent trial of malaria vaccine failed to find a "significant" protective effect against any episode of malaria ($p$ = 0.078), but the estimate of protective efficacy was 67%, with 95% confidence interval – 2.7–89% *(15)*. The appropriate inference from this trial is not that the vaccine does not protect, but that the trial lacked power, as evidenced by the lack of precision of the efficacy estimate.

3. Target and study populations; inclusion and exclusion criteria: The target population is the collection of individuals to whom the vaccine may be administered after licensure. This is distinct from the study population, which comprises those who are invited to participate in the trial. In a trial of acellular DTP vaccine in the United Kingdom, the target population is all children aged 2–4 mo, whereas the study population may be all children who present for routine primary immunization with DTP vaccine in one specific Health District between specific dates.

Members of the study population are recruited into the trial on the basis of selection criteria. Inclusion criteria generally define, in broad terms, the age and other characteristics required of the participants. Exclusion criteria are a detailed list of the operational and medical factors precluding enrollment in the study. These may include a stated intention to move out of the study area before the end of the trial, a relevant previous history of disease or vaccination, or specific contraindications to vaccination. Selection criteria should be objective, and should not be so stringent as to reduce the representativeness of the individuals selected, as compared to the target population. A realistic evaluation of the probable rate is required at an early stage in planning the trial, since this will influence its overall duration (recruitment plus follow-up) and whether or not it is designed as a single or multicenter trial. These issues may have a substantial effect on the cost of the trial.

4. Trial size: The choice of trial size should be based on the primary outcome of interest, with additional calculations illustrating the power and precision available for secondary outcomes. The sample size depends on the significance level and power desired for the vaccine effect that it is required to detect. For Phase II trials, the vaccine effect on the frequency of reactions may be expressed as the difference in reaction rates. For a comparison between two groups, the formula for the sample size in each group ($N$) is then:

$$N = Z\,[p_1(1 - p_1) + p2(1 - p_2)]/(p_2 - p_1)^2 \qquad (2)$$

where $p_1$ and $p_2$ are, respectively, the proportions of unvaccinated and vaccinated with reactions. The quantity $Z$ is a constant that depends on the significance level and power— namely, 7.85 for two-tailed 5% significance and 80% power, and 10.51 for two-tailed 5% significance and 90% power. If the objective of a Phase II trial is to compare post-vaccination antibody levels, the relevant vaccine effect is the difference in log geometric mean titers, and the sample size required in each group is $N = Z.2(s/m)^2$ where $s$ is the standard deviation of the log titers, which may be estimated in earlier trials, and $m$ is the difference in log GMTs to be detected.

Sample size calculations for placebo-controlled Phase III efficacy trials are similar to those for Phase II trials, but require an estimate of the cumulative incidence in the unvaccinated group. This will depend on the planned duration of follow-up. For trials with nonstandard null hypotheses, such as VE <70%, the sample size calculations are more complicated (40). Tables of sample sizes are available for a wide variety of clinical trial designs (41). The numbers to be recruited should allow for such factors as losses to follow-up and insufficient sera. Investigators are often surprised by the large numbers required in clinical trials. Although practical limitations to recruitment clearly cannot be ignored, the consequences of an inadequate sample size should not be underestimated—particularly the ethical implications—since the trial can only be justified if there is a high likelihood that it will yield useful results.

5. Randomization and baselines: The purpose of randomization is twofold: first and most importantly, to remove any subjective bias in the allocation of participants to vaccine groups, and second, to provide a formal statistical basis for significance tests. Randomization does not in itself guarantee that the groups will be comparable, although in large trials they should be roughly balanced. Baseline comparisons should not be undertaken by means of significance tests; whatever the sample size, a proportion of baseline variables are bound to come up as significant. The real issue is whether baseline factors influence outcomes, and by how much. If required, differences in baseline characteristics may be corrected in the analysis by regression techniques (42). However, if important prognostic factors are known prior to the trial, it is far better to achieve balance by block randomization within these categories. In a multicenter placebo-controlled Phase III efficacy trial, the incidence of disease may vary between centers. Thus, balance within trial centers is desirable. This may be achieved by ensuring that, for example, every 10 consecutive study numbers are randomly assigned in equal proportions to vaccine and pla-

cebo, and that blocks of study numbers are assigned to the trial centers. This is a block randomization with block size 10. Note also that a haphazard allocation cannot be described as random—since there is no control over the investigator's prejudices, unconscious or otherwise; randomization lists are best produced using computer-generated random numbers.

In some cases, investigators reject individual randomization for logistical reasons. During a placebo-controlled trial of typhoid vaccine in 81,621 Chilean schoolchildren, the randomization unit was the classroom *(43)*. With this scheme, one might expect local herd immunity effects to magnify slightly the vaccine efficacy.

6. Factorial and parallel group designs: Suppose, as in the example in *(8)*, that it is required to compare antibody responses to DTP and Hib vaccines given i) separately or combined and ii) in the arm or the thigh. In a factorial design, there are four groups, representing all combinations of vaccine formulation and site. The effect of combined vaccine formulation is evaluated by comparing the combined + arm and combined + thigh groups with the separate + arm and separate + thigh groups. The site effect is evaluated by comparing the combined + thigh and separate + thigh groups with the combined + arm and separate + arm groups. Thus, the entire data set is used in both comparisons. In contrast, in a parallel group design, there are three groups: separate + arm (the reference group), separate + thigh (to assess the site effect), and combined + arm (to determine the effect of combined delivery). To obtain the same power for each comparison as in the factorial design, the total sample size in the three-group parallel design is approx 50% greater. Factorial designs usually provide substantial savings, and are recommended whenever practicable.

7. Quality control: The success of a trial—whether Phase I, II, III, or IV—and its impact on medical opinion, will depend to a large extent on its quality. Therefore, special attention to quality control is required at the design stage and throughout the course of the trial. Careful attention to practical details (including the quality of the adhesive used to fix the labels on the vaccine ampoules) is required to reduce protocol violations to a minimum. Procedures and forms should be tested, and for large trials, pilot studies may be required. In trials involving several centers or many staff in the field, it is particularly important to ensure that the protocol is applied consistently. Special training sessions may be required to help ensure this. In trials of long duration, it is particularly important to maintain a high level of enthusiasm and commitment in all participants.

   Auditing procedures to monitor quality should be planned as part of the trial protocol. The numbers recruited, vaccinated, and followed up should be documented at regular intervals. Vaccine-handling procedures, particularly transport and storage, should be closely monitored. Laboratory methods should be standardized prior to testing, and usually require separate protocols. The data should also be scanned for missing information as they are collected.

8. Protocol violations and losses to follow-up: All losses and protocol violations should be accounted for in the final analysis. In Phase III trials, regular contact should be maintained with all participants to document any losses to follow-up. This is particularly important in trials of vaccines requiring multiple doses, in which a reaction to the first or second dose might constitute a contraindication for further doses, and in Phase III trials with extended follow-up.

   The problem of how to handle protocol violations, such as incorrect allocation of vaccines, is complex. One approach, known as the "intention-to-treat" analysis, is to include individuals according to their intended vaccine allocation, regardless of what may have occurred in practice *(44)*. Thus, if an individual was randomized to vaccine, but erroneously received placebo, he or she is still included in the vaccine group. This approach is not valid for vaccine-to-vaccine comparisons, in which the aim is to establish that the vaccines differ by no more than a specified amount, since it could induce a spurious similarity between the groups and would increase the probability of the vaccines being declared equivalent when they are not *(45)*. A reasonable alternative in this case is to exclude incorrectly allocated individuals from the analysis completely.

Analysis of data from Phase III trials involving substantial follow-up times should be performed by survival techniques that correct for losses to follow-up. However, these techniques rely on such losses occurring independently of the vaccine. Thus, the number and pattern of losses in the different groups should be compared, and any differences should be investigated.

9. Biases: In observational studies, the major biases arise from nonrandom allocation of vaccines and biased ascertainment *(21)*. For example, in a highly vaccinated population, estimates of vaccine efficacy based on comparisons of attack rates between vaccinated and unvaccinated people may be biased because individuals who do not receive the vaccine may differ from those who do in some important respects—such as socioeconomic background—which may be related to the probability of exposure. Similarly, in studies of vaccine safety, recent vaccination may increase the likelihood of an adverse event being reported, thus biasing estimates of relative risk against the vaccine.

Clinical trials are not exempt from these types of biases. For example, in the 1964 MRC trial of measles vaccines against unvaccinated controls, 47,041 children were allocated to one of three groups on the basis of their day of birth: killed followed by live vaccines, live vaccine only, or no vaccine *(46)*. In most cases, eligibility for inclusion in the study was assessed when the children presented for vaccination. Children failing to turn up for two vaccination appointments were excluded from the study. Thus, 37% of the 16,884 children allocated to the killed/ vaccine group, 29% of the 13,433 children allocated to the live vaccine group, and only 2% of the 16,724 control children were excluded. Such a large systematic difference between vaccinated and unvaccinated children clearly has the potential to introduce serious bias. In this example, the efficacy of the vaccine was so high that the bias is unlikely to affect the qualitative conclusions of the trial, but the validity of the VE estimate (85%) is still open to question.

10. Multiple significance testing: In the context of significance testing, a false-positive test is known as a Type I error. As the number of independent significance tests increases, the Type I error probability increases: After 14 tests, there is greater than a 50% chance that at least one will turn up significant at the 5% level. Thus, it is important to keep the number of significance tests to a minimum. There are two main implications for clinical trials. First, it is good practice to identify a single primary hypothesis, on which the success of the trial will ultimately be judged. Alternatively, if there is more than one hypothesis, the significance level should be adjusted downward. This was done in a large randomized, double-blind trial of cholera vaccines in Bangladesh involving two vaccine groups and a placebo group *(47)*. In this trial, each vaccine-placebo comparison was judged significant if it produced a one-tailed $p$-value $<0.025$, thus retaining an overall one-tailed 5% significance level for the trial as a whole. Second, it is essential to avoid constant scrutiny of the data as it accumulates, with the intention of stopping recruitment when "significance" is reached; this practice is bound to result in the detection of entirely false "effects." If interim analyses are required—as in many large Phase III trials—these should be carried out by the Data Monitoring Committee at specified intervals, and the choice of stopping guidelines should be discussed with a statistician.

## References

1. Byar, D. P., Schoenfeld, D. A., Green, S. B., Amato, D. A., Davis, R., DeGruttda, V., et al. (1990) Design considerations for AIDS trials. *N. Engl. J. Med.* **323,** 1343–1348.
2. Bellanti, J. A., Zeligs, B. J., Vetro, S., Pung, Y.-H., Luccioli, S., Malvasic, M. J., et al. (1993) Studies of safety, infectivity and immunogenicity of a new temperature-sensitive (ts) 51-l strain of *Salmonella typhi* as a new live oral typhoid fever vaccine candidate. *Vaccine* **11,** 587–590.
3. Costantino, P., Viti, S., Audino, P., Velmonte, M. A., Nencioni, L., and Rappuoli, R. (1992) Development and phase 1 clinical testing of a conjugate vaccine against meningo-coccus A and C. *Vaccine* **10,** 691–698.
4. Gold, R., Leplow, M. L., Goldchneider, I., Draper, T. F., and Gotschlich, E. (1979) Kinet-ics of antibody production to group A and group C meningococcal polysaccharide vac-cines administered during the first six years of life: prospects for routine immunization of infants and children. *J. Infect. Dis.* **140,** 694–697.
5. Rutter, D. A., Ashworth, L. A. E., Day, A., Funnell, S., Lovell, F., and Robinson, A. (1988) Trial of a new acellular pertussis vaccine in healthy adult volunteers. *Vaccine* **6,** 29–32.
6. Bock, H. L., Klockmann, U., Jungst, C., Schindel-Kunzel, F., Theobald, K., and Zerban, R. (1990) A new vaccine against tick-borne encephalitis: initial trial in man including a dose-response study. *Vaccine* **8,** 22–24.
7. Picard, O., Giral, P., Defer, M. C., Fouchard, M., Morel, M., Meyohas, M. C., et al. (1990) AIDS vaccine therapy: phase I trial (letter). *Lancet* **336,** 179.
8. Scheifele, D., Bjornson, G., Barreto, L., Meekison, W., and Guasparini, R. (1992) Con-trolled trial of *Haemophilus influenzae* type B diphtheria toxoid conjugate combined with diphtheria, tetanus and pertussis vaccines, in 18-month old children, including compari-son of arm versus thigh injection. *Vaccine* **10,** 455–460.
9. Miller, E., Ashworth, L. A., Robinson, A., Waight, P. A., and Irons, L. I. (1991) Phase II trial of whole-cell pertussis vaccine versus an acellular vaccine. *Lancet* **337,** 70–73.
10. Pichichero, M. E., Marsocci, S. M., Francis, A. B., Green, J. L., Disney, F. A., Rennels, M. B., et al. (1993) A comparative evaluation of the safety and immunogenicity of a single dose of unbuffered oral rhesus rotavirus serotype 3, rhesus/human reassortant serotypes 1, 2 and 4 and combined (tetravalent) vaccines in healthy infants. *Vaccine* **11,** 747–753.
11. Miller, E., Salisbury, D., and Ramsay, M. (2002) Planning, registration and implementa-tion of an immunisation campaign against meningococcal serogroup C disease in the UK: a success story. *Vaccine* **20,** 558–567.
12. Goldschneider, I., Gotschlich, E. C., and Artenstein, M.S. (1969) Human immunity to the meningococcus. I. The role of humoral antibodies. *J. Exp. Med.* **129,** 1307–1326.
13. Strauss, S. E,, Corey, L., Burke, R. L., Savarese, B., Barnum, G., Krause, P. R., et al. (1994) Placebo-controlled trial of vaccination with recombinant glycoprotein D of herpes simplex virus type 2 for immunotherapy of genital herpes. *Lancet* **343,** 1460–1463.
14. Valero, M. V., Amador, L. R., Galindo, C., Figueroa, J., Bello, M. S., Murillo, L. A., et al. (1993) Vaccination with SPf66, a chemically synthesized vaccine, against *Plasmodium falciparum* malaria in Colombia. *Lancet* **341,** 705–710.
15. Sempertegui, F., Estrella B., Moscoso, J., Piedrahita, L., Hernandez, D., Gaybor, J., et al. (1994) Safety, immunogenicity and protective effect of the SPf66 malaria synthetic vac-cine against *Plasmodium falciparum* infection in a randomized double-blind placebo-con-trolled field trial in an endemic area of Ecuador. *Vaccine* **12,** 337–342.
16. Hall A. J. and Aaby, P. (1990) Tropical trials and tribulations. *Int. J. Epidemiol.* **19,** 777–781.

17. Francis, T., Korns, R. F., Voight, T., Boisen, M., Hemphill, F. M., Napier, J. A., et al. (1955) An evaluation of the 1954 poliomyelitis vaccine trials. *Am. J. Public Health Part 2* **45,** 1–63.

18. Fine, P. E. M. and Clarkson, J. A. (1987) Reflections on the efficacy of pertussis vaccines. *Rev. Infect. Dis.* **9,** 866–883.

19. Vesikari, T. (1993) Clinical trials of live oral rotavirus vaccines: the Finnish experience. *Vaccine* **11,** 255–261.

20. Medical Research Council (1951) The prevention of whooping-cough by vaccination: a Medical Research Council investigation. *Br. Med. J.* June 30, 1463–1471.

21. Farrington, C. P. (1990) Quantifying misclassification bias in cohort studies of vaccine efficacy. *Stat. Med.* **9,** 1327–1337.

22. PHLS Epidemiological Research Laboratory and 21 Area Health Authorities (1982) Efficacy of pertussis vaccination in England. *Br. Med. J.* **285,** 357–359.

23. Storsaeter, J., Hallander, H., Farrington, C. P., Olin, P., Mollby, R., and Miller, E. (1990) Secondary analyses of the efficacy of two acellular pertussis vaccines evaluated in a Swedish phase III trial. *Vaccine* **8,** 457–461.

24. Ad-Hoc Group for the Study of Pertussis Vaccines (1988) Placebo-controlled trial of two acellular pertussis vaccines in Sweden: protective efficacy and adverse events. *Lancet* **April 30,** 955–960.

25. Volberding, P. A., Lagakos, S. W., Koch, M. A., Pettinelli, C., Myers, M. W., Booth, D. K., et al. (1990) Zidovudine in asymptomatic human immunodeficiency virus infection: a controlled trial in persons with fewer than 500 CD4-positive cells per cubic millimeter. *N. Engl. J. Med.* **322,** 941–949.

26. Black, S., Shinefield, H., Fireman, B., Lewis, E., Ray, P., Hansen, J. R., et al., and the Northern California Kaiser Permanente Vaccine Study Center Group, (2000) Efficacy, safety and immunogenicity of heptavalent pneumococcal conjugate vaccine in children. *Pediatr. Infect. Dis. J.* **19,** 187–195.

27. Simanjuntak, C. H., Paleologo, F., Punjabi, N. H., Darmowigoto, R., Soeprawoto, Totosuderjo, H., Haryanto, P., et al. (1991) Oral immunisation against typhoid fever in Indonesia with Ty2la vaccine. *Lancet* **338,** 1055–1059.

28. Storsaeter, J., Olin, P., Renemar, B., Lagergard, T., Norberg, R., Romanus, V., et al. (1988) Mortality and morbidity from invasive bacterial infections during a clinical trial of acellular pertussis vaccines in Sweden. *Pediatr. Infect. Dis. J.* **7,** 637–645.

29. Garenne, M., Leroy, O., Beau, J.-P., and Sene, I. (1991) Child mortality after high-titre measles vaccines: prospective study in Senegal. *Lancet* **338,** 903–907.

30. Medical Research Council Whooping Cough Immunisation Committee (1956) Vaccination against whooping cough: relation between protection and results of laboratory tests. *Br. Med, J.* **2,** 454–462.

31. Orenstein, W. A., Bernier, R. H., Dondero, T. J., Hinman, A. R., Marks, J. S., Bart, K. J., et al. (1985) Field evaluation of vaccine efficacy. *WHO Bulletin* **63,** 1055–1068.

32. Begg, N. and Miller, E. (1990) Role of epidemiology in vaccine policy. *Vaccine* **8,** 180–189.

33. PHLS Whooping-Cough Committee and Working Party (1973) Efficacy of whooping-cough vaccines used in the United Kingdom before 1968. *Br. Med. J.* **Feb. 3,** 259–262.

34. Murphy, T. V., Gargiull, P. M., Massoudi, M. S., Nelson, D. B., Jumaan, A. O., Okoro, C. A., et al. (2001) Intussusception among infants given an oral rotavirus vaccine. *N. Engl. J. Med.* **344,** 564–572.

35. Miller, E., Goldacre, M., Pugh, S., Colville, A., Farrington, P., Flower, A., et al. (1993) Risk of aseptic meningitis after measles mumps and rubella vaccine in UK children. *Lancet* **341,** 979–982.

36. Farrington, P., Pugh, S., Colville, A., Flower, A., Nash, J., Morgan-Capner, P., et al. (1995) A new method for active surveillance of adverse events from diphtheria/tetanus/pertussis and measles/mumps/rubella vaccines. *Lancet* **345,** 567–569.

37. Diamond, A. L. and Laurence, D. R. (1983) Compensation and drug trials (Commentary). *Br. Med. J.* **287,** 676–677.

38. Association of the British Pharmaceutical Industry (1983) Compensation and drug trials. *Br. Med. J.* **287,** 675.

39. Pocock, S. J. (1983) *Clinical Trials: A Practical Approach.* Wiley, Chichester, UK.

40. Farrington, C. P. and Manning, G. (1990) Test statistics and sample size formulae for comparative binomial trials with null hypotheses of non-zero risk difference or non-unity relative risk. *Stat. Med.* **9,** 1447–1454.

41. Machin, D. and Campbell, M. J. (1987) Statistical Tables for the Design of Clinical Trials. Blackwell Scientific, Oxford.

42. Altman, D. G. and Dore, C. J. (1990) Randomisation and baseline comparisons in clinical trials. *Lancet* **335,** 149–153.

43. Levine, M. M., Fereccio, C., Cryz, S., and Ortiz, E. (1990) Comparison of enteric-coated capsules and liquid formulation of Ty21a typhoid vaccine in randomised controlled field trial. *Lancet* **336,** 891–894.

44. Newell, D. J. (1992) Intention-to-treat analysis: implications for quantitative and qualitative research. *Int. J. Epidemiol.* **21,** 837–841.

45 Farrington, C. P. (1993) Intention-to-treat analysis: implications for quantitative and qualitative research (letter). *Int. J. Epidemiol.* **22,** 566.

46. Medical Research Council (1966) Vaccination against measles: a clinical trial of live measles vaccine given alone and live vaccine preceded by killed vaccine. *Br. Med. J.* February 19, 441–446.

47. Clemens, J. D., Sack, D. A., Harris, J. R., Chakraborty, J., Khan, M. R., Stanton, B. F., et al. (1986) Field trials of oral cholera vaccines in Bangladesh. *Lancet* July 19, 124–127.

# 22

## Assuring the Quality and Safety of Vaccines

*Regulatory Expectations for Licensing
and Batch Release*

### Elwyn Griffiths and Ivana Knezevic

### 1. Introduction

Ensuring the consistent safety and efficacy of a vaccine has long been recognized as an essential element in a successful disease-control program. Indeed, the development of appropriate laboratory methods to characterize a vaccine with respect to its component antigens, safety, and potency must be a prerequisite to the routine clinical use of any new bacterial, viral, or antiparasite vaccines. Adequate control measures serve to safeguard vaccinees against both unacceptable adverse events and inadequate protection.

Special considerations apply to the control of vaccines that do not apply to the control of chemical drugs. This is because of the biological nature of the starting materials, the manufacturing process, and the test methods needed to characterize batches of the product. For example, the production of many vaccines involves the culture of cells or microorganisms, and such systems are inherently variable by nature. Also, vaccines are often highly complex products in molecular terms, and there is an incomplete understanding of the relationship between physicochemical characteristics, immunogenicity, and protective efficacy. In addition, some vaccines are made of living organisms. Thus, chemical and physical analyses are generally of only limited value in the characterization of vaccines, and must always be complemented with biological characterization. This is in contrast to chemical drugs, for which definitive chemical analysis of the product can provide an adequate basis for characterization and quality assessment. Nevertheless, the growing sophistication of many procedures for physicochemical

From: *Methods in Molecular Medicine, Vol. 87: Vaccine Protocols, 2nd ed.*
Edited by: A. Robinson, M. J. Hudson, and M. P. Cranage © Humana Press Inc., Totowa, NJ

analysis of biological macromolecules has made their application to some biological products, such as polysaccharide-protein conjugate vaccines, a workable reality (*see* **Subheading 4.3.**). The deleterious effects of drugs are usually based on their chemical composition, but experience with vaccines and other biologicals has shown that major problems or accidents are normally batch-related and not product-related. This emphasizes the need for effective control procedures. Consistency of production is of paramount importance, and the demonstration that the product does not differ from vaccine lots that have been shown to be safe and adequately immunogenic and protective in clinical studies is a crucial component of vaccine evaluation, licensing procedure, and batch release.

A broad range of candidate vaccines derived from novel technologies is now becoming available, raising exciting prospects for the control of infectious diseases that have thus far been difficult to control. However, new products and novel biotechnologies pose new challenges for standardization, quality control, and safety *(1,2)*. Such products require thorough characterization and testing, using the most up-to-date procedures before and during clinical evaluation.

Since the nature of the protective response in humans—which may be cell-mediated, antibody-mediated, or a mixture of both—is not always fully known at the time of licensing, it is vital to ensure that the quality of a vaccine is reproducible at all levels of manufacture. It should be noted that the most easily determined measurement of efficacy, (e.g., antibody responses), may not be the best indicator of protection, and for some antigens there is no correlation between antibody titer and protection. Therefore, successful control of the safety and efficacy of vaccines, as with all biologicals, relies strongly on strict control of the starting materials and manufacturing procedures, as well as that of the end product. Regulatory requirements for biologicals strongly emphasize the in-process control approach. The validation of the ability of certain parts of the manufacturing process to remove unwanted materials, especially potential infectious agents, is also considered essential. However, in some cases it is not possible to reliably detect the infectious agents in starting materials—for example, those that cause bovine spongiform encephalopathy (BSE) or other transmissible spongiform encephalopathies (TSEs). The safety of vaccines with respect to BSE and TSEs is therefore considered to be assured by using materials for vaccine production from safe sources with respect to country/herd/animal. It should be noted that this is a very rapidly evolving field, and particular consideration should be given to obtaining the latest regulatory advice on this issue. Many national and international organizations, such as the World Health Organization (WHO), are updating guidance on precautionary measures to minimize the risk of transmitting BSE/TSEs agents to humans through medicinal products *(3)*. Although the quality, safety, and efficacy of vaccines are the prime responsibility of the manufacturer, in the interest of public health, vaccines are also subjected to independent batch release by national health authorities.

## 2. Standardization, Control, and Regulation of Vaccines

The regulation of biological products, including vaccines, can be divided into three stages: developmental, licensing, and post-licensing. The developmental stage consists of two parts—preclinical research and development, and clinical research and development, which usually consists of three phases: Phase I, II, and III (*see* Chapter 21; **ref. 4**). The preclinical research data include details of the development and production of the vaccine together with reports of control testing, which should be adequate to justify the subsequent clinical testing. The data needed will clearly vary from case to case. In some instances, the justification for a clinical trial might be based on comprehensive laboratory evidence of probable efficacy, supported by a sound understanding of protective mechanisms. In others, mere protection in an animal model may be all that is at hand, and little understanding of protective mechanisms available. It should be noted that there is no requirement for a vaccine to be tested in nonhuman primates before proceeding to human subjects—unless, of course, an appropriate nonhuman primate infection model is available.

The characterization, standardization, and control of vaccine preparations during development are key issues (*see* Chapter 24), and a well-defined candidate vaccine offers by far the best chance of success. If a clinical trial shows a preparation to be protective, then the vaccine subsequently must be made to the same specifications as the successful preparation. In the case of poorly defined materials, it is never certain whether differences in protective efficacy or toxicity are caused by unintentional variations in the vaccine preparations used, suboptimal vaccination schedules, poorly designed trials, or differences in target populations. The fact that it took about 50 yrs from the time of the identification of *Bordetella pertussis* as the causative agent of whooping cough to the licensing of an effective whooping cough vaccine is largely because no attempt was made to standardize the preparations used in the many early trials. Only when some degree of standardization occurred did the development of an effective pertussis vaccine become feasible *(5)*.

In Phase I clinical studies, initial testing of a vaccine is conducted in small numbers of human subjects—usually adults—to test the properties of the vaccine, the levels of toxicity, and, if appropriate, metabolic and pharmacological effects. Phase I studies are primarily concerned with safety. Phase II studies involve larger numbers of subjects, and are intended to obtain preliminary information about a vaccine's ability to produce its desired effect (e.g., immunogenicity or protection) in the target population and relative safety. The final study, Phase III, is an extensive evaluation that fully examines overall safety and protective efficacy. Phase III clinical trials are virtually always randomized double-blind studies, preferably against a placebo, except where there may be ethical difficulties that make such trials impossible. WHO guidelines on the clinical trials of vaccines that emphasize regulatory expectations have recently been developed *(4)*. When, following Phase III trials, a manufacturer has generated sufficient data to demonstrate that a new product is safe and effective for the purpose intended, an application for a market authorization, or license, may be submitted to a national control authority. If approved, the vaccine then becomes available on the market in that particular state.

Following licensing, there is continued surveillance of a product for the more rare adverse events, and it will also be subject to batch release by a national control authority. The monitoring for possible rarer adverse reactions can only be done in very large numbers of subjects, and this is also an important part of overall vaccine evaluation. For all the various types of vaccines discussed here, a comprehensive characterization of the initial batches of a product should be undertaken to establish consistency with regard to identity, purity, potency, and other product characteristics. Thereafter, for the purpose of batch release, a more limited series of tests may be applied. A clear distinction must therefore be made between the tests performed during the development of a vaccine and the tests routinely performed on each production batch of product. An acceptable number (such as 3–5) of successive batches of the bulk-processed product is characterized as fully as possible to determine consistency of composition, and differences between batches should be noted and stated limits set for routine production. The criteria for rejection of harvests and production components should be defined. The tests used in routine batch control should be a selection of the tests used to characterize the vaccine initially and for licensing, and should include tests for identity, purity, and potency. Changes in the production methods at a later date may necessitate further product characterization to demonstrate equivalence, although the extent of re-characterization will depend on the nature of the changes made.

## 2.1. Available Recommendations and Guidelines

The WHO, through extensive international consultation, develops recommendations and guidelines on the production and control of vaccines and other biologicals of significance *(7)*, and these form the basis for assuring the acceptability of products globally. These recommendations and guidelines specify the need for appropriate starting materials, including seed pools and cell banks; strict adherence to established protocols; tests for purity, potency, and safety at specific steps during production; and the keeping of proper records. Examples of available WHO recommendations and guidelines for vaccines are given in **Table 1**; WHO guidelines allow greater flexibility than the recommendations with respect to expected future developments in the field. WHO recommendations are intended to be scientific and advisory in nature, and provide guidance for national regulatory authorities and for vaccine manufacturers. They may be adopted by national health authorities as definitive national regulations, or used as the basis of such regulations. They are also used as the basis for deciding the acceptability of vaccines for purchase by international agencies, such as the United Nations Childrens' Fund (UNICEF) for use in global immunization programs. Regulatory requirements for vaccines and other biologicals are also developed by other bodies, such as the European Agency for the Evaluation of Medicinal Products (EMEA) and Center for Biologics Evaluation and Research (CBER), Food and Drug Administration (FDA), USA, and these documents can be found on the appropriate web sites (www.emea.eu.int and www.fda.gov/cber). In addition, pharmacopoeial requirements, such as those of the European Pharmacopoeia, are also established for vaccines, and are available at the following web site: www.pheur.org.

The increasing development of component vaccines based on highly purified and characterized antigens is likely to lead to vaccines that can in some respects be standardized and controlled much more effectively than before, with specific and relevant

**Table 1**
**Examples of WHO Requirements for Vaccines**

| Guidelines and requirements | WHO Technical Report Series (WHO TRS) |
|---|---|
| Diphtheria, tetanus, pertussis, and combined vaccines | 800 (1990) |
| Acellular pertussis component of monovalent or combined vaccines | 878 (1998) |
| BCG vaccine, dried | 745 (1987), Amendment 771 (1988) |
| *Haemophilus influenzae* type b conjugate vaccines | 897 (2000) |
| Vi polysaccharide typhoid vaccine | 840 (1994) |
| Meningococcal polysaccharide vaccine | 904 (2002), 658 (1981), and 594 (1976) |
| Meningococcal C conjugate vaccines | In press (adopted 2001) |
| Cholera vaccines, oral, inactivated | In press (adopted 2001) |
| Measles, mumps and rubella vaccines and Combined vaccines (live) | 840 (1994) |
| Poliomyelitis vaccine (Inactivated) | 910 (in press) |
| Poliomyelitis vaccine, oral | 904 (2002) |
| Influenza vaccine, inactivated | 814 (1991) |
| Japanese encephalitis vaccine, live | 910 (in press) |
| Hepatitis A vaccine, inactivated | 858 (1995) |
| Hepatitis B vaccines made by recombinant DNA techniques | 786 (1989) Amendment 889 (1999) |
| Use of animal cells, as in vitro substrates for the production of biologicals | 878 (1998) |
| DNA vaccines | 878 (1998) |
| Synthetic peptide vaccines | 889 (1999) |

tests replacing the crude biological tests often used previously. However, where no appropriate animal model exists or where direct serological or immunological correlates of clinical protection are not available, there remains the serious problem of ensuring that each production batch has at least the same protective efficacy as those batches shown to be protective in clinical trials. In such cases, emphasis is increasingly being placed on assuring the consistency of production using modern physicochemical methods that enable characterization of some products to a degree of precision not previously possible. However, as already mentioned, because of a lack of complete understanding of the relationship between the physicochemical properties of a vaccine and its protective efficacy, biological characterization is needed during development, and the choice of lot release tests is critical. In the case of *Haemophilus influenzae* type b (Hib) conjugate vaccine, some lots that had met all lot-release criteria were shown to be poorly immunogenic in humans, and this led to a re-evaluation of requirements for this vaccine (*see* **Subheading 4.3.1.**). There are also problems with the potency testing of combined vaccines containing several new antigens using the present animal models for vaccine potency. Combinations of antigens may interfere with each other in the animal models, but the relevance of this interference for protective efficacy in humans is a topic of considerable current debate. The relevance for clinical protection of antigenic interference in human recipients is thus major issue. For licensing purposes, noninferiority of a vaccine in a combination product to that of the same antigen in an existing licensed formulation will usually need to be established. The multiplicity of antigens in some formulations makes such an evaluation difficult, and establishing noninferiority against clinical end points is impractical. Establishing noninferiority based on serological criteria is also made difficult by the fact that there is sometimes no clear consensus on the level of antibody that predicts whether a vaccine is clinically effective. Such issues remain for complex combination products such as the pneumococcal conjugate vaccine, but further advances are actively being pursued *(8–10)*.

For newly developed products, specific WHO, national, or pharmacopoeial requirements may not be available, and a national regulatory authority must agree on specifications with the manufacturer on a case-by-case basis during licensing. Nevertheless, there may be general guidelines on the production and control of products, such as on DNA and peptide vaccines, as well as recommendations on animal cell substrates used for production, that should be consulted. Also, much useful information about assuring the quality of biologicals in general and on procedures for approving manufacturers and products, and for setting up a national control laboratory, can be found in appropriate WHO guidelines *(11,12)*. For vaccines of global importance, the development of which also involves much international collaboration, it will be essential to ensure the consistency of regulatory approach to novel products, and in 2001, a consultation was organized jointly by the WHO-UNAIDS HIV Vaccine Initiative and the Quality Assurance and Safety of Biologicals Team, WHO, to address scientific considerations for the regulation and clinical evaluation of preventive vaccines against human immunodeficiency acquired immunodeficiency syndrome (HIV/AIDS). The primary objective of this consultation was to identify gaps that must be addressed from a regulatory perspective to ensure an appropriate regulatory framework for the development and evaluation of preventive HIV/AIDS vaccines and their smooth and effective progress toward licensing *(13)*.

### 2.2. Control of Production and Production Facilities

Also significant are recommendations related to establishments in which biological products, including vaccines, are manufactured. These can be found in the WHO document on good manufacturing practice (GMP) for biologicals *(14)*. Particular attention must be given to the training and experience of persons in charge of production and testing, and those assigned to various areas of responsibility in the manufacturing establishments and in the national regulatory authorities. WHO established a Global Training Network in 1996 to facilitate this process, and these details can be found on the following web site: (http://www.who.int/vaccinesaccess/vaccines/Vaccine_Quality/gtn/gtn.htm). It should also be noted that vaccine preparations for clinical trials must be produced under conditions of good manufacturing practice for clinical trial material. Particular attention should be given to developing documented standard operating procedures for both production processes and testing procedures. These should be introduced as early as possible during the development of a vaccine and be well-established by the time Phase III clinical studies are undertaken and an application for marketing authorization has been filed.

Points to consider in relation to good manufacturing practice include:

1. Personnel:
   a. Qualifications/experience;
   b. Organization and reporting relationships;
   c. Training and recording systems;
   d. Health monitoring.
2. Location and construction of the buildings used for manufacture and control.
3. Flow of raw materials, personnel, and product through the facilities.
4. Animal facilities, animal health, and veterinary supervision.
5. Air, water, and steam systems.
6. Electric power and emergency supply.
7. Drainage and effluent systems.
8. Segregation of certain operations.
9. List of major equipment.
10. Maintenance schedules for equipment and buildings.
11. Cleaning.
12. Quality assurance and quality-control procedures.
13. Storage and quarantine procedures.
14. Validation procedures.
15. Documentation.
16. Labeling and packaging facilities and procedures.
17. Recall and retrieval procedures.

## *2.3. Independent Batch Release*

Vaccines represent a group of biologicals that are subject to independent batch release by a national control authority, usually including independent laboratory evaluation by a national control laboratory. The inherent variability of biological production methods has led to the establishment of national and international requirements. These establish procedures for assuring the quality of vaccines and for evaluating consistency, both between manufacturers and over long periods of time. For these products, spot testing is ineffective and has potentially adverse public health consequences. Of course, vaccines are given primarily to large numbers of healthy, often very young, individuals. Therefore, every batch of vaccine must be evaluated independently of the manufacturer before release on the market, especially for trends in quality. However, the extent of laboratory testing by a national control laboratory may vary, ranging from examination of manufacturers' release protocols to complete laboratory testing for the identity, safety, and potency of each lot. The frequency of testing by a national control laboratory depends on the perceived risk to public health, and on knowledge and experience of a manufacturer's ability to consistently produce a particular vaccine of acceptable quality. For example, in some cases the testing of every batch is undertaken, but in others the testing of the fifth or tenth batch may be acceptable. Since

1993, control authority batch release within the European Union has been subject to a standardized procedure, whereby a batch of vaccine released by one member state must be acceptable to other member states. This has involved the harmonization—under the auspices of the European Department on the Quality of Medicines—of the national control tests carried out in the framework of batch release in order to achieve mutual recognition.

## 2.4. Reference Materials

Standards and reference materials play a vital role in the licensing and quality control process, their role ranging from use in specific antigen recognition tests to assays of vaccine toxicity, immunogenicity, and potency. The standardization of the methods used to evaluate vaccines—and to evaluate immune responses to vaccine antigens—is also vital, so that results may be compared directly between laboratories, both within and between countries and between clinical trials.

WHO International Standards and Reference Reagents form the primary standards globally, and individual national regulatory authorities and manufacturers establish their own national or working standards calibrated using the WHO International Standards where available. The national or working standard is used routinely for establishing the quality of each batch. However, with a multiplicity of standard preparations, there is always a danger of drifting away from the International Standard. Therefore, there has been a move to establish regional working standards, and the production of the large number of vials of standard needed for this purpose is now possible with modern technology. The establishment of regional working standards is expected to further harmonize vaccine quality. Thus, in Europe, the European Department for the Quality of Medicines of the Council of Europe is very active in establishing working standards for vaccines, where possible calibrated against the WHO international standards. Examples of currently available WHO International Standards and Reference Reagents for vaccines can be found in **Table 2**. The complete listing of WHO International Standards and Reference Reagents can be found on the WHO web site www.who.int/biologicals.

## 2.5. Stability of Vaccines

Stability evaluation is an essential component of the development of medicinal products, and is used to determine shelf life and set the expiration date. Stability determination is also important in deciding the storage period of starting materials and intermediates. The purpose of stability studies is to guarantee that the medicinal product still has acceptable characteristics supporting quality, safety, and efficacy at the end of its shelf life or storage period. The stability evaluation of vaccines, and other biologicals is a very complex field because the majority of products cannot be well-characterized by physicochemical parameters and, they are by nature, very susceptible to inactivation by environmental factors. The stability of standards and reference materials must also be considered in order to ensure that procedures used to measure relevant parameters are reliably standardized.

**Table 2**
**Examples of WHO International Standards**
**and Reference Reagents for Vaccines**

| Vaccine | WHO reference preparation |
| --- | --- |
| Diphtheria toxoid, adsorbed | Third International Standard (1999) |
| Tetanus toxoid adsorbed | Third International Standard (2000) |
| Hepatitis A | First International Standard (1999) |
| Hepatitis B surface antigen | First International Standard (1985) |
| Poliomyelitis vaccine (inactivated) | First International Reference Reagent (1994) |
| Poliovirus, Sabin, live attenuated types 1, 2, and 3 | First International Reference Reagent (1995) |
| MAPREC analysis of poliovirus type 3 (Sabin) | First International Standard (1996) |
| MAPREC analysis of poliovirus, type 3 (Sabin), high virus reference | First Reference Reagent (1997) |
| MAPREC analysis of poliovirus type 3 (Sabin), low virus reference | First Reference Reagent (1997) |
| Measles vaccine (live) | Second International Reference Reagent (1994) |
| Mumps vaccine (live) | First International Reference Reagent (1994) |
| Rubella vaccine (live) | First International Reference Reagent (1994) |
| Rabies vaccine | Fifth International Standard (1991) |
| BCG vaccine | First International Reference Preparation (1965) |

There is currently very little guidance in the area of stability testing of vaccines. ICH guidelines cover only vaccines based on well-characterized proteins and polypeptides produced by rDNA technology *(15)*. To address this gap, WHO guidelines on the stability testing of vaccines in general are currently being developed and these will focus on the regulatory expectations in this area, covering stability profiles at each stage of vaccine production, including source materials, intermediates, and combination vaccines. These guidelines are intended to assist National Regulatory Authorities and manufacturers in planning, designing, performing, and interpreting stability studies to be used in support of vaccine licensing.

## 2.6. Vaccines of Assured Quality

A vaccine of assured quality can be defined as one that consistently meets appropriate levels of purity, potency, safety and efficacy, as judged through an independent review system competent to take an evidence-based decision on the product for a specified population in a specific context *(16)*. Such a review system would make use of all available information, such as licensing dossiers, surveillance of field performance, lot-by-lot scrutiny, appropriate laboratory testing, GMP inspection of manufacturers, and evaluation of clinical trials, generally assumed by a fully functional regulatory authority. By insisting on competent regulatory oversight, while recognizing the role of risk analysis in the selection of vaccines for use, WHO strongly reiterates the need for a single standard of quality. Only vaccines of assured quality should be considered for use in national immunization programs on the basis of the risk/benefit ratio for the particular population. The risk perception and the risk/ benefit ratio will have a strong impact on the acceptability of the products. This does not necessarily mean that a product is of intrinsically lower quality if it is acceptable in one country and not another. For example, measles vaccines for most public-sector immunization programs are required to meet certain standards of thermostability. Measles vaccines sold to United Nations agencies must meet the WHO recommendation for thermostability at 37°C for 7 d in the lyophilized form. Measles vaccines used in several industrialized countries do not need to meet this criterion, because it is judged that the risk of heat damage through the distribution system is low. This does not mean that a vaccine not confirmed as thermostable is of lower quality.

## 3. General Considerations for Assuring the Quality and Safety of Different Types of Vaccines

The assays used for the characterization and quality control of vaccines should be appropriate and relevant to the nature of the product. Some of the general issues related to different types of vaccines are indicated here.

### 3.1. Control of Classical Killed/ Subunit Bacterial Vaccines

For classical bacterial vaccines that consist of killed whole cells, such as whole-cell pertussis vaccine, or inactivated toxins (toxoids) like diphtheria and tetanus vaccines, the complete "killing" of the organisms, the inactivation of toxins, and the absence of reversion to toxicity are the most important safety factors. Adequate techniques for ensuring the elimination of contaminants derived from host cells or the growth medium are also essential. The potency of such vaccines has generally been estimated using in vivo tests, and a relative potency obtained by using a reference preparation calibrated against its relevant WHO International Standard; potency is expressed in International Units (IU). However, in recent years many attempts have been made to develop more precise in vitro techniques for controlling vaccines such as diphtheria, tetanus, and whole-cell pertussis. When the WHO Requirements for Diphtheria, Tetanus, and Pertussis and Combined Vaccines were last revised in 1989 (*17*), the WHO Expert Committee on Biological Standardization for the first time advised that potency tests could be carried out by animal-sparing methods, provided that consistency of production and testing had already been established for that particular product. For diphtheria and tetanus toxoid vaccines, in vitro serological methods, including toxin neutralization assays, may also now be used to evaluate potency. However, the serological method used must be validated for the vaccines being considered, and much work has been conducted in this area in recent years. Discussion continues about the possibility of developing a simple, robust, and standardized assay suitable for demonstrating consistency of immunological characteristics of diphtheria and tetanus toxoids for batch-release purposes.

Some of the problems with potency assays arise because there are often insufficient data available to permit a correlation between the potency level observed in a laboratory assay and protection in humans. However, potency can be used to measure consistency of production, and a minimum potency level is often used as the basis for lot release. Thus, ensuring that vaccine lots are not released with a potency below an agreed minimum is considered essential in some cases to ensure adequate protection for vaccinees. For example, in the case of the (killed) whole-cell pertussis vaccine, potency is measured by the so-called mouse protection test. The United Kingdom Medical Research Council clinical trials carried out from 1951 to 1959 showed that this test is a good indicator of clinical efficacy, from which it was concluded that vaccines shown to protect mice against intracerebral challenge also protected children against whooping cough (5). The establishment of this correlation between the potency test and efficacy was a milestone in the development of whole-cell pertussis vaccines. In 1964, a WHO International Standard was established together with the requirement that a single human dose should have an estimated potency of not <4 IU and that the lower fiducial limit of error is not <2 IU.

The development of the whole-cell pertussis vaccine illustrates the need to develop procedures to standardize and control the production of vaccines as early as possible during their development and clinical evaluation. For example, it was noted that the production of antibodies and clinical protection following immunization depended on the number of organisms in the vaccine, and methods were therefore developed to measure the bacterial content of preparations. These studies resulted in the use of an opacity reference preparation to measure the bacterial content of whole-cell vaccines. As already mentioned, studies to measure the potency of pertussis vaccines were also undertaken, and resulted in the intra-cerebral challenge mouse potency test, as it is known today. Similarly, a mouse weight-gain test was developed to test for excessive toxicity in preparations. In recent years, more specific tests for active pertussis toxin and endotoxin content of vaccines have been developed. An important factor in the eventual production of a successful whole-cell pertussis vaccine was the discovery by Leslie and Gardner (18) that *B. pertussis* undergoes phase changes. On passage, in vitro smooth (Phase I) strains were found to produce rough (Phase IV) variants that were later shown to be avirulent. Only the smooth form of the organism is suitable for vaccine production. More recent genetic studies have shown that the changes in *B. pertussis* that give rise to Phase IV organisms are chararacterized by the loss of expression of a number of virulence factors. The immunological and pathophysiological activities of *B. pertussis* are also greatly influenced by the composition of the growth medium. Thus, in the production of vaccines, attention must be paid to the growth conditions and to using well-characterized seed strains, this being especially the case when a vaccine has been developed empirically (5). This point is clearly shown in the production of diphtheria toxin for vaccine manufacture, for which toxin synthesis depends on using strains of *Corynebacterium diphtheriae* carrying the tox phage as well as on the use of growth medium containing low levels of iron. Low iron availability is an environmental signal that controls the expression of a number of toxins and virulence determinants, and its molecular mechanism of action is now well-established (19).

The procedures used in the characterization and control of existing traditional vaccines are usually not applicable to newer products developed to protect against the same infection. Each product must be considered on a case-by-case basis. For example, specific guidelines have been developed for the production and control of acellular pertussis vaccines, which differ from those applied to whole-cell pertussis vaccine *(20)*. Likewise, the tests applied to the characterization and control of traditional inactivated cholera vaccine for parenteral use are not necessarily applicable to the new inactivated whole-cell cholera vaccine intended for oral administration, and new control measures have been developed *(21)*.

### 3.2. Control of Live Attenuated Vaccines

Apart from bacillus Calmette-Guérin (BCG), Typhoid vaccine (live Ty21A oral), and more recently, oral cholera vaccine, all other major live attenuated vaccines protect against viral infections, such as oral polio vaccine, measles, mumps, rubella, varicella (chickenpox), and yellow fever vaccines.

For the production of viral vaccines, including inactivated products, the virus is grown in eukaryotic-cell cultures—often in medium containing components of biological origin, such as bovine serum—and the production process also involves other biological materials such as trypsin. Tests are thus undertaken to verify that residual levels of these substances are below a specified amount, and considerable emphasis is also placed on proving the absence of extraneous contaminating agents, such as bacteria, fungi, mycoplasmas and in particular, other viruses. The source of animal—especially bovine—derived materials used in production is also vital in relation to BSE/TSE issues (*see* **Subheading 1.**). The management of concerns associated with the acceptability and use of mammalian-cell substrates for the production of viral vaccines is a major issue. Managing the risks to take advantage of the benefits is done by defining up-to-date criteria and developing guidelines for production and control, as well as international reference materials. Defining appropriate quality controls is the key, and this involves continuous vigilance and regulatory research. New technologies for detecting adventitious agents must be evaluated and standardized, and decisions must be made regarding the interpretation and reliability of the results. Two recent events have raised awareness of the challenge of dealing with potential viral contamination of viral vaccines and its consequences. These are the detection of reverse transcriptase in vaccines produced in chicken embryo cells and the contamination of polio vaccines with simian virus (SV40) *(22–24)*. Tests to detect potential contaminant agents are thus undertaken at different stages of production, such as on the raw materials, cell cultures before production, bulk vaccine pool before clarification, and vaccine in the final containers. Some live viral vaccines are produced in primary cells, and considerable care should be taken to ensure that the cells come from healthy animals, free of specific known infectious agents. Other vaccines are made using diploid or continuous cell lines, and in such cases production is based on well-characterized master and working cell banks shown to be free of potential infectious agents. WHO requirements have been established for primary, diploid, and continuous cell cultures *(25–27)*, in which considerable emphasis is placed on testing for possible viral contaminants. The virus seed pool is also very carefully tested to ensure that it is free of any adventitious agents, and maintains its attenuation.

The immunogenicity of live viral vaccines is based on titration for the minimum infective dose of each lot. The determination of the minimum required titer (virus concentration) is based on dose-range studies carried out during clinical trials of the vaccine. For lot release, the virus content is determined against a reference preparation of the vaccine calibrated against the WHO International Standard or Reference Reagent where available (**Table 2**). Similar considerations of identity and potency apply to the live attenuated bacterial vaccines, BCG and typhoid vaccine (live Ty21A oral), for which potency is again measured by the number of live organisms present.

As previously mentioned, the stability of all vaccines is important, but the thermo-stability of live vaccines is particularly critical. Some of the attenuated viral strains used as live vaccines are especially thermolabile, and therefore stringent requirements for thermostability have been introduced to ensure that the vaccines are sufficiently robust to withstand a certain level of adverse conditions during transport and delivery to recipients. For example, lots of final freeze-dried measles vaccine are incubated at 37°C for 7 d and then tested to ensure that the geometric mean infectious virus titer is equal to or greater than the required minimum number of infective units per human dose, and that the geometric mean virus titer of the vaccine has not decreased by more than $1 \log_{10}$ infectious units.

## 3.3. Control of Vaccines Produced by Recombinant DNA (rDNA) and Other High-Technology Processes

It is well-established that the principles developed for standardizing and control-ling vaccines produced by traditional means apply equally to antigens derived by mod-ern biotechnology, including rDNA technology, although highly characterized products of very high purity can be made in this way. However, additional factors that may compromise safety and efficacy must be taken into consideration. For instance, products from naturally occurring genes expressed in foreign hosts may deviate struc-turally, biologically, or immunologically from their natural counterparts, and may have unexpected and undesirable properties in humans. Also, variations between batches of the product may result from genetic instability during serial cultivation. Some prod-ucts may also contain potentially hazardous contaminants, such as viruses or onco-genic DNA, and the purification process must be shown to be capable of removing them from the final product. Similar considerations may apply to non-rDNA-derived products, such as viral vaccines, produced in continuously growing cell lines. Clearly, the choice of manufacturing process will influence both the nature and range of pos-sible contaminants.

Several guidelines have been produced for assuring the quality of biologicals pre-pared by rDNA technology, including vaccines *(28–30)*. These aim to provide a scien-tifically sound basis for the manufacture and control of medicinal products made by this technology. All guidelines emphasize the need for a flexible approach, so that requirements can be modified in the light of experience of production and use of products and with further development of new technologies. As for traditional vaccines, certain tests are required for every production batch, but others will be required only to establish the validity, acceptability, and consistency of a given manufacturing process. Although such guidelines can be considered to be generally applicable, individual products will exhibit their own peculiarities; thus, production and control of each product must be considered on an individual basis. For example, specific WHO recommendations are available for hepatitis B vaccines made by rDNA technology *(31)*.

Providing guarantees about the safety and efficacy of live vaccines involving attenuated viral or bacterial strains serving as vectors or hosts for the expression and delivery of cloned genes coding for the protective antigens of other pathogens could be more difficult, although it will depend on the system used. Experience in Europe with the live rabies vaccine for foxes, based on an attenuated vaccinia virus as vector for rabies antigen, has shown the vaccine to be extremely successful. Its use has contributed to the control of the disease, with subsequent benefits for both animal and human health. Tests carried out on the target species and on nontarget species have shown no adverse effects resulting from the use of this vaccine, the first to be based on a genetically modified organism (GMO) *(32)*. In some countries, live vaccines based on a genetically modified microorganism are now subject to the rules governing the release of GMOs into the environment *(33)*.

### 3.4. Control of Nucleic Acid and Peptide Vaccines

Guidelines on the production and control of nucleic acid vaccines, and on safety issues related to their clinical use, are available from WHO and several other agencies *(29,30,34)*. The major safety issues posed by DNA vaccines include possible integration events leading to transformation of recipient cells, the potential formation of anti-DNA antibodies, and the unexpected and undesirable effects of long-term expression of a foreign antigen or associate cytokine intended to drive the immune system into producing a strong appropriate response (*see* Chapter 23). These issues have been fully investigated and discussed in recent years, and developments have been monitored closely by the WHO Working Group on Nucleic Acid Vaccines. These reports can be found on the WHO internet site (www.who.int/biologicals).

Another approach to vaccine development is to identify the peptide epitopes on immunogens that elicit protective responses, and to use chemically synthesized versions of these peptides in the production of vaccines (*see* Chapter 8). Unlike traditional and biotechnology-derived vaccines, peptide vaccines are totally synthetic, and do not carry the risk of reversion or incomplete inactivation, or of being contaminated with endogenous microorganisms. However, problems of consistency remain. Peptides are among the most complex of synthetic pharmaceuticals. The synthesis of even a moderate-size peptide involves a very extended sequence of reactions, and the desired product is inevitably contaminated by a wide range of closely related byproducts. Also, peptides themselves have proven to be poor immunogens, and are usually conjugated to a suitable protein or other macromolecular carrier to obtain better and more appropriate immune responses. WHO guidelines for the production and control of peptide vaccines are also available *(35)*, as is a guidance document from the US Food and Drug Administration (FDA) *(36)*.

## 4. Approaches to the Quality and Safety Assessment of Vaccines

The following points, made using specific examples, are designed to provide a framework for organizing the testing and obtaining the evidence needed to support an application to an appropriate licensing authority for the marketing of vaccines. Because of the range of preparations that may be developed as vaccines, it is not possible to give detailed recommendations that cover all situations, and the applicability of these points must be considered in relation to the scientific and medical background of the product concerned.

Regulatory requirements for licensing and batch release of vaccines, excluding clinical efficacy, fall conveniently into three main areas:

1. Control of starting materials, including baseline data on host cells where appropriate.
2. Control of manufacturing process.
3. Control of the final product, including its stability.

The evaluation of vaccine quality and safety should reflect this approach. Current practice is increasingly moving toward the use of more physicochemical and molecular procedures in the characterization and control of vaccines where scientifically justified. There is also a strong initiative to reduce the use of animals in the production and control of vaccines and the European Pharmacopoeia has already relaxed the need to perform an abnormal toxicity test (innocuity) on each lot of product provided certain conditions are met.

### 4.1. Evaluation of Classical Whole-Cell, Inactivated Bacterial Vaccines: Control of Whole-Cell Pertussis Vaccine

Whole-cell pertussis vaccine, in common with other killed bacterial vaccines, such as those for cholera and typhoid, is a biologically complex preparation developed long before the many recent advances in biochemistry, genetics, and immunology. Two factors feature prominently in its quality control: toxicity and potency.

Before release, whole-cell pertussis vaccine must be shown to be potent by the in vivo mouse protection test. A great deal of effort has been put into attempts to obtain greater reproducibility in this. The use of healthy mice selected at random for their place in the test has improved reproducibility of the results, which are also affected by the strain of mice used. Considerable attention is thus given to these particular aspects in WHO requirements for whole-cell pertussis vaccine *(17)*.

An immunizing dose of pertussis vaccine is the minimum number of killed organisms that has been shown to provide an adequate antigenic stimulus and thus protection. The number of killed organisms required for this purpose is indicated by the opacity of the bacterial suspension, estimated before the bacteria are killed.

Tests for toxicity have always posed problems because of the presence of several toxins in the bacterial suspension used to produce the vaccine. The so-called mouse-weight gain test has been adopted widely as an appropriate in-process indicator of toxicity, but more specific tests are now also available (*see* **Subheading 4.1.2.**) and used by many manufacturers and national control laboratories. Here, we list the major control measures that contribute to the production of a safe and effective whole-cell pertussis vaccine.

## 4.1.1. Control of Production

1. Control of source material. Strains of *B. pertussis* are fully characterized, and strain characteristics are verified for each production batch. Strains are chosen so that the final vaccine includes agglutinogens 1, 2, and 3. A seed lot system is employed.
2. Characteristics of the culture medium: Human blood or blood products must not be used in culture media either for bacterial seed or vaccine production. Materials of animal origin should be in accordance with the guidance given in the Report of a WHO Consultation on Medicinal and Other Products in Relation to Human and Animal Transmissible Spongiform Encephalopathies *(3)*.
3. Single harvests are controlled for consistency of growth rate and testing for the presence of agglutinogens. Samples of harvest are tested for purity before killing.
4. Control of opacity. The opacity of each single harvest is measured before the bacteria are killed by comparison with the International Reference Preparation of Opacity. This control procedure standardizes the number of organisms that are present in the final product.
5. *B. pertussis* can be killed and detoxified by a combination of methods, depending on temperature, time, and pH. The methods used should be validated.

## 4.1.2. Control of Final Bulk

1. Final bulk is prepared by pooling a number of single harvests. Detailed records must be kept of lots of single harvest used.
2. Each bulk is tested for the presence of agglutinogens 1, 2, and 3 before adjuvant is added.
3. If the vaccine is to be dispensed into a multidose container, a suitable antimicrobial preservative is added.
4. Adjuvants may be added to the vaccine. Aluminum hydroxide or phosphate is frequently used. The aluminum concentration must not exceed 1.25 mg/single human dose.
5. Sterility: Each final bulk is tested for bacterial and fungal contaminants.
6. Specific toxicity: Each final bulk is tested for toxicity by a validated method, such as the mouse-weight gain test. Other more specific tests are now also used: histamine sensitization assay, Chinese Hamster Ovary Cell (CHO) assay or leukocytosis assay for active pertussis toxin, Limulus Amoebocyte Lysis assay (LAL) for endotoxin.
7. The potency of each final bulk (or of each final lot) is determined by comparison with that of a reference vaccine calibrated against the International Standard for Pertussis Vaccine or equivalent standard. The assay performed is the intracerebral mouse protection test and the potency of the final bulk must not be <4 IU/single human dose and the lower fiducial limit ($P = 0.95$) of the estimated potency should not be <2 IU. Details of the method and how to calculate results can be found in the WHO manual of laboratory methods for potency testing of vaccines *(37)*.

## 4.1.3. Control of the Final Filled Product

1. Identity of the material in the vials is carried out on at least one container from each filled lot.
2. Sterility: Tests for bacterial and fungal contamination should be carried out.
3. Potency test: This is not repeated if done on final bulk, but can be carried out at this stage.
4. Innocuity: Each final lot is tested for abnormal toxicity in five mice and two guinea pigs.
5. Adjuvant content is measured and should be within specifications
6. Preservative content is measured and should be within specifications (if used).
7. pH should meet specifications.
8. Inspection of final containers: each container (vial) is inspected visually for clumping, the presence of particles, or other abnormalities. Faulty containers are discarded.

## 4.1.4. Stability

During development of a vaccine, tests are conducted to determine the loss of potency to be expected during storage. Other parameters should also be evaluated during stability studies. At least three batches obtained from different bulks are tested both in real time and following accelerated stability tests carried out by holding vaccine preparations at temperatures higher than the optimum storage temperature, which is $5 \pm 3°C$. This experimental evidence is submitted during licensing as justification for the shelf-life proposed for the product.

Written records of all of the tests carried out, regardless of results, must be kept. When any changes are made in the production procedure that may affect stability, the vaccine produced by the new method must be shown to be stable.

## 4.2. Evaluation of Classical Live Attenuated Virus Vaccines: Control of Measles Vaccine

Like many other successful viral vaccines, measles vaccine is a preparation of live attenuated virus. The antibody response in people inoculated with the vaccine can be accurately measured, and a number of studies have shown that the presence of detectable levels of appropriate antibodies correlates with protection against disease.

Clearly, it is vital that the strain of virus used to produce live attenuated measles vaccine should show no tendency to produce neurological complications of the type encountered during natural measles. Considerable attention is therefore paid to thoroughly characterizing the vaccine strain; the intracerebral inoculation of monkeys has been used to evaluate neurovirulence *(27)*.

### 4.2.1. Control of Production

1. Control of source materials—strain of measles virus: The strain used in production must be fully characterized, with complete historical records that include information on the origin of the strain, its method of attenuation, and passage level at which attenuation was shown by clinical evaluation. A seed-lot system is employed, and the seed lot—or each of the first five undiluted, clarified virus pools prepared from the same seed lot—must be shown to be non-neuropathogenic in monkeys. In addition, the strain of measles virus used in production should be shown be safe and immunogenic by tests in susceptible humans.

2. Control of source material—cell substrate: Production of vaccine is by propagation of the measles virus in cell substrates. Various cells can be used, such as chicken-embryo cells or human diploid cells. The eggs used as the source of chicken-embryo cells are derived from closed, specific-pathogen-free healthy stocks that are closely monitored for specific pathogens. For diploid cells, a master cell bank and working cell bank are employed, and there are strict requirements for assuring the absence of potential infectious agents and lack of tumorigenicity.

3. Serum used in cell-culture media must be tested to show the absence of bacterial, fungal, and mycoplasmal contamination, as well as the absence of viruses. The use of serum of bovine origin should be in accordance with the guidance given in the Report of a WHO Consultation on Medicinal and Other Products in Relation to Human and Animal Transmissible Encephalopathies *(3)*.

4. Control of cell cultures: Tests are carried out to ensure that no adventitious agents contaminate the system during production. After inoculation of measles virus, cultures for

vaccine production are incubated under controlled temperature conditions. No penicillin or other β-lactam antibiotic should be used at any stage of production.

5. Single harvests are controlled for consistency of virus growth, and are tested for sterility and measles virus content. Single harvests can be pooled to form the virus pool, which again is tested for sterility. The virus pool is clarified to remove cells and cell debris, and the live virus content of the clarified pool is determined.

### 4.2.2. Control of Final Bulk

1. The final bulk, which is prepared from one or more clarified virus pools, is tested for stability and virus content. Sometime substances—such as a diluent or a stabilizer (e.g., human albumin)—are added during the preparation of the final bulk.
2. Each bulk is tested for residual animal serum proteins if serum has been used in the cell culture.
3. Sterility: each bulk is tested for bacterial and fungal contamination.

### 4.2.3. Control of Filled Container

1. The final bulk is distributed into containers and is freeze-dried.
2. Identity tests.
3. Sterility tests: Reconstituted vaccine is tested for bacterial and fungal contamination.
4. Virus concentration and thermostability. The virus content of at least three containers from the freeze-dried lot is determined against a reference preparation of measles vaccine. WHO requires an additional three containers to be incubated at 37°C for 7 d, and the virus content is then measured. The geometric mean infectious virus titer must be equal to or greater than the required minimum number of infective units per human dose, and the geometric mean virus titer must not have decreased by more than $1.0 \log_{10}$ infectious units during the period of incubation. The lowest immunizing dose of virus in the vaccine that induces seroconversion in susceptible individuals is established in dose-response studies *(38)*.
5. Abnormal toxicity tests are carried out in mice and guinea pigs.
6. Residual moisture is determined, and should be within specified limits.
7. Inspection of final containers: carried out visually; those showing abnormalities are discarded.

### 4.2.4. Stability

During the development of the vaccine, tests will have been carried out to show that this particular product is stable at the stipulated storage temperature, which is any temperature below 8°C. However, each lot must pass the thermostability test before being released for use. Written records of all of the tests carried out, regardless of results, must be kept.

## 4.3. Evaluation of Modern Component Bacterial Vaccines: Control of Polysaccharide-Conjugate Vaccines (see Chapter 10)

### 4.3.1. Haemophilus influenzae *Type b*

The production and control of *H. influenzae* type b-conjugate (Hib-conjugate) vaccine illustrates the complexities of the production and control of bacterial polysaccharide - conjugate vaccines. Hib-conjugate vaccines are produced by covalently linking Hib capsular polysaccharide, composed of units of 3-β-D-ribose-f (1 → 1)-ribitol-5-

PO$_4^-$ (PRP), to a protein carrier in order to stimulate, in infants, a T-cell-dependent antibody response that otherwise does not occur with the polysaccharide alone. Conjugate vaccines also induce immunological memory in young children.

WHO recommendations for Hib-conjugate vaccines, first published in 1991, take into consideration important differences in vaccine composition as well as differences in production methods. Thus, these vaccines have been produced using native polyribosylribitol phosphate as well as oligosaccharides, together with different carrier proteins; standard diphtheria toxoid, a nontoxic mutant diphtheria toxin (CRM 197), standard tetanus toxoid, and an outer-membrane protein (OMP) complex of *Neisseria meningitidis* serogroup B have been used as carriers. Clearly, some control tests must therefore be product-specific. Serological correlates of protection in humans exist for Hib-conjugate vaccines, and it is important to show that a conjugate vaccine stimulates a statistically significant serum IgG response. This is in contrast to the case of acellular pertussis vaccines, for which serological correlates of protection have not yet been demonstrated. In the case of *H. influenzae*, the functional activity of the conjugate-induced antibodies is also evaluated by measuring the serum bactericidal activity against *H. influenzae* type b. Consistency of production, and the demonstration that the product does not differ from vaccine lots shown to be safe and adequately immunogenic and protective in clinical studies, are important components in the evaluation and lot-by-lot release of Hib-conjugate vaccines. However, as previously mentioned, certain vaccine lots that had met all established release criteria failed to produce the expected immune responses in infants *(39)*. Unintentional and undetected changes in a vaccine during production emphasize the need for continued post-marketing surveillance, and for further research to develop new strategies and tests to ensure that relevant vaccine characteristics are being properly controlled. WHO recommendations for Hib-conjugate vaccine were revised in 1999 *(40)* to take account of the above problems. Much experience had been gained with the preparation and control of these vaccines since 1991, and it had been shown that the biological assay for potency, the animal immunogenicity test recommended in the original WHO recommendations, does not correlate with the efficacy of the vaccines in infants and did not provide a sensitive indicator of vaccine quality. Thus, although immunogenicity testing in animals remains necessary during vaccine development, the revised Recommendations *(40)* state that an animal immunogenicity test does not need to be used for routine lot release. Instead, the testing focuses on the physicochemical tests to monitor consistency of production of the polysaccharide, the protein carrier and bulk conjugate.

### 4.3.1.1. CONTROL OF PRODUCTION

1. Control of source materials. The strain of *H. influenzae* type b used to prepare the polysaccharide should be well-characterized, and production should be based on a seed-lot system. The culture medium used for production must not contain blood-group substances or polysaccharides of high relative molecular mass. If any materials of animal origin are used in seed production or storage, or in vaccine production, their use should be in accordance with the guidance given in the Report of a WHO Consultation on Medicinal and Other Products in Relation to Human and Animal Transmissible Spongiform Encephalopathies (TSEs) *(3)*.

2. Purification of polysaccharide: Specifications must be set for the purified polysaccharide with respect to the content of moisture, ribose, phosphorus, protein, nucleic acid, and endotoxin. The molecular size of each lot of purified polysaccharide must be determined, and the distribution constant must be shown to be consistent for a given product.

3. Processed polysaccharide: Strict conditions are established for the chemical modification of the polysaccharide in preparation for conjugation to the protein. The processed polysaccharide is evaluated for the number of functional groups introduced for use in the conjugation reaction.

4. Carrier protein: The requirements for the carrier proteins will depend on the particular protein used. If toxoids or inactive variants of a toxin are used, then appropriate tests must be carried out to ensure that these proteins are nontoxic. Test methods to confirm their identity, quality, purity, and safety are carried out. Physicochemical methods that may be used to characterize such proteins include sodium dodecylsulfate-polyacrylamide gel electrophoresis (SDS-PAGE), isoelectric focusing, high-performance liquid chromatography (HPLC), amino acid analysis, amino acid sequencing, circular dichroism, fluorescence spectroscopy, peptide mapping, and mass spectrometry as appropriate. In some conjugation procedures, reactive functional groups or "spacers" may be introduced, and the degree of substitution must be monitored carefully at this stage to ensure consistency.

5. Control of bulk conjugate: A number of multistep conjugation methods are used for production. The method established must be shown to give a reproducible, stable, and safe Hib-conjugate vaccine.

Unreacted functional groups present at the end of conjugation are potentially capable of reacting in vivo. The manufacturing process should therefore be validated to show that it does not produce bulks containing such groups; any remaining groups should be made unreactive by means of "capping reagents." Once the conjugate has been purified, the consistency of manufacture is evaluated by testing for residual reagents, unbound polysaccharide, polysaccharide content, protein content, molecular size, and stability. For example, where appropriate, when tetanus or diphtheria toxoids are used as carriers, the bulk conjugate should also be tested for the absence of specific toxicity. The polysaccharide-to-protein ratio of the conjugate should be within the limits established for that particular conjugate. The final bulk is prepared by mixing an adjuvant and preservative, if used, with a suitable quantity of the bulk conjugate to meet the specifications of the vaccine lots shown to be safe and effective in the clinical trials.

### 4.3.1.2. CONTROL OF FINAL PRODUCT

1. Identity of the material in the vials is carried out on at least one labeled container from each final lot.

2. Sterility: Tests for bacterial and fungal contamination should be carried out.

3. The total PRP content is determined, and must be within + or –20% of the stated content.

4. Each final lot is tested for abnormal toxicity in five mice and two guinea pigs. However, the revised WHO recommendations allow this test to be omitted for routine lot release once consistency of production has been well-established to the satisfaction of the national regulatory authority and when good manufacturing practices are in place. Each lot, if tested, should pass the test.

5. Adjuvant content is measured, and should be within set limits.

6. Residual moisture: If the vaccine is freeze-dried, then the residual moisture content should be within limits sets during development and clinical trial of the vaccine.

7. Pyrogenicity in rabbits or endotoxin content as measured by the LAL test should meet specifications.
8. Preservative content should be measured, and should be within set limits (where used).
9. Stability: The polysaccharide component of conjugate vaccines suffers gradual hydrolysis at a rate that varies with the type of conjugate, type of formulation or adjuvant, type of excipients, and conditions of storage. The depolymerization can result in reduced molecular size of the PRP component, a reduction in the amount of the PRP bound to the carrier protein (e.g., an increase in the free PRP content), and a reduced molecular size of the conjugate. In general, PRP-protein conjugate vaccines are susceptible to gradual hydrolysis, and the expiry date must be established accordingly. Thus, during development, tests must be conducted to determine to what extent the characteristics of the product in question have been maintained throughout the proposed validity period. Final containers from at least three final lots derived from different bulks are tested at the end of the period to evaluate stability during storage. Both unbound polysaccharide and protein are determined, and a vaccine lot must meet specifications for the final product up to the expiration date.

As with all other vaccines, written records of all tests carried out, regardless of results, must be kept. When any changes are made in the production process that may affect stability, vaccine produced by the new procedure must be shown to be stable.

### 4.3.2. Group C Meningococcal Conjugate Vaccine

Following the development of the Hib conjugate vaccines, considerable progress has been made in the development of similar conjugate vaccines based on serogroup C meningococcal capsular polysaccharide. Clinical trials have shown these vaccines to be highly immunogenic in all age groups and to induce immunological memory. In 1999, the Group C meningococcal conjugate vaccines were licensed and introduced into the routine immunization program in the United Kingdom, where they were found to be safe and very effective in decreasing the incidence of Group C meningitis and septicemia. Interestingly, in this case, licensing was based on the proven immunogenicity of the vaccine rather than on clinical efficacy. Following their success in the United Kingdom, other countries have licensed these vaccines and introduced them into their routine vaccination schedules, or are planning to do so. WHO Recommendations for this vaccine were therefore developed and adopted by the WHO Expert Committee on Biological Standardization in November 2001. These are based on the recommendations for the Hib conjugate vaccines, and again emphasize a strategy for the control of the vaccine, which relies heavily on molecular characterization and purity to ensure that each vaccine lot is consistent with the specifications of the vaccine lots used in the definitive clinical trials that confirmed their safety and immunogenicity. Thus, the quality and purity of the polysaccharide, the carrier protein, and the composition of the final protein conjugate are important parameters *(41)*. The immunogenicity of the meningococcal C conjugate vaccines has been evaluated in mice, and such data can provide an indication of the consistency and structural integrity of the vaccine. However, although immunogenicity testing in animals forms a necessary part of vaccine development, experience gained following the licensing of the serogroup C conjugates suggests that, as in the case of Hib vaccine, a routine animal potency test is not necessary when vaccine consistency has been assured by physicochemical criteria.

The amount of free polysaccharide in the final product is an important parameter in the case of the serogroup C meningococcal conjugate vaccine. Only the meningococcal polysaccharide that is covalently bound to the carrier protein—the conjugated polysaccharide—is immunologically significant for clinical protection. Indeed, excessive levels of unbound polysaccharide could potentially result in immunologically hyporesponsiveness to group C polysaccharide, a phenomenon observed in studies of immunized infants and adults. Although the clinical importance of this phenomenon is unclear, for quality-control purposes, each batch of conjugate is tested for unbound or free polysaccharide to ensure that the amount present in the purified bulk conjugate is within the limits of lots shown to be clinically safe and efficacious. Methods that have been used to assay unbound polysaccharide include gel filtration, ultrafiltration, and hydrophobic interaction chromatography, or ultracentrifugation with High-Performance Anion-Exchange Chromatography with Pulsed Amperometric Detection (HPAEC-PAD) or colorimetric detection.

## References

1. Biological Standardization and control. (1997) A scientific review commissioned by the UK National Biological Standards Board. World Health Organization. WHO/BLG/97.1.
2. Biotechnology and world health. (1997) Risks and benefits of vaccines and other medical products produced by genetic engineering. Proceedings of a WHO meeting. WHO/VRD/BLG/97.01.
3. Report of a WHO Consultation on Medicinal and Other Products in Relation to Human and Animal Transmissible Spongiform Encephalopathies, Geneva, 24-26 March, 1997, World Health Organization (WHO/BLG/97.2).
4. WHO guidelines for clinical evaluation of vaccines: regulatory expectations. WHO Technical Report Series (In press).
5. Griffiths, E. (1988) Efficacy of whole-cell pertussis vaccine, in *Pathogenesis and Immunity in Pertussis* (Wardlaw, A. C. and Parton R., eds.), Wiley, Chichester, UK, pp. 353–374.
6. WHO guidelines for good clinical practice (GCP) for trials on pharmaceutical products. (1995) *WHO Technical Report Series* **850**, 97–137.
7. Recommendations and guidelines for biological substances used in medicine and other documents. (2000) *WHO Technical Report Series* **897**, 67–70.
8. Jodar, L., Frasch, C., Carlone, G., Siber, G., Butler, J., Dagan, R., et al. Serological criteria for evaluation and licensure of pneumococcal conjugate vaccines. (In press).
9. Guidance for Industry for the evaluation of combination vaccines for preventable diseases: production, testing and clinical studies. (1997) US FDA.
10. CPMP/BWP/477/97 (1999) —Note for Guidance on Pharmaceutical and Biological aspects of combined vaccines.
11. Guidelines for national authorities on quality assurance for biological products. (1992) *WHO Technical Report Series* **822**, 31–46.
12. Regulation and licensing of biological products in countries with newly developing regulatory authorities. (1995) *WHO Technical Report Series* **858**, 21–35.
13. Scientific considerations for the regulation and clinical evaluation of HIV/AIDS preventive vaccines, (2002) *AIDS* **16**, W15–W25.
14. Good manufacturing practices for biological products. (1992) *WHO Technical Report Series* **822**, 20–30.

15. CPMP/ICH/138/95 Note for Guidance on Quality of Biotechnolocical Products: Stability testing of Biotechnological Products (Q5C) (1995).
16. Milstien J., Dellepiane N., Lambert S., Belgharbi L., Rolls C., Knezevic I., et al. (2002) Vaccine quality—can a single standard be defined? *Vaccine* **20,** 1000–1003.
17. Requirements for diphtheria, tetanus, pertussis and combined vaccines. (1990) *WHO Technical Report Series* **800,** 87–179.
18. Leslie, P. H. and Gardner, A. D. (1931) The phases of *Haemophilus pertussis. J. Hyg.* **31,** 423–434.
19. Bullen J. J. and Griffiths E., eds. (1999) *Iron and Infection: Molecular, Physiological and Clinical Aspects*; 2nd ed., John Wiley & Sons, Chichester, UK.
20. Guidelines for the production and control of the acellular pertussis component of monovalent or combined vaccines. (1998) *WHO Technical Report Series* **878,** 57–76.
21. Guidelines for the production and control of inactivated oral cholera vaccines. Technical Report Series. (In press) .
22. Reverse transcriptase activity in chicken-cell derived vaccine. (1998) *Weekly Epidemiological Record* **73,** No. 28, 209–212.
23. Butel, J. S. (2000) Simian virus 40, poliovirus vaccines and human cancer: research progress versus media and public interests. *Bull. WHO* **78,** (2) 195–198.
24. Vilchez, R. A., Madden, C. R., Kozinetz, C. A., Halvorson, J., White, J. S., Jorgensen, J. L., et al. (2002) Association between simian virus 40 and "non-Hodgkin lymphoma. (2002) *Lancet,* **359,** 817–823.
25. Requirements for the use of animal cells as in vitro substrates for the production of biologicals. (1998) *WHO Technical Report Series* **878,** 19–56.
26. Recommendations for the production and control of poliomyelitis vaccine (oral). (2002) *WHO Technical Report Series* **904,** 31–93.
27. Requirements for measles, mumps and rubella vaccines and combined vaccine (live). (1994) *WHO Technical Report Series* **840,** 100–201.
28. Guidelines for assuring the quality of pharmaceutical and biological products prepared by recombinant DNA technology. (1991) *WHO Technical Report Series* **814,** 59–70.
29. Points to consider on plasmid DNA vaccines for preventive infectious disease indications. Food and Drug Administration. Center for Biologics Evaluation and Research. (1996).
30. CPMP/BWP/3088/99—Note for Guidance on the quality, preclinical and clinical aspects of gene transfer medicinal products (2001).
31. Requirements for hepatitis B vaccines made by recombinant DNA techniques. (1989) *WHO Technical Report Series* **786,** 38–71.
32. Schneider, L. G. (1995) Rabies virus vaccines in non-target effects of live vaccines. *Devel. Biol. Stand.* **84,** 49–54.
33. CPMP/III/5507/94 Note for Guidance on Environmental risk assessment for human medicinal products containing or consisting of GMOs (1994).
34. Guidelines for assuring the quality of DNA vaccines. (1998) *WHO Technical Report Series* **878,** 77–90.
35. Guidelines for the production and quality control of synthetic peptide vaccines. (1999) *WHO Technical Report Series* **814,** 24–43.
36. Guidance for industry for the submission of chemistry, manufacturing and controls information for synthetic peptide substances. Center for Drug Evaluation and Research, and Center for Biologics Evaluation and Research, Food and Drug Administration, Washington, DC. (1994)
37. Manual of laboratory methods for potency testing of vaccines used in the WHO Expanded Programme on Immunization: World Health Organization. WHO/BLG/95.1. (1995).

38. Diaz-Ortega, J. L., Forsey, T., Clements, C. J., and Milstien, J. (1994) The relationship between dose and response of standard measles vaccines. *Biologicals* **22,** 35–44.

39. Egan, W., Frasch, C., and Anthony, B. F. (1995) Lot-release criteria, post licensure quality control and the *Haemophilus influenzae* Type b conjugate vaccines. *JAMA* **273,** 888–889.

40. Recommendations for the production and control of *Haemophilus influenzae* type b conjugate vaccines. (2000) *WHO Technical Report Series* **897,** 27–60.

41. Recommendations for the production and control of Group C meningococcal conjugate vaccine. (2002) *WHO Technical Report Series* (in press).

# 23

## DNA Vaccination

*An Update*

### Douglas B. Lowrie

### 1. Introduction

The volume entitled *DNA Vaccines: Methods and Protocols* was published in this series as recently as 2000, and thus it is no more than 3 yr since the authors of this volume surveyed the scene and prepared their chapters for publication. Yet progress continues to be rapid in this exciting field, and an update is needed. New ways to enhance efficacy in a wide range of applications are being sought, and here the author summarizes the main developments. The subject headings are indicative rather than definitive of the material covered in each section, since developments frequently impact on multiple aspects of DNA vaccinology.

### 2. DNA Uptake, Transcription, and Expression

The main concern in the field of DNA vaccination continues to be the low overall efficiency of the process. Typically, huge amounts of DNA are applied, and minute amounts of antigen are produced. The barriers to efficiency are, to a large extent, physical barriers against entry into the cell and entry into the nucleus. The ballistic approach provides one solution, in which DNA attached to inert particles is fired into the cell and nucleus at high velocity using a gun. However, we might reasonably desire to retain the basic simplicity of the procedure in which injected or even topically applied DNA generates effective immunity.

DNA in extracellular space and in endocytic vesicles is rapidly degraded by enzyme action, but if it gets into the cytosol it is relatively stable. Injection in 150 m$M$ phosphate buffer is reported to enhance stability, presumably by inhibiting enzymic degra-

From: *Methods in Molecular Medicine, Vol. 87: Vaccine Protocols, 2nd ed.*
Edited by: A. Robinson, M. J. Hudson, and M. P. Cranage © Humana Press Inc., Totowa, NJ

dation *(1)*. Plasmid DNA that has entered the cytoplasm has essentially unrestricted access to the nuclear compartment during cell division *(2)*, but in non-dividing cells, special tricks are needed. New techniques for evaluating and enhancing entry into the nucleus have recently been described and reviewed *(3–7)*. Electroporation seems to be highly effective for DNA traverse of both cell and nuclear membranes in non-replicating cells such as muscle in vivo *(8–13)*. An increase in protein expression of up to 70-fold has been seen *(9)*, but electroporation may result in high levels of plasmid integration into cellular DNA that are unacceptable for vaccines. Association of plasmid DNA with nonviral particles continues to be explored as a means of enhancing uptake, into endosomes as well as into the nucleus. Condensation with oligolysine-RGD peptide facilitates entry into the cell as well as into the nucleus *(14)*. Strikingly, linear polyethylenimine particles can be as effective as electroporation *(15)*, perhaps without enhancing the risk of DNA integration.

It is now clear that a large part of the increased expression caused by the SV40 DNA that is commonly present in vaccine plasmids is a result of nuclear targeting. The enhancer region associated with the origin of replication appears to bind a complex of transcription factors and DNA-binding proteins that together mediate nuclear import *(16–18)*. Inclusion of this element can increase expression about 20-fold in injected muscle and in non-dividing cells, but not in dividing cells in which expression is already high *(19)*. This viral dodge of hitching a lift into the nucleus by binding transcription factors has been elegantly exploited by Mesika et al. *(20)*, who incorporated NF$k$B-binding sites into plasmid and increased nuclear localization 12-fold. Depending on the position of the binding sites, they could increase expression by an additional 19-fold by enhancing transcription. As expected, stimuli that increased NF$k$B availability also increased nuclear uptake and expression. Further evidence of the role of transcription factors as nuclear import vehicles has come from studies of a smooth-muscle specific promoter, the promoter of the gamma actin gene *(21)*. Nuclear uptake and expression of plasmid using this promoter was dependent on the availability of the smooth-muscle specific transcription factor SRF. When this protein was expressed in other nondividing cells, they too could import the plasmid into the nucleus and use the promoter.

Evidence that the DNA-binding protein VP22 from herpes simplex virus could enhance uptake of plasmid into the nucleus *(22)* has proven controversial *(23)*. Plasmids that express fusions between antigen and VP22 appear to be much more effective than plasmids expressing the antigen alone in inducing strong CD8+ Th1 immune responses *(24–27)*. Although the phenomenon has been explained alternatively by an increased spreading of the fusion product to adjacent non-transfected cells *(28)*, the evidence for this is drawn from microscopy and may arise from an artefact of methanol-fixed cells *(29)*, so the mechanism awaits definition.

Manipulations of encoded proteins so that they carry amino acid sequences intended to target the antigen to different subcellular compartments—and thus to different antigen presentation pathways and immune responses—have not always had the expected effect. Indeed, totally unexpected subcellular distribution of the protein has been reported *(30)*. Nevertheless, the inclusion of secretion signals tends to preferentially enhance antibody responses *(31–32)*, and targeting proteosomes by including ubiquitin sequences preferentially enhances Th1 cellular immunity *(33)*. The inclusion of both ubiquitin and epitope-flanking sequences to enhance proteolytic processing markedly facilitated tumor eradication in mice by an epitope-string DNA vaccine *(34)*.

Thus far, there are few indications that alternatives to the usual CMV immediate early gene-transcription promoter and enhancer offer much superior responses. However, the ubiquitin B promoter is one candidate, particularly in conjunction with the CMV enhancer, since it resulted in higher and longer-sustained gene expression in mouse lung after intranasal (in) delivery *(35)*. Intradermal (id) gene gun delivery of a plasmid that expresses antigen from a dendritic cell-specific promoter has been found to result in maturation of skin Langerhans cells, migration to draining lymph nodes, and immune responses in mice *(36)*. The efficacy of such a promoter in man might be superior to that of the CMV promoter, particularly if there is a background of pre-existing defense against expression of the human CMV promoter in the face of widespread silent infection with this virus. The safety profile of a promoter expressed only in dendritic cells may also be superior.

## 3. Adjuvants

The importance of stimulation of innate immune responses in vaccination for Th-1 acquired immune responses in general is becoming clear *(37)* and DNA vaccination is no exception. Contaminating LPS and inherent CpG sequences within the plasmid can be potent stimulators through Toll-like receptors. Indeed, it seems likely that some of the variability in efficacy observed in laboratory experiments can be attributed to contamination of plasmid DNA with traces of LPS originating from the *Escherichia coli* in which the plasmid is produced.

CpG and LPS stimulate NF*k*B, TNF-alpha, and Type-1 interferon production through separate receptors and pathways that partially converge, but also have distinct synergistic elements *(38)*. Many known and unknown genes have been detected to be upregulated in spleen cells following stimulation with CpG *(39)*. CpG stimulation of the Type-1 interferon response may be essential for driving the Th1 vs Th2 bias *(40,41)* but CpG oligonucleotides also greatly increased antibody responses to HBV DNA in orangutans *(42)*. It is now known that the stimulatory GTCGTT recognition motif is strongly conserved across ten animal species, but there are differences in the optima *(43)*. Not only are there significant differences in stimulatory sequence optima between mouse and man, complicating the move from preclinical to human clinical trials of DNA vaccines, there are also differences in sequence optima between target cell types and there are antagonistic sequences *(44–46)*. Remarkably, stimulation with CpG sequences has been found to result in functional expression of MHC class II molecules on myocytes, adding fuel to the debate over the relative mechanisms and contributions of myocytes and dendritic cells to immune priming by DNA vaccines *(47)*. Much of the exploratory work on the adjuvant effects of CpG motifs has been done with short, single-strand phosphorothioate molecules. It is evident that although the principles also apply to plasmid DNA, prediction of the outcome of diverse combinations and permutations of CpG motifs in plasmid vaccines is not yet possible *(43)*.

There are alternatives to LPS and CpG sequences for adjuvanticity. Monophosphoryl lipid A (MPL), representing the active component of LPS, can substantially increase primary antibody responses to rabies DNA, regardless of whether the DNA is injected via im or id routes or delivered by gene gun. However, boosting of responses by im or id DNA injections was inhibited by including MPL in the boost *(48)*, perhaps because of enhanced DNA degradation since inclusion of MPL did not inhibit boosting by gene gun delivery of DNA into cells. Co-injection of zymosan as the inflammatory stimulus has been found to enhance the Th-1 antibody and cellular responses to a human immunodeficiency virus-1 (HIV-1) DNA vaccine. The enhancement was complement-dependent, suggesting modulation by recruitment and activation of macrophages or dendritic cells *(49)*. It seems that alterations in the intracellular redox state in antigen-presenting cells (APC) that are responding to CpG or inflammatory stimuli may play a key role in determining the Th-1 to Th-2 balance of the resulting acquired immune response to DNA vaccines *(44,50–53)*.

Co-delivery of DNA that expresses immune signaling molecules continues to show promise for application in vaccines against infections in addition to cancer. For example, DNA expressing either IL-2 or IFN-gamma substantially enhanced specific cell-mediated immunity in rhesus HIV and SIV models *(54)*, and DNA expressing granulocyte-macrophage colony-stimulating factor (GM-CSF) is a safe and well-tolerated adjuvant in DNA vaccines expressing multiple malaria antigens in mice *(55)*. In contrast, although a vaccine made from a random-fragment whole-genome genetic library from SIV and delivered by gene gun substantially protected macaques against challenge with SIV, inclusion of plasmids expressing IL-12 and GM-CSF impaired protection *(56)*. DNA expressing CD40L enhanced both Th1 and Th2 responses to DNA vaccination in a murine HIV-1 model *(57)*. Similarly, DNA expressing either CD40L or CD40 together with plasmid expressing herpes simplex gD antigen enhanced resistance to HSV by promoting CD4+ Th1 responses *(58)*. Co-injection with plasmid expressing LFA-3 enhanced cellular and humoral responses and protection against HSV-2 in mice *(59)*; plasmids expressing IL-8 and RANTES enhanced both antigen-specific CD4+ Th1 cellular immune responses and protection *(60)*; plasmids expressing MCP-1, IP-10 and MIP-1a increased mortality *(60)*. Interestingly, it has been reported that inclusion of human papillomavirus E6 expression in a DNA vaccine against *Leishmania donovani* in order to inhibit *p53*, resulted in higher antigen expression and greater cellular and humoral responses to the co-expressed A2 antigen in mice *(61)*.

## 4. Routes and Delivery Protocols

Bupivacaine has been safely used clinically to enhance the efficacy of DNA vaccines delivered by intramuscular injection *(62,63)*. Although part of the facilitating effect of bupivacaine may be the result of toxicity followed by myocyte replacement/proliferation, the molecule is now seen to form stable liposomal-like structures that enhance DNA stability and perhaps uptake *(64)*. Although delivery of plasmid in association with liposomes and similar lipid formulations has also proven effective in enhancing immune responses, this enhancement is probably not simply the result of increased DNA uptake into target cells, as originally believed. For example, Vaxfectin (Vical Inc., a cationic and neutral lipid formulation) enhanced antibody responses without decreasing cytolytic T-cell responses but it did this without increasing DNA expression in muscle *(65,66)*. It is still not clear to what extent continued production of antigen by transfected myocytes (or any other cell) contributes to the development and maintenance of immune memory, particularly with respect to cytotoxic cellular immunity. The induction of both perforin and antibody-mediated immune destruction of myocytes after im DNA vaccine injection has been demonstrated *(67)*, but presumably not all productive cells are necessarily killed by these responses.

The possibility that DNA vaccines may be applied topically by skin patch has received support from several investigations. For example, immune responses were induced by application of plasmid in saline to normal intact mouse skin *(68)*. Not surprisingly, the process seems much more effective after epidermal stripping. Chitosan-based nanoparticles coated with DNA could elicit significant antigen expression and antibody responses after topical application to abraded mouse skin *(69)*; strong cellular responses against HIV-1 surface antigen expressed from topically applied plasmid were enhanced by co-administered GM-CSF plasmid *(70)*. Similar results were obtained with plasmid-expressing flu matrix gene, and liposomes that included mannan enhanced the responses, as did plasmid expressing GM-CSF *(71)*. Intranasal and aerosol delivery methods continue to be attractive clinical prospects, partially because they target the main route of transmission for many infectious diseases and protective effects can be systemic. Intranasal plasmid delivery to mice was shown to result in mRNA detectable at 2–4 wk in lung, liver, and spleen, and encoded HIV-1 specific protein was detectable in the lung *(72)*.

Although intravenous (iv) DNA delivery during pregnancy may not be acceptable in humans, it is of interest that, in contrast to free plasmid, iv plasmid in liposomes can reach the mouse fetus when given 9.5 d post-coitus, and results in priming for stronger protective responses against influenza challenge *(73)*. Immunization of pregnant goats with in plasmid-expressing *Cryptosporidium parvum* antigen subsequently partially protected the neonates from infection, probably by passive antibody transfer *(74)*. Also intriguing is the observation that plasmid introduced into the oral cavity of lambs *in utero* resulted in substantial antibody and cell-mediated immune responses in neonates *(75)*. Intravulvomucosal delivery of plasmid by gene gun gave stronger cellular and humoral bovine herpes virus (BHV-1) responses in cows than skin delivery *(76)*. This was probably the result of easier access to the Langerhans cells that are the main target of gene gun vaccination, but cost and convenience barriers must be overcome before such delivery technology can be widely accepted *(77)*.

## 5. Applications

A recent review of DNA vaccination against tumor-associated antigens reaffirmed that preclinical studies in animal models support DNA immunization as a potent strategy for mediating antitumor effects in vivo *(78)*. Further evidence that this may be true for at least one category of human tumor, the B-cell lymphoma, has been obtained with the gene sequences encoding the idiotypic determinants linked to a potently antigenic fragment from tetanus toxin to break tolerance and clinical trials are underway (79,80). Malignant melanoma in horses has responded well to direct injection of DNA expressing IL-12 only (81).

Encouragingly, intradermal gene gun delivery of hepatitis B virus DNA on gold into normal human volunteers has resulted in antibody levels that would be expected to be protective, and generated antigen-specific CD8+ cytotoxic T-cells in a Th1 response (82). Less encouragingly, although HIV-1 DNA vaccine plus IL-12 DNA has yielded strong immune responses in infected chimpanzees, only a transient decrease in viral load was obtained (83). Observations that DNA vaccination is superior to viral vectors in generating responses to subdominant epitopes have been confirmed with HIV-1 epitopes in Rhesus monkeys (84). Importantly, it has also been found that there is a lack of antigenic competition for antibody responses following Aotus monkey vaccination with three malaria blood-stage antigens on separate plasmids (85).

Studies in mice have shown that an anti-rabies DNA vaccine is at least as effective as the human diploid-cell vaccine for protection when given 6 h after infection (86). A single dose of the vaccine given either intramuscularly or by gene gun to Cynomologus monkeys gave substantial protection against lethal challenge 1 yr later (87). Antirabies DNA, recombinant vaccinia virus, and human diploid-cell vaccine were equivalent in priming for long-lasting antibody responses. However, recombinant vaccinia virus was ineffective in boosting, regardless of how priming was done (88). In cows, DNA priming enhanced T-cell responses to live BHV without enhancing protection (76). Nevertheless, the prime-boost strategy, in which DNA is used to prime and viral vectors or protein plus adjuvant are used to boost, is gaining ground. For example, DNA vaccination followed by canarypox boosting has been shown to result in a substantially decreased viral load in chronically hepatitis B virus-infected chimpanzees (89). Progress in developing DNA vaccines against pathogens of fish continues (90). The vaccines can be remarkably effective at low doses, and could prove to be cost-effective if suitable delivery procedures can be developed (91,92). The applications of DNA vaccines to the veterinary and fish farming fields have recently been reviewed (93).

It has been suggested that DNA vaccination against intracellular pathogens such as TB and HIV might fail or be unacceptable in regions in which there are high levels of helminthic parasite infestations because of the conflicting requirements for Th1 and Th2 responses. However, it is encouraging that an id plasmid expressing a model antigen (beta-galactosidase) gave a strong Th1 response without affecting the protective schistosome-specific Th2 response in infected mice (94). However, it is clear that DNA vaccination can downregulate Th2 responses. Studies of DNA-based immunotherapeutics of allergic diseases have recently been reviewed (95). Among the notable findings are: plasmids expressing allergens can produce a long-lasting antigen-specific shift of Th2 to Th1, whereas immunostimulatory DNA sequences conjugated to allergen give shorter-lasting but antigen-independent effects (96–99); the effects can be helper-T-cell independent (100); and either CD8 or CD4 cells can mediate the downmodulation of the IgE response seen after therapeutic Derf11 DNA vaccination of sensitized mice (101).

The potential value of plasmids expressing GM-CSF for enhancing production of anti-snake venom by gene gun DNA vaccination has been demonstrated in mice *(102)*. A further broadening of the practical application of DNA vaccines is indicated by a report that DNA immunization with minigenes encoding carbohydrate mimotopes can induce anti-carbohydrate antibody responses *(103)*.

## 6. Safety

There has been no shift in the view that DNA vaccination appears to be safe and clinically acceptable. However, the effects of changes in plasmid backbone and coding sequences are difficult to predict in animal models and thus by extrapolation, in man, each candidate for clinical trial will continue to be evaluated based on its merits. A useful study of the risks of plasmid DNA integration into the genome has been published *(104)*. Three different DNA vaccines were given intramuscularly to mice. At 6 mo the persistent plasmid was down to 200–800 copies/microgram DNA. It was estimated that at worst this could mean integration of 1–8 plasmid copies per 150,000 diploid cells, equating to 1000-fold lower than the spontaneous mutation rate and therefore posing negligible risk.

## References

1. Hartikka, J., Bozoukova, V., Jones, D., Mahajan, R., Wloch, M. K., Sawdey, M., et al. (2000) Sodium phosphate enhances plasmid DNA expression in vivo. *Gene Ther.* **7,** 1171–1182.
2. Brunner, S., Sauer, T., Carotta, S., Cotten, M., Saltik, M., and Wagner, E. (2000) Cell cycle dependence of gene transfer by lipoplex polyplex and recombinant adenovirus. *Gene Ther.* **7,** 401–407.
3. Bremner, K. H., Seymour, L. W., and Pouton, C. W. (2001) Harnessing nuclear localization pathways for transgene delivery. *Curr. Opin. Mol. Ther.* **3,** 170–177.
4. James, M. B. and Giorgio, T. D. (2000) Nuclear-associated plasmid, but not cell-associated plasmid, is correlated with transgene expression in cultured mammalian cells. *Mol. Ther.* **1,** 339–346.
5. Johnson-Saliba, M. and Jans, D. A. (2001) Gene therapy: optimising DNA delivery to the nucleus. *Curr. Drug Targets* **2,** 371–399.
6. Kamiya, H., Tsuchiya, H., Yamazaki, J., and Harashima, H. (2001) Intracellular trafficking and transgene expression of viral and nonviral gene vectors. *Adv. Drug Delivery Rev.* **52,** 153–164.
7. Tachibana, R., Harashima, H., Shinohara, Y., and Kiwada, H. (2001) Quantitative studies on the nuclear transport of plasmid DNA and gene expression employing nonviral vectors. *Adv. Drug Delivery Rev.* **52,** 219–226.
8. Aihara, H. and Miyazaki, J. (1998) Gene transfer into muscle by electroporation in vivo. *Nat. Biotechnol.* **16,** 867–870.
9. Hartikka, J., Sukhu, I., Buchner, C., Hazard, D., Bozoukova, V., Margalith, M., et al. (2001b) Electroporation-facilitated delivery of plasmid DNA in skeletal muscle: Plasmid dependence of muscle damage and effect of poloxamer 188. *Mol. Ther.* **4,** 407–415.
10. Hoover, F. and Kalhovde, J. M. (2000) A double-injection DNA electroporation protocol to enhance in vivo gene delivery in skeletal muscle. *Anal. Biochem.* **285,** 175–178.
11. Maruyama, H., Ataka, K., Gejyo, F., Higuchi, N., Ito, Y., Hirahara, H., et al. (2001) Long-term production of erythropoietin after electroporation-mediated transfer of plasmid DNA into the muscles of normal and uremic rats. *Gene Ther.* **8,** 461–468.

12. Selby, M., Goldbeck, C., Pertile, T., Walsh, R., and Ulmer, J. (2000) Enhancement of DNA vaccine potency by electroporation in vivo. *J. Biotechnol.* **83,** 147–152.

13. Widera, G., Austin, M., Rabussay, D., Goldbeck, C., Barnett, S. W., Chen, M. C., et al. (2000) Increased DNA vaccine delivery and immunogenicity by electroporation *in vivo*. *J. Immunol.* **164,** 4635–4640.

14. Colin, M., Moritz, S., Fontanges, P., Kornprobst, M., Delouis, C., Keller, M., et al. (2001) The nuclear pore complex is involved in nuclear transfer of plasmid DNA condensed with an oligolysine-RGD peptide containing nuclear localisation properties. *Gene Ther.* **8,** 1643–1653.

15. Brunner, S., Furtbauer, E., Sauer, T., Kursa, M., and Wagner, E. (2002) Overcoming the nuclear barrier: cell cycle independent nonviral gene transfer with linear polyethylenimine or electroporation. *Mol. Ther.* **5,** 80–86.

16. Dean, D. A. (2000) Peptide nucleic acids: versatile tools for gene therapy strategies. *Adv. Drug Delivery Rev.* **44,** 81–95.

17. Dean, D. A., Dean, B. S., Muller, S., and Smith, L. C. (1999) Sequence requirements for plasmid nuclear import. *Exp. Cell Res.* **253,** 713–722.

18. Wilson, G. L., Dean, B. S., Wang, G., and Dean, D. A. (1999) Nuclear import of plasmid DNA in digitonin-permeabilized cells requires both cytoplasmic factors and specific DNA sequences. *J. Biol. Chem.* **274,** 22,025–22,032.

19. Li, S., MacLaughlin, F. C., Fewell, J. G., Gondo, M., Wang, J., Nicol, F., et al. (2001) Muscle-specific enhancement of gene expression by incorporation of SV/40 enhancer in the expression plasmid. *Gene Ther.* **8,** 494–497.

20. Mesika, A., Grigoreva, I., Zohar, M., and Reich, Z. (2001) A regulated, NF kappa B-assisted import of plasmid DNA into mammalian cell nuclei. *Mol. Ther.* **3,** 653–657.

21. Vacik, J., Dean, B. S., Zimmer, W. E., and Dean, D. A. (1999) Cell-specific nuclear import of plasmid DNA. *Gene Ther.* **6,** 1006–1014.

22. Elliott, G. and Ohare, P. (1997) Intercellular trafficking and protein delivery by a herpesvirus structural protein. *Cell* **88,** 223–233.

23. Lundberg, M. and Johansson, M. (2001) Is VP22 nuclear homing an artifact? *Nat. Biotechnol.* **19,** 713–713.

24. Cheng, W. F., Hung, C. F., Chai, C. Y., Hsu, K. F., He, L., Ling, M. et al. (2001) Enhancement of Sindbis virus self-replicating RNA vaccine potency by linkage of herpes simplex virus type 1 VP22 protein to antigen. *J. Virol.* **75,** 2368–2376.

25. Hung, C. F., Cheng, W. F., Chai, C. Y., Hsu, K. F., He, L. M., Ling, M., et al. (2001a) Improving vaccine potency through intercellular spreading and enhanced MHC class I presentation of antigen. *J. Immunol.* **166,** 5733–5740.

26. Hung, C. F., Hsu, K. F., Cheng, W. F., Chai, C. Y., He, L. M., Ling, M. et al. (2001b) Enhancement of DNA vaccine potency by linkage of antigen gene to a gene encoding the extracellular domain of Fms-like tyrosine kinase 3-ligand. *Cancer Res.* **61,** 1080–1088.

27. Oliveira, S. C., Harms, J. S., Afonso, R. R., and Splitter, G. A. (2001) A genetic immunization adjuvant system based on BVP22-antigen fusion. *Human Gene Ther.* **12,** 1353–1359.

28. Bennett, R. P. and Dalby, B. (2002) Protein delivery using VP22. *Nat. Biotechnol.* **20,** p. 20.

29. Lundberg, M. and Johansson, M. (2002) Positively charged DNA-binding proteins cause apparent cell membrane translocation. *Biochem. Biophys. Res. Commun.* **291,** 367–371.

30. Ramanathan, M. P., Ayyavoo, V., and Weiner, D. B. (2001) Choice of expression vector alters the localization of a human cellular protein. *DNA Cell Biol.* **20,** 101–105.

31. Li, Z., Howard, A., Kelley, C., Delogu, G., Collins, F., and Morris, S. (1999) Immunogenicity of DNA vaccines expressing tuberculosis proteins fused to tissue plasminogen activator signal sequences. *Infect. Immun.* **67,** 4780–4786.

32. Svanholm, C., Bandholtz, L., Lobell, A., and Wigzell, H. (1999) Enhancement of antibody responses by DNA immunization using expression vectors mediating efficient antigen secretion. *J. Immunol. Methods* **228,** 121–130.

33. Delogu, G., Howard, A., Collins, F. M., and Morris, S. L. (2000) DNA vaccination against tuberculosis: expression of a ubiquitin-conjugated tuberculosis protein enhances antimycobacterial immunity. *Infect. Immun.* **68,** 3097–3102.

34. Velders, M. P., Weijzen, S., Eiben, G. L., Elmishad, A. G., Kloetzel, P. M., Higgins, T., et al. (2001) Defined flanking spacers and enhanced proteolysis is essential for eradication of established tumors by an epitope string DNA vaccine. *J. Immunol.* **166,** 5366–5373.

35. Yew, N. S., Przybylska, M., Ziegler, R. J., Liu, D. P., and Cheng, S. H. (2001) High and sustained transgene expression in vivo from plasmid vectors containing a hybrid ubiquitin promoter. *Mol. Ther.* **4,** 75–82.

36. Morita, A., Ariizumi, K., Ritter, R., Jester, J. V., Kumamoto, T., Johnston, S. A., et al. (2001) Development of a Langerhans cell-targeted gene therapy format using a dendritic cell-specific promoter. *Gene Ther.* **8,** 1729–1737.

37. Schnare, M., Barton, G. M., Holt, A. C., Takeda, K., Akira, S., and Medzhitov, R. (2001) Toll-like receptors control activation of adaptive immune responses. *Nat. Immunol.* **2,** 947–950.

38. Yi, A. K., Yoon, J. G., Hong, S. C., Redford, T. W., and Krieg, A. M. (2001) Lipopolysaccharide and CpG DNA synergize for tumor necrosis factor-alpha production through activation of NF-kappa B. *Intern. Immunol.* **13,** 1391–1404.

39. Uchijima, M., Raz, E., Carson, D. A., Nagata, T., and Koide, Y. (2001) Identification of immunostimulatory DNA-induced genes by suppression subtractive hybridization. *Biochem. Biophys. Res. Commun.* **286,** 688–691.

40. Raz, E. and Spiegelberg, H. L. (1999) Deviation of the allergic IgE to an IgG response by gene immunotherapy. *Int. Rev. Immunol.* **18,** 271–289.

41. Van Uden, J. H., Tran, C. H., Carson, D. A., and Raz, E. (2001) Type I interferon is required to mount an adaptive response to immunostimulatory DNA. *Eur. J. Immunol.* **31,** 3281–3290.

42. Davis, H. L., Suparto, I., Weeratna, R., Jumintarto, Iskandriati, D., Chamzah, S., et al. (2000) CpG DNA overcomes hyporesponsiveness to hepatitis B vaccine in orangutans. *Vaccine* **18,** 1920–1924.

43. Rankin, R., Pontarollo, R., Ioannou, X., Krieg, A. M., Hecker, R., Babiuk, L. A., et al. (2001) CpG motif identification for veterinary and laboratory species demonstrates that sequence recognition is highly conserved. *Antisense Nucleic Acid Drug Dev.* **11,** 333–340.

44. Krieg, A. M. (2002) CpG motifs in bacterial DNA and their immune effects. *Annu. Rev. Immunol.* **20,** 709–760.

45 Verthelyi, D., Ishii, K. J., Gursel, M., Takeshita, F., and Klinman, D. M. (2001) Human peripheral blood cells differentially recognize and respond to two distinct CpG motifs. *J. Immunol.* **166,** 2372–2377.

46. Yamamoto, S., Yamamoto, T., Iho, S., and Tokunaga, T. (2000) Activation of NK cell (Human and mouse) by immunostimulatory DNA sequence. *Springer Semin. Immunopathol.* **22,** 35–43.

47. Stan, A. C., Casares, S., Brumeanu, T. D., Klinman, D. M., and Bona, C. A. (2001) CpG motifs of DNA vaccines induce the expression of chemokines and MHC class II molecules on myocytes. *Eur. J. Immunol.* **31,** 301–310.

48. Lodmell, D. L., Ray, N. B., Ulrich, J. T., and Ewalt, L. C. (2000) DNA vaccination of mice against rabies virus: effects of the route of vaccination and the adjuvant monophosphoryl lipid A (MPL). *Vaccine* **18,** 1059–1066.

49. Ara, Y., Saito, T., Takagi, T., Hagiwara, E., Miyagi, Y., Sugiyama, M., et al. (2001) Zymosan enhances the immune response to DNA vaccine for human immunodeficiency virus type-1 through the activation of complement system. *Immunology* **103**, 98–105.
50. Murata, Y., Amao, M., Yoneda, J., and Hamuro, J. (2002) Intracellular thiol redox status of macrophages directs the Th1 skewing in thioredoxin transgenic mice during aging. *Mol. Immunol.* **38**, 747–757.
51. Pfeilschifter, J., Eberhardt, W., and Huwiler, A. (2001) Nitric oxide and mechanisms of redox signalling: matrix and matrix-metabolizing enzymes as prime nitric oxide targets. *Eur. J. Pharmacol.* **429**, 279–286.
52. Saccani, A., Saccani, S., Orlando, S., Sironi, M., Bernasconi, S., Ghezzi, P., et al. (2000) Redox regulation of chemokine receptor expression. *Proc. Nat. Acad. Sci. USA* **97**, 2761–2766.
53. Wang, F. A., Wang, L. Y., Wright, D., and Parmely, M. J. (1999) Redox imbalance differentially inhibits lipopolysaccharide-induced macrophage activation in the mouse liver. *Infect. Immun.* **67**, 5409–5416.
54. Kim, J. J., Yang, J. S., Nottingham, L. K., Lee, D. J., Lee, M., Manson, K. H., et al. (2001) Protection from immunodeficiency virus challenges in rhesus macaques by multicomponent DNA immunization. *Virology* **285**, 204–217.
55. Parker, S. E., Monteith, D., Horton, H., Hof, R., Hernandez, P., Vilalta, A., et al. (2001) Safety of a GM-CSF adjuvant-plasmid DNA malaria vaccine. *Gene Ther.* **8**, 1011–1023.
56. Sykes, K. F., Lewis, M. G., Squires, B., and Johnston, S. A. (2002) Evaluation of SIV library vaccines with genetic cytokines in a macaque challenge. *Vaccine* **20**, 2382–2395.
57. Ihata, A., Watabe, S., Sasaki, S., Shirai, A., Fukushima, J., Hamajima, K., et al. (1999) Immunomodulatory effect of a plasmid expressing CD40 ligand on DNA vaccination against human immunodeficiency virus type-1. *Immunology* **98**, 436–442.
58. Sin, J. I., Kim, J. J., Zhang, D. H., and Weiner, D. B. (2001) Modulation of cellular responses by plasmid CD40L: CD40L plasmid vectors enhance antigen-specific helper T cell type 1 CD4(+) T cell-mediated protective immunity against herpes simplex virus type 2 in vivo. *Human Gene Ther.* **12**, 1091–1102.
59. Sin, J. I., Kim, J., Dang, K., Lee, D., Pachuk, C., Satishchandran, C., et al. (2000a) LFA-3 plasmid DNA enhances Ag-specific humoral- and cellular-mediated protective immunity against herpes simplex virus-2 in vivo: Involvement of CD4+ T cells in protection. *Cell. Immunol.* **203**, 19–28 (*see* also Erratum, *Cell Immunol.* **204**, p. 150).
60. Sin, J. I., Kim, J. J., Pachuk, C., Satishchandran, C., and Weiner, D. B. (2000b) DNA vaccines encoding interleukin-8 and RANTES enhance antigen- specific Th1-type CD4(+) T-cell-mediated protective immunity against herpes simplex virus type 2 in vivo. *J. Virol.* **74**, 11,173–11,180.
61. Samten, B., Ghosh, P., Yi, A. K., Weis, S. E., Lakey, D. L., Gonsky, R., et al. (2002) Reduced expression of nuclear cyclic adenosine 5'-monophospate response element-binding proteins and IFN-gamma promoter function in disease due to an intracellular pathogen. *J. Immunol.* **168**, 3520–3526.
62. MacGregor, R. R., Boyer, J. D., Ugen, K. E., Lacy, K. E., Gluckman, S. J., Bagarazzi, M. L., et al. (1998) First human trial of a DNA-based vaccine for treatment of human immunodeficiency virus type 1 infection: Safety and host response. *J. Infect. Dis.* **178**, 92–100.
63. Pachuk, C. J., McCallus, D. E., Weiner, D. B., and Satishchandran, C. (2000b) DNA vaccines—challenges in delivery. *Curr. Opin. Mol. Ther.* **2**, 188–198.
64. Pachuk, C. J., Ciccarelli, R. B., Samuel, M., Bayer, M. E., Troutman, R. D., Zurawski, D. V., et al. (2000a) Characterization of a new class of DNA delivery complexes formed by the local anesthetic bupivacaine. *Biochim. Biophys. Acta* **1468**, 20–30.

65. Hartikka, J., Bozoukova, V., Ferrari, M., Sukhu, L., Enas, J., Sawdey, M., et al. (2001a) Vaxfectin enhances the humoral immune response to plasmid DNA-encoded antigens. *Vaccine* **19,** 1911–1923.

66. Reyes, L., Hartikka, J., Bozoukova, V., Sukhu, L., Nishioka, W., Singh, G., et al. (2001) Vaxfectin enhances antigen specific antibody titers and maintains Th1 type immune responses to plasmid DNA immunization. *Vaccine* **19,** 3778–3786.

67. Payette, P. J., Weeratna, R. D., McCluskie, M. J., and Davis, H. L. (2001) Immune-mediated destruction of transfected myocytes following DNA vaccination occurs via multiple mechanisms. *Gene Ther.* **8,** 1395–1400.

68. Fan, H., Lin, Q., Morrissey, G. R., and Khavari, P. A. (1999) Immunization via hair follicles by topical application of naked DNA to normal skin. *Nat. Biotechnol.* **17,** 870–872.

69. Cui, Z. R. and Mumper, R. J. (2001) Chitosan-based nanoparticles for topical genetic immunization. *J. Control. Release* **75,** 409–419.

70. Liu, L. J., Watabe, S., Yang, J., Hamajima, K., Ishii, N., Hagiwara, E., et al. (2001) Topical application of HIV DNA vaccine with cytokine-expression plasmids induces strong antigen-specific immune responses. *Vaccine* **20,** 42–48.

71. Watabe, S., Xin, K. Q., Ihata, A., Liu, L. J., Honsho, A., Aoki, I., et al. (2001) Protection against influenza virus challenge by topical application of influenza DNA vaccine. *Vaccine* **19,** 4434–4444.

72. Tadokoro, K., Koizumi, Y., Miyagi, Y., Kojima, Y., Kawamoto, S., Hamajima, K., et al. (2001) Rapid and wide-reaching delivery of HIV-1 env DNA vaccine by intranasal administration. *Viral Immunol.* **14,** 159–167.

73. Okuda, K., Xin, K. Q., Haruki, A., Kawamoto, S., Kojima, Y., Hirahara, F., et al. (2001) Transplacental genetic immunization after intravenous delivery of plasmid DNA to pregnant mice. *J. Immunol.* **167,** 5478–5484.

74. Sagodira, S., Buzoni-Gatel, D., Iochmann, S., Naciri, M., and Bout, D. (1999) Protection of kids against *Cryptosporidium parvum* infection after immunization of dams with CP15-DNA. *Vaccine* **17,** 2346–2355.

75. Gerdts, V., Babiuk, L. A., Littel-van den Hurk, S. V., and Griebel, P. J. (2000) Fetal immunization by a DNA vaccine delivered into the oral cavity. *Nat. Med.* **6,** 929–932.

76. Loehr, B. I., Pontarollo, R., Rankin, R., Latimer, L., Willson, P., Babiuk, L. A. et al. (2001) Priming by DNA immunization augments T-cell responses induced by modified live bovine herpesvirus vaccine. *J. Gen. Virol.* **82,** 3035–3043.

77. Mumper, R. J. and Ledebur, H. C. (2001) Dendritic cell delivery of plasmid DNA - Applications for controlled genetic immunization. *Mol. Biotechnol.* **19,** 79–95.

78. Haupt, K., Roggendorf, M., and Mann, K. (2002) The potential of DNA vaccination against tumor-associated antigens for antitumor therapy. *Exp. Biol. Med.* **227,** 227–237.

79. Rice, J., Elliott, T., Buchan, S., and Stevenson, F. K. (2001) DNA fusion vaccine designed to induce cytotoxic T cell responses against defined peptide motifs: Implications for cancer vaccines. *J. Immunol.* **167,** 1558–1565.

80. Zhu, D. L., Rice, J., Savelyeva, N., and Stevenson, F. K. (2001) DNA fusion vaccines against B-cell tumors. *Trends Molec. Med.* **7,** 566–572.

81. Heinzerling, L., Feige, K., Rieder, S., Akens, M., Dummer, R., Stranzinger, G., et al. (2001) Tumor regression induced by intratumoral injection of DNA coding for human interleukin 12 into melanoma metastases in gray horses. *J. Investig. Dermatol.* **117,** 899.

82. Roy, M. J., Wu, M. S., Barr, L. J., Fuller, J. T., Tussey, L. G., Speller, S., et al. (2000) Induction of antigen-specific CD8+T cells, T helper cells, and protective levels of antibody in humans by particle-mediated administration of a hepatitis B virus DNA vaccine. *Vaccine* **19,** 764–778.

83. Boyer, J. D., Cohen, A. D., Ugen, K. E., Edgeworth, R. L., Bennett, M., Shah, A., et al. (2000) Therapeutic immunization of HIV-infected chimpanzees using HIV-1 plasmid antigens and interleukin-12 expressing plasmids. *Aids* **14,** 1515–1522.

84. Barouch, D. H., Craiu, A., Santra, S., Egan, M. A., Schmitz, J. E., Kuroda, M. J., et al. (2001) Elicitation of high-frequency cytotoxic T-lymphocyte responses against both dominant and subdominant simian-human immunodeficiency virus epitopes by DNA vaccination of rhesus monkeys. *J. Virol.* **75,** 2462–2467.

85. Jones, T. R., Gramzinski, R. A., Aguiar, J. C., Sim, B. K. L., Narum, D. L., Fuhrmann, S. R., et al. (2002) Absence of antigenic competition in Aotus monkeys immunized with Plasmodium falciparum DNA vaccines delivered as a mixture. *Vaccine* **20,** 1675–1680.

86. Lodmell, D. L. and Ewalt, L. C. (2001) Post-exposure DNA vaccination protects mice against rabies virus. *Vaccine* **19,** 2468–2473.

87. Lodmell, D. L., Parnell, M. J., Bailey, J. R., Ewalt, L. C., and Hanlon, C. A. (2001) One-time gene gun or intramuscular rabies DNA vaccination of non-human primates: comparison of neutralizing antibody responses and protection against rabies virus 1 year after vaccination. *Vaccine* **20,** 838–844.

88. Lodmell, D. L. and Ewalt, L. C. (2000) Rabies vaccination: comparison of neutralizing antibody responses after priming and boosting with different combinations of DNA, inactivated virus, or recombinant vaccinia virus vaccines. *Vaccine* **18,** 2394–2398.

89. Pancholi, P., Lee, D. H., Liu, Q. Y., Tackney, C., Taylor, P., Perkus, M., et al. (2001) DNA prime/canarypox boost-based immunotherapy of chronic hepatitis B virus infection in a chimpanzee. *Hepatology* **33,** 448–454.

90. Heppell, J. and Davis, H. L. (2000) Application of DNA vaccine technology to aquaculture. *Adv. Drug Delivery Rev.* **43,** 29–43.

91. Corbeil, S., LaPatra, S. E., Anderson, E. D., and Kurath, G. (2000) Nanogram quantities of a DNA vaccine protect rainbow trout fry against heterologous strains of infectious hematopoietic necrosis virus. *Vaccine* **18,** 2817–2824.

92. LaPatra, S. E., Corbeil, S., Jones, G. R., Shewmaker, W. D., Lorenzen, N., Anderson, E. D., et al. (2001) Protection of rainbow trout against infectious hematopoietic necrosis virus four days after specific or semi-specific DNA vaccination. *Vaccine* **19,** 4011–4019.

93. LittelvandenHurk, S. V., Gerdts, V., Loehr, B. I., Pontarollo, R., Rankin, R., Uwiera, R., et al. (2000) Recent advances in the use of DNA vaccines for the treatment of diseases of farmed animals. *Adv. Drug Delivery Rev.* **43,** 13–28.

94. Ayash-Rashkovsky, M., Weisman, Z., Zlotnikov, S., Raz, E., Bentwich, Z., et al. (2001) Induction of antigen-specific Th1-biased immune responses by plasmid DNA in Schistosoma-infected mice with a preexistent dominant Th2 immune profile. *Biochem. Biophys. Res. Commun.* **282,** 1169–1176.

95. Horner, A. A., Van Uden, J. H., Zubeldia, J. M., Broide, D., and Raz, E. (2001) DNA-based immunotherapeutics for the treatment of allergic disease. *Immunol. Rev.* **179,** 102–118.

96. Kobayashi, H., Horner, A. A., Martin-Orozco, E., and Raz, E. (2000) Pre-priming: a novel approach to DNA-based vaccination and immunomodulation. *Springer Semin. Immunopathol.* **22,** 85–96.

97. Kobayashi, H., Horner, A. A., Takabayashi, K., Nguyen, M. D., Huang, E., Cinman, N., et al. (1999) Immunostimulatory DNA prepriming: a novel approach for prolonged Th1-biased immunity. *Cell. Immunol.* **198,** 69–75.

98. Tighe, H., Takabayashi, K., Schwartz, D., Marsden, R., Beck, L., Corbeil, J., et al. (2000a) Conjugation of protein to immunostimulatory DNA results in a rapid, long-lasting and potent induction of cell-mediated and humoral immunity. *Eur. J. Immunol.* **30,** 1939–1947.

99. Tighe, H., Takabayashi, K., Schwartz, D., Van Nest, G., Tuck, S., Eiden, J. J., et al. (2000b) Conjugation of immunostimulatory DNA to the short ragweed allergen Amb a 1 enhances its immunogenicity and reduces its allergenicity. *J. Allergy Clin. Immunol.* **106,** 124–134.

100. Cho, B. K., Lian, K. C., Lee, P., Brunmark, A., McKinley, C., Chen, J. Z., et al. (2001) Differences in antigen recognition and cytolytic activity of CD8(+) and CD8(–) T cells that express the same antigen-specific receptor. *Proc. Natl. Acad. Sci. USA* **98,** 1723–1727.

101. Peng, H. J., Su, S. N., Chang, Z. N., Chao, P. L., Kuo, S. W., and Tsai, L. C. (2002) Induction of specific Th1 responses and suppression of IgE antibody formation by vaccination with plasmid DNA encoding Der f 11. *Vaccine* **20,** 1761–1768.

102. Harrison, R. A., Richards, A., Laing, G. D., and Theakston, R. D. G. (2002) Simultaneous GeneGun immunisation with plasmids encoding antigen and GM-CSF: significant enhancement of murine antivenom IgG1 titres. *Vaccine* **20,** 1702–1706.

103. Kieber-Emmons, T., Monzavi-Karbassi, B., Wang, B., Luo, P., and Weiner, D. B. (2000) Cutting edge: DNA immunization with minigenes of carbohydrate mimotopes induce functional anti-carbohydrate antibody response. *J. Immunol.* **165,** 623–627.

104. Ledwith, B. J., Manam, S., Troilo, P. J., Barnum, A. B., Pauley, C. J., Griffiths, T. G., et al. (2000) Plasmid DNA vaccines: Investigation of integration into host cellular DNA following intramuscular injection in mice. *Intervirology* **43,** 258–272.

# 24

## From Vaccine Research to Manufacture

*A Guide for the Researcher*

**Nigel Allison and Howard S. Tranter**

## 1. Introduction

Organizations that are involved primarily in research activities, such as academic departments, may often be largely unaware of the economics and regulations related to the production of a biopharmaceutical in a licensed facility using current Good Manufacturing Practice (cGMP). In a research environment, the goal is usually to produce the product of interest to a high level of purity, using whatever methods are available, for use in a particular study. Little consideration may be given to process reproducibility and optimization, since only small quantities of highly purified material are usually required, and at such a scale of operation, economic factors are of little importance. In contrast, GMP manufacture of material for human or veterinary use is subject to regulation by the competent authorities responsible for controlling the quality, safety, and licensure of medicinal products in countries in which the product is to be registered for use (e.g., Medicines Control Agency, UK; European Medicines Evaluation Agency; US Food and Drug Administration. GMP requires that "products are consistently produced and controlled to the quality standards appropriate to their intended use" *(1)*. The costs involved in testing product, raw materials, and monitoring the manufacturing environment to ensure that the product meets its specification, together with those of operating at large scale, may be substantial. Thus, it is essential to keep such costs to a minimum to ensure an economical manufacturing process.

Generally, manufacturing methods should be simpler than those used in the research laboratory because of the necessity of operating at larger scale and under regulatory constraints. A research process will usually have to undergo some development before it can be used in a manufacturing facility. The amount of development work required

From: *Methods in Molecular Medicine, Vol. 87: Vaccine Protocols, 2nd ed.*
Edited by: A. Robinson, M. J. Hudson, and M. P. Cranage © Humana Press Inc., Totowa, NJ

**Table 1**
**Estimate Duration and Costs of Vaccine Manufacture**

| Activity | Duration (yr) | Cost ($) |
|---|---|---|
| Feasibility (Research and Development) | 4 | 4.9 M |
| Preclinical Development | 4 | 14.7 M |
| Build Manufacturing Plant | 3 | 21.4 M |
| Plant/Process Validation | 3 | 7.0 M |
| Clinical Development | 6 | 10.1 M |
| Registration | 3 | 0.7 M |
| Patenting | 5 | 0.7 M |
| Market Research and Preparation | 1.5 | 1.0 M |
| Total Cost | | 60.5 M |

Data from Gregersen *(2)*.

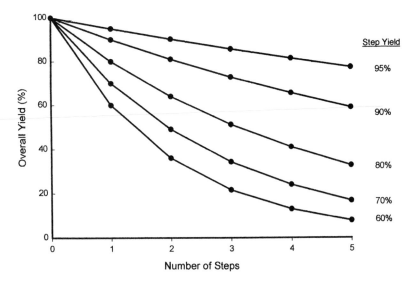

Fig. 1. Loss of process yield with number of process steps.

will make a significant contribution to the overall cost and time of bringing a product into manufacture (*see* **Table 1**). The overriding consideration in designing a new process, therefore, should be to make it as simple as possible with the minimum number of process steps. **Figure 1** shows how the overall product yield decreases with increasing number of steps. Even with a 90% recovery at each step (rarely achievable), a 10-step process will only recover 40% of the product present in the starting material. In addition to the costs of increased manufacturing times and lost product, a large number of process steps will add significantly to future validation costs.

Before embarking upon a new vaccine research project, it is useful to have some idea of what the specification of the new vaccine will be and by what route it will be administered. This will allow the goals of the project to be set from the outset in terms of product purity, number of required doses and approximate scale of operation, and will influence the process methods chosen and determine the level of control for that product. For example, the requirements governing the manufacture of sterile parenteral (injectable) products are considerably more stringent than those pertaining to products for oral application *(1)*. Furthermore, the manufacture of biological/biotechnological products places a greater emphasis on the control of the manufacturing process as a whole, because there is an inherent variability of these products that are tested by bioassay rather than physicochemical methods.

This chapter provides guidance for scientists who are involved in vaccine research on the limitations imposed by GMP on the types of procedures that can be used in medium- to large-scale bioprocessing. In order to minimize development time and to facilitate the technology transfer of processes into manufacture, it is strongly recommended throughout the chapter that techniques that are amenable to scale-up and are compatible with working to GMP, are adopted as early as possible in the research phase. Although the main focus of this article relates to bacterial products, there are generic aspects—particularly in the area of downstream processing—that will apply to many other types of vaccines and biotherapeutics.

## 2. Raw Materials

All materials used in biopharmaceutical manufacture should be purchased from approved suppliers and tested to ensure that they meet the quality specified in the product Certificate of Analysis (CoA). The analytical methods used for such testing must be qualified unless the materials are of pharmacopoeial grade, in which case the raw material tests are specified in one of the pharmacopoeia (e.g., EP, European Pharmacopoeia; USP; United States Pharmacopoeia). Clearly, it is an advantage to purchase pharmacopoeial grades of materials for research and development, if at all possible, to facilitate future technology transfer and reduce the amount of method validation during manufacture. In any event, it is important to obtain and retain the manufacturer's CoA for all materials used during research and development to allow comparable materials of the desired quality to be sourced for manufacture.

Another important consideration is the use of animal products. Regulatory concerns *(3)* over Transmissible Spongiform Encephalopathy (TSE) agents in medicinal products has led to an evaluation of TSE contamination risk in all animal products used in the manufacture of pharmaceuticals. Whenever possible, such products should be replaced with materials of non-animal origin. If a suitable nonanimal product is unavailable, the product should be derived from animals from areas of low TSE risk *(3,4)*. If animal products are used during the research phase of a project, it is almost certain that these will need to be replaced when the process enters development. If the animal substance is a growth-medium component, it is likely to have an effect upon the growth of the production organism and expression of the antigens of interest. The avoidance of such materials during research, or at least the evaluation of alternatives prior to movement into development, can thus save much development time.

## 3. Strain Selection

The selection of a suitable bacterial strain for production of a vaccine antigen(s) or the correct mammalian cell line for virus production is crucial to the success of any vaccine development project. In making the choice, a prime consideration should be the level and stability of antigen expression/viral production that can be achieved. If possible, the bacterial strain or cell line should be obtained from a recognized culture collection with an established and documented provenance. Alternatively, if the chosen vaccine strain is an "in house" clinical isolate, it will be necessary to compile a complete history of the strain, including details of its isolation, identification, and maintenance for product registration. Such information is often neglected during research, making future license submissions difficult. Additional information will be required for recombinant organisms, including the history, sequence, and restriction map of the expression vector and the cloned gene(s). For the vector itself, full details should be maintained of the preparation of the nucleic acid segments, the genes involved, the origin of replication, the fusion product (if any), the characterization of the flanking promoter, enhancer and terminator regions, and the presence of any antibiotic resistance genes. Full details of the requirements surrounding the manufacture of biological products—including vaccines—for human use are to be found in the directives issued by regulatory bodies *(5,6)*. All stock strains should be stored under controlled conditions, and a record should be kept of all subcultures/transfers made *(7)*. This will lay the foundation for the preparation of any future GMP seed banks for manufacture.

Whenever practical, non-pathogenic or attenuated organisms should be used as the containment requirements for the production of pathogenic material will add greatly to the cost of vaccine manufacture and may limit production scale and facility use. Similarly, avoid the use of spore-forming organisms (e.g., *Bacillus* and *Clostridium spp.*) whenever possible, as bacterial spores are extremely resistant to normal cleaning and sanitization regimes, and it is often difficult to validate their total destruction. For this reason, licensing authorities are likely to insist upon dedicated facilities for the growth of such organisms *(1)* which, if the product concerned is of small volume and relatively low value, can prove prohibitively expensive. An alternative to the use of either pathogens or spore-formers would be to express a recombinant form of the required antigen in a non-pathogenic host. This may have the added advantages of increasing the level of antigen expression that can be obtained per unit mass of cells, and will also provide easier routes of product isolation.

### 3.1. Recombinant Expression

A wide variety of bacterial and mammalian expression systems is commercially available (*see* **Table 2**), and it is common practice when commencing the research phase of a new project to evaluate a number of these for optimal expression of the antigen of interest. However, a number of other factors must be considered when choosing an expression system that is compatible with GMP manufacture.

Before commencing any work involving recombinant microorganisms, a mandatory risk assessment is required under the Genetically Modified Organisms Regulations *(8)* to determine the level of containment required for the work. The containment level is

**Table 2**
**Intellectual Property Rights of Commercial Expression-System Components and Associated Protein-Fusion Partners**

| Patent-protected component | Owner of IPR |
| --- | --- |
| The T7 promoter to control recombinant expression (e.g., pET vectors) | Brookhaven National Laboratories |
| The *araBAD* promoter to control recombinant expression (e.g., pBAD vectors) | Xoma Corporation |
| The $P_L$ promoter to control recombinant expression (e.g., pLEX vectors) | Biogen Inc. |
| Vectors containing the His-Tag sequence and Ni-NTA resin for the purification of His-tagged fusion proteins | Hoffmann-La Roche |
| Vectors containing the NusA sequence fused to the protein of interest to aid solubility | University of Oklahoma |
| Vectors containing the thioredoxin reductase sequence fused to the protein of interest to aid solubility | Genetics Institute Inc. |
| Vectors containing the glutathione S-transferase sequence fused to the protein of interest to aid purification (e.g., pGEX vectors) | Chemicon International Inc. |
| Vectors containing sequence encoding a chitin-binding affinity tag that can be removed nonenzymatically (e.g., pTYB vectors) | AMRAD Corporation New England Biolabs |
| Vectors containing the maltose-binding protein sequence fused to the protein of interest to aid purification | New England Biolabs |
| The *Pichia pastoris* expression system, including the AOX1 or GAP promoter | Research Corporation Technologies |
| The NICE Lactobacillus expression system with nisin as inducer | NIZO Food Research |

calculated by taking into account a variety of factors, including the ability of the host to be propagated in humans and animals, the mobility of the vector to other organisms, the nature of the product, and the scale of operation. It is important to remember that manipulations performed during research at small scale may require a much lower level of containment than similar operations at production scale. The advantages of using a non-pathogen to produce the vaccine could well be abolished by inappropriate choice of host organism and expression system. Therefore, there is much to be said for extending the GMO risk assessment to the envisaged production scale to highlight any potential problems at an early stage. A related issue is the use of antibiotics in production facilities. Many manufacturers prohibit the use of β-lactam antibiotics (e.g., ampicillin) in their production suites to avoid the risk of contamination of products and potential allergies in sensitive patients. It is advisable to avoid the use of ampicillin-resistance markers when designing new expression constructs, or alternatively, to determine the stability of recombinant expression in the absence of the antibiotic.

Many expression systems rely upon the addition of an inducer at a specific stage during growth of the organism to "switch on" synthesis of the product of interest. Some of the inducers used may be toxic (e.g., methanol), difficult to remove or expensive (e.g., isopropyl-β-D-thiogalactopyranoside [IPTG]), all factors that could potentially limit the scale of the production operation. Regardless of the inducer used, assays may need to be sourced or developed to validate their removal from the final product. It is thus preferable to use either constitutive expression of product or expression systems that utilize a physiological shift (e.g., temperature) to induce product synthesis.

Products may be expressed intracellularly or extracellularly, depending upon the expression vector used. The mode of expression will greatly influence the downstream processing operations required to isolate the product (*see* **Fig. 2**). There are advantages and disadvantages in both systems, and it is important to choose the one that is most appropriate for the product of interest. In making the choice, the following should be considered:

1. Although extremely high levels of expression can be achieved using yeasts such as *Pichia pastoris*, most yeast cells are difficult to break and may require several passages through a homogenizer. This could damage and reduce the yield of a shear/heat-sensitive protein.
2. Some microorganisms produce extracellular proteases that may rapidly degrade a secreted product. In a pharmaceutical manufacturing process, the addition of highly toxic protease inhibitors to reduce such activity is not an option. However, it may be possible to employ a protease-deficient host strain to minimize this problem (e.g., *E. coli* strains RV308/ATCC 31608 *[9]* and HM125 *[10]*).
3. Some bacteria express certain intracellular recombinant proteins as insoluble, biologically inactive inclusion bodies. Depending upon the particular protein, it may be possible to solubilize and renature such proteins *(11)*; however, the yield is often very poor, and large quantities of aggressive denaturants such as guanidine hydrochloride may be required. Alternatively, it may be possible to manipulate the physiological conditions of growth (e.g., temperature or induction parameters) to favor expression of a soluble product *(12)*.
4. Antigens expressed intracellularly in a soluble form will have to be released from the host cell by some form of mechanical or chemical means before they can be purified. A larger number of purification steps is usually required to separate the product from host proteins when compared with secreted products or proteins expressed in inclusion bodies.

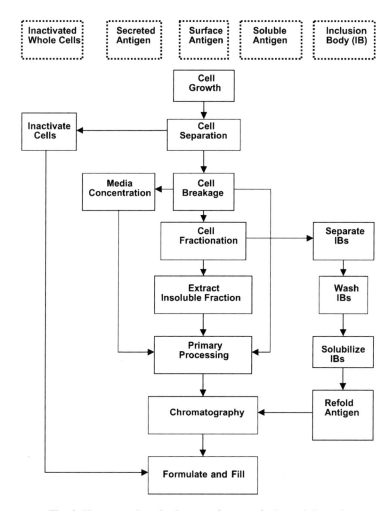

Fig. 2. Key operations in the manufacture of a bacterial vaccine.

If the product of interest is likely to prove refractile to purification, there are a number of commercially available expression systems that use an affinity tag fused to the protein of interest to allow rapid isolation of the product by affinity chromatography. Commonly used fusion partners include hexa-histidine (Novagen), maltose-binding protein (New England Biolabs) and glutathione S-transferase (Novagen). When evaluating such systems during the research phase, it is vital to ensure that the affinity tag can be effectively cleaved from the fusion protein and removed from the product stream subsequent to the affinity chromatography step. Assays may be required to verify the absence of the tag in the final product.

Many commercial expression systems are comprehensively patented (*see* **Table 2**), and their use outside a research environment attracts a heavy royalty. This may involve a significant cost, especially if more than one component of the system (e.g., promoter, vector, or purification tag) attracts intellectual property rights. It is wise to examine such financial implications at an early stage of the research process to avoid costly recloning and re-evaluation prior to or even after development.

## 4. Growth

It is good microbiological practice to prepare a research seed stock of the intended production organism as the primary source for all subsequent research work. This will limit the variation that is sometimes observed between seed stocks, and provide a standard inoculum in a given physiological state for all growth and expression studies. Ideally, the medium in which the seed stock is prepared should be that used for vaccine production. This may not always be possible, since at the beginning of a project the media composition yielding optimal expression may not have been determined.

### 4.1. Media Selection

Media selection is an important aspect of process design, and careful consideration at this stage will be repaid in reduced time and costs for later development stages. The majority of standard media recommended for bacterial expression studies (e.g., L-broth), although useful for early "proof of principle" studies, are not suitable for production purposes because of the presence of animal products and/or low biomass productivity. Selection studies for the growth medium to be used in production should begin as soon as acceptable, and stable levels of antigen expression have been achieved in standard media. The goal should be to produce a simple medium that contains no animal components, and is capable of supporting high biomass production and product yield. The provenance of each medium component will need to be determined to avoid TSE issues, and each will need to be QC-tested to a specification before being introduced into a production area, so it is helpful to avoid using complicated recipes. For example, a medium that requires many amino acids to be added separately could prove expensive and impractical for GMP production. Growth media containing exotic components for which supply may become difficult should be avoided.

### 4.2. Optimization of Growth Conditions

Once a production medium has been chosen, growth experiments using flask culture can be used to begin the optimization of antigen production. Factors that should be examined include: i) temperature, ii) pH control, iii) aeration rate (shaker speed), iv) primary carbon source, v) antifoam requirement, vi) time for initiation of induction (for non-constitutive expression), and vii) time of harvest. Information gained from these studies will provide the basis for transfer of the growth process into small-scale bioreactors where the factors influencing antigen expression can be determined further. Fermenters offer greater control over the physiological factors affecting growth and antigen expression than flask culture, and are capable of increasing production levels several-fold. They may be operated in continuous and fed-batch modes in addition to standard batch culture. If possible, fermentation development should be initiated during the research phase of a vaccine project, instead of — as is often the case — being left until development. The goal should be to produce a scaleable and reproducible process for the growth of the production organism and expression of the vaccine antigens. During this phase, it is important to examine the stability of recombinant expression vectors, by monitoring vector retention during extended growth periods, particularly if the selection pressure for their maintenance (e.g., antibiotic inclusion) has been removed.

## 5. Downstream Processing

The methods chosen for separating the required antigens from the production organism and growth medium will largely be dictated by the host organism, the properties and location of the product, and the specification of the vaccine. Thus, it is helpful to have as much information as possible about these factors before starting. The host organism may contribute a number of unwanted materials into the product stream, such as nucleic acid, protein, and endotoxin. It is better to avoid contamination of the product with such host components rather than to have to remove them at a later stage in the process. For example, although terminating the fermentation and removing the cells at an earlier stage of growth may reduce product yield, it could reduce contamination of a secreted product with cell components arising from lysis. It is common practice in research laboratories to add inhibitors to inactivate host enzymes (e.g., proteases or nucleases) that may compromise the stability of the product. Many of these compounds are highly toxic, and as such cannot be used in the manufacture of human products. Those that can be used must be removed at a later stage, and their absence in the final product must be verified using validated and highly sensitive assays. A better approach is to avoid using such inhibitors in the first place by using protease-deficient hosts, early stage removal, heat or pH inactivation, or by operating under conditions favoring low protease activity (e.g., low temperature).

When designing a purification protocol, consideration should be given to the limitations that the intended production scale may impose. For example, dialysis is a commonly used research method for removing salts and other small molecules from process material. At a large scale, dialysis becomes impractical because of the volumes of dialysis buffer required and the time for the process to reach equilibrium, and is often replaced by tangential flow filtration. Although the latter is more rapid, the high-throughput pumping involved can expose the product to shear forces, and there is also potential for product loss on membranes. A number of manufacturers (e.g., Sartorius, Millipore) market disposable tangential flow units for small volumes that are ideal for evaluation during the research phase, and can be scaled up effectively during process development to manufacture.

### 5.1. Primary Processing

A common feature of many purification protocols designed in research laboratories is an over-reliance on chromatographic steps to remove bulk contaminants. At process scale, chromatographic procedures are generally labor-intensive to perform and validate, and require expensive control equipment. As such, the number of chromatographic steps in a process should be kept to a minimum and reserved for product polishing. Primary processing techniques should be used to remove the majority of unwanted product-stream components.

The first step of any downstream process is the separation of the product from the production organism. In the case of a secreted product, this will involve physical separation of the cells from the culture medium using centrifugation and/or filtration. If the product is not secreted, some method of cell breakage will be required once the cells have been harvested. Generally, mammalian cells are easily lysed using mild techniques (e.g., osmotic shock). Bacteria and yeasts, however, require more aggressive chemical or physical treatments. Chemical methods of cell lysis (e.g. using alkali or surfactants) obviate the need for expensive homogenization equipment, but depend upon the resistance of the product to chemical denaturation. Sonication, although a useful research method, is not widely used for industrial large-scale cell disruption and is usually replaced with high-pressure homogenization or bead mills. All of these methods vary in the efficiency of breakage and their effect upon the product. Material arising from one disruption method may consist of different components, and may thus behave differently during subsequent purification to that generated using another procedure, so it is important during research to use a disruption method as close to that intended for production. The conditions used for cell disruption must be a balance between those that yield optimal product release and those leading to minimal product denaturation. Chromosomal DNA is often a major contaminant, and by virtue of its high molecular mass and viscosity can interfere with later chromatography steps *(13)*. Increasing the degree of nucleic acid shearing by using a higher homogenization pressure or an increased number of passages through the disruption equipment may decrease this problem. Conversely, decreasing shearing will facilitate nucleic acid precipitation using specific precipitants (e.g., streptomycin sulphate or protamine sulphate).

Removal of cell debris is usually accomplished by batch centrifugation in the research laboratory. At a large scale, this may not be practical, and a combination of tangential flow filtration and/or continuous flow centrifugation may be required. Having removed unwanted particulate material, the next priority is to stabilize the product and remove the major contaminants. Water is usually the most abundant contaminant, and concentration is an important part of primary processing. This may be achieved by ultrafiltration using low protein-binding membranes (e.g., polyvinylidene fluoride) with defined mol-wt cut-off pores, precipitants (ammonium sulphate, solvents, pH, heat) or batch binding to an adsorbent. Expanded-bed chromatography is a form of the latter technique, in which a fluidized bed of a specialized chromatographic matrix (usually an ion-exchanger) can be used to capture product directly from a crude, particulate process stream, thus obviating the need for prior clarification *(14)*. A number of manufacturers (e.g., Amersham Biosciences, UpFront Chromatography A/S) supply the necessary equipment suitable for use at a small scale to allow process evaluation. Ammonium sulphate is widely used as a protein precipitant, and has the potential to achieve both concentration and purification in a single step. However, it is important to consider that the high salt concentration of the product stream following this technique will need to be reduced prior to performing chromatographic techniques such as ion-exchange. Precipitation of contaminants and/or product by decreasing the pH of the process stream can be useful if the product is stable under such conditions. For example, acid precipitation can be used effectively to harvest and stabilize botulinum toxin following fermentation in the GMP manufacture of toxoid vaccines *(15)*.

## 5.2. Chromatography

Chromatography workstations (e.g., ÄKTA™, Amersham Biosciences; BioCAD™ At Applied Biosystems) capable of producing complex gradients are often used in the development of product elution conditions from adsorption chromatography matrices in the research laboratory. At large scale, the equipment required to produce such gradients can be expensive, and it is often difficult to reproduce exactly what is achieved at research scale. For these reasons, there is much to be said for using the information obtained from preliminary gradient elution work to develop a simple step-elution method that can easily be adapted to process scale. When designing chromatographic separations, it is easy to forget the benefits of using negative chromatography where, in contrast to traditional methods, the product does not bind to the matrix under the conditions used for application, and is collected in the column flow through fraction. Although this technique does not offer the usual advantages associated with absorption techniques of concentrating the product, it can prove useful in removing persistent contaminants. We have used two consecutive negative chromatographic ion-exchange steps (the first anionic, the second cationic) to great effect in the GMP production of staphylococcal enterotoxin B from culture supernatant fluid following fermentation of *Staphylococcus aureus (16)*.

An important consideration when designing chromatography steps for potential GMP products is the stability of the matrix to cleaning and sanitization procedures. Reputable manufacturers can usually supply details of the physical and chemical stability of chromatography products licensed for GMP use in the form of a dossier, such as a Drug Master File, but it is the responsibility of the vaccine development team to validate product-specific cleaning methodologies. One way of avoiding such costs is to use fresh matrix for each production run if this is economical. The use of chromatography matrices that have been approved for GMP use for process development, should be encouraged whenever possible.

The sequence of individual steps can have a major impact on the economics of the process. The goal should be to combine individual steps in a way that minimizes time-consuming operations such as buffer exchange and concentration. For example, if a process step generates a product stream with high ionic strength (e.g., ammonium sulfate precipitation or ion-exchange chromatography), follow it with a procedure that either requires such starting conditions (e.g., hydrophobic interaction chromatography), or whose operation is unaffected by salt concentration (e.g., gel filtration). In addition to being effective purification tools, adsorption techniques such as ion-exchange chromatography can be used to concentrate material from a dilute product stream (e.g., following protein refolding from solubilized inclusion bodies) much more rapidly and cost-effectively than ultrafiltration methods.

Affinity techniques can yield a phenomenal degree of purification (>1000-fold) in a single step, and are widely used in the purification of recombinant fusion proteins. However, these methods can suffer from a number of disadvantages when applied to production processes. Firstly, the cost of the matrix usually precludes single-use applications. This means that cleaning validation work cannot be avoided. Also, the ligands used are often sensitive to the methods routinely used for sanitization (e.g., treatment with sodium hydroxide or formaldehyde). Information will need to be gathered about the leaching of the affinity ligand from the matrix. If this is significant, methods for its removal will need to be incorporated into the process, and assays for its detection developed and validated. Ligand leaching was a particular problem in our laboratory when using a glutathione-Sepharose matrix in the development of a purification process for a vaccine antigen expressed as a fusion protein with glutathione S-transferase. If the affinity ligand is a biological product (e.g., an antibody), it will have to have been prepared using cGMP and the provenance of the source material established. Finally, several of the commercially produced affinity matrices (**Table 2**) attract a royalty when used in manufacturing processes.

### 5.3. Removal of Host-Specific Contaminants

Endotoxin (lipopolysaccharide), a highly pyrogenic component of Gram-negative bacterial-cell walls, must be reduced to an acceptable level for all parenteral products *(17)*. As the dose may vary from vaccine to vaccine, the endotoxin limit is generally expressed as K/M (K is the threshold pyrogenic dose of endotoxin/kg body mass/h, and M is the maximum recommended dose of product/kg body mass/h). The value of K is usually 5EU/kg/h for parenterals. Elimination of endogenous endotoxin arising from the use of production organisms such as *Escherichia coli* can sometimes prove problematic. Fortunately, because of its high negative charge, endotoxin can be removed using anion-exchange chromatography, provided that it is not co-eluted with the product. Charged nylon-membrane filters (e.g., Zetapor™ from Cuno) use a similar mechanism to reduce endotoxin levels in process streams. Alternative methods include gel-filtration chromatography and ultrafiltration, which depend upon the propensity of endotoxin to form high mol-wt aggregates of 100-1,000 kDa in aqueous solution. The pharmaceutical manufacturing environment aims to minimize exogenous endotoxin contamination by the use of HVAC systems, Laminar Flow Units, cleanroom clothing, depyrogenated glassware, sanitization of equipment and matrices, and use of pharmaceutical-grade water to prepare reagents.

The main concern regarding contamination of vaccines with host-cell DNA is the potential uptake and assimilation of foreign oncogenes by patients' cells. Although this concern relates mainly to products from mammalian-cell culture, the regulatory authorities have adopted a cautionary approach and recommend a level of no more than 10 pg host-cell DNA per therapeutic dose for recombinant products *(18)*. The form of the DNA is more important than the quantity. Fragments of DNA smaller than 250 basepairs represent low risk because they are several times smaller than the size of the average gene. Like endotoxin, DNA can be removed using anion-exchange matrices and filtration devices (e.g., Zetaplus SP™ from Cuno) if it persists beyond the primary processing stage (*see* **Subheading 5.1.**). Alternatively, nucleases may be added to digest nucleic acid, yet, the provenance of such agents and their removal from the final product must be verified prior to manufacture.

Removal or inactivation of endogenous viruses must be verified when animal products (e.g., serum in mammalian-cell-culture media) are used. It is preferable to perform viral inactivation prior to use in the process (e.g., heating to 40–60°C) to avoid degradation/inactivation of the product. Alternatively, most viruses can be separated from soluble protein antigens by gel filtration. Validation of virus removal is normally achieved using appropriate bioassays or immunoassays *(19)*. The best solution is to avoid using potentially contaminated products in the process whenever possible.

## 5.4. Inactivation and Toxoiding

If the vaccine antigen(s) selected retains biological activity that is capable of causing adverse effects in patients (e.g., bacterial toxins, whole-cell vaccines), it will be necessary to inactivate it. For highly toxic substances, it may be beneficial to inactivate early on in the process to avoid the costs and limitations of biological containment. The main drawback of this approach is that some of the methods utilized for inactivation, such as heat or formaldehyde treatment, can cause protein aggregation or crosslinking which may hamper subsequent removal of contaminants. One such example is the diphtheria vaccine, which contains toxin molecules crosslinked to growth-medium peptones *(20)*. The latter are unnecessary antigenic determinants that may cause side effects following the vaccination process.

## 6. Formulation

The presentation of the vaccine is an important consideration that is often neglected in the early stages of a project. Early animal studies should determine whether an adjuvant is required. Preliminary data related to the stability of the product accumulated using research material can be useful in determining whether the final product should be formulated as a sterile liquid or a lyophilized product and whether stabilizing excipients are required. For further details regarding factors influencing vaccine formulation, *see* Chapters 11, 13, and 14.

## 7. Analytical Methods

Apart from generating a prototype production protocol, the research phase of a vaccine program should aim to characterize the physical and biochemical properties of the potential product. In addition to influencing the choice of separation methods used, this data will lay the foundations for the development of quality control tests. These are generally of two types: i) in-process tests that are used to monitor the product, key contaminants, and operating parameters (e.g., pH, temperature or conductivity) throughout the process, and ii) final product tests. Some of the types of assays commonly used for final product testing are detailed in **Table 3**. Foremost of these, particularly with regard to vaccine development, is establishment of a method for evaluating the potency of the active substance(s). This usually involves the development of an animal model for the infection or intoxication the vaccine is designed to protect against, and should occur at an early stage in the research phase, as it is a prerequisite in selecting the vaccine candidate. In selecting an animal model, consider the potential costs involved in routine vaccine batch testing as well as assay validation and stability studies. Several of the methods for quantification, identification, and purity determination, shown in **Table 3**, are in common use in research laboratories but will require validating should the product progress beyond a Phase 1 clinical trial. In choosing a method, consider whether the following validation parameters could be met: reproducibility, accuracy, specificity, range, robustness, and system suitability *(21)*.

**Table 3**
**Methods Used for End-Product Testing of Protein Vaccines**

| Parameter | Test used |
|---|---|
| Efficacy | Animal potency test (product-dependent) |
| Quantity | Protein determination |
| | Immunoassay (e.g., ELISA, Ouchterlony) |
| Identity | Western blotting using monospecific antibody |
| | N-terminal sequencing |
| | Peptide mapping |
| | Mass spectrometry |
| | Amino acid analysis |
| General Safety | Abnormal toxicity test in animals |
| Adjuvant Chemical Test | Dependent upon adjuvant used |
| Stability Tests | Selected from the above and performed over a |
| | range of storage conditions and time intervals |
| Contaminants | |
| Host Protein | Gel electrophoresis (denaturing/non-denaturing) |
| | 2-D electrophoresis |
| | Capillary electrophoresis |
| | Isoelectric focusing |
| | HPLC (reverse phase) |
| | Immunoassays |
| Host DNA | DNA hybridization studies |
| Endotoxin | LAL assay |
| | Rabbit pyrogen test |
| Bacteria/Fungi | Sterility test |
| Viruses | Bioassays |
| | Immunoassays |
| | DNA hybridization studies |
| Process additives | Various (dependent upon analyte) |

## 8. Documentation

It is essential that good records are kept of all work performed during the research phase of a project. These should include the experimental methods and results, analytical procedures and results, the source and batch numbers of all materials, and details of all major equipment used. This information will be required to support any patent application in order to secure possible IPR arising from the work. When the vaccine moves from research into process development, a technology transfer document will

**Table 4**
**Alternative Process Methods Suitable for Scale-Up**
**and/or Use in GMP Production**

| Function | Research method | Possible alternatives for scale-up |
|---|---|---|
| Initiation of expression | Addition of chemical inducer | Constitutive expression<br>Induction by physiological shift |
| Cell growth | Shake-flask culture | Batch or fed-batch fermentation |
| Cell disruption | Sonication | High-pressure homogenizers<br>Bead mills<br>Chemical lysis |
| Decrease proteolytic activity | Use of protease inhibitors | Protease-deficient production strains |
| Removal of host DNA | Use of nucleases | Ion-exchange chromatography<br>Filtration using specialized membranes |
| Removal of particulates | Batch centrifugation | Continuous-flow centrifugation<br>Tangential-flow filtration<br>Expanded-bed chromatography |
| Removal of endotoxin | Polymyxin | Ion-exchange chromatography<br>Filtration using specialized membranes<br>Gram-positive production strains |
| Buffer exchange | Dialysis | Tangential-flow filtration<br>Gel filtration |

be required detailing the research process and analytical methods with representative data from a number of vaccine preparations. This document is valuable even if the research, process development, and subsequent manufacture will take place within the same organization. If future work is to be performed by another organization or contractor, this information assumes an even greater level of importance, as much development time can be wasted in duplicating experimental work omitted from an incomplete technology transfer package. Details of the legalities and additional documentation involved in transferring a process from one commercial organization to another are outside the scope of this article but are reviewed elsewhere *(22)*. The information contained within the technology transfer document, together with data accumulated during process development, is also useful in drafting the documentation required for cGMP manufacture. This will include process flow diagrams, batch manufacturing records, specifications, and standard operating procedures. GMP processes are dependent upon extensive documentation systems to i) prevent errors arising from verbal communication, ii) ensure process reproducibility, and iii) facilitate the tracing of the manufacturing history of any product batch. If the vaccine makes it to the market, the regulatory authorities will require a product development report detailing the history of the vaccine from concept through to manufacture. Research data, together with information from the subsequent process development work, will form a large part of this document.

## 9. Summary

The following key messages summarize the factors that should be considered during a vaccine research project to ensure a smooth and trouble-free technology transfer into process development and manufacture:

- Before pursuing a particular process activity beyond "proof of principle," think ahead to how this will translate into manufacture. If the step is unlikely to scale-up successfully or is not compatible with the principles of GMP, look for alternatives rather than waste time fine-tuning a "nonrunner" (*see* **Table 4**).
- Keep the process as simple as possible to reduce manpower and facility costs, to increase yields and to maximize the potential financial gain.
- Ensure that the process is reproducible at a small scale before technology transfer to avoid high re-development costs.
- Keep good records of all research activities to facilitate preparation of documents for technology transfer, product licensing, and patent application.
- If possible, consult regularly with developmental, safety, quality, and production staff to assess the compatibility of the research process with large-scale GMP manufacture. In this way, mistakes can be rectified at an early stage at low cost.
- Gather as much information as possible on the product to facilitate analytical method development and to guide the selection of suitable separation procedures.
- Develop as many of the analytical methods that will be used for in-process and final product testing as possible along with the research process itself. This will avoid delays in sourcing suitable methods during the late development phase.

## References

1. The Medicines Control Agency (2002) Rules and guidance for pharmaceutical manufacturers and distributors (2002). London: The Stationery Office.
2. Gregersen, J-P. (1997) Vaccine Development: The long road from initial idea to product licensure, in *New Generation Vaccines, 2nd ed.,* (Levine, M. M., Woodrow, G. C., Kaper J. B., and Cobon, G. S., eds.), Marcel Dekker Inc., New York, pp. 1165–1177.
3. European Agency for the Evaluation of Medicinal Products (May 2001) Note for guidance on minimising the risk of transmitting animal spongiform encephalopathy agents via. human and veterinary medicinal products. CPMP/BWP/1230.
4. Center for Biologics Evaluation and Research (April 2000) Letter to manufacturers of biological products: Recommendations regarding bovine spongiform encephalopathy (BSE).
5. International Conference on Harmonisation (1995) Q5B: Quality of Biotechnological Products: Analysis of the Expression Construct in Cells used for Production of r-DNA Derived Protein Products.

6. International Conference on Harmonisation (1997) Q5D: Quality of Biotechnological Products: Derivation and Characterisation of Cell Substrates used for the Production of Biotechnological/Biological Products.

7. Robinson, A., Tranter, H. S., Wiblin, C. N. W., and Hambleton, P. (1995) Development and Production of Vaccines, in *Microbiological Quality Assurance A Guide Towards Relevance and Reproducibility of Inocula.* (Brown, M. R. W. and Gilbert, P., eds.) CRC Press, Boca Raton, FL, pp. 235–246.

8. A Guide to the Genetically Modified Organisms (contained use) Regulations (2000). HSE Books, Sudbury, UK.

9. Maurer, R., Meyer, B. J., and Ptashne, M. (1980) Genetic regulation at the right operator (OR) of bacteriophage $\lambda$-$0_R3$ and autogenous negative control by repressor. *J. Mol. Biol.* **139,** 147–161.

10. Meerman, H. J. and Georgiou, G. (1994) Construction and characterisation of a set of *Escherichia coli* strains deficient in all known loci affecting proteolytic stability of secreted recombinant proteins. *Bio/Technology* **12,** 1107–1110.

11. Rudolph, R. and Lilie, H. (1996) In vitro folding of inclusion body proteins. *FASEB J.* **10,** 49–56.

12. Schein, C. H. and Noteborn, M. H. M. (1988) Formation of soluble recombinant proteins in *Escherichia coli* is favoured by lower growth temperatures. *Bio/Technology* **6,** 291–294.

13. Garg, V. K., Costello, M. A. C., and Czuba, B. A. (1991) Purification and production of therapeutic grade proteins, in *Purification and Analysis of Recombinant Proteins.* (Seetharam, R., and Sharma, S. K., eds.), Marcel Dekker, Inc., New York, pp. 29–54.

14. Draeger, M. N. and Chase, H. A. (1991) Liquid fluidised bed adsorption of proteins in the presence of cells. *Bioseparations* **2,** 67–80.

15. Hambleton, P., Capel, B., Bailey, N., Heron, N., Crooks, A., Melling, J., et al. (1981) Production, purification and toxoiding of *Clostridium botulinum* type A toxin, in *Biomedical Aspects of Botulism.* (Lewis, G. E., ed.), Academic Press, New York, London, pp. 247–260.

16. Allison, N., Brehm, R., Harrison, S., Hiscott, S., Osborne, S., Ridgeway, P., et al. (1999) Large-scale GMP manufacture of staphylococcal enterotoxin B. *Abstracts from 4th International Conference on Separations for Biotechnology.*

17. *European Pharmacopoeia,* 4th ed. (2002) Bacterial Endotoxins, pp. 140–147.

18. Walsh, G. (1998) *Biopharmaceuticals: Biochemistry and Biotechnology.* Wiley, Chichester, UK, pp. 75–157.

19. ICH Guideline CPMP/ICH/295/95 (1997). Quality of biotechnological products: Viral safety evaluation of biotechnological products derived from cell lines of human or animal origin.

20. Rappuoli, R. (1997) New and improved vaccines against diphtheria and tetanus, in *New Generation Vaccines 2nd ed.,* (Levine, M. M., Woodrow, G. C., Kaper, J. B., and Cobon, G. S., eds.), Marcel Dekker, Inc., New York, pp 417–436.

21. ICH Guideline CPMP/ICH/365/96 (1999) Specifications: Test procedures and acceptance criteria for biotechnological/biological products.

22. Biddle, J. A. (1999) Technology transfer: what you always wanted to know but were afraid to ask, in *Vaccines from Concept to Clinic.* (Paoletti, L. C. and McInnes, P. M., eds.), CRC Press, pp. 127–174.

# Index

## A

Adenovirus, recombinant, 37–49
cotransfection (293 cells), 41–43
inflammatory response to, 39, 40
production of replication-deficient
recombinants, 41–44
propagation of, 44
purification and plaque assay, 43, 44
recombinant transfer vector,
construction of, 41
transfection efficiency, 43
Adjuvants, 175–193, 379, 380
Aluminium hydroxide, 176
adsorption of protein to, 181, 182

## B–C

Bacterial toxins,
genetic detoxification, 133–151
Carrier proteins for peptide vaccines,
117–120
choice of, 117–120
coupling to peptide, 119, 120
Cell-mediated immunity 255–277
Cholera toxin,
genetic detoxification, strategy for,
134, 135
immunogenicity testing, 147–149
mucosal adjuvant properties, 245–253
mutant CT, production and
purification of, 147
site-directed mutagenesis, 144–147
structure, 134–136
toxicity test, Y1 adrenal cells, 147, 148
Clinical trials, *see* Trials, clinical
Control of vaccines, 353–376

## D

DNA vaccines, 377–389
adjuvants, 379, 380
application, 381–383
delivery, 380, 381
safety, 283
uptake, transcription, and expression,
377–379

## E

Epitopes in peptide vaccines, 120–123
B-cell epitopes, 120
helper T-cell epitopes,
identification, 121, 122
linkage of epitopes, 122, 123
*Escherichia coli* heat-labile toxin,
genetic detoxification, strategy for,
134, 135
immunogenicity testing, 147–149
mutant LT, production, and
purification of, 144
site-directed mutagenesis, 143, 144
structure, 134–136
toxicity test, Y1 adrenal cells, 147, 148

## F

Formulation, freeze-dried product,
228–231
Freund's adjuvant, 177, 178
complete adjuvant,
general properties of, 177, 178
immunization with, 183
preparation of, 182, 183
incomplete adjuvant,
immunization with, 183
preparation of, 183

Freeze-drying, 223–243
  collapse temperature, 230
  cycle development, 238, 239
  damage during, 234
  equipment, 227, 228
  formulation, 228–231
    biological consequences of,
      231–233
    excipients, 232, 233
  microorganisms, sensitivity to, 233
  primary drying, 225–227
  principles of, 223–227
  safety considerations, 238
  stability, 234–237
    moisture content, determination,
      234, 235
    shelf-life parameters, 235–237
  vaccine characteristics, changes
    during, 237
Functional antibody response,
    assessment of, 289–300

**G**

Genome sequences, use of in vaccine
    design, 301–312
  high-throughput strategy 309
  *Neisseria meningitidis* genome,
    309, 310
  potential gene function, assessment
    of, 303–306
    BLAST and FASTA, 304, 305
  surface protein identification,
    306–308
    protein transport motifs, 307, 308
    transmembrane regions, 306, 307
  vaccine candidates from the genome,
    303–312
    conservation, 310
    selection, 303, 311

**H**

Heterologous antigens expressed in
    lactic acid bacteria, 101–114
  construction of expression vector,
    104–107

expression of cloned genes, 107–112
  immunization with, 110–112
  preparation of protein extracts,
    107–110
  whole cell ELISA for surface
    expression, 110
Heterologous antigens expression in
    *Salmonella*, 83–100
  chromosomal integration, 85–87,
    92–94
  electroporation, 90, 91
  foreign DNA, introduction of,
    90–92
  transduction using P22 lysates,
    91, 92
  plasmid vectors, 84, 85
  recombinant strains,
    characterization of, 94–97
    expression, 95, 96
    heterologous antigen, detection
      of, 96
    lipopolysaccharide analysis by
      SDS-PAGE, 96, 97
    screening by PCR, 94, 95

**I**

Immune response,
  different components of, 10–13
    classes of lymphocytes, 10–12
    differing roles, 12
    recognition patterns, 12
    selective induction, 12, 13
  functional, 289–300
  mucosal, 245–253
  T-cell, 255–277
Immunomodulators, incorporation into
    DNA vaccine, 195–210,
  characterization of expression, 201–206
  expression plasmid, 197–201
  vaccination protocol, 206, 207
Infection, patterns of, 1, 2
  acute, 1
  extracellular, 1
  intracellular, 1
  persistent, 1
ISCOMS, 178, 179

## L

Lactic acid bacteria, development of recombinant strains, *see also* Heterologous antigen expression in lactic and bacteria, 101–114

Liposomes as adjuvants, 179, 180
liposome vaccines, preparation of, storage of, 184
phosphatylyl choline (ovolecithin), preparation of, 183, 184

Live viral vectors, 37–81
adenoviruses, 37–49
Semliki Forest Virus, 69–81
Vaccinia virus, 51–68

Lyophilization of vaccines, *see* Freeze-drying

## M

Manufacture of vaccine, a guide to researchers, 391–407
analytical methods, 403
bacterial growth, 398, 399
bacterial strain selection, 394
documentation, 404–406
downstream processing, 399–403
chromatography, 401, 402
host contaminants, removal of, 402, 403
inactivation, 403
primary processing, 399, 400
formulation, 403
raw materials, 398
recombinant expression 394–398

MHC Class 1-Peptide Tetrameric Complex, construction of, 279–287
cell stain and flow cytometry of tetramers, 285, 286
cloning of MHC class genes into expression vector, 282
expression and purification of heavy chain and $\beta_2$-m proteins, 282

MHC Class 1-peptide complex monomers, 283–286
biotinylation of, 283, 284
ELISA for estimation of, 284, 285
in vitro refolding into, 283
tetramerization of, 285
two-step purification, 284

Microencapsulation of vaccines, 211–222

Moisture content, freeze-dried product, 234, 235

Mucosal immune system, 245, 246

Mucosal immunity, induction of, 245–253
mucosal immunization, 247, 248
oral immunization of humans, 248
oral immunization of mice, 247, 248

Mucosal immunity, measurement of, 248, 249
antibody-secreting cells, isolation from, blood, 249
Peyer's patches, 249
coproantibody levels, 248
ELISPOT assays, 249
IgG and IgA in serum, saliva and stools, 248, 249

Mutagenization, virus, 19–36

## O–P

Opsonophagocytosis assay for *S. pneumoniae* vaccines, 291, 292

Peptide vaccines, synthetic, 115–131
addition of helper T-cell epitopes, 120–123
advantages of, 116
carrier protein, use of, 117–120
coupling to carriers, 119, 120
foot and mouth disease virus peptide vaccine, 124–126
multimeric and cyclic presentation of, 124–126
synthesis of, 117

Pertussis toxin, genetic detoxification, 139–143

PT-deletion mutant,
    construction of, 141–143
    site-directed mutagenesis, 139
    strategy for, 134, 135
    immunogenicity testing, 147–149
    mutant PT, production and
        purification of, 143
    neutralization assay, 148
    structure, 135, 136
    toxicity test, CHO cells, 147, 148
Pneumococcal saccharide conjugate
        vaccine,
    characterization of conjugate, 162–165
    determination of antibodies,
        163, 164
    immunogenicity, 165
    coupling,161, 162
    preparation of, 161, 162
    serotype 19F polysaccharide, 161
Poly (lactide-co-glycolide) (PLG)
        microparticles, 211–222
    encapsulation of proteins, 214, 215
    microparticle diameter,
        determination of, 216
    protein loading, determination of, 215
    rate of protein release from
        microparticles,
        determination of, 216
    structure and general properties,
        211–213
Polysaccharide-conjugate
        vaccines,153–173
    relation of structure to
        immunogenicity, 154–159
    carrier protein, 156, 157
    coupling chemistry, 157, 158
    saccharide chain length, 154–156
    saccharide-to-protein ratio, 158, 159
    saccharide conjugate vaccines,
        examples,
    *Haemophilus influenza* type B
        vaccine, 159
    pneumonococcal serotype 19F
        vaccine, 160–173
Production facilities, control of, 358, 359

Q

Quality assurance of vaccines, 353–376
    batch release, 359, 360
    control of,
        attenuated vaccines, 364, 365,
            369, 370
        killed whole-cell vaccines, 362,
            363, 367–369
        nucleic acid/peptide, 366
        production facilities, 358, 359
        recombinant DNA, 365, 366
        subunit, conjugate, 362–364,
            370–374
    guidelines and recommendations,
        356–358
    reference materials, 360
    regulation of, 361, 362
    stability, 360, 361
Quil A, 178

R–S

Reverse genetics 30–33
*Salmonella*, development of attenuated
        strains, *see also* Heterologous
        antigen expression in
        *Salmonella*, 83–100
Semliki Forest virus, recombinant, 69–81
    analysis of protein expression, 77
    immunization with,
        SFV layered DNA, 78
        SFV particles, 78
        SFV RNA, 78
    infection of target cells, 76
    plasmid, 71–73
    preparation of RNA, 74, 75
    purification and concentration, 76
    titer determination, 77
    transfection of BHK-21 cells by
        electroporation, 75, 76
    vector system, 70, 71
Serum bactericidal assay for Group C
        meningococcal vaccines,
        290–299
    principles, 290, 291

procedure, 294–297
safety, 294–296
Severe Combined Immunodeficient
    (SCID) mice, 313–334
assessing reconstituted mice, 325–328
detection of human antibody,
    325, 326
FACS analysis, 327, 328
histological analysis, 326, 327
immunodeficient mice strains,
    315–320
potential for vaccine studies,
    318–320
SCID, 315–318
SCID-Beige, 315–318
maintenance of, 320, 321
handling, 322, 323
monitoring immunodeficiency,
    323, 324
detection of Beige marker 323, 324
detection of SCID defect, 323
reconstitution with human peripheral
    blood lymphocytes, 324, 325
Stability, freeze-dried product, 234–237

**T**

T-cell responses, techniques for the
    detection of, 255–277
cytotoxic T-cell assays, 271, 272
killing assay, 272
preparation of murine CTL
    effector cells, 271
preparation of target cells, 271
principles, 259–261
ELISPOT assays for cytokine
    secreting cells 270, 271
helper T-cell assays 272, 273
antibody assay, 273
T- and B-cell culture, 272, 273
immunization of mice, 262
alum-adsorbed antigens, 262
immunization, 262
preparation of antigen-presenting
    cells, 265, 266

B-lymphoblastoid cell lines, 266
irradiated murine spleen cells, 265
preparation of mononuclear cells,
    262, 263
human PBMCs 263
spleen cells, 263
viable cell counts, 263
viable mononuclear cells, 263
principles, 259–261
purification of subpopulation of
    lymphocytes, 264, 265
B-cell, 265
CD4+ cells, 265
general principles of, 264
murine T-cells, 264
T-cell proliferation assays, 266, 267
with murine and human cells, 267
with purified cell populations, 267
Th1/Th0/Th2 responses, 268, 269
cytokine bioassay 269
cytokine-conditioned medium, 268
cytokine immunoassay, 268
T-cells, role in immunity, 255–261
factors affecting T-cell responses,
    257–259
antigen, 257
delivery system, 258
immunization schedule, 258, 259
T-cell responses to vaccination,
    257–259
Temperature-sensitive mutants, 19–36
cell substrate of, 22, 23
classical emperical approach, 20, 21
evaluation of vaccine potential, 30
general methods, 22, 25
isolation of, 25–27
mutagenization systems for, 24, 25
continuous mutagenization, 29, 30
low temperature passage, 30
mutant stocks, 27–29
reverse genetics, 30–33
screening of mutants, 26, 27
sequential mutagenization, 28, 29
virus source, 24

Trials, clinical, 335–351
  biases, 348
  design of, 344–348
  ethical considerations, 344, 345
  evaluation process, 335, 336
  hypotheses, estimation power, 345
  Phase I, 336–338
  Phase II, 338–340
  Phase III, 340–343
  Phase IV, 343, 344
  protocol for, 337
  quality control of, 347
  randomization, 346, 347
  significance testing, 348
  targeting population, 345, 346
  trial size, 346

**V**

Vaccine efficacy, 6, 7
Vaccines, future development of, 13, 14
  combination vaccines, 13
  ease of development, 13
  genomic analysis of agents, 14
  mixed vaccine formulations,
    prime/boost, 14, 382

Vaccines, improved and new, 7–10
  new approaches, 8–10
    anti-idotypes, 8
    live vectors, 9, 10
    "naked" DNA 10, 377–389
    oligo/polypeptides, 9, 115–131
    transfected cells, 9
  opportunities, 7
Vaccines, safety, 5, 6
  measles, 5
Vaccines, types of, 2–4
  inactivated, whole microorganisms, 4
  live, attenuated, 3
  subunit, 4
Vaccinia virus, recombinant, 51–68
  cell culture, 55
  characterization of, 62, 63
  chick embryo, fibroblast cells,
    preparation of, 55
  generation of, 58, 59
  isolation of, 59–62
  vaccination in mice, 64
  virus growth, 55–58
Virus mutagenization of, 19–36